Primary Care Mental Health in Older People

Carlos Augusto de Mendonça Lima
Gabriel Ivbijaro
Editors

Primary Care Mental Health in Older People

A Global Perspective

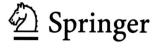 Springer

Editors
Carlos Augusto de Mendonça Lima
Unité de Psychiatrie et de
Psychothérapie
Centre Les Toises
Lausanne
Switzerland

Gabriel Ivbijaro
Mental Health and Population Health
NOVA University Lisbon
Lisbon
Portugal

ISBN 978-3-030-10812-0   ISBN 978-3-030-10814-4   (eBook)
https://doi.org/10.1007/978-3-030-10814-4

This Springer imprint is published by the registered company Springer Nature Switzerland AG
The registered company address is: Gewerbestrasse 11, 6330 Cham, Switzerland

Healing minds

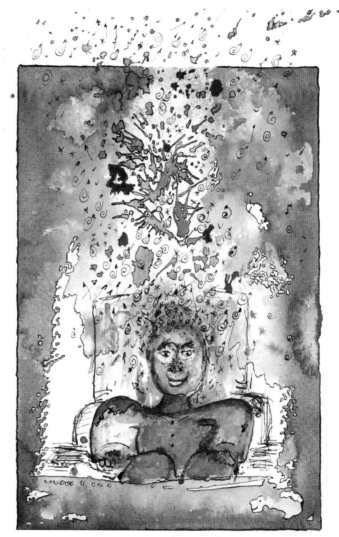

Jean Marie Daunas 2018

Foreword 1

There are three main reasons which are making me welcome this volume. First, it is bringing together primary health-care answers to key mental health problems which people face in older age. The problems to which the answers have been provided have been selected because they are frequent and because there are interventions which have been shown to be effective in reducing their impact. The answers have been provided by an array of experts with vast experience and deal with specific problems such as anxiety disorders and with important background issues such as the frailty of the elderly and the need to maintain and promote their dignity in health and disease.

A second reason for recommending the volume is that the text has not been produced by general practitioners nor by specialists nor by practitioners of allied professions but by all of them working together. There is no other manual where the principle of joint work by specialists, general practitioners, and allied professionals has been applied so rigorously in order to provide answers to problems and advice about action based on a mix of experience and knowledge which these three groups of people usually facing mental health problems in old age have assembled.

A third reason for welcoming this volume stems from its timing. The volume which has been prepared by Professors Ivbijaro and Mendonça Lima makes its appearance at the time when the United Nations have decided to make the fight against the noncommunicable diseases one of their key political as well as humanistic goals. Until recently, the United Nations and the international bodies dealing with health care such as the World Health Organization did not include mental and neurological disorders among their priority concerns: this has happened for the first time 2 years ago when the United Nations adopted their sustainable development goals, including among them the promotion of mental health, and more recently in 2018 when they specifically discussed what could be done to deal with noncommunicable diseases including mental disorders. It is to be expected that the urging of the United Nations will lead to action at country level, and when this happens, it will be particularly important to have materials which can provide guidance for action.

It is thus with much pleasure that I am recommending this volume to the many who have to face mental health and other problems in the elderly and that I am expressing my thanks to its editors who have produced a most valuable text based on evidence and shaped by wisdom and rich practical experience.

Norman Sartorius
President, Association for the Improvement of Mental
Health Programmes (AMH)
Geneva, Switzerland

Foreword 2

It is timely that this valuable book is written when we are faced worldwide with the physical and mental health problems of aging populations. While increasing numbers of older adults are living long and robust lives, many are facing loneliness, frailty, and multimorbidity. Primary health care is particularly well-suited in countries of all types to provide a setting for the coordinated health and social care required by older adults and their families.

The 1978 Declaration of Alma-Ata lays a foundation for primary health care. However, progress over the following decades has been uneven. At least half the world's population lacks access to essential health services—care for communicable and noncommunicable diseases across the life span including mental health. Four decades later, the Declaration of Astana in October 2018 reaffirms the historic 1978 Declaration. Countries around the world have vowed to strengthen their primary health-care systems as an essential step toward achieving universal health coverage. Mental health has a firmer place in this renewed commitment.

The increasing focus on global mental health is linked with this Declaration and with two major policy initiatives related to it. One is the World Health Organization (WHO) call for universal health coverage: to ensure that all people have access to needed health services (including promotion, prevention, treatment, rehabilitation, and palliation) of sufficient quality to be effective, without imposing financial hardship. The first initiative is the World Health Organization (WHO) call for universal health coverage: to ensure that all people have access to needed health services (including promotion, prevention, treatment, rehabilitation, and palliation) of sufficient quality to be effective, without imposing financial hardship. The second initiative is the renewed focus on noncommunicable diseases (NCDs), spearheaded by the WHO Independent High-Level Commission on NCDs and Mental Health.

Primary health care is an important setting for the realization of both these policies—and others, notably the link to health in the UN Sustainable Development Goals—that encourage parity of mental health within health, a holistic approach to health care across the life span, and the engagement and empowerment of communities in health promotion and health care. The holistic approach to health care with a central place for mental health has been championed for decades. The logic and urgency of this approach are undoubted, and no more so than for older adults. Yet, large gaps remain in primary care mental health for this population as for others. There is a need for policy and practice guidance and demonstration of successful approaches to good primary care mental health for older adults at global and local levels.

The editors have responded admirably to the challenge. In a comprehensive volume, they have brought together authors from different disciplines and various parts of the world in a scholarly and humane whole that offers inspiration as well as a practical resource. True to the Declarations of Alma-Ata and Astana, the book is primary care- and community-focused. It covers a number of topics relating to older people that are not commonly found in one volume: improving health, supporting self-care, promoting equity and universal access to care, recognizing the importance of primary care in the treatment of mental health problems of all types, and considering the complex relationship between mental and somatic health. Ensuring that each chapter is written by a combination of primary care doctors, old-age psychiatrists or physicians, and at least one other health professional or family carer gives the book its unusual and special relevance for health professionals, students, and policy-makers as well as interested lay audiences.

I am pleased to note that there are several present and past members of the World Psychiatric Association Section of Old Age Psychiatry among the distinguished authors and editors. I congratulate the editors and contributors on producing this book at a critical time of change in the field.

Helen Herrman
President, World Psychiatric Association
Melbourne, VIC, Australia

Foreword 3

It is with great enthusiasm that I urge you to read this incredibly important work on mental health in the elderly written for primary care. As the global population ages, the practitioner most likely to treat the older person is the primary care physician. Some may lament that there are not enough mental health specialists and particularly not enough specialist in geriatric psychiatry. However, an equally important observation is that person-centered care can effectively be delivered by the provider who cares for the whole person. While there is added challenge because aging persons can have multiple medical problems which need primary care attention, most primary care doctors see large numbers of aging persons and are more experienced than is appreciated. An even bigger challenge comes in the delivery of mental health care. At any age, mental health is undertreated, even in many developed countries. With age, the problem is magnified, often because primary care settings lack confidence in addressing mental health in an aging and often frail population. Serious mental health problems are not assessed because primary care settings have limited resources to address newly identified problems. Additionally, comorbidities of aging may create contraindications to some treatments, and the absence of the specialist may leave the primary care doctor without confidence. Sadly, ignoring diagnosis and treatment may also occur because of the existing nihilism about treating elderly patients in general.

This book offers the perfect antidote to this lack of knowledge, lack of confidence, and the nihilism. Several of the introductory chapters provide a framework for understanding the breadth on influences in aging health including interaction between lifestyle and the physical, social, and economic environment and long-standing individual characteristics. The "how to" of interviewing for mental health and frailty are also offered. While the primary care provider may need a wide referral network for medical specialties, it is of note that more than seven chapters focus on non-pharmacological approaches that provide meaningful benefit. The evidence base that social and behavioral interventions can improve the quality of life of aging persons is well laid out and available to the reader.

I am particularly excited about the focus on promoting dignity in serving elders. Appreciation for the full past of the individuals as well as their present situation can help identify the path for best care and maximize quality of life.

The book has assembled experts for the chapter on pharmacological interventions in geriatric psychiatry and also contains well-constructed chapters on dealing with the most troublesome conditions such as agitation, dementias, and suicide. Written for primary care provider, the text delivers clear description and guidance for diagnosis and management and acknowledges the need to integrate this care delivery with the family and other systems of care.

Dr. Carlos Augusto de Mendonça Lima, who is a giant in the field of geriatric mental health and one of my most respected colleagues, is the editor. After his training at the Federal University of Rio de Janeiro and his equivalence in Portugal and in Switzerland, he specialized in Psychiatry in France and received two Master's degrees and a Doctorate preparing himself not only for a lifetime of work in psychiatry but for a commitment to geriatric mental health. During his time at the World Health Organization, he initiated and then led the Collaborating Centre for Psychiatry of the Elderly. His expertise has been recognized as he has been elected by his peers to many leading professional organizations including the European Association of Geriatric Psychiatry and the International Psychogeriatric Association where I first came to know him. In this past year, he stood up to support patient and physician rights and opportunities to continue to receive approved treatments for dementia. His essay on the "The Old Age Psychiatry Paradox" remains on the IPA website. In it he highlights the growing knowledge in the field of old-age psychiatry, the growing need to serve expanding aging population, and the need to protect aging persons from the stigma of a secular society focused on wealth productivity. He also laments the constant challenges by authorities to undermine this specialty field by denying the need to support geriatric psychiatry specialty care, training, and education of the mental health workforce and by limiting the input of this special expertise in the development of guidelines and care for geriatric conditions. However, not one to simply point to such injustices, Dr. Lima has supported the generalists' need for more information and education to serve aging people because there are insufficient numbers of trained specialists.

Dr. Lima is joined in this effort by Dr. Gabriel Ivbijaro, MBBS, who was trained in Nigeria and has specialties in Neurology and Psychiatry from the United Kingdom. He is a Member of the World Organization of Family Doctors and was President of the World Federation for Mental Health (WFMH). He has been awarded a Member of the Most Excellent Order of the British Empire (MBE) by Her Majesty Queen Elizabeth II. Dr. Ivbijaro is an expert in addressing ways to reducing disparities in mental health services for ethnic minorities, and his psychiatry expertise is further evidenced in his role as Editor in Chief of *Mental Health in Family Medicine*.

Together, through this book, Drs. Lima and Ivbijaro bring their expertise and commitment to serving the mental health needs of elderly patients through their most likely health-care providers, primary care physicians. Because of their leadership, they have been able to assemble international experts to provide this work, written for a wide audience of health-care professionals to provide understanding of the complex problems in geriatric psychiatry. This advocacy in action will serve aging patients by supporting their treating physicians. I am so grateful for the role model these authors provide and this important work. It will make contributions for many physicians and the aging patients they serve.

Mary Sano
President, International Psychogeriatric Association,
Milwaukee, WI, USA

Professor, Department of Psychiatry,
Icahn School of Medicine at Mount Sinai, New York, NY, USA

Foreword 4

Over the past decade, Professor Gabriel Ivbijaro, Dr. Carlos Augusto de Mendonça Lima, and their colleagues have been leading efforts to focus global attention on mental health concerns and to strengthen the role played by primary care clinicians all around the world in the diagnosis and management of mental health problems and in tackling the stigma and discrimination that often accompany a diagnosis of mental illness.

While mental health problems can affect people of all ages, this important new publication focuses attention on an area of clinical practice that is often neglected and poorly managed, and sometimes even ignored: the management of mental health problems in older people.

We are often reminded that "you can judge a society by the way it treats its most vulnerable members." Along with the youngest members of our communities, our most senior members are often among our most vulnerable. And those with mental health problems and disability can be especially vulnerable and at risk of abuse, neglect, and inadequate care.

This area of clinical practice, mental health care for older people, is at last receiving the attention it deserves, and this book provides a timely and very important contribution. As populations age in every country, and as multimorbidity increases, the number of older people with cognitive and other mental health challenges will continue to rise, and our health-care services need to be equipped and supported to support all our older patients.

This book is not afraid to tackle some of the most serious mental health challenges facing older people: neurocognitive disorders, depression and suicide risk, psychosis and agitation, frailty and comorbidity, bereavement and loss, and sexuality and sexual activity.

I especially commend the human rights approach of this publication, advocating for dignity and respect in the clinical treatment of all older people with mental health concerns. As health professionals and carers, we should always treat our patients with the same dignity and respect that we would expect for our own older loved ones, and for ourselves.

I commend the editors, Professor Gabriel Ivbijaro and Dr. Carlos Augusto de Mendonça Lima, and all the contributing authors on this new publication. The important insights and solutions to clinical dilemmas contained in this book will be of great interest to medical students, doctors in training, and established medical practitioners, not only in family medicine and in psychiatry but in all medical specialties. This book will also provide a valuable

resource to all health-care workers involved in working in primary care and
to everyone involved in the care of older people in all settings.

Michael Kidd
Professor and Chair of the Department of Family
and Community Medicine, Past President, World Organization of Family
Doctors (WONCA) 2013–2016, The University of Toronto,
Toronto, ON, Canada

Director, World Health Organization Collaborating
Centre on Family Medicine and Primary Care,
Honorary Professor of Global Primary Care,
Southgate Institute for Health, Society and Equity,
Flinders University, Bedford Park SA, Australia

Director, Beyond Blue, Hawthorn, Australia

Foreword 5

I am honored to be able to introduce this very important book. As the economies of the world develop, education and health systems improve, and people live longer. Hence, the phenomenon of global aging represents a success story for societies and their people. Coming with this though is a dramatic increase in the numbers of older people who have managed to avoid or outlive a wide range of illnesses which in the past would have cut short so many of those lives. This raises significant health challenges for high-, middle-, and low-income economies with an increasingly aging population and a range of chronic illnesses and comorbidities. So for so many countries, primary care needs to be at the forefront of health systems, and the primary care mental health for older people remains much in need of development.

This book is written by a combination of primary care doctors, old-age psychiatrists, physicians, and allied health professionals. It makes an essential contribution to knowledge, and the emphasis on health promotion is particularly welcomed, especially with the need to develop community resilience and self-management strategies in older people. And so important is the human rights approach to respecting autonomy, equity, independence, and universal access for older people. Primary care is likely to continue to be at the forefront of health systems because of the growing need for an emphasis on prevention, tight financial constraints, and a lack of well-developed secondary health-care services in some countries.

I am glad to see that this book addresses the wide range of mental health problems in older people including dementia, depression, and delirium but also has a strong emphasis on comorbidity and polypharmacy. This means that the book should be a reader-friendly practical resource for many clinical services seeking to improve their primary care provision with the most important benefit of also helping improve the care provided to older people.

I congratulate Dr. Carlos de Mendonça Lima and Professor Gabriel Ivbijaro for putting together such a comprehensive and thoughtful book, which, I am sure, will be of great use for many years to come.

Martin Orrell
Director, Institute of Mental Health, President of the
European Association of Geriatric Psychiatry (EAGP),
Nottingham, UK

Mental health is essential for health. Mental and physical problems are interwoven. Mental health problems will be among the leading causes of burden of disease in 2030 and the main causes of disability-adjusted life years. Between 2011 and 2030, the World Economic Forum predicts that mental illness worldwide will cost more than physical ailments such as cancer, heart disease, or diabetes.

Older people live longer and will be the vast majority of the population in the future. It is estimated from community epidemiological surveys that as many as 20–30% of persons meet criteria for mental disorders, but there is a significant gap between the prevalence of mental problems and the number of people receiving care. Primary care helps to close this gap because the majority of people report at least one primary care visit per year and maintain a stable and enduring relationship with their primary care doctors. Therefore, it is no surprise that most mental health treatment is provided in primary care and most psychotropic drugs are prescribed by family physicians. In recent years, there has been a growth in diagnosis and drug treatment, what may represent an increased acceptance of mental illness and improved case finding but may also be the result of overdiagnosis and overenthusiastic treatment, and it is important to have a global perspective of mental health in primary care.

Professor Gabriel Ivbijaro is a very respected professor at Nova University (Lisbon) with a vast experience as Adviser of the World Health Organization, Chair of the World Dignity Project, and Past President of the World Federation for Mental Health. In 2012 in collaboration with an international group of general practitioners, psychiatrists, policy-makers, mental health professionals, and mental health advocates, he edited an unprecedented book providing the best available evidence for the management of patients with mental health conditions in primary care. Following the previous successful model, Professor Gabriel Ivbijaro and Dr. Carlos Augusto de Mendonça Lima coordinated a new fantastic resource to support the delivery of holistic mental health interventions to older adults in the primary care setting.

This book reflects their style, very didactic and complete. It addresses functional mental health problems (such as anxiety, depression, psychotic and personality disorders) and acquired organic mental disorders of old age (such as dementia, cognitive impairments, and delirium) and explores the complex relationship between mental and somatic health and health problems, including aspects of multimorbidity and polypharmacy. Editors and authors are primary care- and community-focused because the main aim of the book is to promote pathways to care for older people with mental health problems respecting their autonomy, independence, and human rights and the importance of the life-course approach.

I am happy to commend this book *Primary Care Mental Health in Older People: A Global Perspective* for use to primary health care professionals, general practitioners, family doctors, community psychiatrists, and trainees, and it should be a standard reference to those providing mental health care.

Isabel Santos
Invited Associated Professor, Medical School,
Universidade NOVA de Lisboa, Lisbon, Portugal

Councilor, Coordination of the Residency in General
and Family Medicine, ARSLVT, Lisbon, Portugal

General Practitioner, UCSP Arruda 1 ACES
Estuário do Tejo, Lisbon, Portugal

Presidente, Colégio da Especialidade de Medicina Geral e Familiar,
Ordem dos Médicos, Lisbon, Portugal

Acknowledgements

Many individuals and researchers who care for older adults have contributed to this book, and we are very grateful to each one of them.

Primary Care Mental Health in Older Adults is based on the current literature and the clinical experience of a group of psychiatrists who care for older adults, family doctors and other mental health professionals, public health professionals, policy makers and mental health advocates with an interest in the mental health of older adults. We would like to thank them all for their invaluable contribution towards the success of this project.

Global mental health is very important. This is why we have brought together experts from all continents of the world who have taken into account current trends in the care of older adults, the current burden of disease, the philosophy of care whilst knowing that primary care can help to improve access to care in an equitable and fair way and ensuring that dignity is at the core of all our clinical encounters with older adults.

We have also included good practice examples to help clinicians, older adults and their families and those who pay for the delivery of services to consider innovative ways to deliver care.

Older adult patients with mental health difficulties, carers and their families matter and we hope that this book will be an additional resource to promote practice that allows them to lead a more fruitful life in the community.

Each chapter in this book was assigned to a team with a team leader/corresponding author who coordinated the contributions of team members to develop the chapter. Each chapter was peer reviewed by a psychiatrist, general practitioner and a public health specialist using the following criteria:

- Will the chapter support primary and community care practitioners caring for older adults with mental health difficulties in their daily practice?
- Will the chapter support dignity in the delivery of care to older adults with mental health difficulties?
- Is the content relevant to the care of older adults with mental health difficulties?
- Are the key messages:
  - consistent with the chapter content?
  - fit for purpose?
- Does the chapter reflect the complexity and systems within primary and community care?
- Are there copyright issues?
- Is the chapter internally consistent?
- Are there any factual errors?
- Are there any chapters that need to be merged to present a more coherent picture?

Additional changes were made by the team and the chapter resubmitted to peer review and accepted once it was considered robust and relevant to primary care and mental health of older adults.

We are grateful to the reviewers for all their efforts. We would also like to thank all the contributors, including the project manager and copy-editors at Springer and all those who contributed in one way or another to produce this book. This work would not have been possible without them.

We learn a lot from our patients, and we are grateful to them.

Contents

Part IV

Part V

Part VI

Contributors

Olatunji Aina College of Medicine of the University of Lagos, Lagos, Nigeria

Şahinde Özlem Erden Aki Department of Psychiatry, Hacettepe University School of Medicine, Altındağ, Turkey

Urska Arnautovska School of Applied Psychology and Mental Health Institute Queensland, Griffith University, Mount Gravatt, QLD, Australia

Sabine Bährer-Kohler International University of Catalonia (UIC), Barcelona, Spain

Dr. Bährer-Kohler & Partners, Basel, Switzerland

Conceição Balsinha CEDOC, Chronic Diseases Research Centre, NOVA Medical School/Faculdade de Ciências Médicas, Universidade Nova de Lisboa, Lisboa, Portugal

Unidade de Saúde Familiar Marginal, São João do Estoril, Portugal

David Baron Keck School of Medicine, University of Southern California, Los Angeles, CA, USA

Karen Bernard Public Health Department, London Borough of Waltham Forest, London, UK

Sergio Luís Blay Department of Psychiatry, Universidade Federal de São Paulo, São Paulo, Brazil

Claire Brooks ModelPeople Inc. Global Insights, Chicago, IL, USA

Christophe J. Büla Service of Geriatric Medicine and Geriatric Rehabilitation, Department of Medicine, University of Lausanne Medical Center (CHUV), Lausanne, Switzerland

Merryl Butters Department of Psychiatry, University of Pittsburgh Medical Center, Pittsburgh, PA, USA

Vincent Camus CHRU de Tours, Tours, France

Université François Rabelais de Tours and INSERM U930, Tours, France

Paulo R. Canineu Laboratory of Neurosciences (LIM-27), Institute of Psychiatry, Faculty of Medicine, University of São Paulo, São Paulo, SP, Brazil

Pontifícia Universidade Católica de São Paulo, Gerontology Program, São Paulo, SP, Brazil

Edmond Chiu Department of Psychiatry, The University of Melbourne, Melbourne, VIC, Australia

David Clarke Center for Ethics, Oregon Health & Science University, Portland, OR, USA

Gastroenterology, Oregon Health & Science University, Portland, OR, USA

Manuel Coroa Department of Psychiatry and Mental Health, Psychogeriatric Unit, Coimbra University Hospital Center, Coimbra, Portugal

Diego De Leo Australian Institute for Suicide Research and Prevention, Griffith University, Mount Gravatt, QLD, Australia

Slovene Centre for Suicide Research, University of Primorska, Koper, Slovenia

Carlos Augusto de Mendonça Lima Unity of Old Age Psychiatry, Centre Les Toises, Lausanne, Switzerland

Thomas Desmidt CHRU de Tours, Tours, France

Anthony Dowell Obstetrics and Gynecology, University of Otago Wellington University of Otago, Wellington, New Zealand

Jenny Downes-Brydon Peninsula Family General Practice, Frankston, VIC, Australia

Monash University Medical School, Clayton, VIC, Australia

Melbourne University Medical School, Melbourne, VIC, Australia

Brian Draper School of Psychiatry, University of New South Wales, Sydney, NSW, Australia

Todd M. Edwards Marital and Family Therapy Program, University of San Diego, San Diego, CA, USA

Yaccub Enum Public Health Department, London Borough of Waltham Forest, London, UK

East London NHS Foundation Trust, London, UK

Partnerships and Sexual Health, Public Health Department, London Borough of Waltham Forest, London, UK

Mercedes Fernández Cabana Servicio de Salud Mental, Hospital Virxe da Xunqueira, A Coruña, Spain

Horácio Firmino Department of Psychiatry and Mental Health, Psychogeriatric Unit, Coimbra University Hospital Center, Coimbra, Portugal

Orestes V. Forlenza Laboratory of Neurosciences (LIM-27), Institute of Psychiatry, Faculty of Medicine, University of São Paulo, São Paulo, SP, Brazil

José Alexandre Freitas CEDOC, Chronic Diseases Research Centre, NOVA Medical School/Faculdade de Ciências Médicas, Universidade Nova de Lisboa, Lisboa, Portugal

Unidade de Saúde Familiar Marginal, São João do Estoril, Portugal

Genevieve Gagnon Department of Psychiatry, McGill University, Montreal, QC, Canada

Department of Psychology, McGill University, Montreal, QC, Canada

Douglas Mental Health University Institute, McGill University, Montreal, QC, Canada

Vinodkumar R. Gangolli Masina Hospital, Mumbai, India

Grand River Hospital, Kitchener, ON, Canada

Department of Psychiatry and Neuro-Behavioral Sciences, McMaster's University, Hamilton, ON, Canada

Alejandro García-Caballero Department of Psychiatry, School of Medicine, University of Santiago de Compostela (USC), Santiago de Compostela, Spain

Department of Psychiatry, EOXI Ourense, Ourense, Spain

South Galician Health Research Institute (IISGS), Ourense, Spain

Bruno Gherman Center for Alzheimer's Disease and Related Disorders, Institute of Psychiatry, Universidade Federal do Rio de Janeiro, Rio de Janeiro, Brazil

David Goldberg King's College, London, UK

Irênio Gomes Instituto de Gerontologia et Geriatria, Pontifícia Universidade Católica do Rio Grande do Sul—PUCRS, Porto Alegre, Brazil

Manuel Gonçalves-Pereira CEDOC, Chronic Diseases Research Centre, NOVA Medical School/Faculdade de Ciências Médicas, Universidade Nova de Lisboa, Lisboa, Portugal

Joana Grave CEDOC, Chronic Diseases Research Centre, NOVA Medical School/Faculdade de Ciências Médicas, Universidade Nova de Lisboa, Lisboa, Portugal

George T. Grossberg Department of Psychiatry and Behavioral Neuroscience, Saint Louis University School of Medicine, St. Louis, MO, USA

John Heafner Department of Neurology and Behavioral Neuroscience, Saint Louis University School of Medicine, St. Louis, MO, USA

Helen Herrman World Psychiatric Association, Melbourne, VIC, Australia

Roger Hilfiker Physiotherapy, School of Health Sciences, HES-SO Valais-Wallis, Leukerbad, Switzerland

Monica Hill Public Health Department, London Borough of Waltham Forest, London, UK

Steve Iliffe Primary Care and Population Health, University College London, London, UK

Centre of Expertise in Longevity and Long-Term Care, Charles University, Prague, Czech Republic

Gabriel Ivbijaro NOVA University, Lisbon, Portugal

Waltham Forest Community and Family Health Services, London, UK

Alicia Beatriz Kabanchik Faculty of Health Science, Maimonides University, Buenos Aires, Argentina

Aleksandra Milicevic Kalasic Department for Social Work, Faculty for Media and Communication, Singidunum University, Belgrade, Serbia

Municipal Institute of Gerontology and Palliative Care, Singidunum University, Belgrade, Serbia

Gustav Kamenski Centre for Public Health, Medical University of Vienna, Vienna, Austria

Michael Kidd Department of Family and Community Medicine, The University of Toronto, Toronto, ON, Canada

Global Primary Care, Southgate Institute for Health, Society and Equity, Flinders University, Bedford Park SA, Australia

Beyond Blue, Hawthorn, Australia

Lucja Kolkiewicz NOVA University, Lisbon, Portugal

East London NHS Foundation Trust, London, UK

Nicolas Kuhne University of Applied Sciences Western Switzerland, Lausanne, Switzerland

Sudhir Kumar Alzheimer's and Related Disorders Society of India, Ernakulam, Kerala, India

Emanuela Sofia Teixeira Lopes Unity of Health and Clinical Psychology, Hospital da Senhora da Oliveira - Guimarães, EPE, Creixomil, Portugal

Valeska Marinho Center for Alzheimer's Disease and Related Disorders, Institute of Psychiatry, Universidade Federal do Rio de Janeiro, Rio de Janeiro, Brazil

Marjolaine Masson Douglas Mental Health University Institute, McGill University, Montreal, QC, Canada

Raimundo Mateos Department of Psychiatry, School of Medicine, University of Santiago de Compostela (USC), Santiago de Compostela, Spain

Psychogeriatric Unit, CHUS University Hospital, Santiago de Compostela, Spain

Brendan McLoughlin Clinical Senior Cognitive Behavioural Therapist, Efficacy, London, UK

Clifton McReynolds Chicago, IL, USA

Christopher NG Department of Neurology and Behavioral Neuroscience, Saint Louis University School of Medicine, St. Louis, MO, USA

Eduardo Nogueira Department of Psychological Medicine, Faculty of Medicine, University of Coimbra, Coimbra, Portugal

Vasco Nogueira Department of Psychological Medicine, Faculty of Médicine, University of Coimbra, Coimbra, Portugal

Taofik Olajobi College of Nursing, Midwifery and Healthcare, University of West London, London, UK

Martin Orrell Institute of Mental Health, European Association of Geriatric Psychiatry (EAGP), Nottingham, UK

António Pacheco Palha Department of Psychiatry, School of Medicine, University of Oporto (Jubilee), Porto, Portugal

World Psychiatry Association (WPA), Geneva, Switzerland

European Federation of Sexology, Tilburg, The Netherlands

Henk Parmentier Woodstreet Medical Center, London, UK

Medical Faculty, Universidade NOVA de Lisboa, Lisbon, Portugal

Jay J. Patel Department of Neurology and Behavioral Neuroscience, Saint Louis University School of Medicine, St. Louis, MO, USA

Jo Ellen Patterson Marital and Family Therapy Program, University of San Diego, San Diego, CA, USA

Marta L.G.F. Pereira Laboratory of Neurosciences (LIM-27), Department and Institute of Psychiatry, Faculty of Medicine, University of São Paulo, São Paulo, SP, Brazil

Manuel Sanchez Perez Unit of Geriatric Psychiatry, Sagrat Cor Hospital, Barcelona, Spain

Janice Richards Waltham Forest Clinical Commissioning Group, London, UK

Jacob Roy Alzheimer's and Related Disorders Society of India, Ernakulam, Kerala, India

Alzheimer's Disease International, London, UK

Joanna Rymaszewska Department of Psychiatry, Wroclaw Medical University, Wroclaw, Poland

Luiz Miguel Santiago Primary Health Care and General Practice of Faculty of Medicine of University of Coimbra, Coimbra, Portugal

Mary Sano International Psychogeriatric Association, Milwaukee, WI, USA

Department of Psychiatry, Icahn School of Medicine at Mount Sinai, New York, NY, USA

Isabel Santos Medical School, Universidade NOVA de Lisboa, Lisbon, Portugal

Coordination of the Residency in General and Family Medicine, ARSLVT, Lisbon, Portugal

UCSP Arruda 1 ACES, Estuário do Tejo, Lisbon, Portugal

Colégio da Especialidade de Medicina Geral e Familiar, Ordem dos Médicos, Lisbon, Portugal

Norman Sartorius Association for the Improvement of Mental Health Programmes (AMH), Geneva, Switzerland

Lilian Scheinkman Department of Psychiatry, State University of Rio de Janeiro, Rio de Janeiro, Brazil

Psychiatry Consultation Liaison Services, Pedro Ernesto University Hospital, Rio de Janeiro, Brazil

Laurence Seematter Bagnoud Service of Geriatric Medicine and Geriatric Rehabilitation, Department of Medicine, University of Lausanne Medical Center (CHUV), Lausanne, Switzerland

Institute of Social and Preventive Medicine, University of Lausanne Medical Center (CHUV), Lausanne, Switzerland

Dale W. Smith Department of Neurology and Behavioral Neuroscience, Saint Louis University School of Medicine, St. Louis, MO, USA

Christopher Soltysiak Mental Health and Joint Planning Waltham Forest Clinical Commissioning Group, London, UK

Wolfgang Spiegel Centre for Public Health, Medical University of Vienna, Vienna, Austria

Florindo Stella Laboratory of Neurosciences (LIM-27), Department and Institute of Psychiatry, Faculty of Medicine, University of São Paulo, São Paulo, SP, Brazil

UNESP – Universidade Estadual Paulista, Biosciences Institute, Campus of Rio Claro, SP, Brazil

Igor Svab Medical Faculty, University of Ljubljana, Ljubljana, Slovenia

Dorota Szcześniak Department of Psychiatry, Wroclaw Medical University, Wroclaw, Poland

Nicoleta Tătaru Department of Psychiatry, Neurology and Psychiatry, Hospital of Oradea, Oradea, Romania

Jessica Uno Keck School of Medicine, University of Southern California, Los Angeles, CA, USA

Armin von Gunten Service de Psychiatrie de l'Age Avancé, Department of Psychiatry, University of Lausanne Medical Center (CHUV), Lausanne, Switzerland

Anne P.F. Wand School of Psychiatry, University of New South Wales, Sydney, Australia

Hakan Yakan School of Medicine, University of Akdeniz, Antalya, Turkey

Part I
Introduction to Primary Care Mental Health in Older Adults

Aims and Concept of Primary Care Mental Health in Older Adults: A Global Perspective

Gabriel Ivbijaro and Carlos Augusto de Mendonça Lima

Primary care mental health in older adults: a global perspective is a resource to support improved care for a growing population of older adults with mental health difficulties that recognises innovative solutions to support the dignity of older adults whilst embracing new technology.

As we celebrate the 40th anniversary of the Alma-Ata Declaration, we need to recognise that not everyone has fully benefitted from the opportunities provided by the move to primary care [1] especially many older adults with mental health difficulties.

We can do better, and the world can do better, but, for this to happen, primary care needs to be more receptive to the special needs of older adults with mental health difficulties and better skilled to address these common problems.

In 1978, the world had a total of 4,287,000,000 habitants; 248,998,000 of them were over 65 years of age representing 5.81% of the total population. Forty years later, the world has a total population of 7,530,000,000 habitants; 654,568,000 of them are over 65 years of age representing 8.70% of the total population. Older adults are now the group with the greatest growth rate [2].

In the context of the rapid growth in numbers of the older adult population, the mental health of older adults has become a huge challenge for all concerned, especially with the high prevalence of mental health issues in this group.

The ageing world population needs to be central in all policies and programmes in order to enable health systems to be more equitable, inclusive and fair. Services need to be designed to respond to the mental health needs of older adults; educational programmes need to be offered for professionals to improve their specific skills to treat and care for this important group.

Carers of older adults with mental health difficulties are an important resource and need to be supported to prevent their own burn out. The population needs to be educated about the ageing process and encouraged to be advocates for older adults with mental health difficulties to combat misconceptions, prejudices, stigma and discrimination [3], and we have provided some resources that can be used to inspect places where older adults with mental health difficulties can be cared for.

Keeping up with technological advances and innovations is very important in delivering quality care to older adults with mental health difficulties to support their continuing independence and dignity, and we have provided some examples of this.

G. Ivbijaro (✉)
NOVA University, Lisbon, Portugal

Waltham Forest Community and Family Health Services, London, UK

C. A. de Mendonça Lima
Unity of Old Age Psychiatry, Centre Les Toises, Lausanne, Switzerland

© Springer Nature Switzerland AG 2019
C. A. de Mendonça Lima, G. Ivbijaro (eds.), *Primary Care Mental Health in Older People*,
https://doi.org/10.1007/978-3-030-10814-4_1

Integrated and collaborative care between primary care, specialists, social services, the voluntary and charitable sector, patients, carers, families and government bodies should always be considered and embraced when developing care packages for older adults with mental health difficulties [4–7].

The WPA-Lancet Psychiatry Commission on the Future of Psychiatry [8] has identified several priority areas for mental health over the next decade including health-care system reform embracing stepped care, increased use of multidisciplinary teamwork, more of a public health approach and the integration of mental and physical health care. The collaboration between primary care teams and other sectors of the health-care system, as well as improving knowledge and skills, will help to improve the mental health care of older adults.

1.1   Structure

The book is structured to enable individuals to understand the complex network of factors that contribute to the mental health of older adults, and each chapter opens with key messages.

- Parts I and II provide an introduction to the foundations of integrated systems to promote good mental health in older adults, including the wide determinants of health, the general concept of frailty and the importance of sometimes complex multimorbidity in this particular population.
- Part III describes the tools for assessment, including neurocognitive assessment.

- Part IV describes therapeutic strategies including the importance of promoting mental and physical health and strategies to advocate for better support for those in need.
- Parts V and VI describes common mental health problems in older adults and how to manage them using a multidisciplinary approach.
- Part VII is focused on psychosocial and neurocognitive rehabilitation.
- Part VIII presents a range of case examples from professionals working with older adults with mental health difficulties.

References

1. World Health Organization. Primary health care: report of the International Conference on Primary Care, Alma-Ata, USSR, 6–12 Sept 1978. Geneva: WHO; 1978.
2. The World Bank. https://data.worldbank.org/indicator/SP.POP.65UP.TO.ZS. Accessed 16 Sept 2018.
3. Graham N, Lindsay J, Katona C, et al. Reducing stigma and discrimination against older people with mental disorders: a technical consensus statement. Int J Geriatr Psychiatry. 2003;18:670–8.
4. WHO, WONCA. Integrating mental health into primary care: a global perspective. Geneva: WHO/WONCA; 2008.
5. WHO, WPA. Psychiatry of the elderly: a consensus statement. Geneva: WHO; 1996. WHO/MNH/MND/96.7.
6. WHO, WPA. Organization of care in psychiatry of the elderly. Geneva: WHO; 1997. WHO/MSA/MNH/MND/97.3.
7. WHO. The world health report 2008: primary care—now more than ever. Geneva: WHO; 2008.
8. Bhugra D, Tasman A, Pathare S, et al. The WPA-lancet psychiatry commission on the future of psychiatry. Lancet Psychiatry. 4:775–818. https://doi.org/10.1016/S2215-0366(17)30333-4.

Epidemiology and the Scale of the Problem

Yaccub Enum, Wolfgang Spiegel, Karen Bernard, Monica Hill, and Taofik Olajobi

Abstract

Population ageing is taking place in nearly all parts of the world. Ageing results from decreasing mortality and declining fertility. Older adults are increasingly playing important roles in society through volunteer work, caring for their families and paid workforce. However, not all older adults enjoy good health. The burden of non-communicable diseases is increasing, and this has now become a major public health issue. Many older adults are living with ill health including poor mental health. Factors that influence older adults' mental and emotional wellbeing include individual characteristics or attributes, socioeconomic circumstances and the broader environment in which they live. With the increasing population of older adults, it is vital that services plan adequately to provide healthcare and wellbeing care to meet the growing demand. This is especially relevant to primary healthcare providers where older adults often seek help in the first instance. Loneliness and social exclusion are important risk factors for poor mental health among older adults. Efforts to improve mental wellbeing of older adults should include tackling loneliness. Collaborative care, bringing together health and social services, is a good way of managing mental health problems in older adults.

Key Points
- Population ageing is taking place in nearly all the countries of the world. The largest increase will occur in Asia, followed by Africa and Latin America, respectively.
- Mental health and emotional wellbeing are equally important in older age as at any other stage of life.
- Factors that influence older adult's mental and emotional wellbeing include individual characteristics or attributes, socioeconomic circumstances and the broader environment in which they live.
- Mental health problems in older adults globally are underestimated and generally under-detected by healthcare professionals.
- Primary care has a very important role to play in detecting mental health problems in older adults.
- Collaborative care is a useful model for providing holistic care for older adults.

Y. Enum (✉) · K. Bernard · M. Hill
Public Health Department, London Borough of Waltham Forest, London, UK

W. Spiegel
Centre for Public Health, Medical University of Vienna, Vienna, Austria

T. Olajobi
College of Nursing, Midwifery and Healthcare, University of West London, London, UK

© Springer Nature Switzerland AG 2019
C. A. de Mendonça Lima, G. Ivbijaro (eds.), *Primary Care Mental Health in Older People*,
https://doi.org/10.1007/978-3-030-10814-4_2

2.1 Introduction

There is no agreed definition of 'older adults' or 'old people', and there are wide variations in what people consider to be old. For the purpose of this paper, we will use the United Nations agreed cut-off numerical criterion of 60+ years to refer to the older population [1].

Population ageing is taking place in nearly all the countries of the world. Ageing results from decreasing mortality and, most importantly, declining fertility. This process leads to a relative reduction in the proportion of children and to an increase in the share of people in the main working ages and of older persons in the population [2].

2.2 Demography of Older Adults

In 2015, there were 901 million people aged 60 or over, comprising 12% of the global population. The population aged 60 or above is growing at a rate of 3.26% per year. The number of older persons in the world is projected to be 1.4 billion by 2030, 2.1 billion by 2050 and 3.2 billion in 2100. Sixty-six per cent of the increase between 2015 and 2050 will occur in Asia, 13% in Africa and 11% in Latin America and the Caribbean. In Europe, 24% of the population is already aged 60 years or over and that proportion is projected to rise to 34% in 2050 [2].

Older persons are projected to exceed the number of children for the first time in 2047. About two thirds of the world's older persons live in developing countries. Because the older population in less developed regions is growing faster than in the more developed regions, the projections show that older persons will be increasingly concentrated in the less developed regions of the world. By 2050, nearly eight in ten of the world's older population will live in the less developed regions [2].

For most nations, regardless of their geographic location or developmental stage, the older population is itself ageing. The population aged 80 and over is growing faster than any younger segment of the older population. At the global level, the average annual growth rate of persons aged 80 years or over (3.8%) is currently twice as high as the growth

rate of the population over 60 years of age (1.9%) [3]. Globally, the number of persons aged 80 or over is projected to increase from 125 million in 2015 to 434 million in 2050 and 944 million in 2100. In 2015, 28% of all persons aged 80 and over lived in Europe, but that share is expected to decline to 16% by 2050 and 9% by 2100 as the populations of other major areas continue to increase in size and to grow older themselves [2].

The older population is mostly female. Because women tend to live longer than men, older women outnumber older men almost everywhere. In 2013, globally, there were 85 men per 100 women in the age group 60 years or over and 61 men per 100 women in the age group 80 years or over. The male to female sex ratios are expected to increase moderately during the next several decades, reflecting a slightly faster projected decline in old-age mortality among males than among females [4].

2.3 Social and Political Participation

Older adults are increasingly playing a critical role in society through volunteer work, caring for their families, paid workforce and transferring experience, skills and knowledge. However, not all older adults enjoy good health. The burden of non-communicable diseases is increasing, and this has now become a major public health issue. Many older adults are living with ill health including poor mental health. Mental and emotional well-being is equally important in older age as at any other stage of life. Approximately 15% of adults aged 60 and over suffer from a mental disorder [5].

2.4 Risk Factors for Poor Mental Health in Older Adults

Factors that influence older adult's mental and emotional wellbeing include individual characteristics or attributes (age, sex, genes), socioeconomic circumstances in which older persons find themselves and the broader environment in which they live. It can be a single aspect or a combination of factors [6].

Older adults are more likely to experience events such as bereavement, a drop in socio-economic status with retirement or a disability that may trigger distorted emotional responses. All of these factors can result in isolation, loss of independence, loneliness and psychological distress which can impact on mental wellbeing. The neurobiological changes associated with getting older (alterations in memory function that are associated with normative ageing), prescribed medication for other conditions and genetic susceptibility (which increases with age) all impact on mental wellbeing [6].

2.4.1 Co-morbidity of Mental and Physical Health Problems in Older Adults

Many people with long-term physical health conditions also have mental health problems. Getting old is a risk for long-term conditions like cardiovascular disease. Cardiovascular disease management has great benefits for older adults' health. Similarly as older adults lose their ability to live independently because of limited mobility, chronic pain or frailty, they are at an increased risk for poor mental wellbeing. Mental health has an impact on physical health and vice versa. For example, older adults with physical health conditions such as heart disease have higher rates of depression than those who are medically well. Conversely, untreated depression in an older adult with heart disease can negatively affect the outcome of the physical illness [7, 8].

2.4.2 Alcohol Abuse

Alcohol abuse is a problem that affects people of all ages, but it is more likely to go unrecognized among older adults [9]. Some reasons for alcohol abuse in older age include loneliness, bereavement and other losses, physical ill health, disability and pain, loss of independence, boredom and depression. Retirement may also provide more opportunities for drinking too much as there is no pressure to go to work each day. According to the Royal College of Psychiatrists,

a third of older adults with alcohol problems (mainly women) develop them for the first time in later life [10].

2.4.3 Medication

Prescribed medications can cause symptoms associated with mental illness in older adults. Many older adults take some kind of medication, and some take several at the same time. There are risks associated with taking multiple medications (both prescribed and over-the-counter medications) due to drug interaction. This can cause problems such as confusion.

2.4.4 Abuse

Older adults are vulnerable to elder abuse—including physical, sexual, psychological, emotional, financial and material abuse, abandonment, neglect and serious losses of dignity and respect. Elder abuse can lead not only to physical injuries but also to serious, sometimes long-lasting, psychological consequences, including depression and anxiety.

2.4.5 Retirement

Retirement from work or career that has been a major part of one's life can affect:

- The social aspect of life through loss of work friendships/relationships
- Sense of self-worth and self-esteem if one felt valued at work
  Financial security

2.5 Mental Health Problems in Old Age: Epidemiology

Older adults aged 60 and over constitute a substantial proportion of vulnerable group of people with an elevated risk of developing mental health problems [11, 12]. They are more likely to have high levels of functional dependency and psychosocial needs which have implications for their health and the delivery of care. According to the World Health Organization (WHO), 6.6% of cases of disability (disability-adjusted life years—DALYs) occurring among older adults aged over 60 is attributable to neurological and mental health problems which account for 17.4% of years lived with disability (YLDs) [13].

It is estimated that about 20% of people at old age have mental health conditions that are not considered as part of "normal" ageing [14]. An earlier report suggests that the number of older adults with major mental health disorders will increase substantially by 2030 [15]. However, it is argued that the true prevalence of mental health problems globally are underestimated and generally underdetected by healthcare professionals [16, 17].

2.5.1 Common Mental Disorders

Common mental disorders (CMD) among the general population include anxiety-related disorders, panic disorder, obsessive-compulsive disorder (OCD), posttraumatic stress disorder (PTSD) and depression [18].

The most common mental disorders reported among older adults are anxiety-related disorders, including phobias and obsessive-compulsive disorder; severe cognitive impairment, including Alzheimer's disease; and dementia, depression and substance use disorders [19–21].

It is estimated that 3.8% of the older population have anxiety related disorders, about 1% are affected with alcohol and drug dependence disorders and in addition about 25% of deaths relating to self-harm and suicides occurred among elderly people aged 60 or above [13]. A meta-analysis of the prevalence of mental disorders in older adults in Western countries shows that the most prevalent mental disorder is dimensional depression (19.5%) followed by lifetime major depression (16.5%). Lifetime alcohol use disorders are estimated to be 11.7%, while drug use disorders, bipolar disorder and current agoraphobia have the lowest prevalence rates [11].

Findings from the Global Burden of Disease Study 2010 indicate that depressive disorders had the highest proportion of total burden among older adults across all regions and accounted for most DALYs (40.5%) caused by mental and substance use disorders. This is followed by anxiety disorders, drug use and alcohol use disorders [22].

2.5.2 Severe Mental Illness (SMI)

Severe Mental Illness is defined according to diagnostic criteria of the International Classification of Mental and Behavioural Disorders, which include major depression, bipolar disorders, schizophrenia, paranoid and other psychotic disorders [23].

A report on the prevalence of serious mental illness among US adults estimated a prevalence of 3.1% for older adults aged 50 years and above [24]. A meta-analysis estimated the prevalence of current bipolar disorder among older adults in 15 different Western countries (Europe and North America) to be 0.5% and 1.1% for lifetime bipolar disorder [11]. Another study estimated the lifetime prevalence of major depression for older adults aged 75 years and older as ranging between 3.7% and 28.0% [20].

2.5.3 Dementia

The prevalence of dementia rapidly increases from about 2% to 3% among those aged 70–75 years to 20% to 25% among those aged 85 years or more [25]. Several studies show the overall prevalence of dementia varies widely among countries, being influenced by cultural and socioeconomic factors [26]. Dementia rates are growing at alarming proportion in all regions of the world and are related to population ageing [27]. The prevalence of dementia is rising with increasing longevity, and this presents a great economic burden [28].

There were an estimated 35.6 million people living with dementia worldwide in 2010, with

58% of them in middle- or low-income countries. The number of people living with dementia is expected to almost double every 20 years, to 65.7 million in 2030 and 115.4 million in 2050. The proportion living in middle- or low-income countries is also projected to increase to 63% in 2030 and 71% in 2050 [29].

However, it has been argued that there is a general trend for overdiagnosis of mild cognitive impairment since the ageing of the population by some is seen as a commercial opportunity [30]. Le Couteur and colleagues point out that the belief that there is value in screening for "pre-dementia" or mild cognitive impairment is creeping into clinical practice, with the resulting overdiagnosis having potential adverse consequences for individual patients, resource allocation and research [30].

The prevalence of dementia in people aged 75 and over in the poorest regions of Latin America was estimated to be higher than in other regions of the world. This may be due to a combination of low to average educational attainment and high vascular risk profile among Latin American elderly population [25].

A systematic review and meta-analysis of the literature on the global prevalence of dementia in people aged 60 and over found that the age-standardized prevalence in most world regions varied between 5% and 7%. The exceptions were in Latin America, with a higher prevalence of 8.5% and a lower prevalence of 2–4% in some sub-Saharan African regions [29].

A meta-analysis of dementia prevalence surveys in the Chinese population found that the prevalence of Alzheimer's disease in the population aged 60 years or older was 1.9% and for vascular dementia was 0.9% [31].

In Europe the number of people with dementia is expected to increase by 90% between 2013 and 2050, from 11 million to 21 million [32].

Current estimates suggest that about 4.2 million adults in the USA have dementia and that the economic cost of their care is about $200 billion per year [33]. This report also estimates that the worldwide prevalence is expected triple to 135.5 million by 2050.

2.6 Suicide in Older Adults

The three most frequent life problems associated with suicide are physical illness, interpersonal problems and bereavement [34]. Long-term conditions and bereavement are common among older adults, and these conditions increase the risk of depression. Social isolation, which is a risk factor for depression, is common among older adults, especially in Europe and the USA. People who are depressed are at a greater risk of suicide and untreated depression can increase the risk of suicide. Even though suicide rates vary by age group in different regions, suicide rates globally are highest in people aged 70 years and over [35]. The primary care setting is an important venue for late life suicide prevention. Primary care providers should be well prepared to diagnose and treat depression in their older patients.

2.7 Conclusion

Population ageing presents challenges for healthcare and social care systems worldwide. However, many older adults are living well. The variability in the prevalence rates reported may be attributed to the use of different diagnostic criteria, geographical and cultural differences in the included studies. Given the demographic transformation taking place in older adults, it is vital that services plan adequately to provide healthcare and wellbeing care to meet the growing demand. This is especially relevant to primary healthcare providers where older adults often seek help in the first instance. Loneliness and social exclusion are important risk factors for poor mental health among older adults. Efforts to improve mental wellbeing of older adults should include tackling loneliness. Collaborative care, bringing together health and social services, is a good way of managing mental health problems in older adults.

References

1. World Health Organization. Definition of an older or elderly person: Proposed Working Definition of an Older Person in Africa for the MDS Project. http://www.who.int/healthinfo/survey/ageingdefnolder/en/. Accessed 15 Dec 2015.
2. United Nations. World population ageing 2013. http://www.un.org/en/development/desa/population/publications/pdf/ageing/WorldPopulationAgeing2013.pdf. Accessed 15 Dec 2015.
3. United Nations. World population ageing 1950–2015: Demographic profile of the older population. http://www.un.org/esa/population/publications/worldageing19502050/pdf/90chapteriv.pdf. Accessed 15 Dec 2015.
4. World Health Organisation. United Nations Department of Economic and Social Affairs ǀ Population Division. World population aging. http://www.un.org/en/development/desa/population/publications/pdf/ageing/WorldPopulationAgeing2013.pdf. Accessed 29 Feb 2016.
5. World Health Organisation. Mental health and older adults, Fact sheet N°381, 2015. http://www.who.int/mediacentre/factsheets/fs381/en/. Accessed 17 Dec 2015.
6. World Health Organisation. Risks to mental health: an overview of vulnerabilities and risk factors. http://www.who.int/mental_health/mhgap/risks_to_mental_health_EN_27_08_12.pdf. Accessed 1 Feb 2016.
7. Egede LE, Ellis C. Diabetes and depression: global perspectives. Diabetes Res Clin Pract. 2010;87(3):302–12.
8. Moussavi S, et al. Depression, chronic diseases, and decrements in health: results from the World Health Surveys. Lancet. 2007;370(9590):851–8.
9. Centre for Substance Abuse Treatment. Substance abuse among older adults. Treatment Improvement Protocol (TIP) Series 26. http://www.ncbi.nlm.nih.gov/books/NBK64422/. Accessed 15 Dec 2015.
10. Royal College of Psychiatrists. Alcohol and older people. http://www.rcpsych.ac.uk/healthadvice/problemsdisorders/alcoholandolderpeople.aspx. Accessed 29 Feb 2016.
11. Volkert J, Schulza H, Härtera M, et al. The prevalence of mental disorders in older people in Western countries—a meta-analysis. Ageing Res Rev. 2013;12:339–53.
12. Challis D, Tucker S, Wilberforce M, et al. National trends and local delivery in old age mental health services: towards an evidence base. A mixed-methodology study of the balance of care approach, community mental health teams and specialist mental health outreach to care homes. Program Grants Appl Res. 2014;2(4):1–479.
13. WHO. Mental health and older adults. 2015. http://www.who.int/mediacentre/factsheets/fs381/en/. Accessed 4 Jan 2016.
14. World Health Organisation. Mental health and older adults, Fact sheet N°381, 2015. http://www.who.int/mediacentre/factsheets/fs381/en/. Accessed 4 Jan 2016.
15. Bartels SJ. Caring for the Whole Person: integrated health care for older adults with severe mental illness and medical comorbidity. J Am Geriatr Soc. 2004;52:S249–57.
16. Kessler RC, Aguilar-Gaxiola S, Alonso J, Chatterji S, Lee S, Ormel J, Üstün TB, Wang PS. The global burden of mental disorders: an update from the WHO World Mental Health (WMH) Surveys. Epidemiol Psichiatr Soc. 2009;18(1):23–33.
17. Baxter AJ, Patton G, Scott KM, Degenhardt L, Whiteford HA. Global epidemiology of mental disorders: what are we missing? PLoS One. 2013;8(6):e65514. https://doi.org/10.1371/journal.pone.0065514.
18. National Institute for Health and Care Excellence (NICE). Common mental health disorders, Guidance and guidelines. NICE. 2011. https://www.nice.org.uk/guidance/cg123. Accessed 25 Jan 2016.
19. Goldberg SE, Whittamore KH, Harwood RH, et al. The prevalence of mental health problems among older adults admitted as an emergency to a general hospital. Age Ageing. 2012;41:80–6. https://doi.org/10.1093/ageing/afr106.
20. Luppa M, Sikorski C, Luck T, et al. Age- and gender-specific prevalence of depression in latest-life—systematic review and meta-analysis. J Affect Disord. 2012;136:212–21.
21. Prince M, Brycea R, Albanese E, et al. The global prevalence of dementia: a systematic review and meta analysis. Alzheimers Dement. 2013;9:63–75.
22. Whiteford HA, Degenhardt L, Rehm J, et al. Global burden of disease attributable to mental and substance use disorders: findings from the Global Burden of Disease Study 2010. Lancet. 2013;382(9904):1575–86.
23. World Health Organisation. The ICD-10 classification of mental and behavioural disorders. Geneva: WHO; 1993.
24. National Institute of Mental Health (NIMH). Serious mental illness (SMI) among U.S. adults. http://www.nimh.nih.gov/health/statistics/prevalence/serious-mental-illness-smi-among-us-adults.shtml. Accessed 29 Jan 2016.
25. Ferri PC, Prince M, Brayne C, et al. Global prevalence of dementia: a Delphi consensus study. Lancet. 2005;366(9503):2112–7.
26. Rizzi L, Rosset I, Roriz-Cruz M. Global epidemiology of dementia: Alzheimer's and vascular type. BioMed Res Int. 2014. http://www.hindawi.com/journals/bmri/2014/908915/. Accessed 5 Jan 2016.
27. Kalaria RN, Maestre GE, Arizaga R, et al. Alzheimer's disease and vascular dementia in developing countries: prevalence, management and risk factors. Lancet Neurol. 2008;7(9):812–26.

28. George-Carey R. An estimate of the prevalence of dementia in Africa: a systematic analysis. J Glob Health. 2012;2(2):020401.

29. Prince M, Bryce R, Albanese E, Wimo A, Ribeiro W, Ferri CP. The global prevalence of dementia: a systematic review and meta-analysis. Alzheimers Dement. 2013;9:63–75.

30. Le Couteur DG, Doust J, Creasey H, Brayne C. Political drive to screen for pre-dementia: not evidence based and ignores the harms of diagnosis. BMJ. 2013;347:f5125.

31. Zhang Y, Xu Y, Nie H, et al. Prevalence of dementia and major dementia subtypes in the Chinese populations: a meta-analysis of dementia prevalence surveys, 1980–2010. J Clin Neurosci. 2012;19(10):1333–7.

32. Alzheimer's Research UK. 10 things you need to know about prevalence. 2015. http://www.alzheimersresearchuk.org/about-dementia/facts-stats/10-things-you-need-to-know-about-prevalence/. Accessed 22 Jan 2016.

33. Langa M. Is the risk of Alzheimer's disease and dementia declining? Alzheimers Res Ther. 2015;7(1):34.

34. Harwood DM, Hawton K, Hope T, Harriss L, Jacoby R. Life problems and physical illness as risk factors for suicide in older people: a descriptive and case-control study. Psychol Med. 2006;36(9): 1265–74.

35. World Health Organisation. First WHO report on suicide prevention. http://www.who.int/mediacentre/news/releases/2014/suicide-prevention-report/en/. Accessed 31 Jan 2016.

Wider Determinants of Health

3

Sabine Bährer-Kohler and Brendan McLoughlin

Abstract

Wider determinants of health are most complex, and there exists a complex interaction between lifestyle and the physical, social, and economic environment and individual characteristics. Wider determinants of health play an important role in the mental health of older adults. During primary care assessment of patients' mental wellbeing, it is important to consider the broader influences on the individual, such as physical health, family/friends and social networks, finances/debts, alcohol and drug use, life events, etc. These wider determinants should be taken into consideration when giving health promotion information. As the wider determinants are often outside the scope of primary care, GPs and others should work with other professionals such as social workers in order to ensure holistic assessment of the older adult's needs and appropriate care planning. Professionals should be mindful of cultural influences, diversities, and differences, maintaining the individual's dignity during the process.

Key Points
- The mental health of older adults is influenced by wider determinants and their life course.
- By considering the wider determinants of health and the concepts of flourishing and languishing involved parties can understand better the impact on health of the interaction between the person and their environment.
- Primary care assessment needs to be holistic and gather information from validated questionnaires and interviews with the person and those close to them.
- Evaluations can be necessary to understand the needs and unmet needs of older adults in primary care settings within their individual situations.
- Evaluations and performance assessments in primary care settings should be explained within national and additional social contexts.
- Heath promotion and intervention needs to be provided by health professionals, local communities, friends, family, and other social networks.

S. Bährer-Kohler (✉)
International University of Catalonia (UIC), Barcelona, Spain

Dr. Bährer-Kohler & Partners, Basel, Switzerland
e-mail: sabine.baehrer@vtxmail.ch,
sabine.baehrer@datacomm.ch

B. McLoughlin
Clinical Senior Cognitive Behavioural Therapist, Efficacy, London, UK

© Springer Nature Switzerland AG 2019
C. A. de Mendonça Lima, G. Ivbijaro (eds.), *Primary Care Mental Health in Older People*,
https://doi.org/10.1007/978-3-030-10814-4_3

- Health promotion consists of modifying specific components of individuals, groups, and populations, with the inclusion of intrapersonal, interpersonal, institutional, environmental, and societal aspects.
- Primary and community health-care teams should have knowledge of the wider determinants of mental health and interventions to promote mental health.
- The role that clients/patients and networks could play in the improvement of health care and primary health care and for an everyday reality in all countries needs to be highlighted.

3.1 Wider Determinants of Health: An Introduction

The UN projected that the proportion of persons aged 60 (+) is expected to double between 2007 and 2050, and their actual number will more than triple, reaching around two billion by 2050 [1]. Developing countries worldwide will see the largest increase in absolute numbers of older persons. Dementia/Alzheimer's disease is strongly associated with increasing age [2, 3].

Wider determinants of health are most complex [4], and there exists a complex interaction between lifestyle and the physical, social, and economic environment and individual characteristics. One of the first works in the field was the Whitehall study published during the 1970s, one of the more current publications is the WHO publication—Social Determinants of health—the solid facts (2003) [5]. The Dahlgren and Whitehead model (1991) [6] as a conceptual background guide underlines the broad and complex content of social determinants. For example, socioeconomic aspects and access to social and health services, health partnerships [7], social involvement, and empowerment are important areas for older adults, besides the improvement and stability of resources [8] of the individual in his individual context. Attention to social determinants during the course of life with the

inclusion of individual's autonomy, independence, and human rights in order to minimize, e.g. risk factors, chronic diseases, and/or multimorbidity [9] and deficiencies of older adults is urgently required.

It is as well very well documented that, e.g. to be part of ethnic minorities [10], living conditions, social participation [11], physical activities, and lifestyle factors are relevant social determinants of health and death amongst older adults [12].

The intersectorial and transsectorial perspective of social determinants with the greatest impact on health-related quality of life (HRQL) must have a high priority in the health sector with sustainable political implementations and with a special focus on management, exploration with diagnostic criteria, and evaluation especially in the primary care settings.

3.2 Nature of the Problem Using a Life Course Approach

The World Health Organization defines mental health as "a state of well-being in which every individual realizes his or her own potential, can cope with the normal stresses of life, can work productively and fruitfully, and is able to make a contribution to her or his community" [13].

When applying this definition to an older person, there may be differences. As someone ages, their potential may change—perhaps through the onset of physical illnesses such as chronic obstructive pulmonary disease can significantly limit activity. Older adults are less likely to work formally, so their fruitfulness may be different to that of someone engaged in traditional employment. They remain in a position to contribute to their communities, for example, through volunteering, and cope with the stresses of normal life. Although the potential of an older person may be different from that of a younger one, they can nonetheless realize it [14].

A further perspective on the definition of health is suggested by Keyes [15]. He has challenged the continuum model of mental health and mental illness, with each being the polar opposite of the other. He proposed that there are two different continua, one measuring the extent of illness and the other with the poles of languishing and flourishing.

The concepts of languishing and flourishing are distinguished by variation in the domains of social acceptance, personal growth, social actualization, purpose in life, social contribution, environmental mastery, social coherence, autonomy (exhibits self-direction and resists unsavoury social pressures), positive (warm and satisfying) relations with others, and social integration.

Using this model, the health continuum (languishing-flourishing) may help to prevent or precipitate a negative movement along the illness continuum. Thus, flourishing may contribute to personal resilience and protect someone developing a mental illness, despite factors which might be associated with onset. Similarly, languishing may make it harder for someone to be able to defend against challenges, leading to illness [15].

Whitehead and Dahlgren's [16] model considers a range of factors which can influence our health known as "the Wider Determinants of Health" [16].

The WHO Commission on Social Determinants of Health [17] reported on socioeconomic and policy influences on health and its wider determinants.

These models for determinants of health will be used to inform the content of this chapter, which will take a life course approach and consider the mediating influence of Keyes work on flourishing and languishing.

Factors which are associated with mental health and wellbeing in later life include [14]:

- Discrimination
- Participation in meaningful activity
- Relationships
- Physical activity
- Poverty

There have been challenges to the applicability of such findings to rural as opposed to urban populations (such as the application of the interaction between health and wealth in rural older women in Canada [18]), but other studies of older rural adults would support them (a relationship existing between health and wealth in rural populations in Vietnam and Brazil [19, 20]).

When older adults themselves were asked what was important in maintaining their wellbeing in Scotland in the UK, they cited [21]:

- Family and friends
- Attitudes (their own and that of society)
- Keeping active
- Maintaining capability and independence
- Negotiating transitions

There are clear overlaps between these, with the most notable difference being that older adults identified transitions as a factor, whereas the previous report included poverty (not having enough income to provide for a decent standard of living and opportunities to participate in society).

Other factors have been identified in different countries and cultures. For example, in Brazil, better self-assessed health was associated with being a widow with independent income [20].

If these are accepted as the prevalent factors once in old age, how can the life course influence them? Within a life course approach, the stages of life which can influence health include:

- Perinatal
- Childhood and young adulthood
- Adulthood
- Old age

Through these stages, a person will be exposed to influences on their health as a result of their own actions and, as noted above, within the context of wider society and culture, systems, economics, and politics. Some of the influences are discussed below.

Perinatal The unborn child can potentially experience undernourishment as a result of a poor and stressed mother. Maternal depression can have a significant impact on a child, affecting weight and bonding and increasing the risk of future depression [22]. Social isolation and self-rated maternal health are often connected with economic deprivation. Social isolation in a mother can pass this disadvantage onto the child [23]. Poor water quality and sanitation [24] and health systems [4] can contribute further risks.

Childhood and Young Adulthood Where children grow up in abusive families, with neglect and violence, they are at increased risk of later health and social problems. This is more likely to occur in lower socioeconomic groups [25]. For those in these lower groups, the impact of poverty and associated issues, e.g. poor access to education, poor nutrition, and infections, contributes to further risks for health [26]. Children who experience social isolation are more likely to have lower educational levels and lower socioeconomic status and are more likely to be obese, smoke, and have psychological problems in the future [27]. Young people are at risk of being bullied for being different in any way, including race, sexuality, and weight. Bullying has adverse social, physiological, and psychological consequences [28]. Adolescence can be a time of increased risk of substance misuse and smoking, which can then continue into adulthood and old age. Levels of physical activity and diet can similarly have significant impacts at this and later stages [29]. Failure to progress in society in developed countries through education and employment deprives young people of the chance to develop social and life skills which contribute to their integration into society and increases the risk of future poor health [30].

Adulthood Unemployment and poor-quality employment are significant risk factors for health problems, a consequence of low income and poverty. These affect diet, living conditions, and the mental health of parents. Unemployment reduces opportunities for social contact through colleagues, etc. and through reduced income and embarrassment about their position. Being out of work makes it harder to find work too, making unemployment a particularly pernicious factor affecting social inclusion and health [31]. It is perhaps unsurprising then that depression and anxiety disorders are two to three times more common in the unemployed [32]. Having experienced depression once, 50% of people will experience it again [33].

Older Age All of the preceding life stages can have an impact on older age, e.g. socioeconomic and educational status [16]. Significantly, by older age, many people have developed long-term physical health conditions, a predictor of mental illness. There is an increasing risk of isolation and perceived loss of status. Transitions were identified by the sample of older adults as a factor effecting their health and wellbeing. Retirement can be a significant transition when contact with friends and colleagues can reduce, together with the sense of participation, capability and independence. Bereavement and the loss of loved ones are inevitable features of older life and can contribute to reduced social contact. These can be compounded by stigma and discrimination—commonly experienced in older age in some communities [17]. Other determinants will influence mental health such as the environment and perceptions of safety [34].

Following on from Keyes' use of the term autonomy [15], increased isolation and reduced participation can contribute to less autonomous behaviour as an older adult may be more dependent on others and less self-directing. This possibly reduced autonomy and dependence on friends, family, and carers and can have implications for their human rights [35] (such as their right to freedom of movement, equality, and access to public services) as they make an older adult vulnerable to a range of abuses (see below).

3.3 Management of the Problem (Topic) Using a Stepped Care Framework to Include

3.3.1 Aspects of Diagnostic Criteria Including Assessment Tools

Evaluations are necessary, for example, to understand the needs and unmet needs of older adults in primary care settings within their individual situations [36], including the possibilities of withdrawal, resignation, and low expectations, not merely to collect information and data. Many older adults and carers do not appear to seek help for their needs for a range of very complex reasons.

It is important to use diagnostic criteria by assessment tools which have a broad spectrum, which include social determinants, which feature liability, comprehensibility, and which are scientifically based and established, means with the possibility of e.g. reliability and validity, self-rated or rated aspects. The strength of social networks has been documented to be one of the biggest determinants in the context.

Around the world, researchers, primary care occupational groups, and others may be able to find assessment tools [37] (APA and others). It is important for a senseful, meaningful, and sustainable manageability in every planned context to find evaluation tools, which are useful, tailored, and aligned to the desired exploration. Primary care workers and others in the health field should be trained to work with scales but also in examining situations for health promotion in a broader, holistic context without any scales. Awareness, effective communication styles, and empathy are substantial content modules.

In the following an extract of possible tools with diagnostic criteria and survey aspects in the broad context of social determinants will be presented, exactly to the following determinants: social networks, social participation, social support, quality of life, agitation, griefs, stress factors, life change events, and social capital.

Name of the test/survey	Abbr.	Authors	Aspects/content
Lubben Social Network Scale and the Lubben Social Network Scale–6	LSNS LSNS-6	Lubben (1988 [38], 2003 [39], 2004 [40])	The Lubben Social Network Scale (LSNS) is a 10-item instrument (or 6 item) to measure social isolation in older adults (aged 65 and above) by measuring perceived social support received by family, friends, and others. It can be used to assess the level of social support. Possible interpretations: isolated, high risk for isolation, moderate risk for isolation, low risk for isolation
Social Participation	WAS	Welin Activity Scale (Welin et al. 1992) [41]	The Welin Activity Scale (WAS) measures the frequency of 32 activities, divided into 3 subcategories: home, outside home, and social activities in the past year
Interpersonal Support Evaluation List	ISEL	Cohen et al. (1997) [42], Cohen and Hoberman (1983) [43]	The 40-item version has 10-item subscales for perceived availability of 4 separate functions of social support: (1) emotional support, (2) instrumental support, (3) companionship support, and (4) self-esteem maintenance through social comparisons
UCLA Social Support Inventory (UCLA-SSI)	UCLA-SSI	Dunkel-Schetter and Bennett (1990) [44], Dunkel-Schetter et al. (1987) [45], Dunkel-Schetter et al. (1986/2015) [46]	The 70-item interview protocol focused on specific stressors. The inventory is based upon a conceptualization of support as interpersonal transactions between people, characterized by several forms. Forms or types of support include: – Information – Advice – Aid – Assistance – Emotional support (cf. Dunkel-Schetter et al. [46])
Arizona Social Support Interview Schedule	ASSIS	Barrera (1980) [47]	The schedule, a 27-item interview guide, provides an assessment of the subject's social network for the past 6 months. However, it requires a skilled interviewer. The schedule assesses six functions: (1) intimate interaction, (2) material aid, (3) physical assistance, (4) guidance, (5) social participation, (7) positive feedback

Name of the test/survey	Abbr.	Authors	Aspects/content
The World Health Organization Quality of Life tool	WHOQOL WHO Bref WHOQOL-SRPB	WHO (2015) [48], WHOQOL-SRPB (2002) [49], WHOQOL Group (1998) [50]	The World Health Organization Quality of Life (WHOQOL) project was initiated in 1991 to develop an international cross-culturally comparable quality of life assessment instrument. Result: The current long version WHOQOL, the short version WHO Bref, and, e.g. an additional 32-item instrument to assess aspects of spirituality, religiousness, and personal beliefs (WHOQOL-SRPB)
Quality of Life Assessment Schedule	QOLAS	Selai et al. (2001) [51]	Dementia QOL instrument—with 10 items—tailored to individual patients. With qualitative and quantitative measurement approaches. Areas: physical, psychological, social/family, usual activities, and cognitive functioning − Self-administered − Caregiver-administered − Interviewer-administered
Cornell-Brown Scale for Quality of Life in Dementia	CBS	Ready et al. (2002) [52]	A global assessment of QOL with 19 items. Reliable and valid measurement of patient QOL. For example, exploration of: − Happiness − Self-esteem − Optimism − Physical complaints − Absence of negative affects
Cohen-Mansfield Agitation Inventory—elderly person	CMAI	Finkel et al. (1992) [53], Cohen-Mansfield (1990) [54], Cohen-Mansfield and Billig (1986) [55]	The Cohen-Mansfield Agitation Inventory (CMAI) is a 29-item scale to assess agitation, exact the frequency of manifestations. A primary caregiver rates the older adult. Measurement: − Physical aggression − Physical nonaggression − Verbal agitation
Inventory of Complicated Grief	ICG	Prigerson et al. (1995) [56]	The Inventory of Complicated Grief with 19-item inventory assesses indicators of pathological grief, to measure maladaptive symptoms of loss, such as anger, disbelief, and hallucinations
The Standard Stress Scale	SSS	Gross and Seebass (2014) [57]	Measuring stress in the life course. 11-item Standard Stress Scale. For example: − Social distress − Social support − Social approval
The Social Readjustment Rating Scale	SRRS	Holmes and Rahe (1967) [58]	One of the most widely cited measurement instruments with 43 items in the stress context to measure a wide range of common stressors and life change events, which have taken place in the last 12 months. For example: • Death of a spouse • Divorce • Marital separation • Death of close family member • Change in financial state • Change in living conditions • Change in residence • Change in sleeping habits

Name of the test/survey	Abbr.	Authors	Aspects/content
General Social Survey items self-rated health social capital	GSS	Kawachi et al. (1999) [59], General Social Survey (GSS) (2015) [60]	Since 1972, the General Social Survey (GSS) has been monitoring societal change and studying the growing complexity. The GSS survey contains a standard core of demographic, behavioural, and attitudinal questions, plus issues of special interest, e.g. the 2014 GSS has modules on, e.g. social identity, social isolation, and civic participation. Kawachi et al. [59] documented a contextual effect of low social capital on risk of self-rated poor health

3.3.2 Specific Issue for Primary Care Assessment

In order for people to get help, they must first come forward for it and be able to access it. Older adults have the same stigmatizing attitudes towards mental illness as the rest of society and can in fact be more stigmatizing. More age appropriate and culturally appropriate services can help with this. The inclusion of a range of stakeholders will contribute to the services and support which will help them to engage [61–63].

Assessment of mental health in older adults by the primary care team needs to be holistic and take into account each person's own life course or story and experiences. This can help to identify and understand the range of influences on that person's health and wellbeing.

In conducting the assessment, the practitioner needs to consider [64]:

- Physical health: Long-term physical health conditions, functional (including visual) limitations, changes in body mass index
- Mental health: Depression and anxiety, cognitive impairment, self-efficacy
- Social health: Frequency and nature of social contact, relationships
- Lifestyle: Levels of physical activity, alcohol use, smoking

These different aspects of someone's health and wellbeing might frequently interact. A long-term physical condition, for example, might reduce functioning, increase social isolation, and reduce self-efficacy and be associated with the development of depression and/or anxiety. These in turn can inhibit management of the long-term condition, and a vicious circle can develop. The interaction between these issues will be idiosyncratic, hence the need for a holistic, personalized assessment.

Health professionals may not be trained or have the time to enable consideration of these broad perspectives. The use of validated scales (see above) may be helpful, but they do require time and training. This can sometimes be mitigated by the person completing questionnaires prior to their consultation with the health professional. Primary care assessment may be most effective if it brings together information from a range of sources [65]. As noted above, the person themselves, any relatives, friends, or carers will be able to supply relevant information for the range of determinants which have been identified above.

They would also need to approach such assessment from perspectives which they are not familiar with. In this case, the views of the older person and any relatives or carers may be more significant than observed symptoms or even rating scales. Such interaction needs time with the conversation steered by knowledge of those factors identified as risk factors for poorer wellbeing and functioning.

What is often required is time and the ability to listen judiciously, being aware of issues and facts to focus on and explore, rather than seeking symptoms which might lead to a diagnosis. This may be carried out effectively by health workers with appropriate basic training and pre-existing social skills, i.e. an understanding of signs and symptoms of disorders and an attitude of understanding of the person, and their world [66]. They could be drawn from local communities and so have a knowledge and understanding of local factors which might contribute to mental health or illness too. This workforce would then consult with other health professionals, pooling the knowledge and information obtained from their respective assessments which can then lead to a more holistic and personalized plan of care, including physical, mental, and social health interventions, and lifestyle advice.

At the population level, where public health bodies are seeking to reduce the incidence or impact of particular conditions, they can undertake screening for such conditions. Given the prevalence of mental health conditions in older adults, and stigmatizing attitudes to mental health and to older adults (from themselves and others), it is good practice to routinely screen for common mental illnesses at each consultation with an older adult. This can be done using the PHQ 4, a validated measure designed as a screening tool for primary care, which asks four questions to predict severity of anxiety or depression [67]. If a system of health checks for older adults is in place, this can be added to them, but this instrument is brief enough to enable routine use in everyday consultations too. Screening in this context is likely to be beneficial as it would identify issues earlier when there are potential interventions which could improve the current situation and possibly prevent deterioration or development of further problems over time [68].

When assessing older adults, practitioners need to be sensitive to the risk of elder abuse. This has been defined as "a single, or repeated act, or lack of appropriate action, occurring within any relationship where there is an expectation of trust, which causes harm or distress to an older person" [69]. Such abuse can take the form of:

- Physical
- Emotional
- Financial
- Sexual
- Neglect

The WHO recognizes this as a significant issue affecting the rights as well as the health and welfare of older adults [70]. This problem can be hard to identify—people (including the abused) will frequently hide such issues through shame and stigma. Where identified in more developed countries, there are often specific services which address such issues. In less developed countries, where such services do not exist, it may be harder to deal with.

3.3.3 Health Promotion

According to the WHO definition, health promotion is "the process of enabling people to increase control over and to improve their health" [71]. The background concepts of health promotion, self-care, and community participation emerged during the 1970s, related to policies promoting, e.g. social justice and social equity. The Ottawa Charter, a very important milestone in health promotion practice worldwide, defines five key strategies for health promotion actions: building a public health policy, creating supportive environments, strengthening community action, developing personal skills, and reorienting health services.

Health promotion in general consists of modifying specific components of individuals, groups, and populations, with the inclusion of intrapersonal, interpersonal, institutional, environmental, and societal aspects. Before considering the implementation of any public health promotion programme, several points such as appropriateness, feasibility, cost-effectiveness, and potential need to be carefully considered [72].

There is documented evidence that intrapersonal factors including beliefs, attitudes, knowledge, skills, self-concepts, motivation, self-control, emotional regulation, coping variables, and resources can have a strong impact [73]. A better socioeconomic position and good housing quality are further important gradients [74, 75]. For older adults, for example, results demonstrated that adults with higher-quality social relationships might be motivated to be engaged in health-promoting behaviours such as leisure activities and, in turn, reap more health benefits [76].

Whenever public health education intervention attempts to modify erroneous values and opinions regarding health promotion, sufficient consultation and conversation time, reminders, and follow-up visits are applied in every case at the intrapersonal level [73].

It has to be faced that primary care professionals are pointing at barriers in the context of primary prevention and health promotion in clinical practice, such as heavy workloads, a lack of skills, competences and knowledge, problems related to the professional-patient relationship, and lack of confidence in the effectiveness of these interventions [77–79]. One reason of the lack of confidence can be the missing knowledge that different segments of the population respond differently to identical public health intervention [80]. Indispensable necessary for health promotion are multidisciplinary knowledge, skill-related competence, and competence with respect to attitudes and personal social characteristics [81].

One aspect of finding solutions to improve the effectiveness of interventions can be to investigate the possibility of using technological innovations. This can be useful in improving patient self-care and care, perhaps using SMS messaging (with reminders) to improve outpatient attendance, or eHealth to improve the clinical management of identified risk factors through provision of tailored feedback, tailored educational materials, and referral to online self-management/empowerment programs [82].

3.4 Self-Care and Interventions

As has been noted above, assessment requires consideration of the older person's life story and their perspective on their lives and health. Many of the influences which have been discussed might be best addressed by the individual with the provision of any support if needed. By old age, some of the damage to health can have already happened. The emphasis needs to be then on what might be done to either mitigate the effects of earlier behaviour and life experience or prevent further problems from developing.

Such interventions might include an increase in physical activity and exercise, stopping smoking, and reducing alcohol intake. If someone is currently engaging in unhealthy behaviour, it can be very hard for them to change those patterns—which may well have become ingrained over many years. Whilst self-care will be central to any improvement in mental health and wellbeing, older adults' capacity to undertake it will vary depending on their physical and mental health and circumstances.

In helping someone to undertake such a behaviour change programme, it is important to work across a range of domains and with a range of supporting organizations [83]. It requires an understanding of the person, their context and circumstances, what barriers to change they may encounter, and how to overcome them. Whilst professional input can contribute to this, professionals are unlikely to be able to provide sufficient time and be available at the right time that someone needs that support. Family members and friends ought to be considered as part of the care and support network for an older person. There is increasing interest in the role and benefits of peer support for people with mental health conditions [84] and some evidence that older adults can help their peers to improve their mental health conditions [85]. Supporting a peer is also good for the supporter, giving them many of the benefits of employment such as a sense of contributing and purpose [84].

Taking a lead from Keyes [15], older adults can be encouraged to focus on, for example, their social contribution, sense of purpose, positive relationships, and social integration. Support from a peer or other sources may be needed to achieve these or other aspects of flourishing such as environmental mastery and autonomy.

3.4.1 Biopsychosocial Interventions

The important role for self-care with aid and support from friends, family and carers, and healthcare teams makes a significant contribution.

In the context of the holistic assessment previously discussed, a number of issues may have been identified which are amendable to intervention. Medical treatments for pain experienced as a result of a long-term condition, for example. This may be restricting someone's activity and having an impact on their social contact. Effective treatment through analgesia might enable someone to go out more, take more physical exercise, and lead them to feel more independent and capable and results in their being more active participants in their communities, reducing social isolation [86].

Similarly, depression, anxiety, and sleep problems can be treated using psychotropic medication. Medication prescribed for mental illness in adults however needs to be used with greater caution in older adults, due to the potential for side effects to be more significant [87]. Tolerance of these drugs is affected by changes in absorption, distribution, metabolism, and excretion of substances which occur with age. Hypotension, for example, is a common side effect of psychotropic medication. This increases the risk of falls. Further caution is advised over polypharmacy and interactions between drugs, especially with older adults being more likely to be taking medication for their physical heath [86]. There is concern over the use of neuroleptic drugs in those with cognitive impairments and challenging behaviour, and high use of psychotropic medication is reported in those in hospital and care homes [88].

This risk of drug interactions adds further emphasis to the need for health-care teams to be communicating effectively.

Where available, the option of taking therapies can reduce the requirement for drug treatments. Psychological therapies such as cognitive behavioural therapy and counselling are effective for older adults and lack any physical side effects. In the major national rollout of psychological therapy services in England [89], recovery rates were generally higher amongst older adults (58% for over 65 years, 45.2% for 36–64-year-olds, and 42.4% for 18–35-year-olds) [90].

Many of the wider determinants of mental health identified above are not amenable to specific health interventions, though those interventions may be useful. Also, thinking back to the Keyes' model [15] interventions might best be tailored to promoting contributions, relationships, and integration. Those beyond the health-care team must therefore contribute to improvement in health. A key function for the health team might be to have knowledge of the wider determinants of health and sources of help to address them. Problems with accommodation, for example, can have a significant impact on health [18] but would be addressed best by a specialist advocate rather than a health professional. Similarly, social isolation may be reduced more by the interventions of a small local charity. The heath-care team therefore would need to signpost people to a range of organizations as indicated by the holistic and person-centred assessment.

The role of primary care might therefore be more about intervening where there are clear treatable health conditions which are having an effect on, for example, social isolation or physical activity and helping people to understand where help with other issues can be found, signposting them to it, and encouraging people to take greater control over influences where they can. By providing greater understanding and support for increased control, they can empower older adults [91].

3.4.2 Evaluation of Interventions

Evaluation, as defined in *The American Heritage Dictionary*, is action "to ascertain or fix the value or worth of" something [92]. As documented, e.g. in patients' experience survey measures, access, interpersonal and intrapersonal communication, coordination, and health promotion in general are important items in the overall context of evaluation in primary health care [93].

Although the lines between intervention research and programme evaluation are not always clearly defined, both are necessary and requested in the context of social determinants [94]. It is generally accepted that better evidence about interventions and brief interventions [95] around the social determinants of health in action are essential [96].

To evaluate social determinants in the broad field of primary care, it is important how primary care is defined, how task shifting is regulated, how interprofessional teams are composed, and how more consistent primary care data to build workforce strategies can be assembled [97].

Social determinants are always embedded in and related to social systems. Any evaluation of interventions including social determinants should reflect and integrate these dependencies and should highlight that the social systems, which make up societies, are not static objects [98].

In general, evaluations and measurements of performance increasingly play an important role in health-care reforms. Stakeholders need quantitative and qualitative information to form and guide their opinions and political will, engagements, decisions, and recommendations in steering health systems in a variety of settings [99]. This requires analysing and evaluating the responsiveness of all participants during interventions as well as the conditions that can impact on behaviour and wellbeing, such as person's internal locus of control [100]. Finally, finding aspects of an answer how care and cure in primary care settings within social determinants can be managed effectively and sustainably.

Further, evaluations and performance assessments in primary care settings should be explained within national and additional social contexts, for example, across countries at similar levels of income and educational attainment.

A final major requirement of evaluations and performance assessments is to start from a proper framework and conditions from which measures are developed, see, e.g. the Primary Care Evaluation Tool (PCET) of the World Health Organization (1990) [101], with access to services, continuity of services, coordination of delivery, and comprehensiveness.

To implement the verified data, to find a good practice model for local communities, and to revitalize primary health care, the comprehensive primary health-care (CPHC) model can be useful and practicable. It is a sound model of health system organization, addressing health issues including effective management and prevention, e.g. of chronic diseases, achieving more equitable health outcomes, and involving communities, other participants, and other network partners in planning and managing services. The operating principles of the model are accessible; locally delivered; community driven; comprised of a mix of direct care, prevention, and promotion; characterized by multidisciplinary teamwork and intersectoral and interagency collaboration; and embedded within ethically and culturally respectful work [102].

3.4.3 Specific Recommendations for Management in Primary Care

3.4.3.1 Part 1

A range of factors determine health. Some of these are individual, such as genetics and less amendable to interventions, whilst others, such as lifestyle are. Beyond this, environmental factors such as housing and community are less open to the influence of the individual. This is true for all ages. Here there is a role for governments. Local governments can encourage increased physical activity or provide opportunities for social contact and engagement, through transport policies and the provision of communal spaces. Central governments determine the provision of pensions. Their policies can influence health throughout the life course and can promote healthier behaviour by individuals (e.g. stop smoking initiatives by governments have had significant impacts on rates of smoking [103]). They can influence the training and practice of health-care professionals and others. They can run publicity campaigns to inform and educate to promote health and to challenge attitudes.

Primary and community health-care teams have knowledge of the wider determinants of mental health and interventions to promote mental health.

- Health-care assessments of older adults should be personalized and holistic and use a life course approach.
- Services need to be accessible (e.g. by public transport) and non-stigmatizing.

- Peer support should be locally promoted and enabled.
- Health-care professionals communicate effectively so all are aware of the range of diagnoses for a person and the treatments being used.
- Evidence-based psychological therapies should be available to older adults with common mental health conditions.
- Primary and community care teams work with their communities to have directories of local services and organizations which deal with the wider determinants of mental health and health.

3.4.3.2 Part 2

Best planned and tailored interventions in the context of wider social determinants and the management in primary care show that the treatment of lifestyle-related conditions can be related to the unwillingness to change habits and opinions. The individual can have, e.g. an insufficient knowledge about health promotion and of the risk of health conditions [104]. Professionals will face the question related to limits of the patients' responsibilities in health counselling and for management in primary care. The participation concept arose from the consumer movement of the 1960s that affirmed the consumer's right to safety, the right to be informed, the right to choose, and the right to be heard. The World Health Organization (WHO) World Alliance for Patient Safety is highlighting the role that clients/patients and networks could play in the improvement of health care and primary health care and for an everyday reality in all countries [105–107].

3.5 Conclusion

Wider determinants of health play an important role in the mental health of older adults. During primary care assessment of patients' mental well-being, it is important to consider the broader influences on the individual, such as physical health, family/friends and social networks, finances/debts, alcohol and drug use, life events, etc. These wider determinants should be taken into consideration when giving health promotion information. As the wider determinants are often outside the scope of primary care, GPs and others should work with other professionals such as social workers in order to ensure holistic assessment of the older adult's needs and appropriate care planning. Professionals should be mindful of cultural influences, diversities, and differences, maintaining the individual's dignity during the process.

References

1. UN. Ageing. http://www.un.org/en/globalissues/ageing/. 2015. Accessed 14 Sept 2015/26 Jan 2016.
2. Alzheimer's Society. 2015. http://www.alzheimers.org.uk/, https://www.alzheimers.org.uk/site/scripts/documents.php?categoryID=200345. Accessed 14 Sept 2015/26 Jan 2016.
3. Qiu C, Kivipelto M, von Strauss E. Epidemiology of Alzheimer's disease: occurrence, determinants, and strategies toward intervention. Dialogues Clin Neurosci. 2009;11(2):111–28.
4. Tsouros AD/WHO, editor. Social determinants of health- the solid facts. Geneva: World Health Organization; 2003.
5. WHO. Social determinants of health- the solid facts. Geneva: World Health Organization; 2003.
6. Dahlgren G, Whitehead M. Policies and strategies to promote social equity in health. Stockholm: Institute for Futures Studies; 1991.
7. Mitchell SM, Shortell SM. The governance and management of effective community health partnerships: a typology for research, policy, and practice. Milbank Q. 2000;78(2):241–89. 151.
8. American Society of Ageing, Wallace SP. Equity and social determinants of health among older adults. American Society of Ageing, Generations. http://www.asaging.org/blog/equity-and-social-determinants-health-among-older-adults. Accessed 21 Sept 2015/26 Jan 2016.
9. Parker L, Moran GM, Roberts LM, Calvert M, McCahon D. The burden of common chronic disease on health related quality of life in an elderly community-dwelling population in the UK. Fam Pract. 2014;31(5):557–63. https://doi.org/10.1093/fampra/cmu035.
10. Stone JR. Elderly and older racial/ethnic minority healthcare inequalities—care, solidarity, and action. Camb Q Healthc Ethics. 2012;21(3):342–52.
11. Rainer S. Social participation and social engagement of elderly people. Procedia Soc Behav Sci. 2014;116(21):780–5.
12. Silva Vde L, Cesse EÂP, de Albuquerque Mde F. Social determinants of death among the elderly: a systematic literature review. Rev Bras Epidemiol. 2014;17(Suppl 2):178–93.

13. World Health Organization. What is mental health? Geneva: World Health Organization; 2013. http://www.who.int/features/qa/62/en/.

14. Lee, M. Promoting mental health and well-being in later life: a first report from the UK inquiry into mental health and well-being in later life. London: Age Concern and the Mental Health Foundation; 2006. http://www.apho.org.uk/resource/item.aspx?RID=70413.

15. Keyes CLM. Mental illness and/or mental health? Investigating axioms of the complete state model of health. J Consult Clin Psychol. 2005;73(3): 539–48.

16. Whitehead M, Dahlgren G. What can be done about inequalities in health? Lancet. 1991;338(8774):1059–63.

17. Solar O, Irwin A. A conceptual framework for action on the social determinants of health. Social Determinants of Health Discussion Paper 2 (Policy and Practice). Geneva: World Health Organization; 2010.

18. Wanless D, Mitchell BA, Wister AV. Social determinants of health for older women in Canada: does rural–urban residency matter? Can J Aging. 2010;29(2):233–47.

19. Hoi V, et al. Health-related quality of life, and its determinants, among older adults in rural Vietnam. BMC Public Health. 2010;10:549. http://www.biomedcentral.com/1471-2458/10/549

20. Bos AM, Bos AJ. The socio-economic determinants of older adults's health in Brazil: the importance of marital status and income. Ageing Soc. 2007;27:385–405.

21. Health Scotland. Mental health and wellbeing in later life; older adults' perceptions. Edinburgh: Health Scotland; 2004. http://www.healthscotland.com/documents/186.aspx.

22. Surkan PJ, et al. Maternal depression and early childhood growth in developing countries: systematic review and meta-analysis. Bull World Health Organ. 2011;89(8):608–15.

23. Eastwood JG, et al. Relationship of postnatal depressive symptoms to infant temperament, maternal expectations social support and other potential risk factors: findings from a large Australian cross-sectional study. BMC Pregnancy Childbirth. 2012;12:148. http://www.ncbi.nlm.nih.gov/pubmed/23234239.

24. Water Aid. The sanitation problem: what can and should the health sector do? London: Water Aid; 2011.

25. Ford E, Clark C. The influence of childhood adversity on social relations and mental health at mid-life. J Affect Disord. 2011;133(1–2):320–7.

26. Hanson M, Chen E. Socioeconomic status and health behaviors in adolescence: a review of the literature. J Behav Med. 2007;30(3):263–85.

27. Lacey R, Kumari M, Bartley M. Social isolation in childhood and adult inflammation: evidence from the National Development Study.

Psychoneuroendocrinology. 2014;50:85–94. http://www.ncbi.nlm.nih.gov/pubmed/25197797.

28. Takizawa R, Maughan B, Arseneault L. Adult health outcomes of childhood bullying victimization: evidence from a five-decade longitudinal British birth cohort. Am J Psychiatry. 2014;171(7):777–84.

29. Stein C, Moritz I. A life course perspective of maintaining independence in older age. Geneva: World Health Organization; 1999.

30. The Marmot Review Team. Fair society, healthy lives: strategic review of health inequalities in England post-2010. London: Marmot Review Team; 2010.

31. Marcus G, Neumark T, Broome S. Power lines. London: RSA; 2011.

32. Royal College of Psychiatrists. Mental health and work. London: Royal College of Psychiatrists; 2008.

33. Burcusa SL, Iacono WG. Risk for recurrence in depression. Clin Psychol Rev. 2007;27(8):959–85.

34. Roh S, et al. Perceived neighborhood environment affecting physical and mental health: a study with Korean American older adults in New York city. J Immigr Minor Health. 2011;13(6):1005–12.

35. United Nations. The universal declaration of human rights. 1948. http://www.un.org/en/universal-declaration-human-rights/.

36. Walters K, Iliffe S, Orrell M. An exploration of help-seeking behaviour in older adults with unmet needs. Fam Pract. 2001;18(3):277–82.

37. APA (American Psychological Association). The American Psychological Association. http://www.apa.org/about/index.aspx. Accessed 18 Sept 2015.

38. Lubben J. Assessing social networks among elderly populations. Fam Community Health. 1988;11(3):42–52.

39. Lubben J, Gironda M. Centrality of social ties to the health and well-being of older adults. In: Berkman B, Harootyan L, editors. Social work and health care in an aging society. New York: Springer; 2003.

40. Lubben J, Gironda M. Measuring social networks and assessing their benefits. In: Phillipson C, Allan G, Morgan D, editors. Social networks and social exclusion: sociological and policy perspectives. Hampshire: Ashgate Publishing; 2004. p. 20–35.

41. Welin L, Larsson B, Svardsudd K, Tibblin B, Tibblin G. Social network and activities in relation to mortality from cardiovascular diseases, cancer and other causes: a 12-year follow up of the study of men born in 1913 and 1923. J Epidemiol Community Health. 1992;46(2):127–32.

42. Cohen S, Doyle WJ, Skoner DP, Rabin BS, Gwaltney JM. Social ties and susceptibility to the common cold. JAMA. 1997;277(24):1940–4.

43. Cohen S, Hoberman H. Positive events and social supports as buffers of life change stress. J Appl Soc Psychol. 1983;13:99–125, 277: 1940–4.

44. Dunkel-Schetter C, Bennett TL. Differentiating the cognitive and behavioral aspects of social support. In: Sarason BR BR, Sarason IG, Pierce GR, editors.

Social support: an interactional view. New York: Wiley; 1990. p. 267–96.

45. Dunkel-Schetter C, Folkman S, Lazarus RS. Correlates of social support receipt. J Pers Soc Psychol. 1987;53(1):71–80.

46. Dunkel-Schetter C, Feinstein L, Call J. UCLA Social Support Inventory (UCLA-SSI/1986). 1986. http://www.cds.psych.ucla.edu/.../. Accessed 17 Sept 2015.

47. Barrera M. A method for the assessment of social support networks in community survey research. Connect. 1980;3:8–13.

48. WHO. The World Health Organization Quality of Life (WHOQOL). http://www.who.int/mental_health/publications/whoqol/en/. Accessed 18 Sept 2015.

49. WHO. WHOQOL Spirituality, Religiousness and Personal Beliefs (SRPB), WHOQOL-SRPB. 2002. http://www.who.int/mental_health/media/en/622.pdf. Accessed 21 Sept 2015.

50. The WHOQOL. Group. The World Health Organization Quality of Life Assessment (WHOQOL). Development and psychometric properties. Soc Sci Med. 1998;46:1569–85.

51. Selai CE, Trimble MR, Rossor MN, Harvey RJ. Assessing quality of life in dementia: preliminary psychometric testing of the quality of life assessment schedule (QOLAS). Neuropsychol Rehabil. 2001;11:3–4. 219–43

52. Ready RE, Ott BR, Grace J, Fernandez I. The Cornell-Brown Scale for quality of life in dementia. Alzheimer Dis Assoc Disord. 2002;16:109–15.

53. Finkel SI, Lyons JS, Anderson RL. Reliability and validity of the Cohen-Mansfield Agitation Inventory in institutionalized elderly. Int J Geriatr Psychiatry. 1992;7:487–90.

54. Cohen-Mansfield J. Agitation in older adults. In: Billig N, Rabins P, editors. Abstracts in social gerontology. vol. 33, no 1. 1990. p. 114.

55. Cohen-Mansfield J, Billig N. Agitated behaviors in older adults I. a conceptual review. J Am Geriatr Soc. 1986;34:711–21.

56. Prigerson HG, Maciejewski PK, Reynolds CF III, Bierhals AJ, Newsom JT, Fasiczka A, Frank E, Doman J, Miller M. The inventory of complicated grief: a scale to measure maladaptive symptoms of loss. Psychiatry Res. 1995;59(1–2):65–79.

57. Gross C, Seebass K. The Standard Stress Scale (SSS): measuring stress in the life course. NEPS Working Paper No. 45. 2014.

58. Holmes TH, Rahe RH. The social readjustment rating scale. J Psychosom Res. 1967;11:213–8.

59. Kawachi I, Kennedy BP, Glass R. Social capital and self-rated health: a contextual analysis. Am J Public Health. 1999;89(8):1187–93.

60. GSS. General social survey. 2015. http://www3.norc.org/gss+website/. Accessed 21 Sept 2015/26 Jan 2016.

61. Palinkas LA, et al. Unmet needs for services for older adults with mental illness: comparison of views of different stakeholder groups. Am J Geriatr Psychiatry. 2007;15(6):530–40.

62. Conner K, et al. Mental health treatment seeking among older adults with depression: the impact of stigma and race. Am J Geriatr Psychiatry. 2010;18(6):531–43.

63. Akincigil A, et al. Racial and ethnic disparities in depression care in community-dwelling elderly in the United States. Am J Public Health. 2012;102(2):319–28.

64. Frost H, Haw S, Frank J. Promoting health and wellbeing in later life. Interventions in primary care and community settings. Scottish Collaboration for Public Health Research and Policy. 2010. http://www.scphrp.ac.uk/wp-content/uploads/.

65. Hunter CL, et al. Integrated behavioral health in primary care: step-by-step guidance for assessment and intervention. Washington, DC: American Psychological Association; 2009.

66. World Health Organisation. Integrating mental health into primary care: a global perspective. Annex One: Improving the practice of primary care for mental health. Geneva: World Health Organisation and WONCA; 2008.

67. Kroenke K, et al. An ultra-brief screening scale for anxiety and depression: the PHQ-4. Psychosomatics. 2009;50(6):613–21.

68. US National Library of Medicine. Benefits and risks of screening tests. 2013. http://www.ncbi.nlm.nih.gov/pubmedhealth/PMH0072602/.

69. Action on elder abuse. What is elder Abuse? 2015. http://elderabuse.org.uk/what-is-elder-abuse/.

70. Cook-Daniels, L., 2003 is the year elder abuse hits the international state. Victimiz Old Adults Disabled. 2003;5:65–6, 76.

71. World Health Organization. The Ottawa charter for health promotion: 1st international conference on health promotion. Ottawa; 1986. http://www.who.int/healthpromotion/conferences/previous/ottawa/en/. Accessed 31 Jan 2016.

72. Bhuyan KK. Health promotion through self-care and community participation: elements of a proposed programme in the developing countries. BMC Public Health. 2004;4:11.

73. Moreno-Peral P, Conejo-Cerón S, Fernández A, Berenguera A, Martínez-Andrés M, Pons-Vigués M, Motrico E, Rodríguez-Martín B, Bellón JA, Rubio-Valera M. Primary care patients' perspectives of barriers and enablers of primary prevention and health promotion-a meta-ethnographic synthesis. PLoS One. 2015;10(5):e0125004. https://doi.org/10.1371/journal.pone.0125004.

74. Graham H. Unequal lives: health and socioeconomic inequalities. Maidenhead: Open University Press; 2007.

75. Acheson D. Independent inquiry into inequalities in health (the Acheson Report). London: HMSO Her Majesty's Stationery Office; 1998.

76. Chang PJ, Wray L, Lin Y. Social relationships, leisure activity, and health in older adults. Health Psychol. 2014;33(6):516–23.

77. Fairhurst K, Huby G. From trial data to practical knowledge: qualitative study of how general practitioners have accessed and used evidence about statin drugs in their management of hypercholesterolaemia. Br Med J. 1998;317:1130–4.

78. Lambe B, Collins C. A qualitative study of lifestyle counselling in general practice in Ireland. Fam Pract. 2010;27:219–23.

79. Rubio-Valera M, Pons-Vigués M, Martínez-Andrés M, Moreno-Peral P, Berenguera A, Fernández A. Barriers and facilitators for the implementation of primary prevention and health promotion activities in primary care: a synthesis through meta-ethnography. PLoS One. 2014;9(2):e89554.

80. Kelly MP, Bonnefoy J, Morgan A, Florenzano F. The development of the evidence base about the social determinants of health. 2006. p. 17. http://www.who.int/social_determinants/resources/mekn_paper.pdf. Accessed 23 Sept 2015.

81. Kemppainen V, Tossavainen K, Turunen H. Nurses' roles in health promotion practice: an integrative review. Health Promot Int. 2013;28(4):490–501.

82. Carey M, Noble N, Mansfield E, Waller A, Henskens F, Sanson-Fisher R. The role of eHealth in optimizing preventive care in the primary care setting. J Med Int Res. 2015;17(5):126.

83. National Institute for Health and Care Excellence. Behaviour change, general approaches. Guideline. Public Health Guideline 6. 2007. nice.org.uk/guidance/ph6.

84. Repper J, et al. Peer support workers; theory and practice. London: Centre for Mental Health; 2013.

85. Chapin R, et al. Reclaiming joy: pilot evaluation of a mental health peer support program for older adults who receive Medicaid. The Gerontologist. 2013;53(2):345–52.

86. Karp J, et al. Advances in understanding the mechanisms and management of persistent pain in older adults. Br J Anaesth. 2008;101(1):111–20.

87. Varma S, Sareen H, Trivedi JK. The geriatric population and psychiatric medication. Mens Sana Monogr. 2010;8(1):30–51.

88. Lindsey P. Psychotropic medication use among older adults: what all nurses need to know. J Gerontol Nurs. 2009;35(9):28–38.

89. Improving access to psychological therapies. http://www.iapt.nhs.uk/.

90. Health and Social Care Information Centre. Psychological therapies: annual report on the use of IAPT services England, 2014/15. Health and Social Care Information Centre; 2015.

91. World Health Organisation Regional Office for Europe. User empowerment in mental health—a statement by the WHO Regional Office for Europe. Copenhagen: World Health Organisation Regional Office for Europe & European Commission; 2010. http://www.euro.who.int/en/health-topics/noncommunicable-diseases/mental-health/publications/2010/userempowerment-in-mental-health-a-statement-by-the-who-regional-office-for-europe.

92. American Heritage Dictionary of the English Language. 2015. https://www.ahdictionary.com/. Accessed 21 Sept 2015.

93. Wong ST, Haggerty J. Measuring patient experiences in primary health care. 2013. http://www.chspr.ubc.ca/sites/default/files/publication_files/Patient%20experiences%20in%20PHC%202013_0.pdf. Accessed 17 Sept 2015/26 Jan 2016.

94. Doll L, Bartenfeld T, Binder S. Evaluation of interventions designed to prevent and control injuries. Epidemiol Rev. 2003;25(1):51–9. https://doi.org/10.1093/epirev/mxg003.

95. Burge SK, Amodei N, Elkin B, Catala S, Andrew SR, Lane PA, Seale JP. An evaluation of two primary care interventions for alcohol abuse among Mexican-American patients. Addiction. 1997;92(12):1705–16.

96. Bambra C, Gibson M, Sowden A, Wright K, Whitehead M, Petticrew M. Tackling the wider social determinants of health and health inequalities: evidence from systematic reviews. J Epidemiol Community Health. 2010;64:284–91. https://doi.org/10.1136/jech.2008.082743.

97. MacLean L, Hassmiller S, Shaffer F, Rohrbaugh K, Tiffany Collier T, Fairman J. Scale, causes, and implications of the primary care nursing shortage. Annu Rev Public Health. 2014;35:443–57.

98. Kelly MP, Bonnefoy J, Morgan A, Florenzano F. The development of the evidence base about the social determinants of health. 2006. p. 19. http://www.who.int/social_determinants/resources/mekn_paper.pdf. Accessed 23 Sept 2015.

99. Murray CJL, Frenk J. A WHO framework for health system performance assessment. Evidence and Information for Policy. 1990. Geneva: World Health Organization, Technical Documents. http://www.who.int/healthinfo/paper06.pdf. Accessed 23 Sept 2015/26 Jan 2016.

100. Berglund E, Lytsy P, Westerling R. The influence of locus of control on self-rated health in context of chronic disease: a structural equation modeling approach in a cross sectional study. BMC Public Health. 2014;14:492. https://doi.org/10.1186/1471-2458-14-492.

101. WHO. Primary care evaluation tool (PCET). http://www.euro.who.int/__data/assets/pdf_file/0004/107851/PrimaryCareEvalTool.pdf. Accessed 18 Sept 2015/26 Jan 2016.

102. Lawless A, Freeman T, Bentley M, Baum F, Jolley G. Developing a good practice model to evaluate the effectiveness of comprehensive primary health care in local communities. BMC Fam Pract. 2014;15:99. https://doi.org/10.1186/1471-2296-15-99.

103. Levy D, Chaloupka F, Gitchell J. The effect of tobacco control policies on smoking rates; a tobacco control scorecard. J Public Health Manag Pract. 2004;10(4):338–53.

104. Jallinoja P, Absetz P, Kuronen R, Nissinen A, Talja M, Uutela A, Patja K. The dilemma of patient responsibility for lifestyle change: perceptions

among primary care physicians and nurses. Scand J Prim Health Care. 2007;25(4):244–9.

105. Kennedy JF. Special message to the Congress on protecting the consumer interest. Public Papers of the Presidents of the United States March 15, 1962, vol. 93. Washington, DC: US Government Printing Office; 1962, p. 236.

106. World Health. World alliance for patient safety. Global patient safety challenge 2005–2006: Clean Care is Safer Care. Geneva: World Health Organisation; 2005. p. 1–25. http://www.who.int/ patientsafety/events/05/GPSC_Launch_ENGLISH_ FINAL.pdf. Accessed 23 Sept 2015.

107. Longtin Y, Sax H, Leape LL, Sheridan SE, Donaldson L, Pittet D. Patient participation: current knowledge and applicability to patient safety. Mayo Clin Proc. 2010;85(1): 53–62.

Part II

Foundation Principles to Promote Mental Health in Older Adults

Frailty

4

Christophe J. Büla, Manuel Sanchez Perez, and Laurence Seematter Bagnoud

Abstract

Frailty is a common clinical syndrome in older adults, usually resulting from the accumulation of decline in physiological processes, function, and reserve in multiple organs or systems. Its prevalence among community-dwelling older adults ranges from 5% to 7% in persons aged 65–74 years to more than 20% in those aged 85 years and over. Through increased vulnerability to stressors, frailty is associated with numerous adverse outcomes such as falls, functional decline, hospital admission, nursing home admission, and death. The frailty process often remains undetected until later stages, when reversibility is no longer possible. Therefore, several definitions of frailty have been proposed, without reaching consensus, and most are too cumbersome to be implemented in clinical routine. Thus, another way of screening for frailty in practice is to rely on comprehensive geriatric assessment. The comprehensive geriatric approach, although not specific to frailty, allows setting up interventions targeting underlying health problems related to frailty and has shown beneficial in preventing the occurrence and consequences of this syndrome. Among specific interventions tested to prevent or reverse frailty, exercise and, to a lesser extent, nutrition appear as the most effective ones, while no pharmacological treatment showed conclusive benefit.

C. J. Büla (✉)
Service of Geriatric Medicine and Geriatric Rehabilitation, Department of Medicine, University of Lausanne Medical Center (CHUV), Lausanne, Switzerland
e-mail: Christophe.Bula@chuv.ch

M. S. Perez
Unit of Geriatric Psychiatry, Sagrat Cor Hospital, Barcelona, Spain

L. Seematter Bagnoud
Service of Geriatric Medicine and Geriatric Rehabilitation, Department of Medicine, University of Lausanne Medical Center (CHUV), Lausanne, Switzerland

Institute of Social and Preventive Medicine, University of Lausanne Medical Center (CHUV), Lausanne, Switzerland

Abbreviations

HR   Hazard ratio (from Cox proportional models analysis)
OR   Odds ratio (from logistic regression analysis)

© Springer Nature Switzerland AG 2019
C. A. de Mendonça Lima, G. Ivbijaro (eds.), *Primary Care Mental Health in Older People*,
https://doi.org/10.1007/978-3-030-10814-4_4

Key Points
- Frailty is a common clinical syndrome in older adults, usually resulting from the accumulation of decline in physiological processes, function, and reserve in multiple organs or systems.
- Several definitions of frailty, often relying on a physical concept, have been proposed without reaching consensus on a gold standard.
- Frailty results in increasing vulnerability to even minor stressors that can trigger disproportionate consequences.
- Frailty has been associated with numerous adverse outcomes such as falls, functional decline, hospital admission, nursing home admission, and death.
- As a non-specific approach targeting underlying health problems related to frailty, comprehensive geriatric assessment and management is beneficial in preventing frailty and its consequences.
- Exercise and, to a lesser extent, nutrition appear as the most effective interventions to prevent as well as to reverse frailty occurrence, while no pharmacological treatment showed conclusive benefit.

4.1 Introduction

Life expectancy has been steadily increasing over the last century in most countries around the world. As individuals age, one of their major concern is to keep a good quality of life, which means for most of them to remain independent and autonomous. However, the very same segment of the older population (i.e., those aged 80 and over) that is growing at fastest speed is hit hard by incident chronic diseases. The concept of frailty was born from observations that older adults do not age at the same pace, with resulting discrepancy between chronological and biological ages. Frailty is an age-related syndrome which might explain the heterogeneity of health statuses in older adults of similar age. Several risk factors, including

chronic diseases, concur to progressively alter physiological functional reserves, ending in a reduced ability to cope with physical or psychological stressors.

Health professionals often claim to easily identify frailty in their older patients. However, this syndrome is less obvious to detect in its initial stages, when it might still be best reversible. Frailty places older adults at increased risk for poor health outcomes, notably disability. Therefore, it is crucial to better understand its determinants and natural history, as well as to develop screening tools and, most importantly, to implement effective interventions aiming at preventing or postponing frailty in aging populations. This chapter first discusses the different definitions of frailty, considered as a physical concept. Then, the epidemiology of frailty and its relationship with chronic diseases, including mental disorders, as well as associated health consequences is reviewed. Finally, the potential clinical usefulness of the concept of frailty in primary care and its management are discussed.

4.2 Definitions and Epidemiology

4.2.1 Definitions

The term "frailty" is commonly used as much by laypeople and by health professionals to usually describe elderly persons with chronic diseases who appear at risk for further deterioration in their health. Likewise, numerous definitions of frailty have been proposed over time in the field of gerontology, but a universally accepted definition is still lacking. Even though clinicians, researchers, and epidemiologist share a consensus on several characteristics of the frailty concept, definitions still differ according to domains considered in this concept. This chapter focuses on frailty as a physical concept, in accordance to a 2006 consensus conference defining frailty as "a state of increased vulnerability to stressors due to age-related decline in physiologic reserve across neuromuscular, metabolic, and immune systems" [1]. As a consequence, when facing an

Fig. 4.1 Vulnerability of frail elderly people to a sudden change in health status after a minor illness [2]

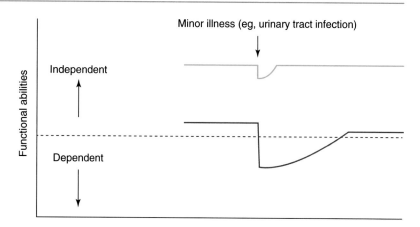

Fig. 4.2 Cycle of frailty, adapted from Fried (1998) [3]

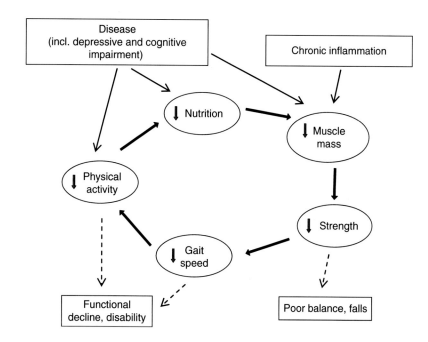

acute illness or even an apparently small insult, frail older adults are likely to experience a greater loss in functional ability as their non-frail counterparts, as well as to have slower and incomplete recovery of their functional status, as shown in Fig. 4.1 [2].

Frailty is a syndrome, i.e., a constellation of symptoms and signs traducing this underlying reduced physiological reserve in physiological systems. Although less frequently admitted, frailty can certainly also result from alteration in physiological reserve in only one system. Numerous attempts have also been made to investigate biological mechanisms underlying the concept of frailty. For instance, studies of inflammatory and

neuroendocrine biomarkers did not yet identify any that would be specific enough to be helpful in identifying frailty. As will be discussed later in this chapter, frailty differs from aging as, even though it affects a substantial proportion of elderly persons as they age, many others are not and will not become frail over their aging path.

In the absence of a gold standard, several researchers proposed an operationalization of the frailty concept. Among other definitions, Fried's frailty phenotype relies on a biological model that postulates a vicious circle of poor nutrition leading to sarcopenia, diminished strength, exhaustion, and very low physical activity (Fig. 4.2) [3]. According to this

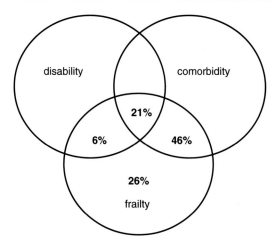

Fig. 4.3 Overlap of frailty, comorbidity, and disability, adapted from Fried (2004) [3]. The diagram shows the distribution of the participants to the Cardiovascular Health Study assessed as frail (*n* = 368) according to the presence of disability and comorbidity

definition, frailty relies on measuring five criteria: (1) unintentional weight loss, (2) low grip strength, (3) slow walking speed, (4) low physical activity, and (5) fatigue. Subjects without any criterion are considered as robust, those with one or two criteria are considered as pre-frail (i.e., with a high risk of progressing to frailty), and those meeting three to five criteria are considered as frail.

Frailty, disability, and comorbidity are considered to be overlapping but distinct entities. As shown in Fried's study, about two-thirds of frail older adults have comorbidity, among whom one in five is additionally disabled [3]. In other words, about three out of four older adults qualifying as frail also presented comorbid conditions, disability, or both. Inversely, frailty was detected in the absence of comorbidity and disability in one in four persons, suggesting that these three health outcomes are different (Fig. 4.3) [4].

Fried's phenotype is widely used in clinical research settings, because only five criteria have to be measured. However, it requires specific material (dynamometer) and is not suitable in care settings. Therefore, several adaptations of Fried's criteria have been operated to overcome these difficulties [5]. Fried's phenotype has also been criticized for excluding the mental health

dimension, even though several criteria (weight loss, slow gait, fatigue) might undeniably be linked to either depressive symptoms or cognitive decline. This criticism appears even more substantiated as cross-sectional studies uniformly indicate that cognitive impairment is more frequent among pre-frail and frail older adults than robust ones and shows a dose-dependent association across the stages of frailty [6]. A consensus panel thus proposed the concept of cognitive frailty to distinguish individuals with both frailty and cognitive impairment without dementia, a subgroup particularly at risk for adverse outcomes [7]. An additional argument supporting the incorporation of an explicit measure of cognitive impairment into Fried's phenotype comes from a study which demonstrated that adding this criterion improved the predictive validity of the model for adverse outcomes [8, 9].

In the meantime, other researchers developed a different approach by evaluating the accumulation of deficits: Rockwood's frailty index uses a count of diseases, geriatric syndromes, physical, cognitive, social, and psychological impairments, as well as abnormal laboratory values, depending on which data are available. It requires that at least 20–30 items are at hand [10]. This more comprehensive approach probably better reflects the multidimensional nature of frailty. It is grounded on the hypothesis of an underlying dynamic process that results in deficits accumulation and challenges the stability of the human body complex system, putting the person at risk for adverse outcomes. The frailty index was conceptualized as a continuous score that should reflect the spectrum of frailty severity rather than an index to categorize older adults into frail and non-frail subgroups. Nevertheless, studies have shown that a score of 0.25 or more (i.e., a quarter or more of measured items shows impairments) can be used as a cutoff to identify frail elderly persons [11].

Because several single measures have been associated with adverse outcomes similar to those associated with frailty, their ability to identify physical frailty has also been examined [12]. For instance, slow gait speed and low grip strength perform well in predicting mortality, and both have also been associated with subsequent cognitive impairment, even a decade earlier, and might therefore be useful to detect preclinical dementia [6].

There is no agreement on the best way to screen for frailty in the clinical context. Both the frailty phenotype and the frailty index are too cumbersome to be implemented in clinical routine. Overall, most simple measures developed to identify frailty tend to have a high sensitivity, even shorter tools adapted to a clinical use. However, their specificity is lower as compared to Fried's frailty phenotype, i.e., there are too many false-positive [12]. For example, a timed-up-and-go test >10 s identifies 93% of subjects meeting Fried's definition for frailty, but about 30% of the individuals with a timed-up-and-go test >10 s are not frail. A similar observation applies for gait speed ≤0.8 m/s. Such a test could be useful to exclude frailty in case of a normal performance (i.e., gait speed >0.8 m/s, or timed-up-and-go-test <10 s, with a negative predictive value of 0.99) [12].

Another way of screening for frailty is to use the information issued from a comprehensive geriatric assessment [2].

4.2.2 Prevalence

The prevalence of frailty varies greatly according to the age of the population under study and is usually about twice higher in women than men.

This prevalence also varies according to the definitions applied in the studies, as well as according to the specific operationalization, in each specific study, of criteria used in these definitions. Frailty is of course much more prevalent among persons who live in long-term care institutions, with 20–75% of residents classified as frail [13]. This paragraph focuses on studies in community-dwelling older adults who have the greatest potential for frailty postponement or reversal.

A systematic review published in 2012 included 21 community-based studies reporting on frailty prevalence, most often using Fried's frailty index [14]. Frailty was found to be more common when criteria of weakness and slow gait were self-reported, rather than objectively assessed. Overall, weighted average prevalence among older adults aged 65 years and over amounted to 44% for pre-frailty and 10% for frailty. However, frailty prevalence increased as age increased, from 5% to 7% in persons aged 65–74 years to 15% in those aged 80–84 years and more than 20% in those aged 85 years and over. These figures are quite close to the estimates of the Cardiovascular Health Study, in which Fried initially quantified the prevalence of the phenotype (Fig. 4.4) [3].

Regarding differences across countries, a European multicountry survey found that the age- and gender-adjusted prevalence of frailty in

Fig. 4.4 Overall and gender-specific prevalence of frailty in the Cardiovascular Health Study, adapted from Fried (2001) [3]

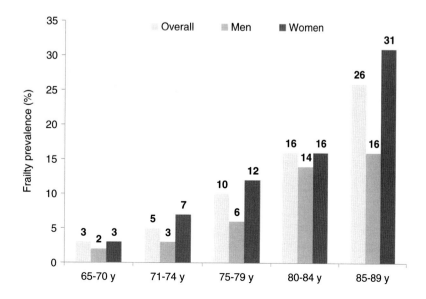

community-dwelling persons aged 65 years and over increased from the north to the south, ranging from less than 10% in Sweden and Switzerland to 27% in Spain [15]. Likely some of this variation might be explained by different perceptions of health, as well as by differences in socioeconomic conditions across Europe.

Studies on the prevalence of frailty in South America and Asia found inconsistent estimates, some observing greater figures compared to Europe and the USA, while other reported lower ones. This might be due to poorer survival of frail older adults in low- and middle-income countries, as compared to wealthier countries with better social and health systems [16].

As previously mentioned, prevalence of frailty strongly depends on the definition used, as indicated by two analyses that retrospectively applied different definitions on the same study population. One study reported that the prevalence of frailty was 9% using the frailty phenotype and 18% using the frailty index [17]. A systematic review specifically examined the impact of modifying the operationalization of the frailty phenotype's criteria, such as using self-reported rather than objectively measured information, or changing the cutoff points. Applying a set of 262 modified definitions of the frailty phenotype, prevalence ranged from 13% to 29% [5].

4.2.3 Incidence and Transitions Between Frailty States

Numerous studies examined the ability of a frailty score to predict poor health outcomes such as disability, hospitalization, and death. There are less data about the impact of changes in frailty status on the risk of these outcomes. However, frailty is a dynamic process, and even though it is more often directed toward worsening frailty, improvement occurs in as much as a third of individuals, especially in the early stages of frailty.

Transitions across frailty states have been examined in a few population-based studies [18–21]. Over 4–8 years of follow-up, these studies showed that:

- Frailty transitions are observable in 50–80% of the population under study, depending on the duration of follow-up and baseline frailty status.
- Most of the transitions occurred between adjacent frailty status (e.g., from non-frail to pre-frail or from pre-frail to frail).
- Transitions are most frequent between the non-frail and pre-frail states, with transitions toward greater frailty (about 40%) being twice more frequent than reverse transitions.
- Complete reversal from frail to non-frail status was exceptional.
- Transitions from non-frail to frail states were uncommon in the absence of a hospitalization.

As mentioned previously, whereas frailty predicts cognitive decline, several studies indicated that cognitive impairment also aggravates the frailty process [6]. Finally, other risk factors (see Sect. 4.2.4 below) for frailty such as lower socioeconomic status are susceptible to accelerate the transition toward more frailty.

4.2.4 Risk Factors and Determinants

Frailty is thought to result most frequently from impairments in multiple systems, including neuromuscular, immune, or metabolic systems. Therefore, a large number of risk factors might be included in its causation. First of all, chronic diseases play an important role in promoting frailty, but social conditions, education, lifestyle, mood, and cognitive disorders modulate the effects of diseases and age-related deficits, ending up in a vicious cycle of fragilization [22]. The life course theory suggests that the negative influence of these factors on the development of frailty might be more pronounced when they occur in an early life sensitive period, by reducing the ability to reach full capacity in adulthood [23].

4.2.5 Relation with Psychological, Cognitive, and Social Functioning

Frailty has reciprocal relationships with psychological, cognitive, and social functioning. These findings suggest that these dimensions have to be taken into account when caring for frail older patients, as quality of life might be threatened by all of these three dimensions as well as by frailty itself [24].

As mentioned previously, evidence from longitudinal studies indicates that frailty and cognition influence each other. A recent review explored the underlying mechanisms of this association [6]. First, it is worth noting that frailty and cognitive impairment share common risk factors, notably cardiovascular diseases which are highly prevalent in older populations. Chronic systemic inflammation might also contribute to both frailty and cognitive decline directly and through vascular disease, notably small vessel alteration.

Further, mood disorders are linked to both frailty and cognition: depressive symptoms sometimes impair cognition and double the odds of incident frailty. Frailty has been shown to increase the risk of new-onset depressive symptoms up to four times [25]. Several processes might be causally implicated, including a reduction in physical activity and a poor nutritional intake. Moreover, personality and perception of aging also influence frailty and cognition through their effects on mood, physical activity, and social participation. Indeed, social network and support seem to narrow over time among frail older adults, who face increasing loneliness, and decreased social activities with sedentarity [7, 26]. Moreover, the onset of frailty is a critical and challenging period for the older adult, but only limited attention has been given to the relationship between physical frailty and psychological vulnerability. The concept of "frailty identity crisis" has been proposed to characterize a psychological syndrome that may accompany the transition from robustness to frailty [27]. While research on this topic is still scarce, this concept suggests that the perception of loss in physical ability might generate anxiety about declining opportunities, changing social role, increasing loneliness, and nearing of death. Transitioning to frailty should be considered a significant negative event in an older adult's life and may cause a psychological process similar to grief. As such, high levels of psychological resources are needed to cope with frailty, and the risk for depression as

well as for entering a vicious cycle of increasing physical frailty is high in case of a maladaptive response [27]. The psychological and social dimensions seem therefore quite closely intertwined to the physical and cognitive ones in modifying the process leading to frailty.

These observations lend support to a frequent criticism about the frailty concept as it neglects the importance of coping through personal and social resources. Therefore, similarly to models of vulnerability developed in the social sciences domain, it has been suggested to incorporate coping into models of frailty. Taking coping resources into account is claimed to better estimate the risk for harm in older adults [28]. Other researchers concluded that social vulnerability was a concept related to frailty, but distinct from it, and demonstrated that social vulnerability was associated with higher mortality, independently from and additionally to frailty [29].

As discussed later in this chapter, addressing appropriately the frailty process in primary care patients requires to also incorporating their social, psychological, and cognitive functioning.

4.2.6 Implication for Independence and Autonomy

Whereas frailty itself does not automatically threaten one's independent and autonomous living, the consequences of frailty on functional decline and hospital admission do have a negative impact. Several studies aimed to produce summarized evidence regarding the consequences of frailty (Fig. 4.5), some of them having their results pooled in meta-analyses. Notably, falls incidence has been shown to be about twice higher in frail older adults (pooled odds ratio from seven studies: OR 1.8) [31]. Frailty also conveys a risk for imminent future falling, even in older adults who still seem to age well, a finding of importance for health professionals [32].

Frailty significantly increases the risk of disability in activities of daily living (OR about 1.8–5) and of nursing home admission, even when adjusted for covariates such as age, gender, and comorbidity [2, 33]. According to a meta-analysis, frailty is associated with a

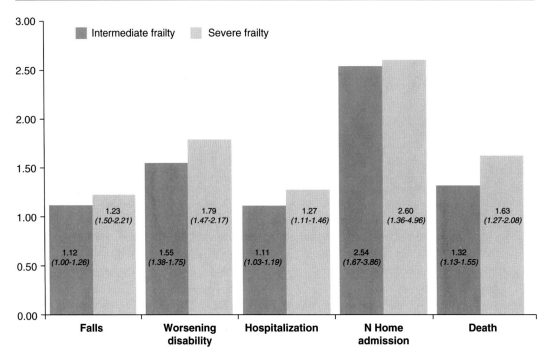

Fig. 4.5 Association between frailty severity and adverse outcomes in the Cardiovascular Health Study (hazard ratios for falls, worsening disability, hospitalization, and death) [3] and the Canadian Study of Health and Aging (odds ratio for nursing home admission) [30]

higher risk for hospital admission (pooled OR from ten studies = 1.9) [34]. For all outcomes, weaker but still significant associations were also found when comparing pre-frail to non-frail individuals. Moreover, each of these outcomes further increases the risk to experiencing another one, e.g., fall-related hospitalization may cause functional decline leading to nursing home admission.

therefore spend time in this state [35]. This time period will theoretically offer a unique window of opportunity to potentially reverse the frailty process. However, important gaps still remain in our ability to reliably detect frailty as well as to effectively manage frailty. Although promising, evidence from trials is still scarce, and application of the frailty concept within the daily clinical practice remains therefore largely empirical.

4.3   Frailty Management

Before presenting in more details the specifics of frailty management in the next sections, it seems important to further discuss why frailty is a relevant concept in primary care. In most countries, gains in life expectancy have triggered growing concerns about the disability burden in the future. Frailty might precede disability by several years in older adults who do not experience catastrophic disability [3], and a large proportion of older adults transitioning to disability will

4.3.1   Frailty in Primary Care: A Useful Concept?

The high prevalence of frailty in community-dwelling older adults is in itself a strong factor that supports its relevance for primary care physicians [14]. Indeed, most primary care physicians are intuitively very familiar with the notion of frailty. Moreover, the five components of Fried's phenotype (weakness, poor endurance, weight loss, reduced physical activity, and slow gait speed) belong to stereotypes frequently associated with aging. Many older adults who suffer multiple chronic diseases are also frail, and addressing frailty should therefore be considered a hallmark of caring for older adults. Yet, because of its close association with chronic diseases, frailty remains frequently undetected in many older adults. Furthermore, it is precisely so among those who suffer from chronic diseases because their physician's attention is monopolized by these diseases' management. This observation has led several national and international bodies to strongly recommend active and systematic search of frailty in older adults aged 70 years or over as a first step toward implementing better adapted management of these chronic diseases [36, 37]. Yet, scientific evidence supporting these guidelines remains relatively weak.

Frailty is also an appealing concept in primary care because it helps us to better understand the heterogeneity of the association between age and health among older adults. Primary care and specialists physicians frequently report their observation that older adults of the same chronological age and—apparent—health status may respond very differently to similar interventions. Frailty is therefore a useful concept not only because it illustrates this heterogeneity but also because it helps to understand as well as to predict these older patients' response to specific treatments, such as chemotherapy or surgery. Indeed, frailty identifies among older adults a subgroup at high risk for adverse outcomes. Markers of frailty have been shown to add to the capacity of chronic diseases to predicting adverse outcomes such as disability or death [37].

Finally, frailty is also an important concept because frailty might precede by several years the development of non-catastrophic disability in a large proportion of older adults. Moreover, observational studies have shown that frailty is reversible in early stage. Although definitive evidence are lacking, some interventions, such as exercise or nutritional support, have been shown to have some effectiveness in preventing frailty. This makes frailty a meaningful target for interventions to prevent functional decline and future disability.

4.3.2 Frailty as a Prognostic Indicator: Preoperative and Pre-treatment Assessment

As previously mentioned, one of the important potential clinical applications of the concept of frailty is to identify vulnerable patients who might need adjustment of their treatment. More and more medical specialties are confronted with an increasing number of very old persons for whom therapeutic decisions are difficult. Identifying among these patients those who need these adjustments because of their frailty is of utmost importance. However, it must be recognized that, even though we are able to identify frailty at a population level, its recognition at the individual level and its translation into adapted management still remain unsatisfactory. For instance, frailty screening was tested to identify cancer patients subsequently found with significant impairments at a comprehensive geriatric assessment [38]. Unfortunately, none of the seven screening methods did perform well in terms of sensitivity (ranging from 31% to 92%) and specificity (ranging from 47% to 97%), resulting in a negative predictive value of only 60%, largely insufficient to be clinically useful at the individual level. In another study in older patients undergoing transcatheter aortic valve replacement, a frailty index based on measures of cognition, mobility, and nutritional status better identified those who experienced functional decline in basic activities of daily living after a 6-month follow-up period, as compared to traditional surgical risk scores [39].

The concept of frailty appears also theoretically useful in helping primary care physicians to identifying, among their patients who are surgery candidates, those who might bear a higher risk for complicated postoperative courses. Frailty is increasingly applied in surgical populations as it precisely helps to better determine the extent of remaining physiological reserve and to assess a patient's capacity to overcome the stress of surgery [40]. Indeed, numerous studies have shown that, even when undergoing elective surgery, frail surgical patients have increased risk of complications, longer stay, and more frequent discharge disposition other than home, as well as increased mortality [41, 42]. However, as in other areas of health care, the implementation of frailty assessment into routine surgical preoperative assessment remains to be seen. Moreover, further studies are needed to show how much, once identified, frail surgical patients benefit from pre- and postoperative interventions to minimize peri- and postoperative risks. Among older surgical patients, frail ones are likely to be those who benefit most from interventions such as neuraxial anesthesia and avoidance of benzodiazepines that proved beneficial in decreasing delirium as well as other postoperative complications and 30-day mortality.

4.3.3 Prevention

Although observational studies suggest the reversibility of the frailty process, strategies to prevent and/or reverse frailty are still lacking. As frailty has been associated with several diseases such as cardio- and cerebrovascular diseases, interventions targeting risk factors for these diseases are likely to be effective. Indeed, evidence from observational studies strongly suggests that exercise is probably the single most effective intervention to prevent frailty incidence. This seems especially true if started in earlier age. For instance, one study showed that, over a 26-year follow-up, active middle-aged adults with the best fitness level had about 34% more time spent without or with only one chronic disease and about 50% less time spent with four or more chronic diseases than sedentary adults [43]. Similarly, obesity has been associated with increased risk of frailty and strategies to reduce weight are likely to also affect subsequent frailty incidence [44].

Overall, these observations suggest that multi-faceted interventions are best suited to address the complex challenge of frailty prevention. A recent large Japanese study precisely implemented such multimodal strategy to prevent or delay frailty incidence. Using a public health approach, physical activity, nutrition, and social participation were promoted through a health education program targeting citizens aged 70 years or older [45]. After a 10-year follow-up, results showed benefits in terms of functional health that corresponded to a gain in healthy life expectancy of 1.2 and 0.5 years in women and men, respectively.

Despite these promising results, it remains unclear whether traditional, disease-oriented, preventative strategies will be sufficient to impact on frailty dynamics. Furthermore, the interplay between such strategies and those aiming at reducing social vulnerability needs further investigation to determine whether such interaction could add to frailty prevention.

4.3.4 Interventions

Currently, scientific evidence supporting interventions to manage frailty is weak. Well-designed interventions that specifically address frailty management are still needed because most studies did not use validated models of frailty to select their population, as well as to measure frailty evolution over time in participants. Despite these limited evidence, two main approaches are still advocated.

The first approach refers to the observed benefits from comprehensive geriatric assessment and management programs in community-dwelling elderly population [36]. These programs have shown their efficacy in maintaining function, increasing the likelihood to remain at home, and decreasing the probability to be institutionalized. Even though some evidence suggest that these programs might actually be less effective among the frailest older adults, the complex, multimodal, interventions they proposed appear especially appropriate to address the multifactorial etiology underlying the frailty concept.

Other countries, such as the UK, are already implementing dedicated frailty care pathways that combine home visits, comprehensive geriatric assessment, targeted interventions, and follow-up monitoring [36]. These programs appear very promising as they combine health and social

Fig. 4.6 Conceptual description of the link between exercise interventions, several chronic diseases, and functional impairments in the disability pathway (adapted from [51])

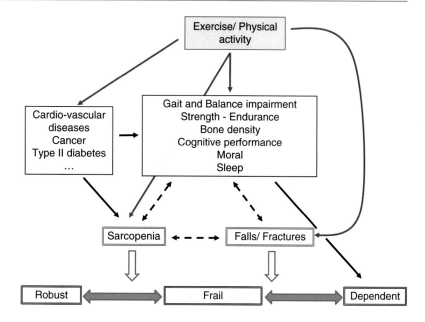

care interventions to provide a better integrated approach. Their effectiveness remains however to be demonstrated.

The second main approach refers to specific interventions designed to treat frailty. Evidence from these targeted interventions is however very limited and comes mostly from exercise interventions. Several systematic reviews have been recently published about the benefits of exercise in frail older adults [46–48]. Results from these studies were mixed but suggest that exercise may improve specific functions, such as transferring or mobility performance. For instance, a structured, moderate-intensity physical activity program that included aerobic, resistance, and flexibility training activities resulted in about 20% (hazard ratio [HR], 0.82; 95% CI, 0.69–0.98, $P = 0.03$) and 30% (HR, 0.72; 95% CI, 0.57–0.91, $P = 0.006$) lower probability over 2.6 years of major disability and mobility impairment, respectively, than a control intervention [49].

Similarly, benefits in reversing frailty have been found in a recent randomized controlled study [50]. Intervention consisted in a multicomponent exercise program including balance, strength, endurance, and stretch exercise training performed 5 days a week over 24 weeks. Only three persons needed to be treated over 24 weeks

to prevent incidence of frailty in one, whereas no frailty reversal was observed among the control group. Interestingly, consistent with the associations described in Fig. 4.6, significant and clinically meaningful improvements were also observed in cognition, depressive symptoms, activities of daily living performance, as well as quality of life of participants who benefited from this multicomponent exercise program. Overall, exercise programs appear to provide benefits to frail older adults, but questions remain about the best combination to propose in terms of type (resistance, endurance, balance, and/or flexibility training), frequency, duration, and intensity.

Because weight loss is considered a major determinant of frailty in older adults, nutritional support appears a logical intervention to propose. Surprisingly, evidence supporting nutritional intervention is very limited, mostly indirect, and not conclusive [52]. For instance, although several randomized controlled trials of vitamin D supplementation reported improvement in muscle strength and decreased in fall risk [53], its role in frailty management remains controversial [54].

Clinical evidence is also still lacking for several pharmacological agents (statins, angiotensin converting enzyme inhibitors, beta-blockers, etc.) and other hormonal supplementation (tes-

Table 4.1 Six-step frailty management (NHS England) [55]

Step	Activity
1. Identification	Use the Electronic Frailty Index (eFI) (or other validated tool PRISMA-7, gait speed) or clinical judgment to establish presence of frailty for all patients aged 65 and over
2. Clinical confirmation	Undertake secondary check using direct assessment with Clinical Frailty Scale (CFS), clinical knowledge of patient, or information available in the healthcare record to validate eFI result
3. Coding	Severe frailty—code Moderate frailty—code Mild frailty—consider coding
4. Summary Care Record (SCR)	Seek consent to share information via enriched SCR
5. *For those with severe frailty* Undertake falls assessment and medications review	Annual review of medications and (see guidance and best practice) code activity Annual direct review to establish if patient has fallen in last year. Code outcome No fall in the last 12 months—no further action required One or more falls in the past 12 months
6	Use clinical judgment for other relevant and appropriate interventions

tosterone, growth hormone, selective androgen receptor modulators, etc.). These have been discussed to manage frailty because they improved some components (mostly muscle wasting and sarcopenia) of the frailty phenotype. Research is still needed in this area, as in several other fields of frailty in older adults.

Finally, strategies such as educating patients and their caregivers about physical frailty and its functional as well as prognostic implications, promoting patients' social engagement, and supporting those experiencing the frailty identity crisis through psychological counseling may all be useful to maximize these patients' functional health and quality of life, as well as their caregivers' well-being [27].

In England frailty identification and frailty care have been incorporated into the GP contract. It outlines a six-step process as shown in Table 4.1.

sicians should be aware of the main symptoms (exhaustion, fatigue, low physical activity) and signs (weight loss, decreased grip strength and walking speed) of frailty. Identifying frail patients has two main implications for their care. First, it allows better adapting pharmacological and/or surgical interventions to prevent complications in these high-risk patients. Second, once diagnosed these patients could benefit from timely interventions aiming at treating—ideally reversing—frailty, even though evidence is still scarce. Nevertheless, comprehensive geriatric assessment and management programs, exercise, and, to a lesser extent, nutritional support interventions have been shown to improve clinical outcomes in frail older population. Further research is however still needed to improve our understanding of frailty, to improving its prediction, as well as the management of frail older adults.

4.4 Conclusions and Recommandations for Primary Care

Frailty is increasingly recognized as an important concept when caring for older patients. In particular, assessing frailty in primary care allows to identifying a subgroup of patients at increased risk of morbidity and mortality. Primary care phy-

References

1. Walston J, Hadley EC, Ferrucci L, Guralnik JM, Newman AB, Studenski SA, et al. Research agenda for frailty in older adults: toward a better understanding of physiology and etiology: summary from the American Geriatrics Society/National Institute on Aging research conference on frailty in older adults. J Am Geriatr Soc. 2006;54(6):991–1001.

2. Clegg A, Young J, Iliffe S, Rikkert MO, Rockwood K. Frailty in elderly people. Lancet. 2013;381(9868):752–62.
3. Fried LP, Tangen CM, Walston J, Newman AB, Hirsch C, Gottdiener J, et al. Frailty in older adults: evidence for a phenotype. J Gerontol A Biol Sci Med Sci. 2001;56(3):M146–M56.
4. Fried L, Walston J. Frailty and failure to thrive. In: Hazzard W, Blass J, Ettinger W, Halter J, Ouslander J, editors. Principles of geriatric medicine and gerontology. 4th ed. New York: McGraw Hill; 1998. p. 1387–402.
5. Theou O, Cann L, Blodgett J, Wallace LM, Brothers TD, Rockwood K. Modifications to the frailty phenotype criteria: systematic review of the current literature and investigation of 262 frailty phenotypes in the survey of health, ageing, and retirement in Europe. Ageing Res Rev. 2015;21:78–94.
6. Robertson DA, Savva GM, Kenny RA. Frailty and cognitive impairment--a review of the evidence and causal mechanisms. Ageing Res Rev. 2013;12(4):840–51.
7. Kelaiditi E, Cesari M, Canevelli M, van Kan GA, Ousset PJ, Gillette-Guyonnet S, et al. Cognitive frailty: rational and definition from an (I.A.N.A./I.A.G.G.) international consensus group. J Nutr Health Aging. 2013;17(9):726–34.
8. Avila-Funes JA, Helmer C, Amieva H, Barberger-Gateau P, Le GM, Ritchie K, et al. Frailty among community-dwelling elderly people in France: the three-city study. J Gerontol A Biol Sci Med Sci. 2008;63(10):1089–96.
9. Avila-Funes JA, Amieva H, Barberger-Gateau P, Le Goff M, Raoux N, Ritchie K, et al. Cognitive impairment improves the predictive validity of the phenotype of frailty for adverse health outcomes: the three-city study. J Am Geriatr Soc. 2009;57(3):453–61.
10. Mitnitski AB, Mogilner AJ, Rockwood K. Accumulation of deficits as a proxy measure of aging. Sci World J. 2001;1:323–36.
11. Rockwood K, Mitnitski A. Frailty defined by deficit accumulation and geriatric medicine defined by frailty. Clin Geriatr Med. 2011;27(1):17–26.
12. Clegg A, Rogers L, Young J. Diagnostic test accuracy of simple instruments for identifying frailty in community-dwelling older people: a systematic review. Age Ageing. 2015;44(1):148–52.
13. Kojima G. Prevalence of frailty in nursing homes: a systematic review and meta-analysis. J Am Med Dir Assoc. 2015;16(11):940–5.
14. Collard RM, Boter H, Schoevers RA, Oude Voshaar RC. Prevalence of frailty in community-dwelling older persons: a systematic review. J Am Geriatr Soc. 2012;60(8):1487–92.
15. Santos-Eggimann B, Cuenoud P, Spagnoli J, Junod J. Prevalence of frailty in middle-aged and older community-dwelling Europeans living in 10 countries. J Gerontol A Biol Sci Med Sci. 2009;64(6):675–81.
16. Harttgen K, Kowal P, Strulik H, Chatterji S, Vollmer S. Patterns of frailty in older adults: comparing results from higher and lower income countries using the survey of health, ageing and retirement in Europe (SHARE) and the study on global AGEing and adult health (SAGE). PLoS One. 2013;8(10):e75847.
17. Widagdo IS, Pratt N, Russell M, Roughead EE. Predictive performance of four frailty measures in an older Australian population. Age Ageing. 2015;44(6):967–72.
18. Gill TM, Gahbauer EA, Allore HG, Han L. Transitions between frailty states among community-living older persons. Arch Intern Med. 2006;166(4):418–23.
19. Gill TM, Gahbauer EA, Han L, Allore HG. The relationship between intervening hospitalizations and transitions between frailty states. J Gerontol A Biol Sci Med Sci. 2011;66(11):1238–43.
20. Lee JS, Auyeung TW, Leung J, Kwok T, Woo J. Transitions in frailty states among community-living older adults and their associated factors. J Am Med Dir Assoc. 2014;15(4):281–6.
21. Espinoza SE, Jung I, Hazuda H. Frailty transitions in the San Antonio longitudinal study of aging. J Am Geriatr Soc. 2012;60(4):652–60.
22. Bortz WM 2nd. A conceptual framework of frailty: a review. J Gerontol A Biol Sci Med Sci. 2002;57(5):M283–8.
23. Kuh D, New Dynamics of Ageing Preparatory Network. A life course approach to healthy aging, frailty, and capability. J Gerontol A Biol Sci Med Sci. 2007;62(7):717–21.
24. Kojima G, Iliffe S, Jivraj S, Walters K. Association between frailty and quality of life among community-dwelling older people: a systematic review and meta-analysis. J Epidemiol Community Health. 2016;70(7):716–21.
25. Vaughan L, Corbin AL, Goveas JS. Depression and frailty in later life: a systematic review. Clin Interv Aging. 2015;10:1947–58.
26. Hoogendijk EO, Suanet B, Dent E, Deeg DJ, Aartsen MJ. Adverse effects of frailty on social functioning in older adults: results from the longitudinal aging study Amsterdam. Maturitas. 2016;83:45–50.
27. Fillit H, Butler RN. The frailty identity crisis. J Am Geriatr Soc. 2009;57(2):348–52.
28. Schroeder-Butterfill E. Le concept de vulnérabilité et sa relation à la fragilité. La Fragilité des Personnes Agées. Rennes: Presses de L'EHESP; 2013. p. 205–28.
29. Andrew MK, Mitnitski AB, Rockwood K. Social vulnerability, frailty and mortality in elderly people. PLoS One. 2008;3(5):e2232.
30. Rockwood K, Howlett SE, MacKnight C, Beattie BL, Bergman H, Hebert R, et al. Prevalence, attributes, and outcomes of fitness and frailty in community-dwelling older adults: report from the Canadian study of health and aging. J Gerontol A Biol Sci Med Sci. 2004;59(12):1310–7.
31. Kojima G. Frailty as a predictor of future falls among community-dwelling older people: a systematic review and meta-analysis. J Am Med Dir Assoc. 2015;16(12):1027–33.

32. Kojima G, Kendrick D, Skelton DA, Morris RW, Gawler S, Iliffe S. Frailty predicts short-term incidence of future falls among British community-dwelling older people: a prospective cohort study nested within a randomised controlled trial. BMC Geriatr. 2015;15:155.

33. Macklai NS, Spagnoli J, Junod J, Santos-Eggimann B. Prospective association of the SHARE-operationalized frailty phenotype with adverse health outcomes: evidence from 60+ community-dwelling Europeans living in 11 countries. BMC Geriatr. 2013;13:3.

34. Kojima G. Frailty as a predictor of hospitalisation among community-dwelling older people: a systematic review and meta-analysis. J Epidemiol Community Health. 2016;70(7):722–9.

35. Hardy SE, Dubin JA, Holford TR, Gill TM. Transitions between states of disability and independence among older persons. Am J Epidemiol. 2005;161(6):575–84.

36. Turner G, Clegg A, British Geriatrics S, Age UK, Royal College of General Practioners. Best practice guidelines for the management of frailty: a British Geriatrics society, Age UK and Royal College of general practitioners report. Age Ageing. 2014;43(6):744–7.

37. Morley JE, Vellas B, van Kan GA, Anker SD, Bauer JM, Bernabei R, et al. Frailty consensus: a call to action. J Am Med Dir Assoc. 2013;14(6):392–7.

38. Hamaker ME, Jonker JM, de Rooij SE, Vos AG, Smorenburg CH, van Munster BC. Frailty screening methods for predicting outcome of a comprehensive geriatric assessment in elderly patients with cancer: a systematic review. Lancet Oncol. 2012;13(10):e437–44.

39. Schoenenberger AW, Stortecky S, Neumann S, Moser A, Juni P, Carrel T, et al. Predictors of functional decline in elderly patients undergoing transcatheter aortic valve implantation (TAVI). Eur Heart J. 2013;34(9):684–92.

40. Anaya DA, Johanning J, Spector SA, Katlic MR, Perrino AC, Feinleib J, et al. Summary of the panel session at the 38th annual surgical symposium of the association of VA surgeons: what is the big deal about frailty? JAMA Surg. 2014;149(11):1191–7.

41. Makary MA, Segev DL, Pronovost PJ, Syin D, Bandeen-Roche K, Patel P, et al. Frailty as a predictor of surgical outcomes in older patients. J Am Coll Surg. 2010;210(6):901–8.

42. Kim SW, Han HS, Jung HW, Kim KI, Hwang DW, Kang SB, et al. Multidimensional frailty score for the prediction of postoperative mortality risk. JAMA Surg. 2014;149(7):633–40.

43. Willis BL, Gao A, Leonard D, Defina LF, Berry JD. Midlife fitness and the development of chronic conditions in later life. Arch Intern Med. 2012;172(17):1333–40.

44. Hubbard RE, Lang IA, Llewellyn DJ, Rockwood K. Frailty, body mass index, and abdominal obesity in older people. J Gerontol A Biol Sci Med Sci. 2010;65(4):377–81.

45. Shinkai S, Yoshida H, Taniguchi Y, Murayama H, Nishi M, Amano H, et al. Public health approach to preventing frailty in the community and its effect on healthy aging in Japan. Geriatr Gerontol Int. 2016;16(Suppl 1):87–97.

46. Theou O, Stathokostas L, Roland KP, Jakobi JM, Patterson C, Vandervoort AA, et al. The effectiveness of exercise interventions for the management of frailty: a systematic review. J Aging Res. 2011;2011:569194.

47. Cadore EL, Rodriguez-Manas L, Sinclair A, Izquierdo M. Effects of different exercise interventions on risk of falls, gait ability, and balance in physically frail older adults: a systematic review. Rejuvenation Res. 2013;16(2):105–14.

48. Gine-Garriga M, Roque-Figuls M, Coll-Planas L, Sitja-Rabert M, Salva A. Physical exercise interventions for improving performance-based measures of physical function in community-dwelling, frail older adults: a systematic review and meta-analysis. Arch Phys Med Rehabil. 2014;95(4):753–69.e3.

49. Pahor M, Guralnik JM, Ambrosius WT, Blair S, Bonds DE, Church TS, et al. Effect of structured physical activity on prevention of major mobility disability in older adults: the LIFE study randomized clinical trial. JAMA. 2014;311(23):2387–96.

50. Tarazona-Santabalbina FJ, Gomez-Cabrera MC, Perez-Ros P, Martinez-Arnau FM, Cabo H, Tsaparas K, et al. A multicomponent exercise intervention that reverses frailty and improves cognition, emotion, and social networking in the community-dwelling frail elderly: a randomized clinical trial. J Am Med Dir Assoc. 2016;7(5):426–33.

51. Seematter-Bagnoud L, Bize R, Mettler D, Büla C, Santos-Eggimann B. Promotion de l'activité physique: projet "Bonnes pratiques de promotion de la santé des personnes âgées". Lausanne: Centre for Ageing Studies (COAV), Lausanne University Hospital; 2011.

52. Malafarina V, Uriz-Otano F, Iniesta R, Gil-Guerrero L. Effectiveness of nutritional supplementation on muscle mass in treatment of sarcopenia in old age: a systematic review. J Am Med Dir Assoc. 2013;14(1):10–7.

53. Bischoff-Ferrari HA, Dawson-Hughes B, Staehelin HB, Orav JE, Stuck AE, Theiler R, et al. Fall prevention with supplemental and active forms of vitamin D: a meta-analysis of randomised controlled trials. BMJ. 2009;339:b3692.

54. Campbell SE, Szoeke C. Pharmacological treatment of frailty in the elderly. J Res Pharm Pract. 2009;39:5.

55. NHS England. Supporting routine frailty identification and frailty care through the GP Contract 2017/2018.

Comorbidity, Multi-Morbidity, Stepped Care and Skill Mix in the Care of the Older Population

5

Gabriel Ivbijaro, David Goldberg, Yaccub Enum, and Lucja Kolkiewicz

Abstract

One of the consequences of an ageing population is the increasing prevalence of people living with more than one long-term condition (multi-morbidity). The coexistence of more than one long-term condition often has poorer outcomes for older adults and makes them more likely to access care from different health and social care providers concurrently. As a result, the overall cost of managing these individuals increases. Collaborative care is a useful way of providing care for such patients, utilising the skills and expertise of different disciplines in primary, secondary care and other settings in a coordinated way. Stepped care ensures that interventions match the severity and complexity of presentation so that effort is not wasted.

Key Points

- Many older adults live with some kind of long-term condition or functional impairment.
- Multi-morbidity affects the management of illness and often results in poorer outcomes.
- Older adults with multi-morbidity are more likely to be accessing more than one caregiver at any time.
- Depression has a detrimental effect on coexisting physical conditions; therefore management of the physical condition should include management of depression.
- Collaborative care is a useful model for organising the care of older adults with multi-morbidity.

G. Ivbijaro (✉)
NOVA University, Lisbon, Portugal

Waltham Forest Community and Family Health Services, London, UK

D. Goldberg
King's College, London, UK

Y. Enum
Public Health Department, London Borough of Waltham Forest, London, UK

East London NHS Foundation Trust, London, UK

L. Kolkiewicz
NOVA University, Lisbon, Portugal

East London NHS Foundation Trust, London, UK

5.1 Introduction

Improvements in science, medical and social care have resulted in increasing life expectancy and a growing population of older adults in almost all regions of the world. In spite of the technological advances, many older adults live with chronic conditions and functional impairment. This presents a challenge to commissioners and providers of health services.

© Springer Nature Switzerland AG 2019
C. A. de Mendonça Lima, G. Ivbijaro (eds.), *Primary Care Mental Health in Older People*,
https://doi.org/10.1007/978-3-030-10814-4_5

5.2 Multi-Morbidity and Comorbidity

It is common for older adults living with long-term conditions to have more than one condition or multi-morbidity, which is the coexistence of two or more long-term conditions [1]. Comorbidity is often used to describe the presence of a defined index condition with other linked conditions, for example, diabetes and depression, and multi-morbidity refers to instances where any condition could be included [2, 3].

Comorbidity affects clinical management of a condition as well as patient self-care. This results in poorer outcomes for patients in terms of morbidity and mortality [4, 5]. Patients with multi-morbidity are more likely to have lower perception of health status and have poorer quality of life. Due to the presence of multiple health issues and lower perception of health status, they are more likely be admitted to hospital [6–8]. A study of the impact of comorbidity on disability found that disability increases rapidly with increasing number of chronic conditions [9]. In addition, certain health conditions and impairments contribute independently to the risk of falling or experiencing a fall injury [10, 11]. Older adults with multi-morbidities are likely to be taking a number of medicines for different conditions. This increases the risks of adverse drug reactions [12].

5.3 Impact of Multi-Morbidity

A case study in the UK (London Borough of Waltham Forest) showed disproportionate use of emergency department and significantly increased cost of treatment for comorbid depression and other long-term conditions such as cancer, hypertension and coronary heart disease (CHD). In this case the average cost per patient with asthma and depression, for example, was found to be almost three times the cost per patient with asthma alone [13]. Furthermore, this study found that general practices with high prevalence of depression also had high prevalence of long-term medical conditions—heart failure and hypertension had the strongest associations.

As depression increases the perceived severity and cost of the management of other long-term health conditions [14, 15], it is necessary to manage both the depression and the long-term physical condition to achieve the best outcomes.

Older adults with multi-morbidities are more likely to be accessing health services from different professionals/disciplines. An individual may be receiving care from primary care, other specialists in secondary care and social care who may not be communicating effectively with each other. This leads to fragmentation of care [16] and a need for a collaborative approach for dealing with comorbid long-term conditions.

5.4 Management of Comorbidity and Multi-Morbidity

A systematic review to determine the effectiveness of interventions designed to improve outcomes in people with multi-morbidity in primary care and community settings [2] identified health service and patient-oriented interventions as follows:

- *Professional interventions*: for example, education designed to change the behaviour of clinicians by increasing professionals' awareness of multi-morbidity or providing training/education to equip clinicians with skills in managing these individuals.
- *Financial interventions*: for example, financial incentives to providers to reach treatment targets.
- *Organisational interventions*: for example, any changes to care delivery such as case management or the addition of different healthcare workers such as a pharmacist to the healthcare team. These interventions may work by changing care delivery to match the needs of people with multi-morbidity across a range of areas such as coordination of care, medicines management or use of other health professionals such as physiotherapists and occupational therapists to address needs relating to physical and social functioning. However, this has to be carefully negotiated to

ensure clarity of roles and payment mechanisms.

- *Patient-oriented interventions*: this would include any intervention directed primarily at individuals, for example, education or support for self-management. These interventions might work by improving self-management, thus enabling people to manage their conditions more effectively and to seek appropriate health care.

5.5 Collaborative Care

Collaborative care is an effective model for integrating mental health care into primary care medical settings. It aims to develop closer partnerships between primary care professionals and secondary care and provides both clinical and cost-effectiveness [17–19]. It is a useful model for ensuring that the care of older adults with multimorbidity, who might be accessing different health and social care services, is well coordinated for the benefit of the patient.

A meta-analysis of practice-based interventions for depression comorbid with a range of long-term conditions concluded that collaborative care interventions improved outcomes for depression and quality of life in primary care patients with a variety of medical conditions, although the effect was modest in diabetes care [20]. In another meta-analysis of collaborative care for depression and diabetes, the authors noted that collaborative care led to better depression outcomes and improved adherence to treatment for both conditions [20].

Ivbijaro et al. [13] set out practical steps for developing a collaborative/integrated service. This includes:

- A need to understand the population you are serving and the existing pathways to care including the range of third sector or non-government organisations and existing secondary care providers.
- Development of a business model and a project plan which includes the workforce, skill mix and training required to deliver the model.

You have to deal with physical and mental health conditions together, as part of a stepped care approach.

- Collaborative/integrated care requires accountability from all the organisations involved in the partnership or collaboration. It requires clear clinical leadership, information sharing protocol with a clear methodology of payments or incentives that are clearly established and understood.
- Clinical protocols and guidelines which clarify when to refer to secondary care and when secondary care should discharge back to primary care.

5.6 Stepped Care

Stepped care is a model used to organise the provision of care for people with common mental health disorders, their families and carers. The model helps healthcare professionals to choose the most effective interventions [21].

Stepped care is collaborative in nature. To progress through the stages, there is a need for some form of collaboration between primary and secondary care. A randomised controlled trial in the Netherlands to evaluate the effectiveness of collaborative stepped care in the treatment of common mental disorders concluded that treatment within a collaborative stepped care model resulted in an earlier treatment response compared with care as usual [22]. The authors emphasised that the organisation of care in the Netherlands, and other countries, may benefit from the rapid provision of low-intensity treatments in primary care and improved collaboration between healthcare providers.

However, if resources are stretched, many of the low-intensity treatments may be hard to provide. The low-intensity treatments are very useful where there are patients receiving a high-intensity treatment which can be replaced by a low-intensity treatment. It is also necessary for primary care physicians and nurses to be trained in these low-intensity treatments.

A qualitative study to gain insight into the perceptions of clinicians on implementing stepped

Table 5.1 The stepped care model [24]

Focus of the intervention	Nature of the intervention
Step 1: All known and suspected presentations of depression	Assessment, support, psychoeducation, active monitoring and referral for further assessment and interventions
Step 2: Persistent subthreshold depressive symptoms; mild to moderate depression	Low-intensity psychosocial interventions, psychological interventions, medication and referral for further assessment and interventions
Step 3: Persistent subthreshold depressive symptoms or mild to moderate depression with • Inadequate response to initial interventions • Moderate and severe depression	Medication, high-intensity psychological interventions, combined treatments, collaborative care[a] and referral
Step 4: Severe and complex[b] depression; risk to life; severe self-neglect	Medication, high-intensity psychological interventions, electroconvulsive therapy, crisis service, combined treatments, multi-professional and inpatient care

[a]Only for depression where the person also has a chronic physical health problem and associated functional impairment

[b]Complex depression includes depression that shows an inadequate response to multiple treatments, is complicated by psychotic symptoms and/or is associated with significant psychiatric comorbidity or psychosocial factors

care for depression found that stepped care is received positively in primary care. While it is difficult to fully implement a stepped care approach within a short time frame, clinicians can make incremental progress towards achieving a stepped care approach. Creating a shared understanding of depression within multidisciplinary teams and reaching a consensus about the care to be provided and the allocation of tasks are important when addressing the implementation process [23].

In stepped care the least intrusive, most effective intervention is provided first. If this intervention does not benefit the individual, an appropriate intervention from the next step should be offered [24]. Table 5.1 illustrates the stepped care model.

The appropriate skill mix is essential in any collaborative work, particularly with stepped care. For example, as step 1 involves case identification and recognition, it is important that if depression is suspected, a practitioner who is competent in mental health assessment reviews the person's mental state and associated functional, interpersonal and social difficulties [24].

Services need to ensure they have appropriately trained staff with skills in delivering evidence-based treatments, access to telephony and efficient patient management information systems. With these in place, stepped care can facilitate supported self-management [25].

5.7 Conclusion

Older adults are more likely to have multi-morbidity, which leads to poorer outcomes for the patient. Those with multi-morbidity are more likely to be accessing more than one health service provider, sometimes in addition to social services. Accessing multiple service providers results in increased overall cost of management. Collaborative care provides a useful model for the management of multi-morbidity in older adults. It can be entirely within primary care or in collaboration with a provider outside primary care. Stepped care is a good model for managing depression accompanying other disorders. It is a way of ensuring that interventions match the severity and complexity of presentation so that effort is not wasted.

References

1. Fortin M, Bravo G, Hudon C, Vanasse A, Lapointe L. Prevalence of multimorbidity among adults seen in family practice. Ann Fam Med. 2005;3(3):223–8.
2. Smith SM, Wallace E, O'Dowd T, Fortin M. Interventions for improving outcomes in patients with multimorbidity in primary care and community settings. Cochrane Database of Syst Rev. 2016;3:CD006560. https://doi.org/10.1002/14651858.CD006560.pub3.
3. Valderas JM, Mercer S, Fortin M. Research on patients with multiple health conditions: different constructs, different views, one voice. J Comorb. 2011;1(1):1–3.

4. Rushton CA, Satchithananda DK, Kadam UT. Comorbidity in modern nursing: a closer look at heart failure. Br J Nurs. 2011;20(5):280–5.

5. Hindmarsh D, Loh M, Finch CF, Hayen A, Close JC. Effect of comorbidity on relative survival following hospitalisation for fall-related hip fracture in older people. Australas J Ageing. 2014;33(3):E1.

6. Payne RA, Abel GA, Guthrie B, Mercer SW. The effect of physical multimorbidity, mental health conditions and socioeconomic deprivation on unplanned admissions to hospital: a retrospective cohort study. Can Med Assoc J. 2013;185(5):E221–8.

7. Brettschneider C, Leicht H, Bickel H, Dahlhaus A, Fuchs A, MultiCare Study Group. Relative impact of multimorbid chronic conditions on health-related quality of life – results from the MultiCare Study Group. PLoS One. 2013;8(6):e66742.

8. Martín-García S, Rodríguez-Blázquez C, Martínez-López I, Martínez-Martín P, Forjaz MJ. Comorbidity health status, and quality of life in institutionalized older people with and without dementia. Int Psychogeriatr. 2013;25(7):1077–84.

9. Verbrugge LM, Lepkowski JM, Imanaka Y. Comorbidity and its impact on disability. Milbank Q. 1989;67(3–4):450–84.

10. McClure RJ, Turner C, Peel N, Spinks A, Eakin E, Hughes K. Population-based interventions for the prevention of fall-related injuries in older people. Cochrane Database of Syst Rev. 2005;1:CD004441. https://doi.org/10.1002/14651858.CD004441.pub2.

11. Vu T, Finch CF, Day L. Patterns of comorbidity in community-dwelling older people hospitalised for fall-related injury: a cluster analysis. BMC Geriatr. 2011;11:45.

12. Duerden M, Avery T, Payne R. Polypharmacy and medicines optimisation. https://www.kingsfund.org.uk/sites/files/kf/field/field_publication_file/polypharmacy-and-medicines-optimisation-kingsfund-nov13.pdf. Accessed Dec 2016.

13. Ivbijaro GO, Enum Y, Khan AA, Lam SS-K, Gabzdyl A. Collaborative care: models for treatment of patients with complex medical-psychiatric conditions. Curr Psychiatry Rep. 2014;16:506.

14. Ivbijaro G. Mental health: a resilience factor against both NCDs and CDs. In: Commonwealth health partnerships 2012. Cambridge: Nexus Strategic Partnerships; 2012. p. 17–20.

15. World Health Organization. The global burden of disease: 2004 update. Geneva: The World Health Organization; 2008.

16. Wallace E, Salisbury C, Guthrie B, Lewis C, Fahey T, Smith SM. Managing patients with multimorbidity in primary care. BMJ. 2015;350:176.

17. Katon W, Russo J, Lin EHB, Schmittdiel J, Ciechanowski P, Ludman E, et al. Cost-effectiveness of a multicondition collaborative care intervention. Arch Gen Psychiatry. 2012;69(5):506–14.

18. Huang Y, Wei X, Wu T, Chen R, Guo A. Collaborative care for patients with depression and diabetes mellitus: a systematic review and meta-analysis. BMC Psychiatry. 2013;13:260–71.

19. Unützer J, Harbin H, Schoenbaum M, Druss B. The collaborative care model: an approach for integrating physical and mental health car in Medicaid Health Homes. Center for Health Strategies and Mathematica Policy Research; 2013.

20. Watson LC, Amick HR, Gaynes BN, Brownley KA, Thaker S, Viswanaathan M, et al. Practice-based interventions addressing concomitant depression and chronic medical conditions in the primary care setting: a systematic review and meta-analysis. J Prim Care Community Health. 2013;4(4):294–306.

21. National Institute for Health and Care Excellence. Common mental health problems: identification and pathways to care. NICE clinical guideline 123. NICE 2011. https://www.nice.org.uk/guidance/cg123.

22. Oosterbaan DB, Verbraak MJPM, Terluin B, et al. Collaborative stepped care v. care as usual for common mental disorders: 8-month, cluster randomised controlled trial. Br J Psychiatry. 2013;203:132–9.

23. Franx G, Oud M, de Lange J, et al. Implementing a stepped-care approach in primary care: results of a qualitative study. Implement Sci. 2012;7:8.

24. National Institute for Health and Care Excellence. Depression in adults: recognition and management (Updated 2016) NICE clinical guideline 90. NICE 2009. https://www.nice.org.uk/guidance/cg90.

25. Richards DA. Stepped care: a method to deliver increased access to psychological therapies. Can J Psychiatr. 2012;57(4):210–5.

Part III

Accessing the Essential

History Taking and Assessment

6

Orestes V. Forlenza, Marta L. G. F. Pereira, Paulo R. Canineu, and Florindo Stella

Abstract

The clinical history is a fundamental part of the medical semiology. It requires assessing the patient with a holistic approach and demands special attention to specific elements that may allow a deeper understanding of disease process and its progression over time. In the present text, we emphasize some of the most relevant aspects of history taking in geriatric psychiatry, including the characterization of premorbid features, personal and family history, and the establishment of an accurate estimate of cognitive/functional status and behavioral symptoms both in primary (functional) and secondary (organic) psychiatric disorders. The identification of risk factors for neuropsychiatric disorders associated to general medical conditions is another important element, for the modification of these factors (whenever possible) may be crucial for overall response and prognosis. We further propose that use of psychometric scales in clinical practice not only yields the objective measurement of baseline cognitive/functional state for diagnostic purposes but also enables the clinician to monitor changes during follow-up, particularly those related to treatment response.

O. V. Forlenza (✉) · M. L. G. F. Pereira
Laboratory of Neurosciences (LIM-27),
Institute of Psychiatry, Faculty of Medicine,
University of São Paulo, São Paulo, SP, Brazil
e-mail: forlenza@usp.br

P. R. Canineu
Laboratory of Neurosciences (LIM-27),
Institute of Psychiatry, Faculty of Medicine,
University of São Paulo, São Paulo, SP, Brazil

Pontifícia Universidade Católica de São Paulo,
Gerontology Program, São Paulo, SP, Brazil

F. Stella
Laboratory of Neurosciences (LIM-27),
Institute of Psychiatry, Faculty of Medicine,
University of São Paulo, São Paulo, SP, Brazil

UNESP – Universidade Estadual Paulista,
Biosciences Institute, Campus of Rio Claro,
SP, Brazil
e-mail: florindo.stella@hc.fm.usp.br

Key Points
- To elaborate a diagnosis of mental disorder in older adults, the search for information related to the current complaint is an active process directed by the clinician. It comprises the identification of initial symptoms and its evolution, as well as the aggravating or improvement factors.
- One of the key aspects of psychiatric history is to identify the patient's cognitive profile and its level of functional performance in daily life activities.
- A crucial step toward the diagnosis of dementia is the description of *when* and

C. A. de Mendonça Lima, G. Ivbijaro (eds.), *Primary Care Mental Health in Older People*,
https://doi.org/10.1007/978-3-030-10814-4_6

how the cognitive and functional impairments have appeared and if this is a persistent and progressive process.

- The elaboration of a clinical interview directly with the patient, followed by an interview with family members or caregivers, decisively contributes to establish a diagnosis and to suggest an etiological hypothesis.
- The nature and onset of the clinical condition and also the context where the condition has emerged, which factors can improve or deteriorate the symptoms, number and reasons for hospital admissions, as well as the recurrences of symptoms and response pattern to previous treatments, constitute elements that should be carefully investigated.
- Clinicians must be aware of particular cultural concepts that misleadingly consider mental disorders among the elderly as "normal" or that attribute other specific conditions, such as depression, apathy, or memory loss, as due to aging.
- Scales with a good reliability rate allow to accurately measure the frequency and severity of cognitive decline, changes in functional and neuropsychiatric symptoms, and, also, the follow-up of treatment results.

6.1 Clinical History of the Current Disease

The purpose of the clinical history is to obtain detailed information about the onset of mental health disease and its progression over time. Each psychopathologic symptom should be carefully investigated based on its appearance, temporal evolution, current manifestations, and functional impairment.

In addition, detailing the clinical history also implies to clarify eventual pathological antecedents, premorbid socio-occupational skills level, family history of neuropsychiatric conditions, as well as the surrounding psychosocial context and all the prescribed drugs.

In order to better understand the complexity of the current medical condition, the clinician should try to understand *when* and *how* the symptoms evolved throughout the course of the disease and to identify aggravating or improvement factors, as well as to be able to recognize any similarities and dissimilarities between the events.

The search for information related to the current complaint is an active process lead by the clinician that helps to contextualize the conditions in which the clinical condition has emerged. This way, memory or depression symptoms may be related to cerebrovascular events. Over time, these occurrences can converge into physical disabilities or vascular dementia. Moreover, current complaints of persistent anergy, bradypsychia, anhedonia, or a sense of worthlessness may be associated with the presence of depression. This correlation can occur in degenerative diseases such as cancer, chronic obstructive pulmonary disease, heart failure, Parkinson's disease, or other general medical illnesses that lead to reduced physical ability, mental performance, and autonomy loss.

6.1.1 Personal Antecedents

Identifying specific neuropsychiatric conditions, such as traumatic brain injury, neuroinfections, central nervous system tumors, depression, anxiety, and sleep disturbances, among other disorders, is one of the most important steps in the clinical history.

Aggressive or uninhibited behavior is very common among patients with bipolar disorder in a manic phase or in patients with frontal syndromes related to cerebrovascular accidents and brain injury. It is also frequent in neurodegenerative conditions, among them, the frontotemporal lobar degeneration—behavioral variant, a condition also known as frontotemporal dementia. Reports of psychotic symptoms like hallucinations and delusions, when associated with bizarre or aggressive behaviors, need to be thoroughly investigated. These events can be mistakenly interpreted as being against the law, under a forensic approach, and not always are understood from a medical point of view.

In addition, clinicians must be aware that history of previous depression, especially with a late onset, when accompanied by cognitive alterations or impairments in daily life activities, can constitute a progression risk to dementia or, eventually, represents a prodromal stage of neurodegenerative disease [1]. Also, previous depression episodes with psychotic symptoms, cognitive impairment, insomnia, anorexia, or suicide attempts can predict the current episode severity.

It must be considered that history of rapid mood cycling, with clinically relevant fluctuations, is an alert sign of extra care when dealing with elderly patients in either a depressive or manic phase. Psychiatric admissions, psychotic symptoms, and episodes of severe agitation suggest that the current bipolar disorder episode deserves close clinical monitoring.

In this scenario, one of the key functions of psychiatric history is to define a cognitive profile and a level of performance in instrumental activities of daily living, in particular, the most complex ones. It is crucial to characterize the onset of memory and other cognitive domain alterations and if there has been any functional decline or if the changes have been persistent and progressive.

6.1.1.1 Alcohol and Other Psychoactive Substances Abuse Pattern

The abuse pattern of alcohol, tobacco, and other nonmedical psychoactive substances deserves special attention from the clinician. Criteria such as age of onset, quantity, frequency, episodes of intoxication, time of use, and addiction must be evaluated. Individuals with a history of alcohol dependence usually show symptoms like mental disorders, abstinence syndrome, altered levels of consciousness, delirium, anxiety episodes, memory, and other cognitive impairments, as well as dementia.

In addition, with the increase in average life expectancy, it is estimated an increase in the rates of individuals with conditions related to alcohol abuse. Listed below are some extended comments on alcohol dependence (see Sect. 6.5).

6.1.1.2 Use of Medical Drugs

The use of drugs, especially those acting on the central nervous system, deserves careful investigation. Benzodiazepines are often used by older adults and is not uncommon the occurrence of dependency associated with them. These drugs have been widely used by patients whose treatment could be conducted using other strategies. Thus, it is not rare an initial prescription of benzodiazepine for long-term treatment of depression, insomnia, or anxiety, with a high inherent risk of sedation, daytime sleepiness, and falls, apart from the tolerance risk and possible addiction. The indiscriminate use of benzodiazepines in elderly patients, especially when they already have mild cognitive impairment, has an adverse impact on memory and other areas of cognition and constitutes a risk of progression to dementia.

6.1.2   Family History

Unlike what happens with young patients, obtaining family history related to the elderly patient becomes a difficult task due to the fact that people who could possibly provide accurate information have already passed away.

This way, the current informants are usually spouses or children, who were close to the patient early in the clinical course of the disease. However, due to their lack of proximity with the patient's predecessors, it is not always possible to collect sufficient information about the emergence and clinical course of the disease. Still, these people represent important references when gathering information about the medical history, especially when similar symptoms are observed in any of these family members at the present moment. Accordingly, researchers have confirmed that suicidal behavior has a strong familial component and people with suicidal history in the family tend to exhibit personality traits compatible with high risk of self-injurious behaviors [2].

6.2   Clinical Interview

The first interview is a crucial moment for the establishment of an interpersonal relationship that will lead to a precise psychiatric clinical history. It is also essential for subsequent assessments, which are invaluable tools to reach a conclusive diagnosis and posterior treatment [3].

Information obtained when interviewing the patient and, additionally, family members or caregivers greatly contributes to achieve a diagnosis and, sometimes, to outline an etiological hypothesis. Aspects such as the nature and onset of the clinical condition, context within which the symptoms have began, aggravating or improvement factors, number and reasons for hospital admissions, frequency and severity of recurrent symptoms, as well as the response pattern to drug interventions, need to be carefully assessed.

Initially, it is important to create a friendly and serene environment where the patient feels encouraged to express, verbally and non-verbally, his complaints. This is usually a useful strategy for the semiotics of the subject's mental disorder.

The clinician needs to guarantee that the patient is able to attend the interview alone and that he has cognitive competence enough to provide reliable answers. Cognitive impairment, lack of confidence, and emotional stress can affect the clarity of semiological data. In any case, it is relevant to promote an active engagement of the patient during the interview. Thus, direct questions, with short and easy to understand sentences, may facilitate an engaged attitude, specially among patients with cognitive deficits.

Another important element to consider during the interview is the alertness and anxiety level shown by the patient, because they can have a significant impact on the quality of his answers. Therefore, it is crucial for the clinician to maintain an open and dialoguing posture, being able at the same time to appreciate each patient's complaint, in order to establish an effective interpersonal communication.

Also, different cultural elements can greatly affect the interview. Particularly in socioeconomically disadvantaged countries, a vast number of clinical conditions are often attributed to aging per se, as if they were not clinically relevant and,

therefore, would not need appropriate clinical assessment and treatment. The notion that certain clinical manifestations can be "normal" or certain prevailing beliefs within the patient's social context may compromise the quality of information. As an example, the cultural misconception that depression is a feature of the aging process or that memory loss is part of the natural course of life leads the informant to underestimate depressive manifestations and not to consider that dementia may be in its early course.

In addition, symptoms like lack of interest, indifference toward surrounding events, reduced response to affective and emotional appeals from the group, phenomena such as insomnia or daytime sleepiness, and conditions like constipation, urinary incontinence, or mental confusion can be interpreted by uninformed family members or caregivers as inherent to natural course of aging and not as possible clinical conditions that deserve appropriate diagnosis and treatment.

Regarding possible approaching methods, when possible, the clinician should be able to interview both the patient and his family members or caregiver, separately. It is important to point out that the informant should be someone living with the patient and who is knowledgeable about his symptoms.

6.2.1 Idiosyncrasies of the Clinical Interview

The way the patient presents himself during the interview can provide elements such as general appearance, overall attitude, facial expressions, body language, costumes, tidiness, and hygiene that will be very helpful when trying to understand his clinical condition. Also, the clinician must ascertain eventual recent changes in his life, like loss of family members or friends, declining socioeconomic conditions, social isolation, and inability to autonomously perform basic health care.

Moreover, a further investigation must be carried out to assess the onset of symptoms. It is not infrequent that family members associate specific events with the onset of disease, when in fact, they must be merely concomitants. A pertinent example is the association of a sudden onset of Alzheimer's disease with a hospital admission for prostate resection or a case of sudden memory loss after a wife's death. Although it is known that stressful events and mourning periods have an adverse impact on cognitive condition, this is not a cause-effect association [3]. Nonetheless, although the emergence of Alzheimer's disease has been observed by family members in the context of a relevant event, most certainly, memory decline would have been insidious and progressive over time, due to a neurodegenerative process.

Finally it is convenient to underline that the search for additional information from other sources—within the patient's personal relationship circle—tends to clarify this issue.

However, it should be noted that a sudden impairment of cognitive abilities is usually associated with an episode of *delirium* as part of a general medical condition (urinary tract infection, drug toxicity, subdural hematoma, acute cerebrovascular event, etc.). A major depressive episode with psychotic symptoms may also favor the emergence of cognitive decline in the elderly, in a relatively short amount of time.

Some psychological factors may compromise the accuracy of information provided by the patient. Individuals with personality disorders may "disguise" behaviors or consciously/unconsciously "deny" certain psychopathological symptoms they consider embarrassing or that may reveal personal weaknesses. Nonetheless, the clinician needs to be aware of the fact that changes in personality, especially the impulsive, socially inadequate, or apathetic types, may represent the first manifestations of frontotemporal dementia.

Also, the speech style of a patient who is uninhibited or without social judgment, combined with socially inadequate attitudes and also difficulty to logically organize answers to the clinician's questions, suggests certain neuropsychiatric conditions, among them, frontotemporal dementia.

6.2.2 Recommendations

During the clinical interview, several recommendations can promote a fruitful relationship between the clinician and the patient, which will lead to a more efficient data research and to more accurate information. The clinician should resist the urge to "infantilize" his relationship with the patient, since this can leave him with a feeling of incompetence or even to lower his self-esteem.

It is the clinician's responsibility to outline a cognitive profile for the patient. However, it must be taken into consideration that specific cognitive impairments, such as attention, thought processing, and motor and semantic aphasia, may compromise the accuracy of information. In accordance, it cannot be overemphasized that at least one informant should be present during the interview, in order to achieve a better data accuracy.

General medical comorbidities tend to become the focus of concerns shown by the patient and his family. The professional must be careful not to underestimate any systemic complaint, in particular those that impact the central nervous system. Additionally, emaciated patients with walking problems, psychomotor retardation, and without any interest in environmental stimuli require additional care from the consultant in order to investigate the general medical conditions underlying the current complaints. On the other hand, the clinician who is conducting the interview aims to achieve a diagnosis of a neuropsychiatric condition.

6.3 Cognitive and Functional Assessment

Specially in patients with dementia—currently designated as major neurocognitive disorder—particular clinical alterations involving cognition, functionality, and behavior can be observed. These changes interact with each other, given that memory deficits and other cognitive domains affect the performance of daily life activities and

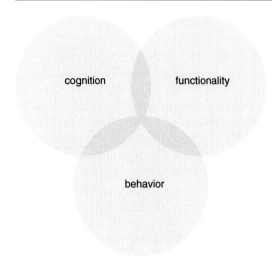

Fig. 6.1 Interaction between cognition, functionality, and behavior

induce, at the same time, disorganized behavior, a phenomena also referred as neuropsychiatric disorders (Fig. 6.1).

6.3.1 Cognitive Screening

For the initial cognitive assessment, several tools are available to measure cognitive domains such as memory, attention, language, executive functions (abstraction, calculation, logical thinking, decision-making, and self-monitoring), working memory, perception, recognition, and praxis. The clinician may use multiple tests: *Mini-Mental State Examination* (MMSE) [4], *Montreal Cognitive Assessment* (MoCA) [5], *Semantic and Phonemic Verbal Fluency Tests* [6], *Boston Naming Test* [7], *Test Clock Drawing* [8], and *Trial Making Test* [9].

Also available is the *Cambridge Cognitive Test* (CAMCOG)—a cognitive section of the *Cambridge Examination for Mental Disorders of the Elderly*—Revised Version (CAMDEX-R) [10]. CAMDEX-R is a structured and comprehensive interview that aims to identify mental disorders in older adults, with a special focus on dementia. The test also aims to assess the impact of cognitive deterioration on daily life activities.

CAMCOG covers a wide range of cognitive domains such as orientation, language, memory, attention, praxis, calculation, abstraction, and perception. Also as part of the instrument is an interview with the informant, in order to complement the existent clinical data.

In more recent years, several computerized tests have been developed such as the *Cambridge Neuropsychological Test Automated Battery* (Cantab) [11] and the *Computer-Administered Neuropsychological Screen for Mild Cognitive Impairment* (CANS-MCI) [12], with the purpose of identifying subjects with mild cognitive impairment.

In general, cognitive screening test have been consistently used by practitioners and represent a useful tool for health professionals working in primary health-care centers to screen the most obvious cognitive alterations. Furthermore, cognitive screening underpins a clinical decision about referring the patient to a more comprehensive neuropsychological assessment in order to clarify the existence of a possible early stage dementia.

6.3.2 Functional Screening

Regarding functional assessment, different strategies have been reported, such as the *Direct Assessment of Functional State, Revised* (DAFS-R) [13], and the *Pfeffer Functional Activities Questionnaire* (Pfeffer) [14]. These instruments allow to screen the ability shown by the patient to carry out instrumental activities of daily living. The value of this type of assessment is directly related to global cognitive ability. When diagnosing dementia, it is critical to determine how much memory impairment and other cognitive domains interfere with the ability to perform instrumental activities of daily living. Table 6.1 summarizes the most common tools for cognitive and functional screening of elderly patients often used in primary mental health-care centers.

Table 6.1 Instruments for cognitive and functional screening in primary mental health care

Global cognitive screening		
Modality	Test	Author
Cognitive assessment	Mini-Mental State Examination, Montreal Cognitive Assessment	Folstein et al. [4]
	Clock Drawing Test	Nasreddine et al. [5], Sunderland et al. [8]
	Verbal Fluency (semantic and phonemic)	Lezak et al. [6]
	Boston Naming Test	Kaplan et al. [7]
	Trial Making Test	Tombaugh [9]
	Cambridge Cognitive Test (CAMCOG)	Roth et al. [10]
Functional assessment	Direct Assessment of Functional State, Revised (DAFS-R)	Loewenstein and Bates [13]
	Pfeffer Functional Activities Questionnaire	Pfeffer [14]

6.4 Assessment of Neuropsychiatric Manifestations

The prevalence of Alzheimer's disease in developing countries reaches 60% of cases [15]. Neuropsychiatric symptoms in this type of dementia have a frequency of up to 80% [16–18] and manifest themselves mainly as depression, apathy, anxiety, delusions and hallucinations, irritability, agitation, aggression, and sleep disturbances [19], even in the early stages of the disease [20, 21]. These manifestations are a source of distress for the patient, and also they anticipate institutionalization, predispose to increased medical comorbidity, increase mortality risk, and cause emotional burden and high workload to families and caregivers [19].

Many scales have been developed with the purpose of evaluating these neuropsychiatric symptoms in patients with dementia. The *Neuropsychiatric Inventory* (NPI) [22] has been one of the most used resources. This instrument considers 12 groups of symptoms considered as "domains," and each domain consists of specific items that clarify the psychopathological condition in dementia patients. Each domain is assessed on the basis of scripted questions administered to the caregiver about the patient's symptoms. The caregiver is asked to rate the frequency and severity of these symptoms in each domain and the level of distress associated with each symptom. It is up to the caregiver to rate a final score for each domain.

De Medeiros et al. [23], in collaboration with JL Cumming (responsible for creating the NPI), have developed a new version of this instrument designated as *Neuropsychiatric Inventory-Clinician Rating Scale* (*NPI-C*). This restructured version includes expanded items within various syndromic domains. Also, *agitation/aggression* domain was split into two new specific domains, with an inclusion of new items in each one of them. From a psychopathological perspective, agitation and aggression are phenomena of a different nature. Generally, patients showing agitation demonstrate wandering behaviors without any defined goal. They also demonstrate uncooperative attitudes or resistance to care; however they do not manifest physical or verbal behaviors against a specific target. On the other hand, an aggressive patient exhibits angry behaviors and presents intentional actions against himself or a particular target or persons, intending to destroy specific objects. In this version, the author added a new domain (*aberrant vocalizations*), more common in advanced dementia conditions.

NPI-C's main feature relies on its accuracy degree. It is the consultant who sets the final score for each item in each domain. Hence, the designation "clinician rating" was chosen for the title of this new version. This way, in order to rate each item's score and each domain's total score, the clinician should take into account all the available information that can help to accurately identify any domain-related neuropsychiatric symptom observed in the past month. Besides the information provided by the caregiver, the patient's interview and direct observations are also important tools when assessing patient's behavior. Furthermore, the clinician can also incorporate any available data from the patient's chart and reports provided by individuals from the patient's inner circle. To sum up, using the expert clinical judgment as part of the rating system increases the assessment's sensitivity and gives a higher accuracy for the diagnosis of neuropsychiatric symptoms [23].

The *Behavioral Pathology in Alzheimer's Disease Rating Scale* (BEHAVE-AD) [24] was developed to investigate psychopathology in patients with Alzheimer's disease, namely, delusions and hallucinations, aggression, sleep and circadian rhythm disturbances, affective disorders, anxiety and phobias, and impairment of activities of daily living. The scale allows for a comprehensive examination of these symptoms and, at the same time, to identify symptom clusters.

Another behavioral assessment tool is the *Cohen-Mansfield Agitation Index* (CMAI) [25]. This inventory is intended to assess episodes of agitation in elderly patients with neuropsychiatric disorders, especially dementia. The consultant completes the test, based on the informant's report, about the frequency of agitation behaviors that occurred within the last 2 weeks. The rating scale ranges from 1 (*never* or *hardly never*) to 7 (*several times an hour*). Also, situations when the instrument is not applicable are taken into consideration, for example, when the caregiver is not able to answer the questions or when the patient does not present agitation, due to a physical disability. A disruptiveness scale was added to the test, and the informant is asked to give information as to how disruptive each behavior is, on a scale from 1 (*never*) to 5 (*extremely*).

Depression is a common condition among older patients. Around 27% of the elderly living in long-stay institutions have major depression

[26]. In Alzheimer's disease, this condition affects approximately 50% of patients [27].

Regarding depressive symptom's assessment, several instruments have been used with good accuracy rates, for example, the *Beck Depression Inventory* [28], the *Hamilton Rating Scale for Depression* [29], the *Montgomery-Asberg Depression Raging Scale* [30], the *Cornell Scale for Depression in Dementia* [31], and the *Geriatric Depression Scale* [32]. These last two scales have been widely used to measure depressive symptoms in elderly patients.

The *Cornell Scale for Depression in Dementia* [31] is an instrument originally designed to measure the course of depressive symptoms in dementia patients undergoing psychopharmacological antidepressant treatment. Apart from its use in clinical trials to determine the efficacy of antidepressants, this scale has also been used to assess symptoms of major depression in dementia, including Alzheimer's disease, in ambulatory patients.

The *Geriatric Depression Scale* [32], in its short version of 15 items, has been widely used, with a good reliability rate, to screen depressive symptoms among the elderly, in specialized clinical settings or in primary mental health-care environments [33, 34]. A score greater than 4 points suggests clinically relevant depressive symptoms, and a score equal to or greater than 11 points indicates severe symptoms.

Apathy is another important condition, one of the most common neuropsychiatric impairments in neurodegenerative disorders, like Alzheimer's and Parkinson's disease. It can also be detected co-occurring with depression, although they have distinct psychopathologic manifestations and different neuropathological correlates [35]. Several studies have reported a high prevalence of apathy in patients with Alzheimer's disease, ranging from 55% to 70% of cases [23, 35]. Patients with this syndrome exhibit a reduction or lack of motivation in three clinical dimensions—emotional reactivity, interest, and initiative.

The *Apathy Inventory* [35, 36] measures the abovementioned dimensions. Thus, the inventory examines alterations of motivation related to

(a) reduction or loss of ability to react affectively and emotionally; (b) reduction or loss of cognitive interest toward a particular target; and (c) reduction or loss of initiative, that is, lack of behaviors in response to internal or external environmental stimuli. For each inventory item, the clinician rates a final score based on the following sources of information: caregiver's reports, patient's interview, and observation of behavioral manifestations during the assessment.

Other scales have also been used to measure apathy in elderly patients with neuropsychiatric conditions: the *Apathy Scale* [37] and the *Apathy Evaluation Scale* [38]. However, these are not scored according to the consultant's judgment, as it happens in the Apathy Inventory but according to information reported by the family or caregiver.

The *Global Deterioration Scale* (GDS) [39] is a scale that measures global deterioration in dementia patients. Individuals are rated according to a seven-point scale. Level 1 refers to no cognitive deficit evidences. Levels 2 and 3 refer to very mild and mild cognitive alterations, respectively. Subsequent levels, from 4 to 7, comprise evident global deterioration levels characterized by severe cognitive and functional decline with clinically relevant disorganized behavior.

The *Brief Psychiatric Rating Scale* (BPRS) [40] has been used to investigate the severity of psychopathologic manifestations in patients with chronic psychotic disorders, such as schizophrenia or persistent delusional disorder. This scale has been used in patients whose disease onset happened long before aging or in older adults with late-onset psychotic symptoms. Table 6.2 reports the most commonly used scales to measure neuropsychiatric symptoms in older adults.

Table 6.2 Frequently used scales to assess neuropsychiatric symptoms in primary mental health care

Assessment of global neuropsychiatric symptoms	
Neuropsychiatric scale	*Author*
Neuropsychiatric Inventory (NPI)	Cummings et al. [22]
Neuropsychiatric Inventory-Clinician Rating Scale (NPI-C)	de Medeiros et al. [23]
Behavioral Pathology in Alzheimer's Disease Rating Scale (BEHAVE-AD)	Reisberg et al. [24]
Cohen-Mansfield Agitation Index (CMAI)	Cohen-Mansfield [25]
Global Deterioration Scale (GDS)	Reisberg et al. [39]
Brief Psychiatric Rating Scale (BPRS)	Ventura et al. [40]
Specific modalities	
Assessment of depression	*Author*
Cornell Scale for Depression in Dementia (CSDD)	Alexopoulos et al. [31]
Beck Depression Inventory (BDI)	Beck et al. [28]
Hamilton Rating Scale for Depression (HRSD)	Hamilton [29]
Montgomery-Asberg Depression Raging Scale (MADRS)	Montgomery and Asberg [30]
Geriatric Depression Scale	Yesavage et al. [32]
Assessment of apathy	*Author*
Apathy Inventory (AI)	Robert et al. [35–36]
Apathy Scale	Starkstein et al. [37]
Apathy Evaluation Scale	Marin et al. [38]

6.5 Complementary Clinical Assessments

6.5.1 Alcohol Abuse

Alcohol abuse is a condition that affects a significant percentage of the general population and has been consistently associated with systemic diseases such as liver cirrhosis, pancreatitis, gastric disorders, nutritional deficiencies, head trauma, seizures, peripheral neuropathy, and cerebrovascular diseases. Also, alcohol abuse has a negative impact on social relationships, working skills, road traffic accidents, or domestic violence, among others. Regarding older adults, alcohol abuse has been related to alcoholic dementia, with a prevalence of 10% of cases [41], and to vascular dementia. In these conditions, it is possible to observe a global cognitive decline or specific cognitive deficits, depending on the affected brain areas. Cognitive impairment usually occurs simultaneously with impairments of daily life activities [3]. A vast number of neuropsychiatric manifestations may also appear, such as social inadequacy, agitation, aggression, depression, anxiety, sleep disorders, or disorganized and bizarre behavior. On the other hand, withdrawal symptoms and dependence syndrome are not uncommon phenomena among seniors with a chronic and abusive drinking pattern.

Several scales help the clinician to measure the degree of alcohol consumption, such as the *CAGE Questionnaire* [42] and the *Alcohol Use Disorders Identification Test* (AUDIT) [43]. These instruments are easy-to-administer screening tools and provide valuable information when assessing this clinical condition. CAGE screens drinking habits developed over time and is an acronym of its four questions (C, Have you ever felt you should *cut* down on your drinking?; A, Have people *annoyed* you by criticizing your drinking?; G, Have you ever felt bad or *guilty* about your drinking?; E, *Eye opener*, Have you ever had a drink first thing in the morning to steady your nerves or to get rid of a hangover?). Two positive responses indicate the need for further research. AUDIT is administered to measure the amount and frequency of alcohol consumption. It also aims to assess the occurrence of binge, dependence symptoms, work-related harm, relationship problems, health impairments, and socially inappropriate or violent behaviors.

6.5.2　Cerebrovascular Risk

Another relevant topic in clinical research is the identification of cerebrovascular risk factors. When uncontrolled, these factors can determine vascular dementia occurrence. This is a highly prevalent condition, particularly in developing countries, with incident estimates of 30%, second only to Alzheimer's disease, with occurrences up to 60% of cases [15]. Cerebrovascular disease can only be preventable in most cases and is strongly associated with hypertension, diabetes mellitus, chronic high cholesterol and triglyceride levels, obesity, sedentary lifestyle, and smoking. These factors raise risk for vascular dementia and Alzheimer's disease. The *Hachinski Ischemic Score* [44] is a clinical tool for identifying cerebrovascular risk factors. A score equal or greater than 7 suggests vascular involvement. In the presence of cognitive and functional decline, a diagnosis of vascular dementia can be considered. Table 6.3 shows the clinical scales for assessing alcohol abuse and cerebrovascular diseases.

A useful way of formulating holistic assessment is to consider the "3 P factors":

- Predisposing factors
- Precipitating factors
- Perpetuating factors

This is illustrated in Table 6.4 below.

To undertake a thorough assessment of these factors, the GP must involve the patient and family/carer.

Table 6.3 Other clinical scales

Other clinical assessment tools		
Complementary assessment	Hachinski Ischemic Score	Hachinski et al. [44]
	CAGE Questionnaire	Ewing [42]
	Alcohol Use Disorders Identification Test (AUDIT)	Saunders et al. [43]

Table 6.4 Formulating holistic assessment in older adults

	Physical	Psychological	Social
Predisposing factors	For example. poor eye sight	For example, low mood	For example, isolation
Precipitating factors	For example, acute infection		For example, bereavement
Perpetuating factors	For example, untreated infection and multiple prescription drugs		

6.6 Conclusion

Clinical assessment of elderly patients in primary health-care settings involves a detailed examination of the clinical condition, exploration of eventual circumstances that may have contributed to the disease manifestation, and its triggering factors. It also contemplates the identification of environmental aspects that may have interfered with the severity and progression of symptoms, imminent risks of worsening, chances of clinical recovery, and prevention of recurrence.

Also, involving family members, long-term caregivers, or informants in the evaluation process can improve data accuracy and reliability, making the clinician's practice safer and more effective.

Another structural condition is the existence of clinical centers with well-planned and managed services and also with formally trained professionals that guarantee an adequate assistance to elderly patient with mental disorders.

In addition, interventions aiming to prevent mental disorders among the elderly, or at least to attenuate their worsening when already present, deserve to be the main focus of primary care in mental health.

It is essential to keep accurate and timely records. As older adults are more likely to be under the care of more than one organization or service, there is a need to establish appropriate data sharing agreements between organizations.

Finally, keeping the patient close to his community and interpersonal relationships, encouraging the ability to make decisions, recognizing cultural and religious beliefs, as well as accepting a different ideological thinking—in short, taking into account every aspect of the patient's personal history—constitute a key element of a humanized clinical intervention with elderly patients.

References

1. Rosenberg PB, Mielke MM, Appleby BS, et al. The association of neuropsychiatric symptoms in mci with incident dementia and Alzheimer's disease. Am J Geriatr Psychiatr. 2013;21(7):685–95.
2. Kim CD, Seguin M, Therrien N, et al. Familial aggregation of suicidal behavior: a family study of male suicide completers from the general population. Am J Psychiatr. 2005;162(5):1017–9.
3. Sahu S, Crugel M. Taking a psychiatric history from elderly patients. In: Mohammed T, Abou-Saleh MT, Katona C, Kumar A, editors. Principles and practice of geriatric psychiatry. 3rd ed. West Sussex: Wiley; 2011.
4. Folstein MF, Folstein SE, McHugh P. Mini-Mental State: a practical method for grading the cognitive state of patients for the clinician. J Psychiatr Res. 1975;12:189–98.
5. Nasreddine ZS, Phillips NA, Bédirian V, et al. The montreal cognitive assessment (MoCA): a brief screening tool for mild cognitive impairment. J Am Geriatr Soc. 2005;53:695–9.
6. Lezak MD, Howieson DB, Bigler ED, et al. Neuropsychological assessment. 5th ed. New York: Oxford University Press; 2011.
7. Kaplan E, Goodglass H, Weintraub S. Boston naming test. Philadelphia: Lippincott Williams & Wilkins; 2001.
8. Sunderland T, Hill JL, Mellow AM, et al. Clock drawing in Alzheimer's disease: a novel measure of dementia severity. J Am Geriatr Soc. 1989;37:725–9.
9. Tombaugh TN. Trail making test A and B: normative data stratified by age and education. Arch Clin Neuropsychol. 2004;19:203–14.
10. Roth M, Huppert FA, Mountjou CQ, et al. CAMDEX-R: the revised Cambridge examination for mental disorders of the elderly. 2nd ed. Cambridge: Cambridge University Press; 1999.
11. Wild K, Howieson D, Webbe F, et al. Status of computerized cognitive testing in aging: a systematic review. Alzheimers Dement. 2008;4(6):428–37.
12. Tornatore JB, Hill E, Laboff JA, et al. Self-administered screening for mild cognitive impairment: initial validation of a computerized test battery. J Neuropsychiatry Clin Neurosci. 2005;7(1):98–105.
13. Loewenstein DA, Bates CB. The direct assessment of functional status revised (DAFS-R). Manual for Administration and Scoring. Miami Beach: Neuropsychological Laboratories, Mount Sinai Medical Center, The Wien Center for Alzheimer's Disease and Memory Disorders; 2006.
14. Pfeffer RI. Measurement of functional activities in older adults in the community. J Gerontol. 1982;37:323–9.
15. Kalaria RN, Maestre GE, Arizaga R, et al. Alzheimer's disease and vascular dementia in developing countries: prevalence, management, and risk factors. Lancet Neurol. 2008;7(9):812–26.
16. Lyketsos CG, Steinberg M, Tschanz JT, et al. Mental and behavioral disturbances in dementia: findings from the Cache County Study on Memory in Aging. Am J Psychiatr. 2000;157(5):708–14.
17. Aalten P, Verhey FRJ, Boziki M, et al. Neuropsychiatric syndromes in dementia results from the European

Alzheimer Disease Consortium: Part I. Dement Geriatr Cogn Disord. 2007;24:457–63.

18. Zuidema SU, Derksen E, Verhey FR, et al. Prevalence of neuropsychiatric symptoms in a large sample of Dutch nursing home patients with dementia. Int J Geriatr Psychiatry. 2007;22(7):632–8.

19. Lyketsos CG, Miller DS. For the Neuropsychiatric Syndromes Professional Interest Area of the International Society to Advance Alzheimer's Research and Treatment. Addressing the Alzheimer's disease crisis through better understanding, treatment, and eventual prevention of associated neuropsychiatric syndromes. Alzheimers Dement. 2012;8:60–4.

20. Lyketsos CG, Lopez O, Jones B. Prevalence of neuropsychiatric symptoms in dementia and mild cognitive impairment. JAMA. 2002;288(12):1475–83.

21. Stella F, Radanovic M, Balthazar ML, et al. Neuropsychiatric symptoms in the prodromal stages of dementia. Curr Opin Psychiatry. 2014;27(3):230–5.

22. Cummings JL, Mega M, Gray K, Rosenberg-Thomson S, Carusi DA, Gornbein J. The Neuropsychiatric Inventory: comprehensive assessment of psychopathology in dementia. Neurology. 1994;44:2308–14.

23. de Medeiros K, Robert P, Gauthier S, et al. The Neuropsychiatric Inventory-Clinician rating scale (NPI-C): reliability and validity of a revised assessment of neuropsychiatric symptoms in dementia. Int Psychogeriatr. 2010;22:984–94.

24. Reisberg B, Auer SR, Monteiro IM. Behavioral pathology in Alzheimer's disease (BEHAVE-AD) rating scale. Int Psychogeriatr. 1996;8(3):301–8.

25. Cohen-Mansfield J, Marx MS, Rosenthal AS. A description of agitation in a nursing home. J Gerontol. 1989;44:M77–84.

26. McDougall FA, Matthews FE, Kvaal K, et al. Prevalence and symptomatology of depression in older people living in institutions in England and Wales. Age Ageing. 2007;36(5):562–8.

27. Lee HB, Lyketsos CG. Depression in Alzheimer's disease: heterogeneity and related issues. Biol Psychiatry. 2003;54(3):353–62.

28. Beck AT, Ward CH, Mendelson M, Mock J, Erbaugh J. An inventory for measuring depression. Arch Gen Psychiatry. 1961;4:561–71.

29. Hamilton M. Development of a rating scale for primary depressive illness. Br J Soc Clin Psychol. 1967;6:278–96.

30. Montgomery SA, Asberg M. A new depression scale designed to be sensitive to change. Br J Psychiatry. 1979;134(4):382–9.

31. Alexopoulos GS, Abrans RC, Young RC, Shamoian CA. Cornell scale for depression in dementia. Biol Psychiatry. 1998;23:271–84.

32. Yesavage JA, Brink TL, Rose TL, et al. Development and validation of a geriatric depression screening scale: a preliminary report. J Psychiatr Res. 1983;17:37–49.

33. Almeida OP, Almeida SA. Short versions of the geriatric depression scale: a study of their validity for the diagnosis of a major depressive episode according to ICD-10 and DSM-IV. Int J Geriatr Psychiatry. 1999;14(10):858–65.

34. Blank K, Gruman C, Robison JT. Case-finding for depression in elderly people: balancing ease of administration with validity in varied treatment settings. J Gerontol A Biol Sci Med Sci. 2004;59(4):378–84.

35. Robert PH, Mulin E, Malléa P, et al. Apathy diagnosis, assessment, and treatment in Alzheimer's disease. CNS Neurosci Ther. 2010;16:263–71.

36. Robert PH, Clairet S, Benoit M, et al. The Apathy Inventory: assessment of apathy and awareness in Alzheimer's disease, Parkinson's disease and mild cognitive impairment. Int J Geriatr Psychiatry. 2002;17:1099–105.

37. Starkstein SE, Mayberg HS, Preziosi TJ, et al. Reliability, validity and clinical correlate of apathy in Parkinson's disease. J Neuropsychiatry Clin Neurosci. 1992;4:134–9.

38. Marin RS, Biedrzycki RC, Firinciogullari S. Reliability and validity of the Apathy Evaluation Scale. Psychiatry Res. 1991;38:143–62.

39. Reisberg B, Ferris SH, De Leon MJ. The global deterioration scale for assessment of primary degenerate dementia. Am J Psychiatr. 1982;139:1136–9.

40. Ventura J, Green MF, Shaner A, et al. Training and quality assurance with the brief psychiatric rating scale: "the drift buster". Int J Methods Psychiatr Res. 1993;3:221–4.

41. Gupta S, Warner J. Alcohol related dementia: a 21st-century silent epidemic? Br J Psychiatry. 2008;193:351–3.

42. Ewing JA. Detecting alcoholism: the CAGE questionnaire. JAMA. 1984;252(14):1905–7.

43. Saunders JB, Aasland OG, Babor TF, et al. Development of the Alcohol Use Disorders Identification Test (AUDIT): WHO collaborative project on early detection of persons with harmful alcohol consumption—II. Addiction. 1993;88:791–804.

44. Hachinski VC, Iliff LD, Zilkha E, et al. Cerebral blood flow in dementia. Arch Neurol. 1975;32:632–7.

Neurocognitive Assessment

7

Thomas Desmidt, Merryl Butters, Hakan Yakan,
Wolfgang Spiegel, Gustav Kamenski,
and Vincent Camus

Abstract

Neurocognitive disorders, are frequent in old age, they alter activity of daily living and may be complicated by serious psychological or behavioral symptoms. They also may alter the quality of life of family caregivers. In that context, their early detection is a major issue in primary care. Regarding the use of screening tools in primary care, the present chapter review different points: which screening tools should GP use, when, and how? Answering these questions should help improving an appropriate use of screening tools, the early screening being the first step of the healthcare paths.

Key Points

- The diagnosis of a cognitive disorder is often challenging, particularly distinguishing normal age-related cognitive changes from early Alzheimer's disease and related disorders.
- The term "poor memory" means different things to different people, and a comprehensive neurocognitive assessment will enable a clinician to establish the problem.
- There are limitations in the primary care setting in enabling comprehensive neurocognitive assessment.
- There are tools available for dementia screening. However, none of them is recognized as the most suitable for primary care.
- The MMSE is a reliable test to assess the severity of a patient's overall deficit and has the advantage of assessing various cognitive functions in addition to memory, including attention, orientation, language, and visuospatial orientation.

T. Desmidt
CHRU de Tours, Tours, France

M. Butters
Department of Psychiatry, University of Pittsburgh
Medical Center, Pittsburgh, PA, USA

H. Yakan
School of Medicine, University of Akdeniz,
Antalya, Turkey

W. Spiegel · G. Kamenski
Centre for Public Health, Medical University
of Vienna, Vienna, Austria

V. Camus (✉)
CHRU de Tours, Tours, France

Université François Rabelais de Tours
and INSERM U930, Tours, France
e-mail: vincent.camus@univ-tours.fr

C. A. de Mendonça Lima, G. Ivbijaro (eds.), *Primary Care Mental Health in Older People*,
https://doi.org/10.1007/978-3-030-10814-4_7

7.1 Introduction

In primary care, between 10% and 15% of older adult patients have evidence of cognitive impairment [1], and general practitioners (GPs) are increasingly asked to screen, diagnose, and manage patients suffering from Alzheimer's disease and related disorders (AD&RD). Neurocognitive assessment (NA) is now widely used in the screening and diagnostic process of cognitive disorders, and NA is commonly thought in terms of the standardized neuropsychological tests used to measure cognitive abilities and deficits. Indeed, a comprehensive neuropsychological evaluation, usually performed by a neuropsychologist or equivalent, generally requires several hours to complete. However, shorter and more suitable cognitive tests are now available for the primary care setting. Still, GPs are sometimes reluctant to implement NA [2], either because of lack of time, information, and training or because some of them argue that a formal diagnosis of dementia is not necessary for appropriate management of AD&RD for various reasons, including no currently available disease-modifying treatment (although symptomatic treatments are available). However, recent guidelines [3] recommend that GPs have a central role for systematic screening for cognitive impairments, as growing data tend to show that early diagnosis is significantly associated with more advantages than inconveniences in management of Alzheimer's disease patients. In the following chapters, we review the use of NA in primary care and the role of GPs in the screening and diagnostic processes of cognitive disorders, eventually suggesting practical strategies to implement NA in primary care.

7.2 Cognitive Assessment for the Diagnosis of Neurocognitive Disorders

7.2.1 The Diagnosis of Neurocognitive Disorders

The diagnosis of a neurocognitive disorder is often challenging. GPs are increasingly demanded to identify and characterize cognitive impairments, and, in older adults, distinguishing normal age-related cognitive changes from MCI or from early Alzheimer's disease and related disorders (AD&RD, which include not only Alzheimer's disease but also cerebrovascular diseases, Lewy body disease, frontotemporal lobar degeneration, etc.) may be challenging. Moreover, cognitive complaints may also reflect affective and/or anxiety symptoms or disorders, personality traits, as well as an unstable medical condition (including delirium identified as an acute and sudden change in cognition characterized by a disturbance in attention, awareness, and at least one other cognitive domain) or medication side effects. Studies have shown that late or missed diagnoses of dementia are not uncommon in primary care with less than one-third of cases of mild dementia and 38–71% of moderate to severe cases of dementia being formally diagnosed [4]. Diagnostic challenges include the gap between patients' subjective cognitive complaints and the effective presence of vascular disease or a neurodegenerative disorder [5]. Moreover, complaining of cognitive deficits does not necessarily mean an individual has a dementia, and conversely, a neurodegenerative disorder may develop without an individual being aware and thus voicing any cognitive complaints. On the one hand, cognitive deficits may be due to normal aging or other psychiatric disorders (especially depression which may be challenging to identify in older adults), and on the other hand, cognitive deficits due to underlying neurodegenerative disorders may not be identified as such but rather be considered as normal aging. Informal observation alone by a physician is not sufficient to diagnose AD&RD, which is rather a stepwise, iterative process. The diagnostic strategy generally includes a thorough review of the medical history (to look for other potential etiology of impairment); a clinical interview of the patient and relatives (to ascertain change in everyday function); a medical examination; neuroimaging; blood sampling and, in appropriate cases, CSF testing in appropriate cases and, when available; screening for other psychiatric disorders and differential diagnoses; and eventually neurocognitive assessment (NA) as the core of the diagnosis process. Indeed,

DSM5 AD diagnostic criteria are based on the identification of impairments in at least two cognitive domains (major neurocognitive disorder) among learning and memory, language, complex attention, executive function, perceptual-motor cognition, and social cognition—deficits that progressively evolve for several years and are associated with functional deficits (otherwise, the cognitive disorder may be labeled as a mild cognitive impairment—MCI or a mild neurocognitive disorder). NA not only allows "objective" confirmation of cognitive impairment, but it also provides the opportunity to characterize the type of cognitive impairment, i.e., identify the cognitive functions that are impaired (working memory, episodic memory, executive function, language, visuospatial ability, etc.). Moreover, it can provide an assessment of the severity and the progression of cognitive impairment, and stages of AD are usually based on the use of repeated NA (MMSE score, for instance).

In primary care, patients often report having a "poor memory," but the term "memory" has a variety of meanings such as remembering to perform a task in the future ("prospective memory"), finding misplaced objects (which may reflect attention or organizational skills rather than memory per se), and remembering names ("word finding") or recent events or newly acquired information ("episodic memory"). Even a deficit in episodic memory may underlie a range of different memory-related processes, including difficulties with initial learning, or encoding of information or difficulties in efficiently retrieving information, and actual loss or decay of the memory trace, comprehensive NA (beyond a screening instrument such as the MMSE or MoCA) enables one to make such distinctions. For instance, if a patient shows poor performance on initial learning or recall trials of a test, but after a delay, he is still able to recall most of the information he learned, then his deficit is likely one of learning or encoding rather than forgetting. Similarly, comparison of cued recall to free recall permits the identification of patients with inefficient retrieval rather than actual forgetting, and comparison of immediate free recall to delayed free recall allows for the

identification of decay or loss of the memory trace. These types of distinctions are key in the differential diagnostic process.

7.2.2 The Role of GPs in the Diagnostic Process

Most of the current practice guidelines advocate a central role for the GP who is assumed to be able to detect and diagnose AD&RD [6]. A recent study from the United Kingdom found that GPs appeared mostly concordant with recommendations and perform most of the diagnosis process except NAs that are documented in less than 40% of the patients' records [7]! Yet, a recent Dutch study [8] found that a diagnosis made with and without NA leads to different conclusions: a GP's diagnosis of suspected dementia was confirmed by NA less than half of the time, and conversely NA was associated with cognitive impairments in 12.5% of the GPs' diagnosis of no cognitive impairment. The authors conclude that many of the missed diagnoses of cognitive disorders in primary care may be due to the lack of formal NA. They also note that the lack of awareness of cognitive impairments by GPs was particularly seen in older adults whose cognitive impairments were misattributed to normal aging only.

What could be the limitations for GPs to implement NA in their routine practice? Some studies [9] found various reasons: (1) NA is viewed as time-consuming; (2) some GPs confess a lack of skills or familiarity; (3) direct referral to specialists is sometimes preferred; (4) some GPs argue that provision of good care does not require a diagnosis and some believe the diagnosis may even be harmful to the patient, including stigmatization [10]; and finally, some GPs negatively perceive the importance of early diagnosis [11]. With regard to time consumption, a comprehensive NA indeed usually requires several hours, but much shorter cognitive tests, taking less than 10 min to perform, have been developed and been found to be accurate and suitable for diagnosing dementia in most (although not all—screening instruments often miss mild dementia in highly educated or high-functioning individuals) patients seen in the primary care setting. Besides, in some countries, a specific consultation fee for NA has been recognized by healthcare systems. With regard to familiarity and skills, many authors indeed recommend more NA training for physicians [9]. Although instructions are usually very clear for brief NA tools, they still require training and sometimes supervision to avoid basic mistakes in both administration and interpretation of the results. Notably, some websites provide instructional videos for online NA training, designed by experts, and involve real physicians and real patients [12]. With regard to the specialist referral, most of the memory clinics or specialists have long appointment delays, and pre-assessments by GPs may allow for shorter consultations and eventually reduced delays and inappropriate referrals. Finally, with regard to diagnosis disclosure and to the importance of early diagnosis, studies tend to show both potential benefits and inconveniences [13]. However, a large majority of patients and caregivers claim they prefer to be aware of the diagnosis rather than being left in uncertainty [14]. Moreover, recent recommendations tend to highlight the benefits of an early diagnosis [15], including early provision of available treatments but also implementation of care plans and access to services in order to improve symptoms, help maintain independence, improve quality of life, reduce unfavorable dementia-related behaviors, and reduce caregivers' stress. These recommendations argue then for a screening strategy in the general population.

7.3 Cognitive Assessment for the Screening of Neurocognitive Disorders

7.3.1 Is Systematic Cognitive Screening Associated with Benefits?

The US health reform legislation of 2010 has put an emphasis on early detection of cognitive impairments, and US authorities have recommended a systematic screening for persons 65 and older [16]. NA is now a mandated component of both the initial and annual wellness visit, although the implementation is at the discretion of the provider. Nonetheless, the issue of whether or not to employ systematic cognitive assessment in primary care has been controversial, and some authors have argued that screening has been inappropriately urged because of the lack of efficacy evidence [17]. Their argument is based on the questionable performances of the screening tests, as they may be responsible for as much as 23% of false positives when applied to the general population [18]. Besides, many factors apart from dementia influence the tests, including premorbid intelligence, education, ethnicity, sensory impairment, mood, and both medical and neuropsychiatric comorbidities [19]. In addition, it is argued that an earlier diagnosis has not been shown to reduce morbidity/mortality and screening may be associated with harms, including psychological harms from labeling and direct harms associated with diagnostic tests, early treatment, and overtreatment [20]. A survey in the United Kingdom reported that one in five physicians had received complaints from patients who were unhappy about dementia screening [21]. On the contrary, others have argued that screening is the first step toward improving care [22]. Their argument is based on the potential benefits of early detection, as it may optimize medical management of coexisting conditions that could worsen cognition, as it may help in planning for the future when decision-making capacity is still relatively intact, as this is a necessary step for providing education about symptoms and access to services [23]. Moreover, dementia is not merely a cognitive disorder, but it is significantly associated with behavioral and psychological symptoms, and their diagnosis and management are often challenging and particularly burdensome to caregivers. Knowing the diagnosis of dementia certainly optimizes the clinicians' strategies to prevent or manage behavioral and psychological symptoms of dementia which otherwise could be misidentified and taken for late-life schizophrenia or late-life depression, than rather being psychotic symptoms of AD or apathy, for instance. Obviously, other psychiatric conditions require different treatment strategies, and since patients with dementia are highly sensitive to some psychotropic drugs, a misdiagnosis may imply severe side effects. In addition, as dementia is associated with potentially preventable excess morbidity, early identification of AD may be associated with early interventions to reduce complications, and a prospective study found that more than 40% of hospitalized patients older than 70 years had dementia, but only one-half had been previously diagnosed [24].

7.3.2 The Strategy of the Screening Procedure

Based on expert recommendations [3], the Alzheimer's Association acknowledges the benefits of an earlier diagnosis and argues for a population screening strategy and provides a set of recommendations to incorporate NA within the annual wellness visit on the website of the association [12]. An algorithm for NA implementation is provided. It first suggests not to systematically implement NA if neither the patient nor an informant reports symptoms related to cognitive decline. If the patient or an informant reports suspect symptoms or if no informant is available to confirm, or again if the GP has the clinical impression of a beginning AD, it is recommended to conduct a brief structured NA which should include either a Mini-Cog, a General Practitioner Assessment of Cognition (GPCOG), or a Memory Impairment Screen (MIS) as well as an informant assessment, either a Short (IQCODE), an Eight-item Informant Interview to Differentiate Aging and Dementia (AD8), or a GPCOG, informant part. Finally, the conduction of a full dementia evaluation by the GP himself or the referral to a specialist is recommended if scoring reach a certain threshold (Mini-Cog ≤3, patient GPCOG <5, MIS ≤4, Short IQCODE ≥3.38, AD8 ≥2, informant GPCOG ≤3). The website also provides the tests as well as instructional videos designed for primary care setting on how to assess cognition, disclose an AD diagnosis, and recommend follow-up.

Other groups, including the 10/66 Dementia Research Group, have proposed specific dementia screening tests suitable for cross-cultural studies and for low- and middle-income countries [25]. These tests have been found to identify a much higher incidence of dementia in countries such as Cuba, Venezuela, or rural China, compared to classical tests and DSM-IV criteria [26]. To diagnose dementia, the 10/66 group refers to a probabilistic algorithm based on two cognitive tests, an informant interview and the diagnostic output from a structured clinical interview. The cognitive tests are the Community Screening Instrument for Dementia (CSI-D; 32 items, 20 min) [27] and the modified CERAD 10-word list-learning task with delayed recall [28].

7.4 Choosing Cognitive Assessment Tools for use in Primary Care

7.4.1 The Choice of the Tests

There are more than 40 published tests available for dementia screening. According to guidelines, however, no one tool is recognized as the best suited for primary care [3]. The ten most commonly used screening tests have been recently reviewed for their diagnostic performance to detect dementia [29]. The authors found that the MMSE, certainly the most widely applied test for dementia screening, had a good sensitivity (0.81) and specificity (0.89) for dementia screening, but they also found that several tests had similar performances including the Mini-Cog, the ACE-R, and the MoCA. They concluded that several free tests, which possess good performance characteristics and are easily to administer, are available for dementia screening. Nonetheless, they also pointed out that one issue that remains to be addressed is the cutoff score standardization, including cutoff adjustments for premorbid IQ and functioning, as brief screening cannot be sensitive enough to capture mild impairment in high-functioning people, for example. Still, the most common cutoff score for MMSE is 23–24/30, but some studies refer to a score of 25–26/30.

Likewise, the range of the cutoff score of the Mini-Cog test is also variable across studies, although a majority of them refer to a score below 3 for potential dementia.

The MMSE is a reliable test to assess the severity of a patient's overall deficit and has the advantage of assessing various cognitive functions in addition to memory, including attention, orientation, language, and visuospatial orientation. Moreover, it usually takes less than 10 min to perform. However, the MMSE overemphasizes language and underemphasizes visuospatial and executive functions and has become less accessible and useful since its intellectual property rights were transferred to Psychological Assessment Resources in 2001. Shorter and free tests, usually taking less than 5 min, are available like the MIS and the Mini-Cog, but they assess only memory for the first and also visuospatial and executive functions for the latter. Other various tests with a similar duration of the MMSE (less than 10 min) are also suitable for the primary care setting, like the MoCA and the GPCOG. Compared to the MMSE, the MoCA has the advantage of assessing executive functions and has been shown to reliably detect MCI. The GPCOG also assesses executive functions and daily living functions as well. Other longer tests (10–20 min) are available like the ACE-R or informant-rated questionnaires like the IQCODE and the E-Cog. These may be suitable for the primary care setting, when a more complete NA is required.

According to guidelines [3], NA should be performed both for the screening and the diagnosis of dementia. In the primary care setting, a brief evaluation instrument with a high and well-established sensitivity (especially for screening purpose) and specificity (especially for "positive" diagnosis) would be more appropriate, as GPs' consultation is not limited to NA only and extra time is needed for the global assessment of the patient. Guidelines recommend either MMSE or freely available tests, especially Mini-Cog, MIS, and GPCOG. Mini-Cog has the advantage of being very brief as it only requires that the patient learn three words, draw a clock, and then recall the three words. In addition, Mini-Cog has shown very good sensitivity/specificity in meta-analysis. MIS (or the very

similar test of the five-words screening test) is also very brief and focuses on free and cued recall that helps distinguish episodic memory from executive deficit. GPCOG takes about 10 min to perform and has the advantage of assessing a large panel of cognitive functions, like the MMSE or the MoCA, and is composed of an informant part with a validated interview to assess relative's awareness of the patient's cognitive decline. MoCA is also a reliable and free test, available in many languages, and has multiple alternate forms, to minimize practice effect.

7.4.2   The Implementation of Cognitive Assessment Tools in Primary Care

In primary care, NA takes place within the patient's global evaluation and is usually not the first step of the consultation which would rather typically begin with a thorough clinical interview to precisely characterize the patient's complaints (the nature of the symptoms, frequency and severity, onset and course, degree to which they interfere with regular activities), to review his/her medical history as well as interviewing his/her relatives when available. The patient should also be prepared to undergo NA, and explanations regarding the purpose of the test should be provided, along with a brief overview of the procedure and general instructions. In addition, an appropriate context is required for NA. A simple explanation, that the test will help the physician understand whether there is something going on in their brain that requires treatment, is often very helpful. Still, testing may be disturbing for patients with cognitive decline, and patients may sometimes refuse to cooperate. Physicians should reduce their patient's stress, and it may sometimes require delaying the NA, on a latter appointment if necessary. In particular, a patient's emotional instability may lead to inconclusive results. Moreover, a one-on-one assessment (physician and patient alone) may be necessary if, for any reasons, the relatives' interactions are disturbing. Sometimes, on the contrary, relatives' presence improves the emotional stability.

When the patient is ready to perform the NA, the physician should strictly follow the instructions of the test and should be aware of the appropriate scoring. As an example, instructions may require one to repeat several words in a row and only then to ask the patient to recall them and not to say the first word, ask the patient to recall it, then proceed with the second word, etc. Sometimes a limited time or a limited number of attempts are allowed. Sometimes one may score zero on an item even if the patient has refused to respond, for example. Finally, a single assessment may not be sufficient to accurately detect a cognitive disorder, and complementary NA within a follow-up period may be required. Referral to a specialist may be required, especially in case of an atypical presentation and behavioral/psychiatric symptoms or in young patients. If the patient is depressed or has an acute episode of a psychiatric or medical disorder, NA may be inconclusive, and waiting until the patient has recovered is generally required before proceeding to perform the NA.

The National Institute for Health and Care Excellence (NICE) in England has developed a useful dementia care pathway which provides evidence-based recommendations and information on risk factors, early identification, diagnosis, and assessment [30].

7.5 Conclusion

We reviewed here the available options to face the challenges of the practical implementation of NA in primary care. Recommendations are now available for GPs guidance, and NA tools suitable for primary care setting can be used to avoid both the risk of underestimation (impairments falsely attributed to normal aging only, for instance) and overestimation (diagnosis of AD instead of disorders that mimic cognitive impairments, such as psychiatric disorders or medications, for instance) of cognitive disorders. Although some GPs may be reluctant to implement NA in their practice, because it requires training or it's time-consuming, for instance, NA is an invaluable tool for the diagnosis and the

characterization of cognitive disorders. Besides, evidence-based data tend to show that early detection, which usually falls to GPs, generally contributes to a better management of patients with AD&RD and their relatives.

References

1. Callahan CM, Hendrie HC, Tierney WM. Documentation and evaluation of cognitive impairment in elderly primary care patients. Ann Intern Med. 1995;122(6):422–9.
2. Temple RO, Carvalho J, Tremont G. A national survey of physicians' use of and satisfaction with neuropsychological services. Arch Clin Neuropsychol. 2006;21(5):371–82.
3. Cordell CB, Borson S, Boustani M, Chodosh J, Reuben D, Verghese J, et al. Alzheimer's association recommendations for operationalizing the detection of cognitive impairment during the Medicare Annual Wellness Visit in a primary care setting. Alzheimers Dement. 2013;9(2):141–50.
4. Bradford A, Kunik ME, Schulz P, Williams SP, Singh H. Missed and delayed diagnosis of dementia in primary care: prevalence and contributing factors. Alzheimer Dis Assoc Disord. 2009;23(4):306–14.
5. Purser JL, Fillenbaum GG, Wallace RB. Memory complaint is not necessary for diagnosis of mild cognitive impairment and does not predict 10-year trajectories of functional disability, word recall, or short portable mental status questionnaire limitations. J Am Geriatr Soc. 2006;54(2):335–8.
6. Geldmacher DS, Kerwin DR. Practical diagnosis and management of dementia due to Alzheimer's disease in the primary care setting: an evidence-based approach. Prim Care Companion CNS Disord. 2013;15(4):pii: PCC.12r01474.
7. Wilcock J, Jain P, Griffin M, Thuné-Boyle I, Lefford F, Rapp D, et al. Diagnosis and management of dementia in family practice. Aging Ment Health. 2016;20(4):362–9.
8. van den Dungen P, Moll van Charante EP, van de Ven PM, Foppes G, van Campen JPCM, van Marwijk HWJ, et al. Dutch family physicians' awareness of cognitive impairment among the elderly. BMC Geriatr. 2015;15:105.
9. Kaduszkiewicz H, Wiese B, van den Bussche H. Self-reported competence, attitude and approach of physicians towards patients with dementia in ambulatory care: results of a postal survey. BMC Health Serv Res. 2008;8:54.
10. Vernooij-Dassen MJFJ, Moniz-Cook ED, Woods RT, De Lepeleire J, Leuschner A, Zanetti O, et al. Factors affecting timely recognition and diagnosis of dementia across Europe: from awareness to stigma. Int J Geriatr Psychiatry. 2005;20(4):377–86.

11. Turner S, Iliffe S, Downs M, Wilcock J, Bryans M, Levin E, et al. General practitioners' knowledge, confidence and attitudes in the diagnosis and management of dementia. Age Ageing. 2004;33(5):461–7.

12. Cognitive Tests and Patient Assessment. Alzheimer's Association. Available from: http://www.alz.org/health-care-professionals/cognitive-tests-patient-assessment.asp#alzheimers_screening.

13. U.S. Preventive Services Task Force. Screening for cognitive impairment in older adults: recommendation statement. Am Fam Physician 2015;91(6):Online.

14. Value of Knowing - Research - Alzheimer Europe. Available from: http://www.alzheimer-europe.org/Research/Value-of-Knowing.

15. Borson S, Frank L, Bayley PJ, Boustani M, Dean M, Lin P-J, et al. Improving dementia care: the role of screening and detection of cognitive impairment. Alzheimers Dement. 2013;9(2):151–9.

16. Preventive visit and yearly wellness exams. Medicare.gov. Available from: https://www.medicare.gov/coverage/preventive-visit-and-yearly-wellness-exams.html.

17. Le Couteur DG, Brayne C. Should family physicians routinely screen patients for cognitive impairment? No: screening has been inappropriately urged despite absence of evidence. Am Fam Physician. 2014;89(11):864–5.

18. Mitchell AJ, Meader N, Pentzek M. Clinical recognition of dementia and cognitive impairment in primary care: a meta-analysis of physician accuracy. Acta Psychiatr Scand. 2011;124(3):165–83.

19. Fox C, Lafortune L, Boustani M, Dening T, Rait G, Brayne C. Screening for dementia--is it a no brainer? Int J Clin Pract. 2013;67(11):1076–80.

20. Procedure Manual - US Preventive Services Task Force. Available from: http://www.uspreventiveservicestaskforce.org/Page/Name/procedure-manual.

21. Stirling A. GPs hit by widespread complaints from patients "unhappy" over dementia screening. Pulse Today. Available from: http://www.pulsetoday.co.uk/clinical/more-clinical-areas/elderly-care/gps-hit-by-widespread-complaints-from-patients-unhappy-over-dementia-screening/20005138.fullarticle.

22. McCarten JR, Borson S. Should family physicians routinely screen patients for cognitive impairment? Yes: screening is the first step toward improving care. Am Fam Physician. 2014;89(11):861–2.

23. Vickrey BG, Mittman BS, Connor KI, Pearson ML, Della Penna RD, Ganiats TG, et al. The effect of a disease management intervention on quality and outcomes of dementia care: a randomized, controlled trial. Ann Intern Med. 2006;145(10):713–26.

24. Sampson EL, Blanchard MR, Jones L, Tookman A, King M. Dementia in the acute hospital: prospective cohort study of prevalence and mortality. Br J Psychiatry J Ment Sci. 2009;195(1):61–6.

25. 10/66 Dementia Research Group. https://www.alz.co.uk/1066/.

26. Prince M, Acosta D, Ferri CP, Guerra M, Huang Y, Llibre Rodriguez JJ, et al. Dementia incidence and mortality in middle-income countries, and associations with indicators of cognitive reserve: a 10/66 Dementia Research Group population-based cohort study. Lancet. 2012;380(9836):50–8.

27. Hall KS, Gao S, Emsley CL, Ogunniyi AO, Morgan O, Hendrie HC. Community screening interview for dementia (CSI "D"); performance in five disparate study sites. Int J Geriatr Psychiatry. 2000;15(6):521–31.

28. Fillenbaum GG, van Belle G, Morris JC, Mohs RC, Mirra SS, Davis PC, et al. Consortium to establish a registry for Alzheimer's disease (CERAD): the first twenty years. Alzheimers Dement. 2008;4(2):96–109.

29. Tsoi KKF, Chan JYC, Hirai HW, Wong SYS, Kwok TCY. Cognitive tests to detect dementia: a systematic review and meta-analysis. JAMA Intern Med. 2015;175(9):1450–8.

30. NICE Dementia: supporting people with dementia and their carers in health and social care. Clinical Guidance [CG42]. Sept 2016.

Promoting Dignity in the Care of the Older Adult

8

Gabriel Ivbijaro, Lucja Kolkiewicz, David Goldberg, Claire Brooks, and Yaccub Enum

Abstract

This chapter considers the importance of dignity in the care of older people. It starts with a case vignette to illustrate that dignity is not simply a medical input but a holistic approach to life. It considers the definition of dignity and how this is related to all aspects of care in older people with special reference to clinical syndromes including frailty and dementia and the need for evidence-based care delivery to avoid violations of an individual's dignity. Technology has an increasing role to play in care delivery to older adults, and this is considered through the lens of dignity. Recommendations include:

G. Ivbijaro (✉)
NOVA University, Lisbon, Portugal

Waltham Forest Community and Family Health Services, London, UK

L. Kolkiewicz
NOVA University, Lisbon, Portugal

East London NHS Foundation Trust, London, UK

D. Goldberg
King's College, London, UK

C. Brooks
ModelPeople Inc. Global Insights, Chicago, IL, USA

Y. Enum
Public Health Department, London Borough of Waltham Forest, London, UK

East London NHS Foundation Trust, London, UK

- Maintaining older adults' independence as much as possible should always be at the centre of their care plans. This can be facilitated by giving older adults choice and involving them and their carers in developing and implementing care plans.
- For frail older adults and those with dementia, for example, caregivers should always balance the need for safety with the older adult's independence and autonomy.
- All staff caring for older adults must be suitably trained and supported to maintain dignity in older adults. They must be aware of the older adult's cultural background and respect any cultural sensitivity, demonstrating empathy, respect and kindness while caring for the older adult.
- Older adults are more likely to be receiving care from different agencies due to comorbidities, personal care and social needs. Collaborative care is a good model to ensure that all the agencies/caregivers work together with the older adult at the centre.
- Services that provide care for older adults such as care homes, sheltered housing and hospitals should embrace and invest in new technology to help enhance older adults' independence and quality of life.
- Social isolation is a risk factor for poor mental health, which can affect older adults' self-esteem. Health and social care commissioners should ensure there are facilities in place to

identify and help older adults at risk of social isolation such as befriending schemes and day centres.

Key Points

- Although everybody is entitled to be cared for with dignity, irrespective of age, ethnicity and gender, it is especially important to address the many older people do not feel valued
- Dignity should be central to the development of all health and social care packages provided to the older adult population.
- Older adults should participate in all decisions made to support their health and social care.
- There is a need for a good framework for providing feedback from patients and carers on the care environment such as PLACE used in the UK.
- The use of robots and other assistive technologies to support dignity and independence in older adults should be promoted.
- Providing a range of sheltered living maximises independence.
- More effective transitions of care can prevent homelessness in older adults and should include temporary shelter and assistance while their healthcare and social needs are assessed.

8.1 Introduction

Mr Brown is a 72-year-old gentleman who has become progressively blind as a result of complications of glaucoma and now resides in sheltered accommodation for older adults. Prior to moving into sheltered housing, he was a keen gardener and a cyclist and enjoyed outdoor activities.

During a routine consultation, Mr Brown complained of feeling lonely and hopeless and

said that he wished that he could cycle again. He also told his family doctor that he gained value and self-worth from helping others and found this more difficult to do because of his failing eyesight. He and his family doctor considered possibilities for addressing his loneliness and they came up with the idea of riding tandem with another person who had good eyesight.

On his return to the sheltered housing complex, Mr Brown discussed this idea with the sheltered housing manager who paired him up with another lonely gentleman who was 80 years old and had a diagnosis of diabetes. The two gentlemen were referred to a sports therapist who supported them to buy a tandem bicycle, and they now safely ride around the area together, the 80-year-old gentlemen with good eyesight in front and the 72-year-old gentleman with failing eyesight behind.

When reviewed in their family practice appointment 3 months later, they both expressed how happy they were to be able to help one another, to have the freedom to ride and explore and to feel valued again. They each felt their dignity had been reinstated.

Dignity in mental health and social care is very important especially in older adults. If dignity in care is maintained, it protects against stigma and discrimination, elder abuse and neglect and supports the legal framework to support older adults who may have lost their autonomy as a result of mental illness and other co-morbidities associated with the older adult population [1–3].

Many people are living longer with co-morbidity, dementia and other progressive illnesses [4, 5]. The quality of care provided is important to the older adult population, their families and carers, and dignity in the care of the older adult is very important [6, 7].

Increased longevity is the result of a significant decline in mortality rates across the whole age spectrum, and nations have often not taken this into account in their long-term planning. As a result the older adult population face many more challenges [5, 8].

There is a lot said about dignity in health by health providers, and in health policy in the experience of care described by many older patients, this often does not go beyond rhetoric. Many individuals and reports continue to highlight age discrimination and poor access to health delivery and social care in the older age group [9, 10].

8.2 Definition

The concept of dignity is now central to many policies worldwide to support the delivery of care, but there is often no single agreed definition of dignity in care. Despite this people are usually able to recognise when an individual's dignity is violated and also when dignity in care is enhanced. We therefore require the concept to be clarified into its component parts so that caregivers and care receivers can have a shared understanding of what is being referred to when we talk about dignity in health [11–13].

A good working definition of dignity is that it refers to being of value or having worth [9]. If healthcare professionals can keep this in mind during every encounter with an older adult, then dignity is likely to be maintained and enhanced. Dignity is often included in the code of practice for many professional groups, including nurses [14] and doctors [15], and is included in the Declaration of Human Rights [16].

Research has shown that a sense of personal dignity flows from two components: one internal, "how I see myself", and one external, "how others see me" [17]. These two dimensions reinforce each other. Therefore, it's essential for healthcare professionals to approach an older adult empathetically—*as an individual human being*—while also recognising his or her specific age-related physical and mental health needs. The temptation to stereotype older adults into a single homogenous group takes away their individuality, contributes to the increased stigma associated with older age and increases the risk of denying them their dignity.

8.3 Frailty

An important area in which dignity in care is important is in the management of frail older adults. Frailty is highly prevalent with increasing age and leads to increased dependency, institutionalisation and falls. Traditionally it was thought that the onset of frailty was irreversible resulting in stigma, loss of hope and therefore loss of dignity [18, 19].

Recent evidence has provided hope in the field of frailty and recommends that adults with frailty should be identified early using a validated screening tool. Individuals who are identified as suffering from frailty should be included in a physical activity training programme that includes a resistance training component and investigated for other causes of fatigue and weight loss [20].

In the same way that the management of secondary causes of frailty and fatigue is important in promoting dignity in the older adult, the management of overmedication is also very important. Many older adults in care homes and other types of supported accommodation experience overmedication, and the prevalence can be up to one half of the patients in some care homes [21]. Managing polypharmacy is essential because it will help to reduce falls, improve mobility and decrease multiple medication interactions that lead to side effects and poorer quality of life.

STOPPFrail (Screening Tool of Older Persons Prescription in Frail adults with limited life expectancy) can be used to identify prescribed medication that can be stopped safely, particularly for those older adults who are in end-stage physiological pathological conditions, with a poor 1-year survival prognosis, with severe cognitive and functional impairment and for symptom control rather than prevention of disease progression [22].

The STOPPFrail criteria have been generated using Delphi methodology and can be used by appropriately trained clinicians for medication review, and the instrument is not constrained by copyright as long as it is not used for a commercial purpose.

It highlights four key principles to be taken into account in the review and reduction of medication in adults over the age of 65 years. The four principles that need to be considered are:

(a) Whether the individual have end-stage irreversible pathology
(b) Whether the individual have a poor prognosis for 1-year survival
(c) Whether the individual suffers from severe functional and/or cognitive impairment
(d) Whether symptom control is the priority rather than prevention of disease progression

Keeping these principles in mind during the assessment of the older adult enables the clinician, the patient and their family member/carer to come to a shared understanding and the STOPPFrail screenign tool can support this and has been shown to be very reliable [23]. STOPPFrail has also been used in the management of palliative care in frailty [24].

8.4 Eliminating Unnecessary Medication

Dignity is also supported by offering evidence-based treatment interventions because this reduces unnecessary treatment, including unnecessary medication. The most common medications associated with preventable drug-related admissions to hospital or adverse drug reactions and over-treatment in older adults are antiplatelets (including aspirin when used as an antiplatelet), diuretics, non-steroidal anti-inflammatories (NSAIDs), anticoagulants, opioid analgesics, beta blockers, drugs affecting the renin-angiotensin system, drugs used in diabetes, positive inotropes, corticosteroids, anti-depressants, calcium channel blockers, anti-epileptics and nitrates. Patients who are prescribed these medications need to be thoroughly reviewed to ensure that the medication is (a) required and (b) prescribed in the right dose for the right indication [25, 26].

Treating individuals and teams should become familiar with the most up-to-date guidelines and resources available in the local area in order to provide the best available treatment for the patients.

8.5 Dementia

In addition to the treatment interventions offered, an important goal in the care of dementia is supporting quality of life, dignity and comfort, and this should remain central to treatment and care delivery. Meaningful attention should be paid to the activities of daily living, the choice of treatments offered and the involvement and engagement of the individual and their family to enhance and maintain the individual's dignity [27].

Intervention programme that includes the individual's family network has also been found to be helpful. Family caregiver's health needs should also be considered, because positive health in family caregivers has been found to improve the well-being of the person with dementia. This promotes dignity because it delays the time it takes for people with dementia to be cared for in supported institutional settings [28].

Collaboration with other caregivers, community groups and families is essential, because no one individual or organisation will have all the necessary resources to provide the holistic care that people with dementia and their families require and are entitled to [29, 30].

8.6 Technological Innovation and Robots

The use of technology to support the older adult to maintain independence and personal dignity needs to be accelerated [31]. Simple technology to support independence is already available in some communities and includes telephones and alarm systems.

The proportion of older adults in the population is expected to rise significantly by 2020, and with a reduction in or shortage of caregivers, there is a need to consider the role of assistive robots and technologies that will support patients to continue to live as independently as possible and support some of their daily needs to be met [32, 33].

Robots can assist the older adult and their carer's in a number of ways including daily household and personal care tasks, the monitoring of behaviour and health and the provision of companionship [33–36].

The use of robots to support dignity and independence of the older adult has a lot of potential but ethical issues and concerns have been raised. These include the reduction of human contact resulting in social isolation and the possibility of deception of the older adult with cognitive difficulties [31, 37].

Robotic pets have been found to be effective in care homes, and their use is associated in an improvement in resident's physiological functions, including improved urinary function and improved efficiency in vital organs [38]. Robotic pets can promote relaxation and motivation in care home residents and have social effects such as stimulation of communication among residents and caregivers, similar to live animals [39, 40].

For robots to be deployed properly as part of a personalised care package to support dignity, individuals and their carers should be included in the decision-making about what kind of a robot is necessary and what the function of that robot will be while acknowledging that robots are not a replacement for human contact [41].

There are many robots and the list continues to grow and, with improvements, some are being retired and new ones are coming onto the market. Examples of robot used for therapeutic or assistive purposes, or with a dual assistive and therapeutic function, include Paro, a baby harp seal robot with moving parts covered with pure white fur. It is equipped with four primary senses: visual (light sensor), audio (determination of sound source direction and speech recognition), balance and tactile senses [38]. iCAT is another example, made of hard plastic with a catlike appearance [42]. One of the most studied robots so far is Pearl, a mobile robot that provides functional care by helping older adults to navigate through nursing facilities [43].

8.7 Sheltered Housing, Residential and Nursing Care Homes and Hospitals

Although, in general, older adults prefer to remain at home, it is inevitable that some will require care in sheltered, residential and nursing care homes. In these circumstances, research shows that the older adult residents want a well-trained workforce sensitive to their need that provides care in a safe and clean place. They want reliable key workers and a positive attitude among staff [7].

Similarly research shows that many older adults prefer to die at home, but this is not possible in many cases. If an older adult is to die in any supported setting other than their own home, it is important for them and their family to be involved in planning this. Some of the things that older adults find important to prepare for in these circumstances are pain control, good management of any symptoms that they are experiencing, the avoidance of inappropriate prolongation of life, feeling that they still have control as an individual and closeness to loved ones. Religious, spiritual and cultural values also need to be considered and incorporated into care planning [44–46].

Older adult residential and nursing home residents want to participate in decisions about their own care, the choice of where they live and their daily routine, including what to wear. Older adult residents want good security wherever they are and having someone to talk to [7].

When the factors that contribute to dignity in supported accommodation settings were explored, the themes that emerged were those of independence, autonomy, choice, ability to control your destiny and privacy. More specifically, older adults living in such settings wanted to be recognised as individuals that demand and expect respect, the opportunity to talk to other people and the maintenance of good physical appearance [8]. Some studies have suggested that bringing in pieces of their own furniture and household belongings including photographs supports the recognition of individuality [7, 47].

It is therefore important that those who commission and deliver any kind of supported accommodation to the older adult take this into account if they are to support the dignity of their residents.

One of the greatest challenges to care delivery in sheltered, residential and nursing care settings is that of balancing risk management with privacy while supporting maximum independence. There need to be environmental, relational and procedural structures in place to ensure that the older adult has as much independence and privacy as possible while reducing risk because many people's greatest fear when they enter such accommodation is loss of independence [48].

It has been suggested that there should be a different contracting model for people who are placed in long-term care. In Missouri, USA, a change of language from patients to tenants, and an opportunity for people to remain in the same location as their needs increase to support independence, has been provided. In this model individuals are treated as tenants whatever their level of care need [49].

For a model such as this to work requires a clear and specific contract that includes appropriate quality markers that are regularly monitored. Quality indicators that have been considered relevant include injuries, falls, behavioural symptoms, polypharmacy, bladder and bowel incontinence, prevalence of dehydration and incidence of decline in activities of daily living (ADL) skills. It is essential for the quality markers to be codesigned with residents, carers and those who commission and pay for the services. This requires underpinning by regular inspections with the results published and made available to residents, carers and the general public so that confidence in the system can be maintained and areas for improvement targeted.

Supported accommodation of all types should continue to empower residents through providing the opportunity and supporting an independent residents' council so that resident's views can be actively considered and change and improvement plans taken forward [50].

Some patients will require hospital treatment and care. Patients are more vulnerable to loss of dignity in such settings, and staff should be aware that their interventions can help to promote patient dignity or lead to loss of patient dignity. Hospital managers need to play a role in ensuring that the institution promotes dignity and that staff have the capabilities to provide dignity in care. Ward design can either support privacy, autonomy and dignity or make patients more vulnerable by making it harder to promote individuality [51, 52].

When an older adult is admitted to an inpatient hospital ward, it is important to include them in all the decision-making, and the care plan should contain a section on maintaining dignity so that this can be at the forefront of everybody's mind. Issues that should regularly be considered include personal and oral hygiene, ability to interact and communicate, good nutrition and hydration, opportunity to exercise, privacy and the quality of staff patient interactions [53–56].

Patient-Led Assessments of the Care Environment (PLACE) is an example of good practice in providing institutions with the motivation for improvement by providing clear messages to hospital managers directly from patients and carers.

PLACE was introduced in the UK National Health Service (NHS) in 2013. Organisations train patients and carers to be assessors (patient assessors) to go into hospitals as part of a team to assess how the environment supports the provision of clinical care. PLACE training materials and assessment forms are freely available on the Internet [57]. All hospitals in the public and private sector should engage in patient-led activity with feedback provided to hospital management, patient groups and the local public.

In all supported care settings, good staff communication skills are fundamental to the promotion of dignity in older adults, and this is a skill that can be taught. Patients should routinely be asked about how they would like to be addressed, and there should be meaningful interactions between those who care for the older adult and the older adult being cared for in order to avoid social isolation [58].

8.8 Homelessness

The proportion of older adults among the homeless population is rising sharply, and likely to continue to do so, influenced by demographic, economic and social trends in western societies. For example, in the UK, people over 60 are now more than twice as likely to be homeless than in 2009 [59]. In the USA, late baby boomers, born in 1954–1964, have a higher risk of homelessness than other age cohorts [60], and one third of the chronic homeless are aged 50 years old or over, a number which are likely even higher today [61].

Homelessness goes hand in hand with physical and mental health issues. The homeless older adults are more likely than their housed peers to have chronic conditions, including mental health issues, and face substantial barriers to accessing healthcare [62]. Homeless individuals also suffer from geriatric conditions decades earlier than housed older adults, including cognitive or visual impairment, incontinence and frailty [63].

The homeless older adults often fall between the cracks of government provision because they are not elderly enough to meet the criteria for the type of social programmes they require or face delays and lack of coordination in the transition of care following a hospital admission. Research shows that stigma is endemic in the way the homeless older adult is treated in hospital and on discharge back onto the streets, with little support [64].

Not only are the homeless older adults unable to age with dignity on the harsh streets; they also have a four times higher mortality rate compared to housed older adult [65]. Preventing homelessness is essential to promote dignity in the care of older individuals and ensure equality of health and life expectancy.

8.9 What Patients Want

Many older adults want the same as everybody else in the general population. They want services that are reliable and dependable, easy to access and with competent staff that are sensitive and recognise diversity. When they have health needs, older adult people like to have their needs managed in a collaborative way [7]. This requires a supportive community. Older adult people want to be close to their families if they need to receive treatment in hospital. We need innovation for this to be achieved, taking the patients' view into account, and may have to adapt and use a new technology in an ethical way.

The elderly, as much as the general population, want healthcare professionals to care for them with empathy, seeing the patient as an individual and developing a human connection [66]. There is growing evidence that clinical empathy—the medical professional's cognitive understanding of patients' emotions combined with emotional attunement—directly enhances therapeutic efficacy [67]. Increasingly, the teaching and spreading of empathetic behaviour must be a priority among healthcare professionals caring for the elderly [68].

8.10 Research Opportunities

Dignity is a complex issue and there are areas for futher research including the ethical implications for use of technology including robots and theri acceptability to older adults.

8.11 Recommendations

- Maintaining older adults' independence as much as possible should always be at the centre of their care plans. This can be facilitated by giving older adults choice and involving them and their carers in developing and implementing care plans.
- For frail older adults and those with dementia, for example, caregivers should always balance the need for safety with the older adult's independence and autonomy.
- All staff caring for older adults must be suitably trained and supported to maintain dignity in older adults. They must be aware of the

older adult's cultural background and respect any cultural sensitivity, demonstrating empathy, respect and kindness while caring for the older adult.

- Older adults are more likely to be receiving care from different agencies due to comorbidities, personal care and social needs. Collaborative care is a good model to ensure that all the agencies/caregivers work together with the older adult at the centre.
- Services that provide care for older adults such as care homes, sheltered housing and hospitals should embrace and invest in new technology to help enhance older adults' independence and quality of life.
- Social isolation is a risk factor for poor mental health, which can affect older adults' self-esteem. Health and social care commissioners should ensure there are facilities in place to identify and help older adults at risk of social isolation such as befriending schemes and day centres.
- All healthcare providers should work with older adults, their carers and voluntary sector organisations to ensure that whenever it is appropriate, older adults are cared for in their homes or in the community with the right package of care, instead of in hospital.

References

1. Saxena S, Hanna F. Dignity—a fundamental principle of mental health care. Indian J Med Res. 2015;142(4):355–8.
2. UN General Assembly. International covenant on economic, social and cultural rights. United Nations Treaty Series, vol. 933; 1966. p. 3.
3. WHO. WHO quality rights tool kit to assess and improve quality and human rights in mental health and social care facilities. Geneva: WHO; 2012.
4. Ferri CP, Prince M, Brayne C, Brodaty H, Fratiglioni L, Ganguli M, Hall K, Hasegawa K, Hendrie H, Huang Y, Jorm A, Mathers C, Menezes PR, Rimmer E, Scafuzca M. Alzheimer's disease international. Global prevalence of dementia: a Delphi consensus study. Lancet. 2005;366(9503):2112–7. https://doi.org/10.1016/S0140-6736(05)67889-0.
5. Jacobzone S. Ageing and care for frail older adult persons. An overview of international perspectives,

6. Lothian K, Philip I. Maintaining the dignity and autonomy of older people in the healthcare setting. BMJ. 2001;322:668–70.
7. Levenson R, Jeyasingham M, Joule N. Looking forward to care in old age. Care services inquiry working paper. London: Kings Fund; 2005.
8. Hall S, Dodd RH, Higginson IJ. Maintaining dignity for residents of care homes: a qualitative study of the views of care home staff, community nurses, residents and their families. Geriatr Nurs. 2014;35:55–60. https://doi.org/10.1016/j.gerinurse.2013.10.012.
9. Gallagher A, Li S, Wainwright P, Jones IR, Lee D. Dignity in the care of older people—a review of the theoretical and empirical literature. BMC Nurs. 2008;7:11. https://doi.org/10.1186/1472-6955-7-11.
10. Picker Institute Europe. Improving patients' experience: sharing good care no. 11 stroke care: the National Picture. Oxford: Picker Institute Europe; 2005.
11. Nordenfelt L. Dignity in the care of the older adult. Med Health Care Philos. 2003;6:103–10.
12. Department of Health. A new ambition for old age. London: Department of Health; 2006.
13. Gallagher A. Editorial: what do we know about dignity in care? Nurs Ethics. 2011;18(4):471–3.
14. International Council of Nurses. The ICN code of practice for nurses. Geneva: ICN; 2012.
15. World Medical Association. World Medical Association International Code of Medical Ethics. Adopted by the 3 General Assembly of the World Medical Association, London, England, October 1949 and amended by the 22 World Medical Assembly, Sydney, Australia, August 1968 and the 35 World Medical Assembly, Venice, Italy, October 1983 and the 57 WMA General Assembly, Pilanesberg, South Africa, October 2006. https://www.wma.net/policies-post/wma-international-code-of-medical-ethics/. Accessed 10 July 2018.
16. UN General Assembly. Universal Declaration of Human Rights. Paris: 10 December 1948, 217 A (III). http://www.refworld.org/docid/3ae6b3712c.html. Accessed 10 July 2018.
17. Mann J. Dignity and health: the UDHR's revolutionary first article. Health Hum Rights. 1998;3(2):30–8.
18. Freid LP, Tangen CM, Walston J, Newman AB, Hirsch C, Gottdiener J, Seeman T, Tracy R, Kop WJ, Burke G, McBurnie MA, Cardiovascular Health Study. Frailty in older adults: evidence for a phenotype. J Gerontol. 2001;56A(3):M146–56.
19. Sternberg SA, Schwartz AW, Karunananthan S, Bergman H, Clarfield AM. The identification of frailty: a systematic literature review. J Am Geriatr Soc. 2011;59(11):2129–38. https://doi.org/10.1111/j.1532-5415.2011.03597.x.
20. Dent E, Lien C, Lim WS, Wong WC, Wong CH, Ng TP, Woo J, Dong B, de la Vega S, Poi PJH, Kamaruzzamana SBB, Won C, Chen L-K, Rockwood K, Arai H, Rodriguez-Manas L, Cao L, Cesari M,

Cahn P, Leung E, Landi F, Fried LP, Morley JE, Vellas B, Flicker L. The Asia-Pacific clinical practice guidelines for the management of frailty. J Am Med Dir Assoc. 2017;18:564–75.

21. Onder G, Liperoti R, Fialova D, Topinkova E, Tosato M, Danese P, Gallo PF, Carpenter I, Finne-Soveri H, Gindin J, Bernabei R, Landi F, SHELTER Project. Polypharmacy in nursing home in Europe: results from the SHELTER study. Send to J Gerontol A Biol Sci Med Sci. 2012;67(6):698–704. https://doi.org/10.1093/Gerona/glr233.

22. Lavan AH, Gallagher P, Parsons C, O'Mahoney D. STOPPFrail (Screening Tool of Older Persons Prescription in Frail adults with limited life expectancy): consensus validation. Age Ageing. 2017;46:600–7. https://doi.org/10.1093/ageing/afx005.

23. Lavan AH, Gallagher P, O'Mahoney D. Inter-rater reliability of STOPPFrail (Screening Tool of Older Persons Prescriptions in Frail adults with limited life expectancy) criteria amongst 12 physicians. Eur J Clin Pharmacol. 2018;74(3):331–8. https://doi.org/10.1007/s00228-017-2376-2. Epub 2017 Nov 20

24. Sevilla-Sánchez D, Molist-Brunet N, Espaulella-Panicot J, González-Bueno J, Solà-Bonada N, Amblàs-Novellas J, Codina-Jané C. Potentially inappropriate medication in palliative care patients according to STOPP-Frail criteria. Eur Geriatr Med. 2018;9(4):543–50.

25. Zhang M, D'Arcy C, Price SD, Sanfilippo FM, Preen DB, Bulsara MK. Co-morbidity and repeat admissions to hospital for adverse drug reactions. BMJ. 2009;338:a2752. https://doi.org/10.1136/bmj.a2752.

26. Cresswell KM, Fernando B, McKinstry B, Sheikh A. Adverse drug events in the elderly. Br Med Bull. 2007;83:259–74. https://doi.org/10.1093/bmb/ldm016.

27. Volicer L. Goals of care in advanced dementia: quality of life, dignity and comfort. J Nutr Health Aging. 2007;11(6):481.

28. Smits CHM, de Lange J, Dröes R-M, Meiland F, Vernooij-Dassen M, Pot AM. Effects of combined intervention programmes for people with dementia living at home and their caregivers: a systematic review. Int J Geriatr Psychiatry. 2007;22:1181–93. https://doi.org/10.1002/gps.1805.

29. Funk M, Ivbijaro G, editors. Integrating mental health into primary care: a global perspective. Geneva/London: WHO/Wonca; 2008.

30. Ngo J, Holroyd-Leduc JM. Systematic review of recent dementia practice guidelines. Age Ageing. 2015;44:25–33. https://doi.org/10.1093/ageing/afu143.

31. Sharkey A, Sharkey N. Granny and the robots: ethical issues in robot care for the older adult. Ethics Inf Technol. 2012;14:27–40. https://doi.org/10.1007/s10676-010-9234-6.

32. Lesnoff-Caravaglia G. Gerontechnology: growing old in a technological society. Springfield, IL: Charles C Thomas; 2007.

33. Frennert S, Östlund B, Eftring H. Would granny let an assistive robot into her home? In: Ge SS, Khatib O, Cabibihan JJ, Simmons R, Williams MA, editors. Social robotics. ICSR 2012. Lecture notes in computer science, vol. 7621. Berlin: Springer; 2012.

34. Allen C, Wallach W, Smit I. Why machine ethics? IEEE Intell Syst. 2006;21(4):12–7.

35. Anderson M, Andeerson SL, Armen C. An approach to computing ethics. IEEE Intell Syst. 2006;21(4):56–63.

36. Banks MR, Banks WA. The effects of group and individual animal assisted therapy on loneliness in residents of long-term care facilities. Anthrozoös. 2005;18:396–408.

37. Banks MR, Willoughby LM, Banks WA. Animal-assisted therapy and loneliness in nursing homes: use of robotic versus living dogs. J Am Med Dir Assoc. 2008;9:173–7.

38. Wada K, Shibata T. Living with seal robots – its sociopsychological and psychological influences on the older adult at a care home. IEEE Trans Robot. 2007;23(5):972–80.

39. Baum MM, Bergstom N, Langston NF, Thoma L. Physiological effects of human/companion animal bonding. Nurs Res. 1984;33(3):126–9.

40. Gammonley J, Yates J. Pet projects animal assisted therapy in nursing homes. J Gerontol Nurs. 1991;17(1):12–5.

41. Mordoch E, Osterreicher A, Guse L, Roger K, Thompson G. Use of social commitment robots in the care of older adult people with dementia. Maturitas. 2013;74:14–20. https://doi.org/10.1016/j.maturitas.2012.10.015.

42. Van Breemen A, Yan X, Meerbeek B. iCAT: an animated user-interface robot with personality. Proceedings of the fourth international joint conference on autonomous agents and multiagent systems; 2005. p. 143–4.

43. Pineau J, Montemerlo M, Pollack M, Roy N, Thrun S. Towards robotic assistants in nursing homes: challenges and results. Robot Auton Syst. 2003;42(3-4):271–81. https://doi.org/10.1016/S0921-8890(02)00381-0.

44. Searight HR, Gafford J. Cultural diversity at the end of life: issues and guidelines for family physicians. Am Fam Physician. 2005;71(3):515–22.

45. Prendergast TJ, Claessens MT, Luce JM. A national survey of end-of-life care for critically ill patients. Am J Respir Crit Care Med. 1998;158:1163–7.

46. Dy SM, Shurarman LR, Lorenz KA, Mularski RA, Lynn J. A systematic review of satisfaction with care at the end of life. J Am Geriatr Soc. 2008;56(1):124–9. Epub 2007 Nov 20. https://doi.org/10.1111/j.1532-5415.2007.01507.x.

47. Anttonen A, Haïkïö L. Care 'going market': Finnish older adult-care policies in transition. Nord J Soc Res. 2011;2:70–90. https://doi.org/10.15845/njsr.v2i0.111.

48. Bland R. Independence, privacy and risk: two contrasting approaches to residential care for older people. Ageing Soc. 1999;19:539–60.

49. Marek KD, Rantz MJ. Aging in place: a new model for long term care. Nurs Adm Q. 2000;24(3):1–11.

50. Hendriks N, Truyen F, Duval E. Designing with dementia: guidelines for participatory design together with persons with dementia. In: IFIP conference on human-computer interaction. Berlin: Springer; 2013. p. 649–66.

51. Baillie L. Patient dignity in an acute hospital setting: a case study. Int J Nurs Stud. 2009;46:23–37.

52. Walsh K, Kwanko I. Nurses' and patients' perceptions of dignity. Int J Nurs Pract. 2002;8(3):143–51.

53. Van der Geest S. The toilet: dignity, privacy and care of older adult people in Kwahu, Ghana. In: Stroeken K, Makoni S, editors. Ageing in Africa. London: Routledge; 2002.

54. Wårdh I, Andersson L, Sörensen S. Staff attitudes to oral health. A comparative study of registered nurses, nursing assistants and home care aides. Gerodontology. 1997;14(1):28–32.

55. Stanley SH, Laugharne JDE. Clinical guidelines for the physical care of mental health consumers: a comprehensive assessment of monitoring package for mental health and primary care clinicians. Aust N Z J Psychiatry. 2011;45:824–9.

56. Cederholm T, Barazzoni R, Austin P, Ballmer P, Biolo G, Bischoff SC, Compher C, Correia I, Higashiguchi T, Holst M, Jensen GL, Malone A, Muscaritoli M, Nyulasi I, Pirlich M, Rothenberg E, Schindler K, Schneider SM, de van der Schueren MAE, Sieber C, Valentini L, Yu JC, Van Gossum A, Singer P. ESPEN guidelines and terminology of clinical nutrition. Clin Nutr. 2017;36(1):49–64. https://doi.org/10.1016/j.clnu.2016.09.004.

57. NHS Digital. Patient led assessments of the care environment (PLACE). https://digital.nhs.uk/data-and-information/areas-of-interest/estates-and-facilities/patient-led-assessments-of-the-care-environment-place#assessment-forms. Accessed 14 July 2018.

58. Caris-Verhallen WMCM, Kerkstra A, Bensing JM. The role of communication in nursing care for older adult people: a review of the literature. J Adv Nurs. 1997;25:915–33.

59. Ministry of Housing, Communities & Local Government. Statutory homelessness and prevention and relief, October to December (Q4) 2017: London. 2018.

60. Culhane DP, Metraux S, Byrne T, Steno M, Bainbridge J. The age structure of contemporary homelessness: evidence and implications for public policy. Anal Soc Issues Public Policy. 2013;13:1–17.

61. Hahn JA, Kushel MB, Bangsberg DR, Riley E, Moss AR. The aging of the homeless population: fourteen-year trends in San Francisco. J Gen Intern Med. 2006;21:775–8.

62. Baggett TP, Singer DE, Rigotti NA, O'Connel JJ. The unmet needs of homeless adults. Am J Public Health. 2010;100(7):1326–33.

63. Brown RT, Hemati K, Riley ED, Lee CT, Ponath C, Tieu L, Guzman D, Kushel MB. Geriatric conditions in a population-based sample of older homeless adults. The Gerontologist. 2017;57(4):757–66. https://doi.org/10.1093/geront/gnw011.

64. Healthwatch England. Safely home: what happens when people leave hospital and care settings? Healthwatch England special inquiry findings July 2015. London: Healthwatch England; 2015.

65. O'Connell JJ. Premature mortality in homeless populations: a review of the literature. National Health Care for the Homeless Council; 2005.

66. Sinclair S, Torres M-B, Raffin-Bouchal S, Hack TF, McClement S, Hagen NA, Chochinov HM. Compassion training in healthcare: what are patients' perspectives on training healthcare providers? BMC Med Educ. 2016;16:169. https://doi.org/10.1186/s12909-016-0695-0.

67. Halpern J. What is clinical empathy? J Gen Intern Med. 2003;18(8):670–4.

68. Lee T. How to spread empathy in healthcare. Harv Bus Rev. 2014. https://hbr.org/2014/07/how-to-spread-empathy-in-health-care.

Part IV

Therapeutic Approach of Older Adults with Mental Disorders

Pharmacological Interventions in Older Adults

9

Jay J. Patel, Dale W. Smith, John Heafner, Christopher NG, and George T. Grossberg

Abstract

In this chapter, we discuss the different pharmacological interventions for psychiatric diseases in the geriatric population. We specifically divide these treatments into five categories: anxiolytics and sedative-hypnotics, antipsychotics, antidepressants, mood stabilizers, and cognitive enhancers. These categories are further divided into disease-specific medications. The utility, general recommendations, mechanism of action, dosing, and adverse reactions of drugs are covered for the medications in this chapter. The treatment of mental illness in the geriatric population is a complicated process due to the physiologic changes of metabolism, drug absorption, and drug excretion. These transformations specifically alter the dosing of pharmacological treatments in older adults. The shift in metabolism inherently changes the side effect profile of medications compared to the general adult population, which further complicates the utilization of pharmaceutical interventions for older adults with psychiatric conditions. It is our goal to provide a solid background for clinicians to make prudent decisions in the treatment approach of psychiatric diseases in the geriatric population.

Abbreviations

ACE	Angiotensin-converting enzyme
AD	Alzheimer's disease
ADCS-ADL	Alzheimer's disease cooperative study/activities of daily living inventory score
ADLs	Activities of daily living
AED	Antiepileptic drug
APA	American Psychiatric Association
BADL-S	Bristol Activities of Daily Living score
BUN	Blood urea nitrogen
BZDs	Benzodiazepines
CBC	Complete blood count
CBT	Cognitive behavioral therapy
CKD	Chronic kidney disease
CNS	Central nervous system
ECG	Electrocardiogram
ECT	Electro-compulsive therapy
eGFR	Glomerular filtration rate
GABA	Gamma-aminobutyric acid
GAD	Generalized anxiety disorder
GIS	Global impression score

J. J. Patel (✉) · D. W. Smith · J. Heafner · C. NG
Department of Neurology and Behavioral Neuroscience, Saint Louis University School of Medicine, St. Louis, MO, USA
e-mail: jay.patel@health.slu.edu; jpatel32@slu.edu

G. T. Grossberg
Department of Psychiatry and Behavioral Neuroscience, Saint Louis University School of Medicine, St. Louis, MO, USA

© Springer Nature Switzerland AG 2019
C. A. de Mendonça Lima, G. Ivbijaro (eds.), *Primary Care Mental Health in Older People*,
https://doi.org/10.1007/978-3-030-10814-4_9

HAMD-17	Hamilton Depression Rating Scale score
HIV	Human immunodeficiency virus
LFT	Liver function test
MADRS	Montgomery Asberg Depression Rating Scale
MAOI	Monoamine oxidase inhibitor
MMSE	Mini mental status exam
MNCD	Major neurocognitive disorder
NMDA	N-methyl-d-aspartate
NPI	Neuropsychiatric inventory
OCD	Obsessive compulsive disorder
OSA	Obstructive sleep apnea
PTSD	Post-traumatic stress disorder
SAD-S	Social avoidance and distress scale
SIADH	Syndrome of inappropriate antidiuretic hormone secretion
SIB	Severe impairment battery scale
SJS	Steven-Johnson syndrome
SNRI	Serotonin-norepinephrine reuptake inhibitor
SSRI	Selective serotonin reuptake inhibitor
SSRIs	Selective serotonin reuptake inhibitors
TCA	Tricyclic antidepressant
TENS	Toxic epidermal necrolysis syndrome

Key Points
- The most effective treatment approach toward insomnia in older adults is the non-benzodiazepines, zolpidem, zaleplon, and zopiclone.
- Anxiety disorders are now largely treated with antidepressants, but there are some situations where benzodiazepines can still continue to play a role.
- In older adult patients with major neurocognitive disorder, non-pharmacological methods should be attempted first due to the risk of significant side effects of antipsychotics.

- Antipsychotics for older adults, if necessary, should be chosen based on side effect profile; atypical neuroleptics have less severe side effects than typical neuroleptics.
- SSRIs are the first line for depression in older adults due to favorable side effect profile.
- Depression with co-occurring medical conditions should be treated with monotherapy when possible.
- Mood stabilizers are effective medications for controlling manic and/or depressive symptoms but have significant adverse events and should be monitored appropriately.
- There is limited research on mood stabilizers in the older adult population, so most dosing recommendations are based on younger, healthier individuals.
- Cholinesterase inhibitors are the mainstay of treatment options for mild to moderate Alzheimer's disease, while memantine is first line for moderate to severe Alzheimer's disease.
- New treatment options such as vitamin E are showing promise in slowing the progression of disease, but there are still no treatment options available to prevent, stop, or reverse major neurocognitive disorder.

9.1 Anxiolytics and Sedative Hypnotics in Older Adults

9.1.1 Introduction

Anxiety and insomnia are serious conditions in older adults that deserve ample attention. They can be debilitating disorders which can drastically affect an older adult patient's daily life, and it is important to alleviate these problems with appropriate forms of intervention that carry the least risk. In fact, it is shown that more than 50% of older adults may have insomnia, revealing that it may be a much more prevalent condition than people may suspect [1]. Although insomnia is often mistaken as a normal part of aging and is too frequently ignored, this lack of restorative sleep can worsen other health conditions or impact quality of life, and therefore it is important to develop a strong treatment plan. On the other hand, anxiety is less likely to be a standalone diagnosis and is much more associated with comorbid depression or another general medical or psychiatric disorder [2]. Although many of the anxiety disorders are now being treated with antidepressants, this chapter of the text will focus on various other forms of treatment such as benzodiazepines (BZDs) which still continue to play a role in some treatment approaches. However, before anxiolytics and sedatives can be further elaborated upon, it is important to take a brief step back and understand how they function. This discussion will start with the mechanism of selected anxiolytics and hypnotics before moving onto the treatment approach of prevalent illnesses.

9.1.2 Pharmacology and Adverse Effects

BZDs such as diazepam act as agonists at the gamma-aminobutyric acid (GABA) receptor on postsynaptic neurons [3]. It is important to note that these GABA receptors can be located in various areas of the central nervous system (CNS) including the cerebral cortex, limbic regions, cerebellum, and brainstem [4]. Therefore, the widespread effect of BZDs opens the opportunity for potential unwanted side effects such as cognitive dysfunction including amnesia, confusion, impaired reaction time, and sedation. BZDs are also metabolized by cytochrome P450 3A4 in the liver, and this can lead to interactions with several other drugs that work through the same enzyme in hepatocytes [5]. This includes antiepileptics and some antibiotics such as macrolides, and it logically follows that CYP450 3A4 inducers decrease levels of BZDs, while inhibitors increase their levels. Furthermore, there can be additive sedative effects when BZDs are used

alongside other CNS depressants including alcohol and opioid pain relievers. This can lead to life-threatening sedation [6]. Similarly, the rate of absorption is increased on an empty stomach or with alcohol, whereas it is decreased by food or antacid use [7]. This is why it is important that patients be informed on which conditions to take medications. Lastly, BZDs are lipophilic, and this affects their volume of distribution. Since fatty tissues increase with age, distribution will also increase in older adults [8]. This accounts for the most lipophilic drugs having a short duration of effect due to rapid redistribution to adipose tissue versus the less lipophilic drugs having a longer duration of effect.

To delve deeper into BZDs, it is important to discuss the two different types. The first type is oxidatively metabolized including alprazolam, chlordiazepoxide, diazepam, and others, and they lead to active metabolites. They have very long half-lives and have decreased clearance with age. This can cause daytime sedation and slowed activity, and therefore these BZDs are not recommended in older adults. On the other hand, some BZDs are conjugated such as lorazepam, oxazepam, and temazepam. More specifically, they undergo glucuronidation. They produce no active metabolites and have short half-lives, especially lorazepam and oxazepam. Their clearance is not affected by age, and they are all around a safer option to use in older adults [7].

In case of an overdose on BZDs due to the drug itself or factors like alcohol, it is important to note that there can be extreme sedation. This can lead to falls, immobility, confusion, and incontinence. Flumazenil is a BZD antagonist that can be used for reversal in emergency situations. However, it is important to monitor for seizures, and this therapy should not be used in those with a history of seizure disorders. Furthermore, it is important to taper the use of BZDs in older adults when discontinuing their use, and this could potentially last several weeks [9, 10].

Some non-BZDs that similarly act as anxiolytics include buspirone, gabapentin, and hydroxyzine. Buspirone is a 5HT-1A partial agonist, and it can alleviate anxiety without causing sedation or functional impairment. This is thought to be due to the interaction with multiple neurotransmitters at multiple sites in the brain [11]. Although the mechanism is not fully understood, it is nevertheless an effective drug that can be used for generalized anxiety. However, it is important to note that it takes two or more weeks to take effect, so it would not be a good drug for acute anxiety or panic attacks. Gabapentin has a much vaguer mechanism. It is similar in structure to GABA but does not act on GABA receptors. Instead, it modulates GABA synthesis. Gabapentin has also been shown to bind to voltage-gated calcium ion channels which help with pain alleviation in disorders of hyperalgesia [12]. On the other hand, hydroxyzine has the most well-understood mechanism of action, and it is a first-generation antihistamine thus acting as a H1-receptor antagonist. It has been used in older adults for anxiety relief in generalized anxiety disorder as well as anxiety associated with psychoneurosis. However, due to its highly anticholinergic properties, there is a high risk of adverse effects including confusion, dry mouth, and constipation. This limits its use as an anxiolytic in the older adult population [13–15].

Lastly, there are several types of hypnotics that are popularly used. Ramelteon is a melatonin receptor agonist that operates via circadian rhythms to promote sleep. It has no effect on any of the other CNS receptors, and so it has a low chance of abuse. It acts on MT1 and MT2 [16]. There is also zolpidem, zopiclone, and zaleplon which act on the GABA receptor similar to BZDs. However, they induce less tolerance and dependence than BZDs and therefore are generally preferred [17]. An important consideration to prescribing these medications, though, is the risk of "hangover effects." This includes residual sleepiness, psychomotor retardation, and cognitive impairment in the day following nighttime administration. This is especially harmful in older adults considering the increased risk of falls and subsequent injuries including hip fractures [18]. Nevertheless, trazodone is another drug used for sedation, and it acts as a serotonin antagonist and reuptake inhibitor [19]. This is similar to the mechanism of some antidepressants.

9.1.3 General Recommendations for Selected Syndromes and Disorders

Although the list of anxiety and sleep disorders is extensive, this chapter will discuss some of the most common diseases in older adults. First of all, generalized anxiety disorder (GAD) is at least 6 months of excessive uncontrollable worry. It has a high level of comorbidity with major depression, and anxiety may even be a symptom of the depression itself. Cognitive behavioral therapy (CBT) may be useful in selected older adults with GAD, but more controlled trials are needed in this population. The pharmacotherapy of choice is antidepressants regardless if the patient has depression or not. Some of the more efficacious drugs in this category include citalopram and venlafaxine. BZDs may also be used but are less favored due to their side effect profile, and lorazepam or oxazepam is preferred if necessary. Lastly, buspirone can be used but it is secondary to antidepressants [20].

Another source of anxiety may be specific phobias which cause extreme irrational fear. Studies have found that there is a 10% phobia prevalence in people over 65 years of age, and this is split into agoraphobia which accounts for 7.8%, specific phobia which accounts for 2.1%, and social phobia which accounts for 1.3%. Agoraphobia is an irrational fear of crowded or enclosed spaces, whereas social phobia is an irrational fear of social situations. For all these disorders, the treatment of choice is behavioral therapy and not pharmacotherapy. CBT and progressive desensitization allow for people to lessen the perceived severity of their stressor and therefore experience less anxiety [21].

Another source of stress in older adults is panic attacks, but it is less frequent in older adults and rarely starts for the first time in old age. Therefore, a novel presentation of panic disorder necessitates a full workup in order to ensure another illness or drug is not causing the panic attack symptoms. If a true panic disorder is diagnosed, then various forms of treatment can be applied. Since there are no reliable predictors to the response of certain treatments, there have been no appreciable differences among CBT, antidepressants, or BZDs. It is recommended that the risks and benefits of each type of treatment should drive the treatment selection. Similar to GAD, panic disorder has a high comorbidity with depression, and so first-line treatment is usually selective serotonin reuptake inhibitors (SSRIs). Also, they carry less side effect risks than BZDs [22].

Two other disorders that will be briefly discussed are post-traumatic stress disorder (PTSD) and obsessive compulsive disorder (OCD). PTSD is defined as greater than 1 month of disturbing thoughts, feelings, or dreams after a stressful life event. This may manifest as re-experiencing the trauma, avoidance, and/or hyperarousal. Many contributory factors play a role in recovery from PTSD such as the patient's social support and personality traits. Regardless, the mainstays of treatment have been CBT, antidepressants, and group therapy [23]. On the other hand, OCD involves irrational obsessions which drive compulsive behavior and cause severe anxiety in daily life. Most often it manifests in young adulthood and persists into late life. CBT may be effectively used to deal with obsessions appropriately so that compulsions are not expressed. Also, SSRIs and clomipramine (be wary of anticholinergics) can be used as additional pharmacotherapy and both have proven to be effective [24].

As for sleep disorders, insomnia is by far the most common. It is characterized by an inability to fall and/or stay asleep. To reiterate what was previously mentioned, it is often ascribed to normal aging despite that more than 50% of older adults may have insomnia. A very effective approach is changing maladaptive sleep habits or improving sleep hygiene. This includes relaxation techniques to induce sleep, and sleep restriction can be incorporated to only sleep during specific times of the day in order to maintain a proper sleep-wake cycle. There can also be stimulus control therapy to limit the use of the bedroom to sleeping and sexual activity only. If older adult patients cannot sleep, they are encouraged to leave and read a book or perform another activity until they feel drowsy at which point they can return to the bedroom. Pharmacotherapy can

also be used, and zolpidem, zaleplon, and zopiclone are the most effective non-BZDs which can alleviate insomnia. They do not alter sleep architecture and have no tolerance or rebound insomnia that can be seen with other treatments. Still, there may be a risk of hangover effects, and it is important to exercise caution. Trazodone and ramelteon may also be used. On the other hand, antipsychotics, diphenhydramine, chloral hydrate, barbiturates, and benzodiazepines are not recommended as primary treatments. Furthermore, many older adult patients may try to self-medicate with over-the-counter antihistamines such as Tylenol PM (the PM component is diphenhydramine), but these do not maintain sleep, and there is a risk of tolerance. Anticholinergic side effects of these drugs may include cognitive impairment, daytime drowsiness, constipation, urinary retention, and visual blurring, and therefore these drugs are to be avoided [25].

9.2 Antipsychotics for Older Adults

9.2.1 General Recommendations

In the past, older adult patients with major neurocognitive disorder (MNCD), agitation, and psychosis have been treated with antipsychotic medications. On the contrary, more recent studies have contradicted this approach to behavioral disturbances in these patients. Recent studies have shown that there is modest benefit from using antipsychotic medications in geriatric patients with agitation and psychosis. In fact, these studies have shown that there is an increased risk of mortality, stroke, and neurocognitive decline (black box warning) [26]. These recent findings have led the American Psychiatric Association (APA) to release new guidelines for the use of antipsychotics in older adults.

The APA has most recently suggested that antipsychotics in older adult patients with MNCD should only be used when the symptoms of agitation and psychosis are dangerous and/or can cause harm to others or the patient [27]. It is also recommended that non-pharmacological methods should be attempted prior to starting a geriatric patient on antipsychotics. Prior to starting a patient on antipsychotics, the physician should always weigh the risks and benefits with the patient, their family members, or their surrogate decision-maker. The initial treatment should always be started at a low dose and increased slowly. Patients can experience significant side effects such as Parkinsonism, akathisia, dyskinesia, orthostasis, and sedation, depending on the choice of neuroleptic. If these occur, the physician must assess the risks and benefits to determine if the antipsychotic should be discontinued. The antipsychotic medication should also be discontinued if there has been no significant response after 2–4 weeks. The medication should be tapered off gradually when being discontinued. If the patient does show response to medications, then the drug should be tapered off within 4 months of beginning the drug. The patient's should be monitored on a monthly basis as the antipsychotic is being tapered off. The APA also recommends that all antipsychotic medications should be used in conjunction with other non-pharmacological treatments [28].

The selection of which antipsychotic medication to use is based upon their side effects and how they may affect each individual patient. We will focus on the three most commonly used agents. As previously discussed, antipsychotics in older adults have shown to increase the risk of mortality, stroke, neurocognitive decline, extrapyramidal symptoms, sedation, and a serious but rare condition called neuroleptic malignant syndrome [28]. Atypical and conventional antipsychotics have also shown to have an increased risk of falls. For example, in a meta-analysis of geriatric patients, the odds ratio for any psychotropic use among patients who had one or more falls was 1.73 (95% CI 1.52–1.97) [29].

Conventional antipsychotics work by blocking dopamine (D2) receptors. Atypical antipsychotics work by blocking both dopamine (D2) receptors and serotonin (2A) receptors. Atypical antipsychotics have been preferred over the use of conventional antipsychotics because they have less severe side effects.

9.2.1.1 Olanzapine

Olanzapine is a second-generation antipsychotic that can be used to treat schizophrenia, manic episodes in bipolar I disorder, and agitation associated with schizophrenia and bipolar I and for augmentation in depression. Olanzapine can also be used off-label for delirium, post-traumatic stress disorder, Tourette syndrome, and chemotherapy-associated nausea or vomiting. Olanzapine works by antagonizing serotonin $5\text{-}HT_{2A}$ and $5\text{-}HT_{2C}$, dopamine D_{1-4}, histamine H_1, and alpha$_1$-adrenergic receptors.

Olanzapine Dosing: The dosage for short-acting oral olanzapine in older adults for psychosis should start at a low dose of 2.5–5 mg daily and can be increased to a maximum of 5 mg twice per day. The dosage for short-acting IM is the same as oral olanzapine. If using oral olanzapine off-label, they should be initially started at a dose of 1.25–5 mg daily. The dose can be increased gradually, but should not exceed 10 mg daily. If using olanzapine extended release IM, it is recommended to start at a low dose of 150 mg every 4 weeks. For the off-label use of olanzapine for psychosis and agitation related to MNCD, it is recommended to start with an initial dose of 2.5–5 mg of the short-acting IM. The patient can receive up to two more additional doses of 1.25 or 2.5 mg.

Side Effects of Olanzapine: Olanzapine can affect the cardiovascular system by causing orthostatic hypotension and prolonging the Q-T interval which may cause an arrhythmia [30]. It can also affect the central nervous system by causing drowsiness, extrapyramidal symptoms, and insomnia. The extrapyramidal side effects include akathisia, cogwheel rigidity, tremor, Parkinsonism, and hypertonia. Extrapyramidal side effects are lower when doses are 5 mg per day or less [30]. Olanzapine also has an effect on the metabolic system, which causes weight gain in patients. Patients on olanzapine can have increased appetite and constipation while taking the medication. This medication can also have an impact on the hepatic system by causing patients to have an elevated AST and ALT while having a decreased serum bilirubin. Olanzapine can also cause a rare but serious skin condition called drug reaction with eosinophilia and systemic symptoms (DRESS) [31]. The patient should also be monitored for hyperglycemia and evaluated for cerebrovascular risks that can occur with all antipsychotics [32].

Olanzapine Precautions and Drug Interactions: Olanzapine should be used with caution in patients with certain diseases. Olanzapine should be used with caution in patients with MNCD-Lewy body type because antipsychotics can trigger severe extrapyramidal symptoms in this patient population. Due to possible elevated AST and ALT levels, olanzapine should be used with caution in patients with hepatic impairment.

Olanzapine has interactions with several drugs. Olanzapine when combined with potassium acid phosphate, potassium chloride, potassium citrate, and potassium phosphate may cause constipation. The combination of these drugs may decrease the rate of passage of potassium throughout the gastrointestinal tract, which can cause ulcers and stenosis. Olanzapine should be avoided with bromocriptine because it antagonizes dopamine receptors. Olanzapine should also be avoided with the use of epinephrine because it can cause hypotension due to an unopposed beta agonist effect [33]. CYP1A2 inducers may require dosing adjustments because olanzapine is a CYP1A2 substrate.

9.2.1.2 Risperidone

Risperidone is an atypical antipsychotic that has mixed serotonin and dopamine antagonist activity. It has a more profound effect on 5-HT_2 receptors than dopamine D_2. Risperidone also antagonizes to alpha1, alpha2 adrenergic, and histamine receptors. Risperidone is used to treat manic episodes in bipolar I disorder, schizophrenia, and agitation in patients with autism [34]. It has been used off-label for major depressive disorder, psychosis, and agitation associated with Alzheimer's disease, Tourette syndrome, and post-traumatic distress disorder [34].

Risperidone Dosing: It is recommended that oral risperidone be administered at an initial dose of 0.25–0.5 mg per day. An initial dose of less than 1 mg per day can reduce the incidence of orthostatic hypotension and syncope in older adults. An increase in the dosage should be done slowly and gradually. It should not be increased at an increment greater than 0.5 mg. The dosage of risperidone should be decreased if the patient has any renal or hepatic impairment. If IM/depot risperidone is administered to patients with hepatic and renal impairment, then the patient should be given oral risperidone at 0.5 mg twice per day for the first week and then 2 mg per day for the week after. If this is tolerated, the patient can be started on IM risperidone at 25 mg every 2 weeks, while oral risperidone is continued for the 3 weeks following the initial injection. When risperidone is used off-label for Alzheimer-related neurocognitive disorder, it is recommended to start with a dose of 0.25 mg daily and to increase in increments of 0.25 mg every 2–4 days [35]. The maximum dose should be 2 mg daily divided into two doses per day. Patients usually have the best response at a dose of 0.5 mg twice per day [35].

Risperidone Side Effects: Risperidone has side effects that involve multiple systems that are similar to olanzapine. It can affect the central nervous system by causing sedation, Parkinsonism, akathisia, tremor, insomnia, headache, and anxiety. The side effects of sedation and Parkinsonism are of greater importance in older adults because they can increase the risk of falls. Risperidone can increase appetite and has metabolic effects by causing weight gain. In addition to increased appetite, it may cause constipation, vomiting, nausea, and abdominal pain. It also may cause urinary incontinence, which occurs more often in children. As with the other antipsychotics, it can cause neuroleptic malignant syndrome. Risperidone is contraindicated in patients that have a hypersensitivity reaction to the drug which include symptoms of rash, angioedema, shortness of breath, and wheezing [36].

Risperidone Drug Interactions: Risperidone has similar drug interactions with those of olanzapine due to its antagonism of dopamine and serotonin receptors. Risperidone should be avoided with bromocriptine which also antagonizes dopamine receptors. Haloperidol and risperidone should not be administered together because this combination can increase risperidone levels, which can increase the sedative and extrapyramidal effects of the antipsychotic. Use of vemurafenib should also be avoided with risperidone because it can increase risperidone levels by inhibiting the hepatic metabolism of risperidone [36]. Ginseng is a substance that should be avoided with risperidone because it can worsen psychiatric conditions. Ziprasidone is another drug that should be avoided with risperidone because its additive effects can cause psychomotor impairment in patients [36]. This would especially be of concern in older adult patients because it would increase the risk of falls. CYP2D6 inhibitors may require dosing adjustments because risperidone is a CYP2D6 substrate.

9.2.1.3 Quetiapine

Quetiapine is another atypical antipsychotic that antagonizes dopamine and serotonin. Quetiapine can be used to treat acute episodes of mania in bipolar disorder. It can be used as a monotherapy or used in combination with other drugs such as divalproex or lithium. It can also be used to treat major depressive disorder and schizophrenia. Quetiapine has several off-label uses: psychosis in Parkinson disease, delirium, generalized anxiety disorder, post-traumatic stress disorder, and agitation and psychosis associated with Alzheimer's disease and obsessive compulsive disorder [37].

Quetiapine Dosing: It is recommended to use an initial dose of 50 mg daily of quetiapine when being used as a treatment for schizophrenia or bipolar disorder. The dose can be titrated by increments of 50 mg per day to a dose that achieves desired effects [38]. When quetiapine is used in conjunction with an antidepressant to treat major depressive disorder, it is recommended to start at an initial dose of 50 mg daily and to titrate in increments of 50 mg daily until the desired effect is achieved. When quetiapine is used off-label to treat psychosis in Parkinson disease, it is recommended to start with a dose of 25 mg daily that can be administered in one or split into two doses. The dose can be increased to reach the desired effects, but the maximum dose should be 200 mg daily. When quetiapine is being

used off-label to treat psychosis and agitation related to MNCD and Alzheimer's disease, it is recommended to start with a dose ranging from 12.5 to 50 mg per day [39]. The dose can be increased up to 300 mg daily.

Quetiapine Side Effects: The side effects of quetiapine can involve multiple systems. Quetiapine has an effect on the cardiovascular system by causing hypotension, tachycardia, and prolonged QT. It affects the nervous system by causing sedation, dizziness, agitation, fatigue, and extrapyramidal symptoms. Quetiapine has also been known to cause weight gain, decrease HDL levels, increase LDL levels, and cause hyperglycemia [40]. It affects the gastrointestinal system by causing constipation and increased appetite. Some individuals can develop a hypersensitivity reaction to this drug, and it should be avoided in these patients. Quetiapine has anticholinergic effects; therefore, it should be used with caution in patients with urinary retention, decreased gastrointestinal motility, or vision problems. Agranulocytosis and neutropenia has been shown in patients taking antipsychotics. A patient with a history of a low white blood cell count should have a complete blood count before administration. Quetiapine should be discontinued if the neutrophil count is less than 1000 [40]. Quetiapine may also cause hypothyroidism. TSH and free T4 levels should be checked prior to administration and periodically during follow-up visits.

Quetiapine Drug Interactions: Quetiapine has several interactions with drugs that should be considered when deciding to administer it. As stated earlier, quetiapine can lead to prolongation of the QT; therefore, it is contraindicated with cisapride and dronedarone because they both can cause a prolonged QT leading to additive effects of the two drugs [41]. Quetiapine should be avoided if patients are taking any drugs that can prolong the QT such as amiodarone, clarithromycin, and many other drugs. Azelastine, a central nervous system depressant, should be avoided in combination with quetiapine because it can enhance central nervous depression [41]. CYP3A4 inducers may require dosing adjustments because it can decrease quetiapine concentrations. Likewise, CYP3A4 inhibitors may require dosing adjustment because it can increase levels of quetiapine.

9.2.1.4 Newer Agents

Lurasidone is an atypical antipsychotic that has had minimal research done in the geriatric population. Lurasidone binds to dopamine (D2), norepinephrine (alpha 2A and 2C), and serotonin (1A, 2A, and 7) receptors. The drug acts as an antagonist at all of these receptors except on serotonin 1A receptors. It acts as a partial agonist on serotonin 1A receptors. It is metabolized via CYP 3A4. The bioavailability of lurasidone has been shown to be three times higher when administered with food [42]. It is recommended to start with an oral dose of 40 mg daily. The dose can be increased based off of the patient's response and tolerability. The maximum dose is 160 mg per day. Lurasidone has less metabolic side effects and is less likely to cause an arrhythmia than other antipsychotics.

Cariprazine is another atypical antipsychotic with minimal research in the geriatric population. It is an atypical antipsychotic that displays partial agonist activity at dopamine D_2 and serotonin 5-HT_{1A} receptors and antagonist activity at serotonin 5-HT_{2A} receptors. It is a D3/D2 receptor partial agonist. It has a higher affinity for D3 than D2. It has been recently approved for use in older adults. It is recommended to start with an initial oral dose of 1.5 mg daily and to adjust based on response and tolerability to 3 mg on day 2. Adjustments can be made in increments of 1.5 or 3.0 mg. The maximum dose is 6 mg. It is metabolized via CYP3A4. Cariprazine has similar side effects to the other atypical antipsychotics. It is less likely to cause an arrhythmia than other atypical antipsychotics [43].

Pimavanserin is a recently approved antipsychotic used for psychosis in Parkinson's disease. It has a unique mechanism of action. It is an inverse agonist and antagonist with a high affinity for 5-HT_{2A} receptors and low affinity for 5-HT_{2C} and sigma 1 receptors. It does not have affinity for 5-HT_{2B}, dopaminergic (including D_2), muscarinic, histaminergic, or adrenergic receptors or to calcium channels.

9.3 Antidepressants

9.3.1 Introduction

Pharmacologic treatment for depression in older adults is understudied proportional to the considerable problems that it presents. Few randomized, placebo-controlled trials have focused specifically on antidepressant use in the geriatric population. This research is important because side effects and comorbidities make treatment of depression in older adults different from treatment in other populations. The problem of late life mood disorders is not insignificant.

Although depression rates are lower in this population [44], there is a possibility of underreporting. This is due to the stigma of seeking treatment and the silent presentation of this disorder in older adults [45]. Independent of prevalence, and possibly more concerning, is an increased risk of suicide in this population when compared to younger patients [46]. Another factor that increases morbidity and mortality in these patients is depression's danger when combined with comorbidities. Depression has been linked with poor outcomes in pneumonia, coronary heart disease, and nonalcoholic fatty liver disease [45, 47, 48], but these are only some examples in a wide sea of research on the topic. The purpose of this section is to outline treatment strategies for depression specific to older adult patients in the primary care setting with particular attention to side effects and comorbidities.

9.3.2 Treatment Concerns

Treatment of depression in older adults comes with unique challenges. Meta-analyses have shown that antidepressants are effective in older adults, but have not shown differences in efficacy between classes of antidepressants [49]. Therefore, medication choices should be made on an individualized basis with side effects in mind. They are more susceptible to side effects and have pre-existing medical conditions that may complicate antidepressant treatment. Given these issues, individualized medication plans are essential for safe and effective treatment.

9.3.3 Dosing

American Psychiatric Association (APA) guidelines recommend lower starting doses and slowing the process of titrating the medication up to an effective dose [50]. They also recommend weekly visits in the acute phase of depression to monitor for improvement and side effects. The acute phase may also last longer in older adults irrespective of titration speed. For example, in younger patients, signs of improvement may be seen in 2–4 weeks, whereas in older adults it may take 6–8 weeks [49, 50]. Even more care needs to be taken with patients with co-occurring renal or hepatic dysfunction. While most drugs will still require a decrease in starting dose, selective serotonin reuptake inhibitors (SSRIs) seem to be the safest in these patients [50, 51]. Once the patient is titrated to an effective dose, management seems to mirror younger patients as effective doses appear to be similar to younger adults [49, 52, 53].

9.3.4 Side Effects in the Context of Comorbidities

Specific medication interactions and contraindications for specific comorbidities will be discussed later, but overall, older patients are more likely to experience side effects even at "lower" doses [49]. This is the most important factor informing medication choice and will dominate the rest of this section.

Comorbidities increase the risk of side effects with certain antidepressants. Epidemiological studies have found increased rates of depression in patients with chronic diseases so it is important to know which drugs can be prescribed safely [54]. Geriatric patients are also more likely to suffer from chronic medical conditions and have more medications in general. Therefore, they should require even more attention when prescribing psychoactive drugs. Dementia and anticholinergic sensitivity are among the most important comorbidities to keep in mind in older adults because of their prevalence and relatively poor outcomes when combined with cholinergic blockade. This blockade commonly occurs with TCAs, and the subsequent delirium is a dangerous and common occurrence [55]. One consultation and liaison service at a hospital examined the 1-year mortality rate of older adult inpatients with either dementia, delirium, or depression. Of the three, delirium had a significantly higher mortality rate of 35.5% [56]. Given this increased risk, the implications for treatment are clear: delirium is a poor trade-off for the treatment of geriatric depression. Therefore, TCAs should be used with extreme caution in older adults. Other pre-existing conditions can be worsened by cholinergic blockade. The most important of these includes benign prostatic hyperplasia and glaucoma with risk of developing urinary retention and acute angle closure glaucoma, respectively [50].

Cardiovascular risk in a patient is another reason to carefully examine medication choice. TCAs are associated with higher risks in these patients due to induction of dangerous arrhythmias [57]. SSRIs, on the other hand, are considered safe and may even improve mortality [58]. Hypertension is yet another condition worsened by antidepressants, but in this case, SNRIs are the culprit. These drugs tend to raise blood pressure [59] and should be avoided in patients with uncontrolled hypertension [50]. Antidepressants worsening obesity is another problem [50]. The greatest weight changes have been seen with mirtazapine, TCAs, and monoamine oxidase inhibitors (MAOIs), but there is evidence that most antidepressants with the notable exception of bupropion cause weight gain [60]. TCAs can also worsen glycemic control in some diabetic patients [61]. Obstructive sleep apnea (OSA) is another common condition in older adults that may influence treatment of depression [50]. This is not only because OSA can mimic depression but because for OSA patients whose depression is confirmed and treated, the sedating effects of some antidepressants may increase daytime sleepiness [62]. Mirtazapine, trazodone, and TCAs seem to have the most sedating effects [63–65].

Comorbidities may also present an opportunity to choose the best drug for a patient. If a patient has depression along with other conditions that can be treated with a certain antidepressant, it's better to use that one medication than to add two or more. A good example of this is an older patient who is losing weight, depressed, and having trouble sleeping. A concise medication in this situation is mirtazapine at bedtime [50]. It is associated with weight gain and sedation and is as effective as SSRIs in depression studies [66–68]. Smoking cessation in the setting of depression is another opportunity to combine medications. Bupropion by itself or as an adjunct is effective in this situation [69]. Obesity can be another indication for use of bupropion because it seems to be the most weight neutral of all antidepressants [70].

Many examples of chronic pain in the setting of depression can be treated with one concise antidepressant. The most well-known example of this is duloxetine, the serotonin-norepinephrine reuptake inhibitor, used for pain and depression. While this benefit may not reach clinical significance in studies, it has been shown to help [71]. This marginal effect is particularly important to keep in mind for risk-benefit analysis. Though TCAs and serotonin-norepinephrine reuptake inhibitors (SNRIs) have been shown to improve chronic pain and neuropathic pain [72], there is a question as to whether this is worth the side effects in some patients. A depressed older adult patient with chronic pain, dementia, glaucoma, and benign prostatic hypertension may not benefit from the cholinergic blockade seen in TCAs. Likewise, a depressed older adult patient with chronic pain and uncontrolled hypertension may not benefit from an SNRI. Fibromyalgia co-occurring with depression is much the same although duloxetine and amitriptyline have been shown to be the most effective [73]. This comes with the same weighing of risks. Chronic headache can also be treated with a TCA such as amitriptyline, but again, aging patients may be at higher risk for side effects due to the anticholinergic properties of these medications [50, 74]. The specific comorbidities that may preclude use of certain medications will be discussed next.

9.3.5 Medication Classes

9.3.5.1 SSRIs

Various classes of antidepressants have their unique side effects. Each class has medications that may be better tolerated in this vulnerable population. The first class is the SSRIs. SSRIs are superior to placebo in older adults [75] and are considered first line due to their favorable side effect profile. Dropout rates due to side effects for SSRIs are lower in multiple systematic reviews [49, 76]. Two caveats to this statement are the drugs paroxetine and fluoxetine. According to the Beer's Criteria, paroxetine has the most anticholinergic activity of any SSRI and should be treated with the same caution as a TCA [77]. Fluoxetine's use in older adults is likewise discouraged because of its long half-life [78]. Paroxetine, fluoxetine, and fluvoxamine also have a higher risk of drug-drug interactions owing to their inhibition of the cytochrome P450 system [50, 79]. Sertraline, citalopram, and escitalopram have less interactions so are the preferred SSRIs in older adults, although no study has found significant differences in efficacy. Side effects may be relatively mild compared to other classes, but there are several serious side effects specific to older adults that merit discussion. The first of these is the syndrome of inappropriate antidiuretic hormone (SIADH) secretion which is common only in older adults. While this can occur with any antidepressant [77], the risk is highest for SSRIs and venlafaxine (an SNRI) for which the rate has been reported to be between 10 and 28% [80, 81]. The relative frequency with which this occurs makes periodic measurements of sodium levels prudent in the acute phase [50]. Increased falls and fractures are other adverse outcomes researched with SSRI use. In nursing home studies, SSRI use significantly increased the fall risk [82, 83]. The mechanism of this increased fall risk is not known. The risk of fracture was also increased with one study reporting

90% increase in risk [84]. Fall risk may increase fracture risk in this situation, but there may be another component. Functional serotonin receptors have been found in the bone that suggested a direct effect by SSRIs on bone mineral density [85]. However, these findings may be exaggerated by the fact that depressed patients may have lower bone mineral density in the first place [85]. It may be beneficial to assess fall risk when first prescribing SSRIs. SNRIs are similar to SSRIs in efficacy and most of their side effect profile. SNRIs differ in that they may raise blood pressure [69] and should be used with caution in patients with uncontrolled hypertension.

9.3.5.2 TCAs

TCAs are a good example of the need for further research in geriatric psychopharmacology. They are widely considered to be inferior to SSRIs due to their side effect profile and have shown higher treatment withdrawal rates in a systematic review [49]. This is in stark contrast to a recent cohort study in which it was found that SSRIs were actually linked with increased risk of several adverse outcomes compared to TCAs [86]. There are several reasons for this. One possible reason is that this study found that TCAs were often prescribed at a lower dose in older adults and this may account for the decreased side effects. Low-dose TCAs may be a future direction of research as some studies have found little difference in efficacy between high- and low-dose TCAs [86]. Another encouraging avenue in the use of TCAs is the secondary amines, nortriptyline, and desipramine. They have decreased anticholinergic activity compared to the tertiary amine TCAs, but further research is needed to assess their risk in geriatric populations [50, 79]. These are the encouraging aspects of TCAs that must be taken in context with the considerable negatives.

Most adverse outcomes with TCAs have already been addressed with the most obvious being anticholinergic activity and arrhythmia induction. As discussed earlier, cholinergic blockade can lead to delirium, acute angle closure, and urinary retention in high-risk patients. For patients with cardiovascular risk factors, they should be given a pretreatment electrocardiogram

(ECG) to assess for arrhythmias and QT prolongation [50, 57, 87]. Another equally important complication is their lethality in overdose [57]. At a usual therapeutic dose, taking only a 10 day supply may be lethal [50]. This is especially important in older adults given their increased suicide rates.

9.3.5.3 MAOIs

MAOIs have in large part been replaced by TCAs and SSRIs in older adults. This is due to serious side effects (including the need for washout period when switching to and from other antidepressants) and comparable efficacies. The most important of these side effects is hypertensive crisis with ingestion of tyramine [88]. This is usually prevented with dietary restrictions, but with the prevalence of neurocognitive impairment in older adults, it may make these hard to follow.

9.3.5.4 Atypicals and Future Directions

Mirtazapine is an atypical antidepressant that is commonly used in older adults. It acts as an antagonist on alpha-2 receptors. It is used so often because mirtazapine has comparable effects with other antidepressants, may work faster, and can be used effectively as an adjunct with SSRI treatment [66, 67]. Another favorable aspect is its sedating effect, useful for treating depression and co-occurring insomnia. It also causes weight gain which may be beneficial for some older adult patients experiencing weight loss.

Bupropion is another atypical antidepressant that has shown efficacy in certain situations. It has lower rates of sexual side effects, can help with lethargy [89], and has shown to be an effective adjunct therapy in the general population [69]. It's most serious side effect in older adults is its propensity to lower seizure threshold. A thorough seizure history should be taken before introduction of bupropion [90].

Trazodone is an atypical antidepressant that works much like SSRIs but has different efficacies and side effects. Trazodone may not work as well as other antidepressants [91]. The most serious side effect is priapism [92]. Sedation is the most common side effect of trazadone and is one reason why it is used [93]. If, for example, a depressed patient has developed a dependence on benzodiazepines, then trazodone may be helpful in the withdrawal period to encourage sleep.

One future direction for depression treatment involves the use of ketamine, an N-methyl-D-aspartate (NMDA) antagonist. Ketamine's activation of glutamatergic receptors is hypothesized to increase excitatory activity in the CNS in depressed patients. A randomized trial of ketamine therapy for treatment refractory depression yielded short-term results. Hamilton depression scales were significantly lower from 110 min to 7 days, but after that, there was no difference from placebo [94]. The significance of this study is that depression may be more complicated than just a serotonin imbalance, and novel treatments may be developed to address this.

Other possible treatments in the future include the drugs levomilnacipran, vilazodone, and vortioxetine. While it is true that only vortioxetine has proven efficacious in older adult patients, the other novel treatments introduce new pathways to improvement for patients. Levomilnacipran appears to improve functioning. There is inconclusive evidence that vilazodone may have a faster onset of action and may have less sexual side effects. Vortioxetine appears to have a cognitive enhancement effect that is not entirely explained by mood improvement. More evidence is needed to prove efficacy against established antidepressants [95].

9.3.6 Conclusion

In conclusion, pharmacological treatment for depression in older adults requires special attention given to each individual's risks and benefits. Antidepressants seem to work as well in older adult patients as in the general population, and there is no difference in efficacy between classes. The choice is therefore made by side effect profiles and comorbidities. While SSRIs are generally considered the safest, their use comes with risks that are specific to and common in older adult. TCAs have a poor side effect profile in older adult including induction of arrhythmias, anticholinergic activity, and lethality in overdose.

Table 9.1 Averse effects of antidepressants

Drug classes	Pertinent side effects in older adults
SSRI	CYP 450 inhibitor Anticholinergic effects with paroxetine Risk of fracture Risk of falls Serotonin syndrome with MAOI Anorgasmia/erectile dysfunction Weight gain Discontinuation syndrome Risk of bleeding with NSAIDs
SNRI	Hypertension
TCA	Sedation Orthostatic hypertension Cholinergic blockade Weight gain Arrhythmia induction Lethality in overdose
MAOI	Serotonin syndrome with SSRI Hypertensive crisis
Mirtazapine	Weight gain Sedation Increased cholesterol
Bupropion	Seizure risk
Trazodone	Priapism Sedation Orthostasis
Nefazodone	Liver failure Sedation

Atypicals can be used in special circumstances and to treat conditions co-occurring with depression. Antidepressants often require dose adjustments due to both renal and hepatic dysfunction but also due to age-related metabolic slowing. Depression in older adults is of special concern given its risks when combined with comorbidities. Careful antidepressant use is essential in treatment, though more research is needed to elucidate details of treatment (Tables 9.1 and 9.2).

9.4 Mood Stabilizers

Mood stabilizers are utilized for the management of bipolar I and bipolar II disease and hypomania. Individuals with bipolar I and II or hypomania should also be assessed for psychotic or mixed features, which would require the use of antipsychotics. This section will only focus on mood stabilizers, while antipsychotics are useful therapies for mood stabilization; their efficacy

Table 9.2 Dosing for antidepressants

Selected drugs	Starting dose (mg/day)	Usual dose (mg/day)
Citalopram [96]	10	10–20 FDA issued warning to not exceed 20 mg/day due to risk of arrhythmia in older adults
Escitalopram	5	5–10 FDA issued warning to not exceed 10 mg/day due to risk of arrhythmia in older adults
Sertraline	25	50–150
Desvenlafaxine	25	50
Venlafaxine	37.5	75–300
Duloxetine	20–30	30–120
Nortriptyline	25	25–50 (serum level useful)
Desipramine	25–50	100–200 (serum level useful)
Selegiline transdermal	6	6
Mirtazapine	7.5–15	15–60
Bupropion, XL, SR	75	150–300
Trazodone	25–50	150–300

will be discussed in a different section of this chapter. The mainstay mood stabilizers are lithium, valproate, and lamotrigine with other antiepileptic medications used as adjunctive, secondary, or tertiary treatment. Before beginning any medication regimen, patients should be assessed for comorbid conditions such as renal impairment, substance abuse, or anxiety disorders.

9.4.1 Lithium

Lithium is the treatment of choice for acute mania, acute depressive episodes, and bipolar II disorder and for maintenance treatment of bipolar I and II disorder. Lithium's mechanism of action is not completely understood in the treatment of mania. For the acute phase, lithium can be used in conjunction with antipsychotics or benzodiazepines for optimal treatment. Based on a systematic review of 22 randomized trials, lithium demonstrated better control of mania symptoms than chlorpromazine and placebo. In the same review, there were no significant differences in efficacy or adverse effect profile when comparing lithium to haloperidol, valproate, and carbamazepine [97]. Lithium and divalproex both showed a significant difference from placebo for the treatment of mania with 49 and 48% response, respectively, compared to 25% response in placebo group [98]. Lithium compared to olanzapine had better outcomes in controlling frequency and intensity of symptoms in a small, 3 week, controlled trial [99]. Treatment with lithium is also associated with decreased successful suicides and all-cause mortality, but not decreased suicide attempts [4]. Dosing for lithium is shown in Table 9.3 [100–103].

Screening and Monitoring Before treating with lithium, patients must have weight/BMI, BUN, electrolytes, calcium, estimated glomerular filtration rate (eGFR), thyroid function, and complete blood count (CBC) checked. Electrocardiogram (ECG) should be checked for individuals with a predisposing heart condition. When first starting patients on lithium, check levels at the first week and then every week and every dose change until blood levels are stable. Once the patient is on maintenance dosing, their weight/BMI, BUN, electrolytes, calcium, eGFR, thyroid function, and CBC should be checked every 3 months for the first year and then 6 months moving forward if there are no abnormalities [100–103].

Interactions As with all medications, lithium has interactions with other medications. Those on lithium should avoid nonsteroidal anti-inflammatory drugs, diuretics, angiotensin-converting enzyme (ACE) inhibitors, and angiotensin receptor blockers. All of these may increase serum lithium levels causing potential toxicity [100–103].

Adverse Effects The common adverse effects of lithium are listed in Table 9.4 [100–103]. Individuals on lithium are at specifically high risk for chronic kidney disease (CKD) and hypothyroidism. Women, older adults, and those on prolonged treatment are particularly susceptible to CKD and hypothyroidism [105, 106].

Table 9.3 Dosing for mood stabilizers [100–103]

	Lithium	Valproate/divalproex	Carbamazepine	Lamotrigine [104][a]
Starting dose	300 mg/twice daily and adjust every 2–3 days until 900–1800 mg/day oral	15–20 mg/kg loading for acute mania or 500–750 mg/day increasing as needed every 2–3 days	Begin at 200 mg twice daily and increase by 200 mg daily as tolerated	Oral: 25 mg/day for 2 weeks and then increase to 50 mg/day for 2 weeks and then to 100 mg/day for 1 week, and then maintain at 100–200 mg/day
Desired blood serum level	Acute-phase serum level > 0.8 mEq/L Maintenance between 0.6 and 0.75 mEq/L	50–125 µg/mL	4–12 µg/mL	Levels not useful/needed

[a]Dosing depends on concurrent use of valproate, carbamazepine, phenytoin, phenobarbital, primidone, rifampin, and oral contraceptives

Table 9.4 Common adverse effects of mood stabilizers [100–103]

	Lithium	Valproate/divalproex	Carbamazepine	Lamotrigine
Thirst	x			
Polyuria	x			
Cognitive effects	x			
Sedation	x	x		
Tremor	x	x		x
Weight gain	x	x		
Diarrhea	x	x		
Polyuria	x			
Nausea	x			x
Hypothyroidism	x			
Diabetes insipidus	x			
Hair loss		x		
Leukopenia		x		x
Thrombocytopenia		x		x
Elevated liver transaminase levels		x		
Hepatic failure		x		
Pancreatitis		x		
Headache			x	x
Fatigue			x	
Nystagmus			x	
Ataxia			x	
Rash (SJS/TENS)			x	x
Pancytopenia				x
Aseptic meningitis				x
Dry mouth				x
Dizziness				x
Somnolence				x

Treatment Cessation Lithium treatment needs to be tapered over a 4-week time period but preferably 3 months while continuously monitoring for recurrence of mania or depressive symptoms. Tapering over 15–30 days rather than 1–14 showed benefit in a small retrospective study of roughly 100 women. Women who were tapered quickly had relapse of symptoms in two-thirds cases, while women who were slowly tapered only had a relapse of symptoms in one third of cases [107].

9.4.2 Valproate/Divalproex

Valproate and divalproex are similar medications that are both metabolized to the active ingredient valproic acid. Divalproex comes in an extended, enteric-coated capsule formulation, while valproate is a slow-release formula used for intravenous use. The mechanism of action of valproic acid is unknown but is believed to exert its effects through increasing GABA within the brain. Both are approved for the treatment of acute mania or mixed episodes associated with bipolar disorder with or without psychotic symptoms. A Cochrane review demonstrated valproate more effective than placebo, but no different than lithium or carbamazepine; however, it was less effective than olanzapine but had better adverse effect profile in regard to weight gain and sedation. Symptoms for patients were measured with the Young Mania Rating Scale and the Social Avoidance and Distress Scale (SAD-S) [108]. For individuals not in an acute episode, divalproex ER is effective for ambulatory hypomania and bipolar I and II at 15–30 mg/kg/day for 8 weeks when compared to placebo [109]. For older adults, usual maintenance doses of divalproex are 500–1500 mg/day.

Screening and Monitoring Before beginning valproate/divalproex treatment, patients need to have their weight/BMI, CBC, and liver function test (LFT) checked [5–8]. If there are no abnormalities at baseline, then weight/BMI, CBC, and LFTs should be checked at 6 months and then annually assuming there are no abnormalities [100–103].

Interactions As with all medications, valproate has interactions with other medications. Anticonvulsants, including carbamazepine and lamotrigine, olanzapine, and smoking are not recommended while using valproate or any of its derivatives. Patients that develop signs of blood or liver disorders should seek medical attention immediately [100–103].

Adverse Effects The common adverse effects of valproate are listed in Table 9.4 [100–103]. More serious adverse effects include thrombocytopenia. Reproductive issues in younger adults and suicide. Suicide risk is discussed at the end of the section along with the rest of the AEDs.

9.4.3 Carbamazepine

Carbamazepine is an AED used for acute mania or mixed episodes with bipolar I. Carbamazepine acts on voltage-gated sodium channels leaving them less excitable until the drug dissociates. It also acts as a GABA receptor agonist. Traditionally carbamazepine is utilized for the treatment of seizures; however, significant evidence exists for its use as a mood stabilizer. A systematic review of seven randomized control trials demonstrated therapeutic effects similar to lithium and for trial withdrawal due to adverse effects, number of adverse effects, and improved Global Impression Score (GIS) [110]. No screening tests or regular monitoring is needed before prescribing carbamazepine. The most common adverse effects of carbamazepine are listed in Table 9.4 [100–103]. Unfortunately, due to the need for monitoring blood levels, monitoring for agranulocytosis, and its multiple effects on the CYP-450 system, carbamazepine is infrequently use in older bipolar patients. Its active metabolite oxcarbazepine is easier to use, has less drug interactions, and has no need for monitoring serum levels. Its major liability is hyponatremia.

9.4.4 Lamotrigine

Lamotrigine is an AED utilized for maintenance therapy for individuals diagnosed with bipolar I disorder who are receiving standard therapy. Lamotrigine is a sodium channel blocker that inhibits voltage-sensitive sodium channels resulting in stabilization of neuronal membranes. While lamotrigine is traditionally used for seizures and has an FDA approval for maintenance therapy of bipolar I, there is evidence to support its use in treating hypomania or depressive symptoms of bipolar II. A randomized trial of 102 patients showed no significant differences between lamotrigine and lithium on the Hamilton Depression Rating Scale (HAMD-17) score or the Montgomery Asberg Depression Rating Scale (MADRS) [15]. In post hoc analysis of two other randomized trials, lamotrigine was shown to have a significant effect on weight loss when compared to lithium and placebo for obese patients. There were no weight loss effects for nonobese individuals [16]. The most common adverse effects of lamotrigine are listed in Table 9.4 [100–103].

Screening Before beginning treatment with lamotrigine, individuals should have a CBC, LFTs, BUN level, and electrolytes checked. Rashes are a serious concern and should be monitored closely. Individuals of Asian ancestry should consider screening for *HLA-B1502* to avoid increased risk of Steven-Johnson syndrome (SJS) [100–103].

Treatment Cessation When stopping treatment with lamotrigine, similar to lithium, the medication should not be stopped immediately. Taper off treatment over a 4-week period [100–103].

9.4.5 Suicide Risk with Mood Stabilizers

When evaluating suicide risk, there is mixed evidence from the literature about mood stabilizers. Lithium appears to decrease suicide mortality compared to valproate, but does not decrease the number of suicide attempts when compared to 11 different antiepileptic drugs (AEDs). A retrospective study of greater than 20,000 patients indicates a significant increase in suicide 1.7/1000 life years for valproate vs 0.7/1000 for lithium. Carbamazepine and combo therapies showed no significant differences compared to lithium [17]. However, another cohort study of greater than 47,000 patients indicates that there is no significant difference when comparing AED use to lithium in bipolar patients in terms of suicide attempts. However, there was a decrease in suicide attempts between individuals post AED treatment when compared to pretreatment num-

bers. Lastly, AEDs were shown to be protective against suicide when compared to the group taking no medications [110]. More evidence is needed to confirm the relationship between lithium, AEDS, and suicide.

9.5   Cognitive Enhancers

Currently there are no medications that will reverse or cure cognitive decline. Older adults diagnosed with cognitive decline have options as to possibly slowing the progression of their disease based on clinical presentation and symptomatology. These medications have been used traditionally to treat dementia, which is now classified as major neurocognitive disorder (MNCD).

As with any age group, but specifically older adults, medication adverse effects need to be seriously considered before writing prescriptions. The clinician should discuss the risk and benefits with the patient and family to determine whether benefits of the drug outweigh the possible adverse effects. The main classes and/or drugs under the domain of cognitive enhancers are cholinesterase inhibitors (donepezil, rivastigmine, galantamine), memantine, and herbal therapies (ginkgo biloba and huperzine A). These drugs are focused on delaying or improving function within the realm of cognition, behavior, mood, global function, quality of life, and activities of daily living (ADLs).

9.5.1   Cholinesterase Inhibitors

Cholinesterase inhibitors have been shown to have a benefit for those with mild, moderate, and severe Alzheimer's disease (AD). Cholinesterase inhibitors mechanism of action is through binding and irreversibly inhibiting cholinesterase, which increases the availability of acetylcholine in cholinergic synapses. All cholinesterase inhibitors should be started at the time of diagnosis unless otherwise indicated. As a class, cholinesterase inhibitors have shown overall benefits, improving Mini Mental Status Exam (MMSE) scores and neuropsychiatric inventory (NPI) scores, ADLs, and behavior at 6-month and year-long assessments [111]. Currently, not enough evidence exists to demonstrate superiority among the cholinesterase inhibitors; however, when compared donepezil, rivastigmine, and galantamine show no significant differences in effect on cognition, functioning, or behaviors [111]. Weak evidence indicates that donepezil is associated with fewer adverse effects than oral rivastigmine and galantamine [112].

For all cholinesterase inhibitors, greater benefits have been shown for increased dosing; however, as the dose increases, the number and severity of adverse events increase [113]. The most common adverse effects of cholinesterase inhibitors are nausea, vomiting, and diarrhea [111]. Other studies indicated that cholinesterase inhibitors have also been associated with an increased risk of bradycardia and syncope [114], worsened incontinence [115], and truncal dystonia [116]. The Society of Geriatric Physicians recommends periodic assessment of cholinesterase inhibitors for clinical benefit and possible adverse effects.

After initiation of cholinesterase inhibitors, systematic reviews have shown benefits in continuing cholinesterase inhibitors as opposed to ceasing therapy. Upon stopping cholinesterase inhibitors in five separate trials, the patients experienced worsening neuropsychiatric and cognitive function [117].

Donepezil Donepezil is a centrally acting cholinesterase inhibitor, which is dosed depending on the severity of the diagnosis. See Table 9.1 for all cholinesterase inhibitor dosing. Individual trials and systematic reviews have shown benefits in cognition, functioning, and behavior with the use of donepezil with benefits in quality of life, health resource use, and associated costs [111]. At 10 mg per day dosing, donepezil was effective in improving MMSE and Bristol Activities of Daily Living score (BADL-S) at 52 weeks even after progression to moderate or severe AD [118].

While donepezil has its benefits and may slow the progression of AD, studies have demonstrated that institutionalization or progression of the dis-

ease is unaffected compared to no medication usage at 3 years [119].

Rivastigmine Rivastigmine is a centrally acting cholinesterase inhibitor, which is dosed depending on the severity of the diagnosis. Two routes exist for rivastigmine dosing, oral and transdermal. Regardless of the dose or route of administration, rivastigmine demonstrated lower rates of deterioration on measures of global impression in seven different trials. At lower doses (1–4 mg), patients showed improvements in cognition, but not ADLs. At higher doses (6–12 mg), patients showed improvements in ADLs and cognition, although not surprisingly the patients suffered worse adverse events compared to placebo. While there were differences in effect based on the dosing, the route of administration (patch vs capsules) showed no differences in cognition, behavior, and ADLs when compared to high-dose rivastigmine; however, the transdermal route produced fewer adverse effects [120, 121].

Galantamine Galantamine is a centrally acting cholinesterase inhibitor, which is dosed depending on the severity of the diagnosis. Two formulations exist for galantamine dosing, immediate and extended release. Both have similar effects just at different dosages. If treatment is stopped for any reason for longer than 3 days, then the dosing regimen should be restated with the lowest dose. See Table 9.1 for all cholinesterase inhibitor dosing. At higher doses, 16–24 mg/day galantamine improved global impression score, cognitive function [1], and impairment scores, but not in ADLs [122].

Tacrine For completeness sake, tacrine will be mentioned in this chapter, but it is no longer on the market within the United States as of 2012 due to hepatotoxicity. Tacrine is associated with decreased cognitive decline and improved global impression scores over the first 3 months of usage [123] (Tables 9.5 and 9.6).

Memantine Another drug used for the treatment of MNCD is memantine, which is an NMDA receptor antagonist that impacts the glutamater-

Table 9.5 Dosing for cognitive enhancers

	Donepezil	Rivastigmine oral	Rivastigmine transdermal	Galantamine ER	Galantamine IR	Memantine XR	Memantine
Starting dose	5 mg; increase to 10mg at 4-6 weeks; increase to 23 mg at 3 months or later, if needed	1.5 mg twice daily; increase by 1.5 mg twice daily at 2 weeks intervals up to 12 mg twice daily	4.6 mg; increase to 9.5 mg/day at 4 weeks; increase to 13.3 mg 4 weeks later if indicated	8 mg am; increase to 16 mg am at 4 weeks; increase to 24 mg at 8 weeks or later, if needed	4 mg twice daily; increase to 8 mg twice daily at 4 weeks; increase to 12 mg twice daily at 8 weeks or later, if needed	7 mg daily; increase by 7 mg/week up to 28 mg/day	5 mg; increase by 5 mg/week to 20 mg/day
Mild	5–10 mg/day	3–6 mg BID	9.5 mg/day	Titrate according to adverse effects	Titrate according to adverse effects	Not used for mild disease	Not used for mild disease
Moderate	5–10 mg/day or 10–23	3–6 mg BID	9.5 mg/day	Titrate according to adverse effects	Titrate according to adverse effects	7–28 mg/day	5–20 mg/day
Severe[a]	10–23 mg/day	9–12 mg BID	Up to 13.3 mg/day	Titrate according to adverse effects	Titrate according to adverse effects	7–28 mg/day	5–20 mg/day

[a]Take medications as tolerated due to increased adverse effect profile at higher doses [111]

Table 9.6 Adverse effects of cognitive enhancers

	Donepezil	Rivastigmine	Galantamine	Memantine
Nausea	X	X	X	
Vomiting	X	X	X	X
Diarrhea	X	X	X	X
Muscle cramps	X[a]			
Fatigue	X[a]			
Headache	X	X	X	X
Insomnia	X			
Any GI complication	X	X	X	X
Dizziness	X	X		X
Confusion			X	X

[a]Adverse effects worsen as dose increases [111, 124]

gic system. Dosing regimens for memantine can be seen in Table 9.5. In six different controlled trials, memantine showed benefits for cognition, ADLs, and behavior in comparison to placebo for individuals with moderate-severe AD. Although effective for moderate-severe AD, memantine may have decreased effectiveness for individuals with mild AD [125].

One double-blind, placebo-controlled trial utilizing the MMSE and BADL-S tools did not demonstrate a significant difference in the use of memantine or memantine plus donepezil for individuals who have progressed to moderate or severe dementia [8]. However, another randomized control trial showed benefits of adding memantine 10 mg to donepezil on ADLs and the severe impairment battery (SIB) scale [126]. Currently, there is not enough data to support the additive effects of memantine and cholinesterase inhibitors for individuals with mild AD. However, adding memantine to a cholinesterase inhibitor has been shown to delay time to nursing home admissions at 2.5 years when compared to cho-linesterase inhibitors alone and individuals on no medications [127].

Other Medications and Herbal Remedies Along with the traditional treatments for MNCDs, other remedies have been tried mainly focusing on cognitive function. First, based on Cochrane reviews of statins [128] and omega-3 fatty acids [129], there is no existing evidence to support the use of these substances for prevention or treatment of AD or vascular dementia. These agents have not been researched in the treatment of other types of MNCD in any substantial trials. Along with statins and omega-3 fatty acids, there is limited to no evidence to support the use of vitamins for prevention or treatment of AD. Research has been done into the effect of various vitamins (B6, B12, folic acid, and E). Based on Cochrane reviews, limited to no evidence supports the use of vitamins B6 [130], B12 [131], and folic acid [132]. High-dose vita-min supplementation (folic acid, B6, and B12) compared to placebo was shown to have no effect on cognition or ADLs but increased depression-related adverse events [133].

While high-dose vitamin supplementation (folic acid, B6, and B12) did not prove to have desired benefits, a randomized control trial evalu-ating the effects of vitamin E on AD showed promising results. At 2000 IU of vitamin E, indi-viduals with mild to moderate AD had slower functional cognitive decline as tested by the Alzheimer's Disease Cooperative Study/ Activities of Daily Living (ADCS-ADL) Inventory score. Over the 2-year follow-up, the ADCS-ADL scores declined by 3.15 units more in the placebo group compared to the vitamin E group; therefore, vitamin E can be utilized in dosages of 2000 IU to treat mild to moderate AD. However, when vitamin E was used in con-junction with memantine, there was no statistical significance in ADCS-ADL scores when com-pared to placebo [134].

Other over-the-counter herbal remedies that have been researched are *Ginkgo biloba* and huperzine A. For *Ginkgo*, there is mixed evi-dence with no conclusive results on its effects on cognition. Based on 3 systematic reviews of 36 randomized trials with multiple methodolog-ical flaws, there is evidence that ginkgo in doses greater than 200 mg may show improvements in clinical global impression (CGI) scores and ADLs at 6 months. At any dose *Ginkgo* was associated with improved cognition at 3 months but not 6 months [135, 136]. Huperzine A has a similar mechanism of action as cholinesterase inhibitors and is derived from Chinese Club Moss. Recommended dosing is 0.2–0.8 mg twice daily. Huperzine A compared to placebo showed improvements in MMSE and ADLs; however, when compared to trials with galan-tamine and donepezil, there were no significant differences shown in MMSE, ADLs, or adverse effects [137]. With the exception of vitamin E, more research is needed in order to make any recommendations for use in treatment of MNCD.

9.6 Conclusion

Treating mental illness in older adults is a chal-lenging yet necessary endeavor that merits careful decision-making. Whether it is insom-nia or depression, serious psychiatric ailments in older adults often compound co-occurring diseases and increase overall morbidity. The physiologic changes associated with aging, including differences in drug absorption, metabolism, and excretion, also change the side effect profile compared to the adult popu-lation and further complicate treatment. Although it may appear difficult, it is impor-tant that the physician is willing to learn and adapt according to the patient's presentation and response to treatment, and diligence must be practiced to avoid all harmful medicine effects. Overall, patience and persistence are important characteristics of any physician treating mental health in older adults, and the information presented in this chapter is a good basis from which to expand as more research and data is collected.

References

1. Kamel NS, Gammack JK. Insomnia in the elderly: cause, approach, and treatment. Am J Med. 2006;119(6):463–9.
2. Fiske A, Wetherell JL, Gatz M. Depression in older adults. Annu Rev Clin Psychol. 2009;5:363–89.
3. Gallager DW. Benzodiazepines: potentiation of a GABA inhibitory response in the dorsal raphe nucleus. Eur J Pharmacol. 1978;49(2):133–43.
4. Young AB, Chu D. Distribution of GABAA and GABAB receptors in mammalian brain: potential targets for drug development. Drug Dev Res. 1990;21(3):161–7.
5. Ogu CC, Maxa JL. Drug interactions due to cytochrome P450. Proc (Bayl Univ Med Cent). 2000;13(4):421–3.
6. Gudin JA, et al. Risks, management, and monitoring of combination opioid, benzodiazepines, and/or alcohol use. Postgrad Med. 2013;125(4):115–30.
7. Greenblatt DJ, Shader RI. Effects of age and other drugs on benzodiazepine kinetics. Arzneimittelforschung. 1980;30(5):886–90.
8. Griffin CE, et al. Benzodiazepine pharmacology and central nervous system–mediated effects. Ochsner J. 2013;13(2):214–23.
9. Treatment of benzodiazepine overdose with flumazenil. The Flumazenil in Benzodiazepine Intoxication Multicenter Study Group. Clin Ther. 1992;14(6):978–85.
10. Sheikh JI. Anxiolytics, sedatives, and older patients. Prim Psychiatry. 2004;11(8):51–4.
11. Eison AS, Temple DL Jr. Buspirone: review of its pharmacology and current perspectives on its mechanism of action. Am J Med. 1986;80(3B):1–9.
12. Taylor CP. Mechanisms of action of gabapentin. Rev Neurol. 1997;153(1):S39–45.
13. American Geriatrics Society 2015 Beers Criteria Update Expert Panel. American Geriatrics Society 2015 updated Beers Criteria for potentially inappropriate medication use in older adults. J Am Geriatr Soc. 2015;63(11):2227–46.
14. Llorca PM, Spadone C, Sol O, Danniau A, Corruble E, Faruch M, Macher JP, Sermet E, Servant D. Efficacy and safety of hydroxyzine in the treatment of generalized anxiety disorder: a 3-month double-blind study. J Clin Psychiatry. 2002;63(11):1020–7.
15. Schram WS. Use of hydroxyzine in psychosis. Dis Nerv Syst. 1959;20(3):126–9.
16. Zammit GK. Ramelteon: a novel hypnotic indicated for the treatment of insomnia. Psychiatry (Edgmont). 2007;4(9):36–42.
17. Sanger DJ. The pharmacology and mechanisms of action of new generation, non-benzodiazepine hypnotic agents. CNS Drugs. 2004;18(1):9–15.
18. Vermeeren A. Residual effects of hypnotics: epidemiology and clinical implications. CNS Drugs. 2004;18(5):297–328.
19. Frecska E. Trazodone-its multifunctional mechanism of action and clinical use. Neuropsychopharmacol Hung. 2010;12(4):477–82.
20. Flint AJ. Generalised anxiety disorder in elderly patients: epidemiology, diagnosis and treatment options. Drugs Aging. 2005;22(2):101–14.
21. Pachana NA, Woodward RM, Byrne GJA. Treatment of specific phobia in older adults. Clin Interv Aging. 2007;2(3):469–76.
22. Flint AJ, Gagnon N. Diagnosis and management of panic disorder in older patients. Drugs Aging. 2003;20(12):881–91.
23. Weintraub D, Ruskin PE. Posttraumatic stress disorder in the elderly: a review. Harv Rev Psychiatry. 1999;7(3):144–52.
24. Jackson CW. Obsessive-compulsive disorder in elderly patients. Drugs Aging. 1995;7(6):438–48.
25. Kamel NS, et al. Insomnia in the elderly: cause, approach, and treatment. Am J Med. 2006;119(6):463–9.
26. Gill SS, et al. Antipsychotic drug use and mortality in older adults with dementia. Ann Intern Med. 2007;146(11):775–86.
27. Kales HC, et al. Mortality risk in patients with dementia treated with antipsychotics versus other psychiatric medications. Am J Psychiatry. 2007;164(10):1568–76.
28. Masand PS. Side effects of antipsychotics in the elderly. J Clin Psychiatry. 2000;61(Suppl 8):43–9.
29. Leipzig RM, Cumming RG, Tinetti ME. Drugs and falls in older people: a systematic review and meta-analysis: II. Cardiac and analgesic drugs. J Am Geriatr Soc. 1999;47(1):40–50.
30. Leucht S, et al. Efficacy and extrapyramidal side-effects of the new antipsychotics olanzapine, quetiapine, risperidone, and sertindole compared to conventional antipsychotics and placebo. A meta-analysis of randomized controlled trials. Schizophr Res. 1999;35(1):51–68.
31. Prevost P, et al. Hypersensitivity syndrome with olanzapine confirmed by patch tests. Eur J Dermatol. 2012;22(1):126–7.
32. Wooltorton E. Olanzapine (Zyprexa): increased incidence of cerebrovascular events in dementia trials. Can Med Assoc J. 2004;170(9):1395.
33. Ereshefsky L. Pharmacokinetics and drug interactions: update for new antipsychotics. J Clin Psychiatry. 1996;57:12–25.
34. Katz IR, et al. Comparison of risperidone and placebo for psychosis and behavioral disturbances associated with dementia: a randomized, double-blind trial. J Clin Psychiatry. 1999;60(2):107–15.
35. Yu F. Behavioral management in long-term care. Enc Adulthood and Aging. 2016. https://doi.org/10.1002/9781118521373.wbeaa098.
36. Boettger S, Jenewein J, Breitbart W. Haloperidol, risperidone, olanzapine and aripiprazole in the management of delirium: a comparison of efficacy, safety, and side effects. Palliat Support Care. 2015;13(4):1079–85.

37. Hahn M, Sylvia Gomes S, Remington GJ. Low-dose, off-label quetiapine use, metabolic syndrome and impaired fasting glucose in an elderly man: a case report. Brain Disord Ther. 2015;4:149.
38. Vieta E, et al. Quetiapine in the treatment of acute mania: target dose for efficacious treatment. J Affect Disord. 2007;100:S23–31.
39. Maher AR, et al. Efficacy and comparative effectiveness of atypical antipsychotic medications for off-label uses in adults: a systematic review and meta-analysis. JAMA. 2011;306(12):1359–69.
40. Garver DL. Review of quetiapine side effects. J Clin Psychiatry. 2000;61:31.
41. Kennedy WK, Jann MW, Kutscher EC. Clinically significant drug interactions with atypical antipsychotics. CNS Drugs. 2013;27(12):1021–48.
42. Guay D. Comment on the potential utility of the new atypical antipsychotic lurasidone in the geriatric population. Consult Pharm. 2011;26(8):579–82.
43. Mattingly G, Anderson R. Cariprazine for schizophrenia and bipolar I disorder: as a dopamine D3-preferring D3/D2 partial agonist, cariprazine offers an alternative to antipsychotics that preferentially modulate D2 receptors. Curr Psychiatr Ther. 2016;15(2):34.
44. Gum AM, King-Kallimanis B, Kohn R. Prevalence of mood, anxiety, and substance-abuse disorders for older Americans in the national comorbidity survey-replication. Am J Geriatr Psychiatry. 2009;9:769–81.
45. Tomeno W, Kawashima K, Yoneda M, et al. Nonalcoholic fatty liver disease comorbid with major depressive disorder: the pathological features and poor therapeutic efficacy. J Gastroenterol Hepatol. 2015;30(6):1009–14.
46. Conwell Y, Thompson C. Suicidal behavior in elders. Psychiatr Clin North Am. 2008;2:333–56.
47. Carney RM, Freedland KE. Depression, mortality, and medical morbidity in patients with coronary heart disease. Biol Psychiatry. 2003;3:241–7.
48. Kao LT, Liu SP, Lin HC, Lee HC, Tsai MC, Chung SD. Poor clinical outcomes among pneumonia patients with depressive disorder. PLoS One. 2014;9(12):e116436.
49. Mottram P, Wilson K, Strobl J. Antidepressants for depressed elderly. Cochrane Database Syst Rev. 2006;1:CD003491.
50. Gelenberg AJ, et al. Practice guideline for the treatment of patients with major depressive disorder. Washington, DC: American Psychiatric Association; 2010.
51. Wilson K, et al. Antidepressant versus placebo for depressed elderly. Cochrane Database Syst Rev. 2001;2:CD000561.
52. Hedayati SS, Yalamanchili V, Finkelstein FO. A practical approach to the treatment of depression in patients with chronic kidney disease and end-stage renal disease. Kidney Int. 2011;3:247–55.
53. Mauri MC, et al. Pharmacokinetics of antidepressants in patients with hepatic impairment. Clin Pharmacokinet. 2014;12:1069–81.
54. Wells KB, Golding JM, Burnam MA. Psychiatric disorder in a sample of the general population with and without chronic medical conditions. Am J Psychiatry. 1988;8:976–81.
55. Bains J, Birks J, Dening T. Antidepressants for treating depression in dementia. Cochrane Database Syst Rev. 2002;(4):CD003944.
56. Tsai MC, et al. One-year mortality of elderly inpatients with delirium, dementia, or depression seen by a consultation-liaison service. Psychosomatics. 2012;5:433–8.
57. Thanacoody HK, Thomas SH. Tricyclic antidepressant poisoning: cardiovascular toxicity. Toxicol Rev. 2005;3:205–14.
58. Taylor CB, et al. Effects of antidepressant medication on morbidity and mortality in depressed patients after myocardial infarction. Arch Gen Psychiatry. 2005;7:792–8.
59. Thase ME. Effects of venlafaxine on blood pressure: a meta-analysis of original data from 3744 depressed patients. J Clin Psychiatry. 1998;10:502–8.
60. Zimmermann U, et al. Epidemiology, implications and mechanisms underlying drug-induced weight gain in psychiatric patients. J Psychiatr Res. 2003;37(3):193–220.
61. Lustman PJ, et al. Effects of nortriptyline on depression and glycemic control in diabetes: results of a double-blind, placebo-controlled trial. Psychosom Med. 1997;59(3):241–50.
62. Lu B, Budhiraja R, Parthasarathy S. Sedating medications and undiagnosed obstructive sleep apnea: physician determinants and patient consequences. J Clin Sleep Med. 2005;4:367–71.
63. Merck & Co., Inc. Remeron tablets: prescribing information. http://www.fda.gov/Drugs/default.htm. 2016.
64. Mylan Pharmaceuticals Inc. Amitriptyline tablets: prescribing information. http://www.fda.gov/Drugs/default.htm. 2016.
65. Labopharm Europe Limited. Oleptro XR tablets: prescribing information. http://www.fda.gov/Drugs/default.htm. 2010.
66. Papakostas GI, Homberger CH, Fava M. A meta-analysis of clinical trials comparing mirtazapine with selective serotonin reuptake inhibitors for the treatment of major depressive disorder. J Psychopharmacol. 2008;8:843–8.
67. Gartlehner G, et al. Comparative benefits and harms of second-generation antidepressants: background paper for the American College of Physicians. Ann Intern Med. 2008;10:734–50.
68. Davis R, Wilde MI. Mirtazapine : a review of its pharmacology and therapeutic potential in the management of major depression. CNS Drugs. 1996;5:389–402.
69. Thase ME, et al. Remission rates following antidepressant therapy with bupropion or selective serotonin reuptake inhibitors: a meta-analysis of original data from 7 randomized controlled trials. J Clin Psychiatry. 2005;8:974–81.

70. Croft H, et al. Effect on body weight of bupropion sustained-release in patients with major depression treated for 52 weeks. Clin Ther. 2002;4:662–72.

71. Krebs EE, et al. Treating the physical symptoms of depression with second-generation antidepressants: a systematic review and metaanalysis. Psychosomatics. 2008;49(3):191–8.

72. Saarto T, Wiffen PJ. Antidepressants for neuropathic pain: a Cochrane review. J Neurol Neurosurg Psychiatry. 2010;12:1372–3.

73. Carville SF, et al. EULAR evidence-based recommendations for the management of fibromyalgia syndrome. Ann Rheum Dis. 2007;4:536–41.

74. Rampello L, et al. Evaluation of the prophylactic efficacy of amitriptyline and citalopram, alone or in combination, in patients with comorbidity of depression, migraine, and tension-type headache. Neuropsychobiology. 2004;4:322–8.

75. Schneider LS, et al. An 8-week multicenter, parallel-group, double-blind, placebo-controlled study of sertraline in elderly outpatients with major depression. Am J Psychiatry. 2003;7:1277–85.

76. Anderson IM. Selective serotonin reuptake inhibitors versus tricyclic antidepressants: a meta-analysis of efficacy and tolerability. J Affect Disord. 2000;1:19–36.

77. American Geriatrics Society 2012 Beers Criteria Update Expert Panel. American Geriatrics Society updated Beers Criteria for potentially inappropriate medication use in older adults. J Am Geriatr Soc. 2012;60(4):616–31.

78. Malach F, Wilson K. Canadian Coalition for Seniors' Mental Health 2nd National Conference. Aging Health. 2007;3(6):707–10.

79. Sandson NB, Armstrong SC, Cozza KL. An overview of psychotropic drug-drug interactions. Psychosomatics. 2005;46(5):464–94.

80. Fabian TJ, et al. Paroxetine-induced hyponatremia in older adults: a 12-week prospective study. Arch Intern Med. 2004;2004(3):327–32.

81. Kirby D, Harrigan S, Ames D. Hyponatraemia in elderly psychiatric patients treated with Selective Serotonin Reuptake Inhibitors and venlafaxine: a retrospective controlled study in an inpatient unit. Int J Geriatr Psychiatry. 2002;3:231–7.

82. Thapa PB, et al. Antidepressants and the risk of falls among nursing home residents. N Engl J Med. 1998;13:875–82.

83. Arfken CL, Wilson JG, Aronson SM. Retrospective review of selective serotonin reuptake inhibitors and falling in older nursing home residents. Int Psychogeriatr. 2001;1:85–91.

84. Prieto-Alhambra D, et al. Excess risk of hip fractures attributable to the use of antidepressants in five European countries and the USA. Osteoporos Int. 2014;3:847–55.

85. Rabenda V, et al. Relationship between use of antidepressants and risk of fractures: a meta-analysis. Osteoporos Int. 2012;1:121–37.

86. Coupland C, et al. Antidepressant use and risk of adverse outcomes in older people: population based cohort study. BMJ. 2011;343:d4551.

87. Miller MD, et al. Long-term ECG changes in depressed elderly patients treated with nortriptyline. A double-blind, randomized, placebo-controlled evaluation. Am J Geriatr Psychiatry. 1998;1:59–66.

88. Pfizer Inc. Nardil tablets: prescribing information. http://www.fda.gov/Drugs/default.htm. 2009.

89. Papakostas GI, et al. Resolution of sleepiness and fatigue in major depressive disorder: a comparison of bupropion and the selective serotonin reuptake inhibitors. Biol Psychiatry. 2006;12:1350–5.

90. Fava M, et al. 15 years of clinical experience with bupropion HCl: from bupropion to bupropion SR to bupropion XL. Prim Care Companion J Clin Psychiatry. 2005;3:106–13.

91. Cunningham LA, et al. A comparison of venlafaxine, trazodone, and placebo in major depression. J Clin Psychopharmacol. 1994;2:99–9106.

92. Thompson JW, Ware MR, Blashfield RK. Psychotropic medication and priapism: a comprehensive review. J Clin Psychiatry. 1990;1990(10):430–3.

93. Mendelson WB. A review of the evidence for the efficacy and safety of trazodone in insomnia. J Clin Psychiatry. 2005;4:469–76.

94. Zarate CA, et al. A randomized trial of an N-methyl-D-aspartate antagonist in treatment-resistant major depression. Arch Gen Psychiatry. 2006;8:856–64.

95. Deardorff WJ, Grossberg GT. A review of the clinical efficacy, safety and tolerability of the antidepressants vilazodone, levomilnacipran and vortioxetine. Expert Opin Pharmacother. 2014;17:2525–42.

96. US Food and Drug Administration, FDA Drug Safety Communication: abnormal heart rhythms associated with high doses of Celexa (citalopram hydrobromide) (August 24, 2011). http://www.fda.gov.ezp.slu.edu/Drugs/DrugSafety/ucm269086.htm. Accessed 12 Feb 2012.

97. Poolsup N, Li Wan Po A, de Oliveira IR. Systematic overview of lithium treatment in acute mania. J Clin Pharm Ther. 2000;25:139–56.

98. Bowden CL, Brugger AM, Swann AC, Calabrese JR, et al. Efficacy of divalproex vs lithium and placebo in the treatment of mania. The Depakote Mania Study Group. JAMA. 1994;271:918–24.

99. Shafti SS. Olanzapine vs. lithium in management of acute mania. J Affect Disord. 2010;122:273–6.

100. Price AL, Marzani-Nissen GR. Bipolar disorders: a review. Am Fam Physician. 2012;85:483–93.

101. Mohammad O, Osser DN. The psychopharmacology algorithm project at the Harvard South Shore Program: an algorithm for acute mania. Harv Rev Psychiatry. 2014;22:274–94.

102. Yatham LN, Kennedy SH, Parikh SV, Schaffer A, et al. Canadian Network for Mood and Anxiety Treatments (CANMAT) and International Society for Bipolar Disorders (ISBD) collaborative update of CANMAT guidelines for the management of

patients with bipolar disorder: update 2013. Bipolar Disord. 2013;15:1–44.

103. Grande I, Berk M, Birmaher B, Vieta E. Bipolar disorder. Lancet. 2016;387:1561–72.

104. Abou-Khalil BW. Making sense of lamotrigine serum levels. Epilepsy Curr. 2005;5:115.

105. Shine B, McKnight RF, Leaver L, Geddes JR. Long-term effects of lithium on renal, thyroid, and parathyroid function: a retrospective analysis of laboratory data. Lancet. 2015;386:461–8.

106. Bocchetta A, Ardau R, Fanni T, Sardu C, et al. Renal function during long-term lithium treatment: a cross-sectional and longitudinal study. BMC Med. 2015;13:12.

107. Viguera AC, Nonacs R, Cohen LS, Tondo L, Murray A, Baldessarini RJ, Baldessarini RJ. Risk of recurrence of bipolar disorder in pregnant and nonpregnant women after discontinuing lithium maintenance. Am J Psychiatry. 2000;157:179–84.

108. Macritchie K, Geddes JR, Scott J, Haslam D, de Lima M, Goodwin G. Valproate for acute mood episodes in bipolar disorder. Cochrane Database Syst Rev. 2003;(1):CD004052.

109. McElroy SL, Martens BE, Creech RS, Welge JA, et al. Randomized, double-blind, placebo-controlled study of divalproex extended release loading monotherapy in ambulatory bipolar spectrum disorder patients with moderate-to-severe hypomania or mild mania. J Clin Psychiatry. 2010;71:557–65.

110. Gibbons RD, Hur K, Brown CH, Mann JJ. Relationship between antiepileptic drugs and suicide attempts in patients with bipolar disorder. Arch Gen Psychiatry. 2009;66:1354–60.

111. Birks J. Cholinesterase inhibitors for Alzheimer's disease. Cochrane Database Syst Rev. 2006;(1):CD005593.

112. Lockhart IA, Mitchell SA, Kelly S. Safety and tolerability of donepezil, rivastigmine and galantamine for patients with Alzheimer's disease: systematic review of the 'real-world' evidence. Dement Geriatr Cogn Disord. 2009;28:389–403.

113. Wang J, Yu JT, Wang HF, et al. Pharmacological treatment of neuropsychiatric symptoms in Alzheimer's disease: a systematic review and meta-analysis. J Neurol Neurosurg Psychiatry. 2015;86:101–9.

114. Kim DH, Brown RT, Ding EL, Kiel DP, Berry SD. Dementia medications and risk of falls, syncope, and related adverse events: meta-analysis of randomized controlled trials. J Am Geriatr Soc. 2011;59:1019–31.

115. Starr JM. Cholinesterase inhibitor treatment and urinary incontinence in Alzheimer's disease. J Am Geriatr Soc. 2007;55:800–1.

116. Sink KM, Thomas J 3rd, Xu H, Craig B, Kritchevsky S, Kritchevsky S, Sands LP. Dual use of bladder anticholinergics and cholinesterase inhibitors: long-term functional and cognitive outcomes. J Am Geriatr Soc. 2008;56:847–53.

117. O'Regan J, Lanctot KL, Mazereeuw G, Herrmann N. Cholinesterase inhibitor discontinuation in patients with Alzheimer's disease: a meta-analysis of randomized controlled trials. J Clin Psychiatry. 2015;76:e1424–31.

118. Howard R, McShane R, Lindesay J, Ritchie C, et al. Donepezil and memantine for moderate-to-severe Alzheimer's disease. N Engl J Med. 2012;366:893–903.

119. Courtney C, Farrell D, Gray R, Hills R, et al. Long-term donepezil treatment in 565 patients with Alzheimer's disease (AD2000): randomised double-blind trial. Lancet. 2004;363:2105–15.

120. Birks JS, Chong LY, Grimley Evans J. Rivastigmine for Alzheimer's disease. Cochrane Database Syst Rev. 2015;(4):CD001191.

121. Winblad B, Cummings J, Andreasen N, Grossberg G, et al. A six-month double-blind, randomized, placebo-controlled study of a transdermal patch in Alzheimer's disease—rivastigmine patch versus capsule. Int J Geriatr Psychiatry. 2007;22:456–67.

122. Burns A, Bernabei R, Bullock R, Cruz Jentoft AJ, et al. Safety and efficacy of galantamine (Reminyl) in severe Alzheimer's disease (the SERAD study): a randomised, placebo-controlled, double-blind trial. Lancet Neurol. 2009;8:39–47.

123. Qizilbash N, Whitehead A, Higgins J, Wilcock G, Schneider L, Farlow M. Cholinesterase inhibition for Alzheimer disease: a meta-analysis of the tacrine trials. Dementia Trialists' Collaboration. JAMA. 1998;280:1777–82.

124. Dunn NR, Pearce GL, Shakir SA. Adverse effects associated with the use of donepezil in general practice in England. J Psychopharmacol. 2000;14:406–8.

125. McShane R, Areosa Sastre A, Minakaran N. Memantine for dementia. Cochrane Database Syst Rev. 2006;(2):CD003154.

126. Tariot PN, Farlow MR, Grossberg GT, Graham SM, McDonald S, Gergel I. Memantine treatment in patients with moderate to severe Alzheimer disease already receiving donepezil: a randomized controlled trial. JAMA. 2004;291:317–24.

127. Lopez OL, Becker JT, Wahed AS, Saxton J, et al. Long-term effects of the concomitant use of memantine with cholinesterase inhibition in Alzheimer disease. J Neurol Neurosurg Psychiatry. 2009;80:600–7.

128. McGuinness B, Craig D, Bullock R, Malouf R, Passmore P. Statins for the treatment of dementia. Cochrane Database Syst Rev. 2010;(8):CD007514.

129. Burckhardt M, Herke M, Wustmann T, Watzke S, Langer G, Fink A. Omega-3 fatty acids for the treatment of dementia. Cochrane Database Syst Rev. 2016;4:CD009002.

130. Malouf R, Grimley Evans J. The effect of vitamin B6 on cognition. Cochrane Database Syst Rev. 2003;(4):CD004393.

131. Malouf R, Areosa Sastre A. Vitamin B12 for cognition. Cochrane Database Syst Rev. 2003;(3):CD004326.

132. Malouf R, Grimley Evans J. Folic acid with or without vitamin B12 for the prevention and treatment

of healthy elderly and demented people. Cochrane Database Syst Rev. 2008;(4):CD004514.

133. Aisen PS, Schneider LS, Sano M, Sano M, Diaz-Arrastia R, et al. High-dose B vitamin supplementation and cognitive decline in Alzheimer disease: a randomized controlled trial. JAMA. 2008;300:1774–83.

134. Dysken MW, Sano M, Asthana S, et al. Effect of vitamin E and memantine on functional decline in Alzheimer disease: the TEAM-AD VA cooperative randomized trial. JAMA. 2014;311:33–44.

135. Birks J, Grimley Evans J. Ginkgo biloba for cognitive impairment and dementia. Cochrane Database Syst Rev. 2007;(2):CD003120.

136. Weinmann S, Roll S, Schwarzbach C, Vauth C, Willich SN. Effects of Ginkgo biloba in dementia: systematic review and meta-analysis. BMC Geriatr. 2010;10:14.

137. Yang G, Wang Y, Tian J, Liu J-P. Huperzine A for Alzheimer's disease: a systematic review and meta-analysis of randomized clinical trials. PLoS One. 2013;8:e74916.

Psychological Interventions in Older Adults

10

Todd M. Edwards, Anthony Dowell, David Clarke, Vinodkumar R. Gangolli, and Jo Ellen Patterson

Abstract

As older adults grow increasingly dependent on their adult children, family roles shift, and multiple unfamiliar demands are placed on caregivers, which puts older adults and caregivers at increased risk for mental illness. When older adults are able to overcome barriers to accessing mental health services (e.g. stigma), psychological therapies are effective when used on their own or in combination with psychotropic medication. This chapter describes a variety of psychological therapies for older adults coping with depression, anxiety, dementia/cognitively impaired disorders, and personality disorders. In addition, numerous resources are offered to help older adults and their family members clarify the necessary changes that must be made to cope with losses and preserve meaning and hope. The chapter highlights several ways to deliver care, including upskilling of existing primary care staff, stepped care, collaborative care, and referral to a mental health specialist in the community.

T. M. Edwards (✉) · J. E. Patterson
Marital and Family Therapy Program,
University of San Diego, San Diego, CA, USA
e-mail: tedwards@sandiego.edu;
joellen@SanDiego.edu

A. Dowell
Obstetrics and Gynecology, University of Otago
Wellington University of Otago,
Wellington, New Zealand
e-mail: tony.dowell@otago.ac.nz

D. Clarke
Center for Ethics, Oregon Health & Science
University, Portland, OR, USA

Gastroenterology, Oregon Health & Science
University, Portland, OR, USA
e-mail: DrDave@stressillness.com

V. R. Gangolli
Masina Hospital, Mumbai, India

Grand River Hospital, Kitchener, ON, Canada

Department of Psychiatry and Neuro-Behavioral
Sciences, McMaster's University,
Hamilton, ON, Canada

Key Points
- The combination of extended years of shifting roles in families as older adults gradually grow increasingly dependent on their adult children and the multiplying demands on caregivers suggests that both older adult family members and caregivers will be at increased risk for depression and anxiety.
- When older adults are able to overcome barriers to accessing mental health services (e.g., stigma), psychological therapies are effective when used on their own or in combination with psychotropic medication in older adults who

suffer from common disorders, such as depression, anxiety, dementia/cognitively impaired disorders, and personality disorders.

- Psychological intervention for bodily distress syndrome in older adults is based on accurate assessment of the underlying psychosocial issues, which are often not evident to the patient or present in the medical record.
- The psychological treatment of dementia/cognitively impaired disorder is specifically focused on specific targets, which include global quality of life, affective states, disruptive behavioral symptoms, functional impairment, and prevention of self-harm.
- Numerous resources exist to help older adults and their family members clarify the necessary changes that must be made to keep the losses in their place and protect other sources of meaning and hope.
- Psychological therapy for older adults can be delivered in a variety of ways. These include upskilling of existing primary care staff to provide psychological interventions: stepped care, collaborative care, and referral to a mental health specialist in the community.

10.1 Introduction

The afternoon of human life must also have a significance of its own and cannot merely be understood as a pitiful appendage to life's morning.—Carl Jung

Between 2015 and 2050, the proportion of the world's population over 60 years will nearly double, from 12% to 22%. Identifying and implementing effective, community-level psychological interventions for older adults are essential. To date, mental health problems of older adults have been under-identified by healthcare professionals, family members, and patients themselves. The stigma surrounding mental illness contributes to older adults' reluctance to seek help. When older adults do seek help, there is evidence that a variety of psychosocial interventions are effective in alleviating distress for the patient and family [1].

A chapter on psychological interventions for older adults can never capture all of the salient issues for older adult patients and their family members. We have chosen to address treatments for common presentations in primary care, including depression, anxiety, and bodily distress syndrome, and secondary care, including dementia and personality disorders. We also discuss the universal experience of loss. Although we do not address preventive programs, it is important to note that there are many strategies to promote mental health well-being, including adequate housing, social support for older adults coping with illness and their caregivers, and education to prevent elder abuse, among others.

10.2 General Considerations

Ageism and generational values, both on the part of the service user, the practitioner and society in general, can be major barriers to a good therapeutic outcome. Ageism may be expressed as beliefs such as "too old to change," which may prevent older adults from seeking help or getting referred for help and also reduces expectations about therapy outcomes. Patients may feel that they do not deserve psychological therapy and it should be reserved for those who are younger. However, many older adults express a preference for a talking treatment [2].

When older adults do get referred and participate in therapy, age-specific adaptations of standard therapy procedures are advisable. For example, the pace of therapy should be slower, and fonts for written material should be larger. Providing memory aids such as handouts and session summaries also can be very helpful. Accounting for unique cohort-based differences (e.g., sociohistorical environment, norms and commonly held beliefs, role expectations, illness beliefs, culture) and age-specific stressors (e.g., chronic illness and disability, loss of loved ones and, consequently, sources of support, caregiving responsibilities) is also advisable. In-home mental health services may be a valuable option for those who lack reliable transportation and/or have a medical or physical disability.

Most empirical evidence has shown some effectiveness of psychological therapies when used alone or in combination with psychotropic medication in older adults who suffer from common disorders such as depression, anxiety, dementia/cognitively impaired disorders, and personality disorders. Generally, there are two types of psychotherapies: (1) those used in adults which are modified for use in older patients, most prominent among them are cognitive behavioral therapy (CBT), problem-solving therapy (PST), dialectical behavior therapy (DBT), interpersonal therapy (IPT), and family therapy; and (2) those devised specifically for older adults which include psychosocial, behavioral, and cognitive stimulation therapies in cognitively impaired patients.

Psychological treatments can be offered to older patients and/or their caregivers with the following indications:

- Patient preference, as an alternative treatment to medication (e.g., in the treatment of an anxiety disorder)
- Augmenting the effect of psychotropic medication (e.g., in the treatment of a depressive disorder)
- To avoid the use of potentially harmful medication (e.g., in managing behavioral symptoms of dementia)
- To foster adherence to medication (e.g., in the treatment of depression)
- To help distressed caregivers (e.g., treating a dementia caregiver experiencing depressive and anxiety symptoms)
- To alleviate psychological problems related to aging (e.g., to help achieve contentment and acceptance of aging or to resolve disputes within a family brought on by the illness of an older family member)

- As part of a collaborative care intervention in the treatment of depression, anxiety, and/or bodily distress syndrome
- To provide the clinician and patient with a psychological formulation to the patient's problems [3]

Deficits in verbal reasoning, speed of responses, and sensory function may result in difficulty understanding the complex verbal content of some psychological treatments. Therefore, evaluation for psychological treatment should include at least a brief assessment to look for possible deficits [4].

10.3 Interventions for Common Disorders in Primary Care

10.3.1 Anxiety and Depression

The combination of extended years of shifting roles in families as older adults gradually grow increasingly dependent on their adult children and the multiplying demands on caregivers suggests that both older adult family members and caregivers will be at increased risk for depression and anxiety. Symptoms of anxiety and depression are common in all countries throughout the lifespan, with up to 13.5% of older adults having depression and between 1 and 15% diagnosed with anxiety disorders [5–7]. How depression and anxiety manifest will vary greatly by culture.

It is important to recognize that in primary care settings, the most common mental disorders encountered are various mixtures of anxious, depressive, and somatic symptoms, and in many cases, a diagnosis of "anxious depression" will be appropriate [8]. These symptom clusters have been documented in all global populations and countries in which they have been studied and are consistently found to be more prevalent among women than among men [9].

Although there are fewer studies available for other therapies in older age groups, the available evidence suggests that, as in younger people, most therapies will have some efficacy compared with no intervention. In the treatment of late-life depression, psychotherapy may be the only available modality, if the antidepressant pharmacotherapy is poorly tolerated. An expert consensus guideline from 2001 favored cognitive behavioral therapy (CBT), problem-solving therapy, interpersonal therapy, and supportive psychotherapy over psychodynamic psychotherapy. The consensus among the experts was to recommend psychotherapy as an adjunctive treatment to pharmacotherapy, except in the case of mild depression or dysthymia, for which psychotherapy alone was seen as an alternative to medication [10, 11].

Pharmacotherapy is quite effective in the management of late-life anxiety; however, unwanted side effects can limit the use of psychotropic medication. CBT appears to be the best form of psychotherapy to manage the diagnosis and treatment issues that exist within the older population with generalized anxiety disorder [12]. Also, CBT can be used to augment psychotropic medications.

Other forms of psychotherapy for anxiety include psychoeducation, relaxation training, cognitive restructuring, and exposure to anxiety-provoking stimuli. Relaxation training, which is based on behavioral psychology, is most frequently used and is also the most well-substantiated treatment for anxiety in older adults. Work by DeBerry showed that progressive muscle relaxation and meditation relaxation techniques reduced anxiety symptoms more effectively than treatment control condition in older adults [13]. These strategies can be taught in brief individual or group sessions.

While the overall effectiveness of psychological therapies in the management of these conditions is recognized, debate continues about any differences in effectiveness between therapies, the best way to deliver psychological therapies in primary care settings, and the relative merits of psychological versus drug therapies. The overall costs of providing psychological therapies to large numbers of patients are also an important issue, particularly given the rapid growth in the aging population.

10.3.1.1 Stepped Care for Anxiety and Depressive Symptoms

The delivery of psychological therapy for anxiety and depression is increasingly aligned to the concept of stepped care. Stepped care delivers the simplest and most effective intervention first. If the patient fails to benefit from the initial intervention, then a more complex intervention from the next "step" is considered [14, 15].

Although a firm evidence base for a stepped care approach is lacking, it is recommended in evidence-based guidelines as the approach to take in the management of depression in a number of high-income countries. Examples of this approach have also been described in the treatment of depression and anxiety disorders in primary care in low- and middle-income countries, including India and Chile [16]. Psychological therapies lend themselves to a stepped care approach as they can be tailored to the availability of local resources.

A range of specific therapies has been assessed for the psychological management of anxiety and depression. They range from low-intensity modifications to lifestyle (e.g., exercise) and social connectedness to more specific therapies such as CBT, which require more intensive input. All psychological therapies have their effectiveness increased by a good therapeutic relationship between the health provider, the patient, and family. We describe the range of therapies below.

10.3.1.2 Exercise

There is good evidence for exercise as a low-intensity input treatment for mild to moderate depression. It is likely that it is also effective for the relief of symptoms of anxiety [17]. A recent meta-analysis which specifically assessed nine trials with older adult patients, suggested that, for older adults who present with clinically meaningful symptoms of depression, prescribing structured exercise tailored to individual ability will reduce depression severity [18].

10.3.1.3 Enhancing Social Contact (Befriending)

Befriending may also be useful in the management of mild depression in older adults [19].

There is significant literature suggesting that social support affects the onset, course, and outcome of depression and individuals with distress appreciate emotional and social support. One way of providing this support is through befriending, where a relationship between two or more individuals is initiated, supported, and monitored by an external agency. A systematic review of 24 studies showed that compared with usual care or no treatment, befriending had a modest but significant effect on depressive symptoms in both the short and long term [19].

While low-intensity interventions are effective in the management of depressive symptoms, there may be little difference between their effectiveness. In a recent randomized controlled trial, for example, while overall mood scores improved with intervention, no differential effect was observed between a physical activity intervention and social visits on mood in a group of older primary care patients with depressive symptoms [20].

10.3.1.4 Cognitive Behavioral Therapy (CBT)

The most commonly prescribed psychotherapies are those derived from cognitive therapies, which focus on overly negative beliefs the patient possesses that lead to low mood and low self-esteem [21]. CBT, and the associated problem-solving therapy (PST), emphasizes behavioral techniques, repetition, a slower pace, identifying a highly specified focus, and giving homework assignments for practice. For example, PST explicitly trains patients to select and solve daily problems that seemed insurmountable to them initially, with the goal of increasing their self-efficacy and overcoming feelings of helplessness, which form the core of depression. With continued rounds of problem-solving with highly specific action plans arrived at through patient-therapist collaboration, self-esteem and confidence rises, thereby countering demoralization and lowering overall depressive symptoms [22]. Planned termination takes place when 6–8 sessions are completed. In PST, the hoped-for result is that the newfound confidence in problem-solving will continue to additional problems,

which, if also successfully handled, will maintain the patient's confidence and continue to relieve depressive symptoms over the long term [11].

There is considerable literature outlining the efficacy of CBT for anxiety and depression in many different populations and different countries. WHO recommends it as a treatment for depression in adults. The evidence base for CBT is more developed than for other therapies. It seems likely this is due to a lack of research evidence rather than a lack of potential benefit from other therapies. It should also be considered that in many cases the comparator used to assess the effectiveness of a specific intervention was "treatment as usual." This is something that is likely to vary widely across settings. Furthermore, research trials take place in a highly controlled environment that is unlikely to accurately reflect day-to-day clinical practice. In pragmatic observational studies where patients have had access to a wide range of different therapies, there is often little difference between them [23].

In the most recent meta-analysis, 23 randomized controlled trials were included. At the end of the intervention period, CBT was shown to be significantly more effective at reducing depressive symptoms (irrespective of whether rated by clinicians or participants) than treatment as usual or being on a waiting list but not than active controls. The same pattern of results was found for 6-month follow-up. Clinician-rated outcome measures resulted in larger effect sizes in favor of CBT than self-rated measures. No significant differences in efficacy were found between CBT and other treatment (pharmacotherapy and other psychotherapies) [24].

A similarly conducted meta-analysis and regression explored the effect of CBT on anxiety in community settings. Twelve studies were included. CBT was significantly more effective than treatment as usual or being on a waiting list at reducing anxiety symptoms at the end of the intervention, with the effect size being moderate, but when CBT was compared with an active control condition, the between-group difference in favor of CBT was not statistically significant, and the effect size was small. At 6- but not 3- or 12-month follow-ups, CBT was significantly more effective at reducing anxiety symptoms than an active control condition, although the effect size was again small. The review confirmed the effectiveness of CBT for anxiety disorders in older adults but was suggestive of lower efficacy in older than working-age people [25].

10.3.1.5 Additional Therapies

Interpersonal psychotherapy (IPT) was empirically derived from attachment theory and social psychology as a specific treatment for depression. It is a manual-based treatment that focuses on one of four specific areas: (1) grief, (2) role transition (such as retirement or ceasing to drive), (3) role disputes (e.g., with spouse, boss, or adult children), and (4) interpersonal deficit (those with more chronic trouble maintaining mutually satisfying relationships) [26]. The work of IPT is carried out in a real-world setting of patients' current interpersonal relationships, which are explored in depth with problem-solving strategies to help make currently available relationships more satisfying and in the process reduce depressive symptoms. A monthly maintenance version is particularly useful for maintaining gains in those with chronic role disputes [27].

Reminiscence or life review therapy helps patients to either accept past negative events and resolve past conflicts or recollect past coping strategies. A number of studies involving older adult patients with depression demonstrate that those receiving reminiscence therapy showed fewer depressive symptoms, less hopelessness, and improved life satisfaction [28, 29].

10.3.2 Bodily Distress Syndrome

Many terms and labels have been applied to patients experiencing pain or other physical symptoms that are not fully explained by organic or structural abnormalities, including body distress syndrome (BDS), psychophysiologic disorder, medically unexplained symptoms, and chronic functional syndromes (fibromyalgia, irritable bowel syndrome, etc.). Diagnostic tests in these patients typically reveal either no abnormalities or findings that are found just as fre-

quently in asymptomatic people. An estimated 25–30% of primary care outpatients fall into this category.

Presenting symptoms may affect almost any organ system and often more than one simultaneously. Gastrointestinal symptoms; chronic joint, limb, and spine pain; headache; and problems referable to the neurologic, ENT, cardiac, pulmonary, urologic, or gynecologic systems are common. Fortunately, in most of these patients symptoms are linked to one or more forms of psychosocial stress. Intervention directed at these issues leads to relief of symptoms, sometimes dramatically, and at other times only after months or years of psychotherapy.

Psychological intervention for BDS is based on accurate assessment of the underlying psychosocial issues, which are often not evident to the patient or present in the medical record. Therefore, it is helpful to mention the possibility of psychosocial stress as a cause of symptoms during the initial encounter with patients who lack an obvious organic etiology for their illness. Most patients accept this more readily than when stress is brought up only after extensive diagnostic testing. It is important to emphasize that physical symptoms linked to stress are just as "real" as symptoms with an organic or structural etiology and that there is no suspicion of symptoms being imaginary, self-inflicted, or due to malingering, psychosis, or psychological "weakness."

10.3.2.1 The Stress Checkup

Stress checkup is a term readily accepted by patients for the process of uncovering the links between psychosocial issues and physical symptoms. In an integrated practice, the stress checkup can be initiated by a doctor and, if needed, completed by the mental health professional. The latter may also provide initial treatment and, where indicated, referral for mental health follow-ups.

The stress checkup consists of six parts as follows. This information may be gathered over multiple visits when time is limited:

(a) Illness chronology: The stress checkup begins with acquiring a detailed chronology of the patient's illness. Knowing when and where the symptoms began and their pattern over time is essential to recognizing links to stressful events in the patient's life that are discovered later in the process. It is also important to look for patterns in the symptoms that don't correspond to an organic or structural etiology, for example, a 75-year-old man with 25+ years of daily spine pain that was completely absent during his annual 2-week fly-fishing holiday.

(b) Current stresses: Almost any source of ongoing life stress is capable of causing physical symptoms. A personal crisis, problems with a spouse or partner, difficulty with children or parents, workplace issues, financial problems, or a dilemma involving a friend or neighbor are worthy of inquiry. Another common theme in this category is a lack of self-care skills. A good question here is "Are you the kind of person who takes care of those around you but has difficulty finding time for yourself?" Corroboration of the patient's answer to this question from a spouse/partner/friend is often helpful. Along similar lines, the question, "What do you do for enjoyment and how often?" can be revealing. For many patients with limited self-care skills, their childhood environment presented problems that prevented them from focusing on their own needs. Consequently they failed to develop self-care skills, and now, as adults, their lives lack space for personal fulfillment and recreation.

(c) Childhood stress: Surprisingly, childhood stress can lead to symptoms years and even decades after the patient has left the family of origin. Symptoms may begin during childhood or adolescence but may also emerge for the first time in mid-life. Symptoms may be mild or severe and could persist for years or decades. Good questions to ask are the following: Were you under stress as a child? If you learned that a child you care about was growing up exactly as you did, would that make you feel sad or angry? On a scale of 1–10, 10 being worst, how much stress did you experience as a child? and Can you tell me a little more about why you chose that number for the last question? In listening to the response to the last question, be aware that the common denominator in childhood stress capable of causing physical illness in adults is treatment of the child that adversely impacts their self-esteem in a lasting way. This may result from physical, sexual, or verbal/emotional abuse. Many patients found it nearly impossible to elicit praise or support from their parents. Others were emotionally or physically neglected. Still others grew up in homes where one or both parents were physically violent with each other and/or were substance abusers. It is helpful to be aware of two significant barriers that hinder accurate assessment in this population. The first is that to survive childhood adversity, many patients suppressed their emotional reaction to their early experience and as adults are not consciously aware of the magnitude of their suffering. Consequently, they may appear to minimize the adversity of their early lives. Detailed questioning combined with empathic skills is often needed for an accurate assessment. The second significant barrier is that physical illness may arise during the process of recovering from childhood stress. Consequently, patients may be skeptical about stress causing their illness because their lives are noticeably improved in relation to the past.

(d) Depression often presents with a somatic chief complaint. Further complicating the diagnosis, the majority of my patients denied feeling depressed though they often admitted to feeling stressed or exasperated. Other clues to depression are a vague, non-specific description of the symptoms and desperation to find relief that is out of proportion to the findings on a physical exam. Confirmation follows inquiry into early morning awakening, anhedonia, fatigue, anorexia, tearfulness, thoughts of self-harm, and loss of hope for the future.

(e) Post-traumatic stress: The link between a terrifying or horrifying event and an unexplained illness is clear when symptoms begin soon after the trauma accompanied by typical manifestations of post-traumatic stress disorder (flashbacks, nightmares, avoidance of reminders of the trauma, emotional numbness, vigilance). More challenging, but not rare, is onset of the illness long after the trauma. In this situation, the onset of symptoms typically follows a triggering event linked to the trauma, as demonstrated below:

A 57-year-old woman with severe, focal (3 cm diameter) right upper quadrant (RUQ) abdominal pain for 3 weeks. At age 45 she suffered a violent abduction and sexual assault by three men who left her tied to a tree in a remote area. Symptoms began the day after her first visit to a therapist to discuss PTSD symptoms, during which she vomited uncontrollably at one point.

(f) Anxiety may also present with a somatic chief complaint. The most common clue to this etiology is that symptoms are significantly less severe, less common, or absent when the patient is in what they consider to be a safe environment. A patient who had diarrhea attacks only away from home is a typical example. Another patient experienced progressive stiffness and discomfort in the neck and shoulders the longer he was away from home. It was not surprising to learn that he worked on the night shift where he was the only person in the building and shopped for groceries at nearly vacant all-night markets. A variant of this condition is social anxiety disorder where symptoms are triggered by certain social conditions such as public speaking or being with large numbers of people. Patients often worry about embarrassing themselves or being judged by others.

10.3.2.2 Treatment

A useful diagnostic technique that also initiates treatment is to ask the patient, between their initial and follow-up visits, to compile a list of all the stresses in their life, both the past and present. This has value for several reasons:

- Patients who would like to discuss their stresses over more time than is available during their appointment can work on this list instead.
- Many patients are surprised at the number of items on the list.
- Many will notice that their stresses tend to cluster in certain areas, such as with their spouse or in the workplace.
- Often patients will find solutions to a few of the items, and notice this is associated with an improvement in their symptoms.

Patients who are symptomatic due to a lack of self-care skills should, ideally, set aside 2–5 h per week (best as a block) for trial and error in a search for an activity whose major purpose is enjoyment. This process may require months, often induces guilt (at first) and benefits from support by other members of the patient's household. But once the patient acquires the ability to self-indulge on a regular basis, their symptoms often respond in a gratifying way.

Depression, PTSD, and anxiety can be managed with counseling and/or medication depending on the patient's preference and local expertise. They are discussed elsewhere in this book. Patients with physical symptoms resulting from adversity in childhood often benefit from psychotherapy, but there are several techniques applicable in a medical setting (implemented by a behavioral health practitioner or medical clinician) that can be surprisingly beneficial.

The first step is to support greater conscious awareness of emotions about childhood maltreatment that have persisted to the present. For example, even patients who deny ongoing issues with past adversity may reconsider when asked to imagine their own child (or a child they care about) enduring the same experience, as demonstrated below:

- A 74-year old man with a 55-year history of a variety of unexplained symptoms described being physically abused by his father as a boy in a flat, unemotional tone using few words.

He appeared to be skeptical that this experience could be relevant to his illness after so many years. But after I asked him to imagine his grandson enduring the same treatment, he agreed to visit a support group for adults abused as children. He quickly recognized that he was, by far, the oldest person in the room. However, after keeping silent for the first two meetings, in the third he unburdened himself among those highly supportive survivors for nearly 45 min. His physical symptoms resolved soon after.

Another benefit of having the patient imagine a child enduring the same maltreatment is to better appreciate the magnitude of physical and mental challenges that they have overcome. This can help them overcome the poor self-esteem that is so often a long-lasting effect of having been abused. One might suggest that the patient was "born on the far side of a dangerous mountain, but climbed up and over it to become an adult." This emphasizes their lack of culpability for their family situation as well as the credit they can take for having survived.

Once the patient has greater conscious recognition of the magnitude of their anger, fear, or grief, a helpful next step is to reduce the somatic expression of emotion (which causes symptoms) by writing about it. In effect, we are trying to convert somatic expression of emotion into verbal expression:

- When the patient feels ready, writing a letter to the person(s) who perpetrated the maltreatment (not to be mailed, typically) can be cathartic.
- Other patients prefer to write in a journal as ideas occur to them.
- Another helpful exercise is to imagine a child enduring what the patient experienced and write about what they would like to communicate to such a child.

If perpetrators of childhood maltreatment are still active in the patient's life, it can be helpful to discuss setting boundaries to limit the degree or change the nature of their interaction.

10.4 Interventions for Common Disorders in Secondary Care

10.4.1 Dementia/Cognitively Impaired Disorders

The development of psychosocial therapies for dementia/cognitively impaired disorders is complicated because these disorders are progressively deteriorating conditions which are unlikely to remit as a result of psychotherapy. The treatment is specifically focused on typical targets, which include global quality of life, affective states, disruptive behavioral symptoms, functional impairment, and prevention of self-harm.

Cognitive stimulation therapy is a psychotherapeutic technique that helps patients cope with the cognitive symptoms of dementia. Usually these symptoms can cause distress and injury in patients and increased stress in caregivers. It derives from reality-orientation therapy, which aims to continually orient patients' attention to the current situation and surroundings by repeating who they are and where they are. Cognitive stimulation therapy focuses on improving information-processing abilities. Treatment can take place in formal groups or through training of professional or lay caregivers to administer intervention activities during the course of day-to-day activities [30].

Two manual-based psychotherapies have been modified to target the particular needs of older patients with cognitive impairment and depression. Problem-solving therapy (PST) has been modified to include in-house assistance with very practical problem-solving that can include caregivers as well. PST has been shown to improve depression and disability measurement scores. Interpersonal therapy has been modified to incorporate the caregiver into the treatment process at every level. There is a heavy emphasis on psychoeducation tailored individually to identified patients as well as caregivers concerning executive dysfunction, with a flexible use of individual or joint problem-solving sessions to seek optional coping strategies that may need to be adjusted further in the face of continued cognitive decline [27].

Another set of empirical treatments for caregivers with growing empirical support is based on the progressively lowered stress threshold (PLST) theory [31]. From this perspective, the disease process underlying dementia progressively lowers the patient's ability to cope with stressors such as fatigue, change in routine, or physical illness. Treatment consists of educating and training caregivers in managing the patient's environment to minimize such stressors. PLST-based training is effective in reducing problem behaviors and caregiver distress about patient's behavior problems [32]. In dementia, the PLST approach shows great promise.

10.4.2 Personality Disorders

The prevalence rate of personality disorders in the older adult community is between 10% and 20%, analogous to the 13% prevalence rate among younger age groups [33, 34]. Overall, the emotionally constricted/risk-averse disorders in Cluster A (paranoid and schizoid personality disorders) and Cluster C (obsessive-compulsive, avoidant, and dependent personality disorders) are the most commonly diagnosed conditions in late life [33].

Most empirical evidence suggests that older adult patients with depression and comorbid personality disorder are generally less responsive to treatments for depression including antidepressants and psychotherapy, respond more slowly to these treatments, report more severe depressive symptoms, and are more likely to experience depressive recurrence. Older adults with a personality disorder diagnosis are also more likely to report suicidal ideation and experience more severe anxiety symptoms. They also report having less social support, worse interpersonal functioning after antidepressant treatment, are less likely to be married, and are more likely to report occupational difficulties. Older patients with personality disorder experience a lower quality of life and greater functional impairment and disability after treatment of depression [11].

Dialectical behavioral therapy (DBT) has shown to be effective in reducing suicidal ideation, improving interpersonal skills, and increasing coping skills, and coping. DBT consists of regular sessions of group therapy and additional sessions of specific training that strive to improve emotion-regulation skills and distress tolerance. The skills for delivering this therapy require intensive training and a commitment of several hours per week for at least 6 weeks.

10.5   Interventions for Transitions and Losses in Later Life

Whether they're coping with a specific mental health disorder or not, all older adults are coping with a variety of transitions (e.g., retirement, moves) and losses (e.g., friends, physical decline). Four areas that deserve special attention by healthcare professionals include health, finances, social ties, and purpose/meaning. If an older adult has adequate resources in these four broad areas, aging need not be a period of depression and hopelessness. However, for most people, aging gradually involves multiple losses in each of these areas. In addition, the cultural context of the older adult strongly influences his resources and how he and his caregivers respond to losses.

An appropriate metaphor to guide responses to these losses comes from the family literature on coping with chronic illness [35]. "Finding the place for the illness and keeping it in its place" recognize that losses, whether they are illness, death of loved ones, retirement from meaningful work, physical frailty, or other losses, can change a person's life forever. However, the patient and his family have some influence over the ultimate effects of the losses. "Keeping it in its place" suggests that losses do not have to always spill over into every area of well-being. Sources of pleasure and meaning can be protected with thoughtful planning and an understanding of the patient's wishes.

In *Being Mortal*, Dr. Atul Gawande illustrates how often the wishes of the patient are missed or overlooked as caregivers, family members, and medical providers respond to inevitable changes

[36]. Dr. Gawande suggests that the patient is the expert on the place of the loss in her life. Also, with help, she can often identify the areas of her life that most need protecting against the incursion of the loss. Activities like the card game Go Wish can help clarify what is most important to the patient.

One reason the patient's preferences might be overlooked is that the losses lead to increasing dependence on others. The patient may begin to feel that she has little to contribute and may even feel like she is only a burden. She may feel increasingly isolated. As the patient faces losses, family members may need to compensate for the losses in some ways, such as driving the loved one to her doctor's appointments or providing financial support. Thus, family members often want to participate in decisions about how to respond to changes from aging. Balancing the patient's needs and the family's needs can be challenging and renegotiation of roles and responsibilities can be explicit or implicit. Qualls discusses the many tasks of aging adults and their family members [37]. Some of the common areas that need restructuring include roles, authority, flexibility, closeness/distance, and responsibilities. While most patients and their families will not attend family therapy, the physician can use other resources, such as those found in Table 10.1 to help patients and their families negotiate the inevitable changes.

Table 10.1 identifies some of the numerous resources on the web to help older adults clarify adaptations that must be made to keep the losses in their place and protect other sources of meaning and hope. Table 10.1 also lists resources that healthcare professionals, aging adults, and their family members could use. Encouraging patients to use these resources can create a sense of agency as the patient comes to terms with necessary transitions and simultaneously identifies what he values most about his life.

10.6 Methods of Therapy Delivery

Psychological interventions for older adults can be delivered in a variety of ways. These include:

- Upskilling of existing primary care staff to provide psychological interventions
- Stepped care, which was described earlier
- Collaborative care, which is described below
- Referral to a mental health specialist, who is responsible for the patient's presenting problem and its treatment (e.g., a course of psychotherapy)

Collaborative care is a growing movement around the world that links doctors and mental health specialists, either through a traditional referral system or by immediately assisting with care in coordination with other healthcare professionals as they are in the process of seeing their patients. When a doctor detects emotional stress, a formal mental health diagnosis, or a health behavior change need, they can perform a "warm handoff" during the visit to the onsite mental health professional, which is more likely to result in patients receiving timely mental health services compared with usual referral to similar, but distant, services. Additional potential benefits of collaborative care include (1) improved sensitivity and accuracy of mental health problem identification; (2) contributions to increased screening, detection, and intervention; and (3) possibly earlier prevention of mental health and substance use issues. While more studies are needed to deepen the support for collaborative services across the full range of mental health needs, there is strong evidence from the USA and UK that such care improves outcomes for older adults with depression [38]. Two of these initiatives are described below.

IMPACT—A primary care physician and depression care manager (nurse, social worker, psychologist, family therapist) implement a shared treatment plan and consult with a psychiatrist as needed. The care manager provides education about depression, provides problem-solving therapy, and monitors depressive symptoms. A study of 1801 patients showed that IMPACT significantly reduces depressive symptoms in comparison with usual care and change persists after 1 year [39].

PROSPECT—To prevent suicide among older primary care patients by reducing suicidal

Table 10.1 Resources to help older adult patients

Resources for healthcare professionals	Resources for patients	Resources for caregivers and families
Supporting someone who is grieving This brochure is helpful to understand how to approach and communicate with someone who is grieving. It can also be used as a tool when supporting family members who are caring for others who are grieving. http://www.caringinfo.org/files/public/brochures/Supporting_Someone_Who_is_Grieving.pdf	*National Institute of Health: Senior Health* This website gives great tips for aging adults who need exercise help, up to date medical information on specific aging issues, as well as videos that make the information easy to attain. http://nihseniorhealth.gov/	*Aging parents and common sense—A practical guide for you and your parents* This online booklet gives great advice for parents who may be struggling with financial planning, living situations, and understanding their parent's aging process. It also gives tips on healthy communication for caregivers and how to deal with some tough conflicts that are associated with aging. http://www.caringinfo.org/pdf/resources/Aging%20Parent-Guide_5thEd.pdf
Caregiver family therapy CFT is a form of therapy aimed to improve family functioning for those involved in family caregiving and institute problem-solving methods in reducing burden on the family. This website gives a brief summary of the therapy, as well as resources including online training links. http://www.apa.org/pi/about/publications/caregivers/practice-settings/intervention/family-therapy.aspx	*Transitions in Later Life* This website is sponsored by a British foundation that offers collections of journal articles specific to learning about emotional well-being when transitioning to later life, including topics on retirement and increasing physical frailty. https://transitionsinlaterlife.wordpress.com/resources-journal-articles/journal-articles-on-emotional-well-being-in-transitions-in-later-life/	*There is No Right or Wrong Way to Grieve After a Loss* This pamphlet explains what grief is, how to experience grief, and how to know when grief is ending. http://www.caringinfo.org/files/public/brochures/There_is_no_Wrong_or_Right_Way_to_Grieve_After_a_Loss.pdf
Caregiver family therapy: Empowering families to meet the challenges of aging by Sara Honn Qualls and Ashley Williams This book explains the concepts behind CFT and gives clinical examples to help providers care for the needs of caregiving families. This link directs you to a brief summary of the book and where to purchase it. http://www.apa.org/pubs/books/4317295.aspx	*BenefitsCheckUp* A great resource for patients to research what benefits they are eligible for such as Medicare, food programs, and more. https://www.benefitscheckup.org/	*National Hospice and Palliative Care Organization* This website gives a lot of resources on advance care planning, end of life care, grief and loss, and other resources on caring for a loved one. http://www.caringinfo.org/i4a/pages/index.cfm?pageid=3406

Go Wish Go Wish card game is an intervention that gets people thinking about what is most important in life if it were to be shortened by severe illness. One, two, or more people can play it. http://www.gowish.org/article.php/how_to_play	*The Positive Aging Newsletter* This site, sponsored by the Taos Institute, offers readable newsletters, which provide summarized research, news stories, and books related to positive aging. Both caregivers and patients can benefit. http://www.taosinstitute.net/positive-aging-newsletter	*Family Caregiver Alliance* Based in California, this organization gives great advice on educating caregivers on their loved one's needs as well as where to find support groups to take care of themselves as well. https://www.caregiver.org/resources-health-issue-or-condition
Evidence-based practices with older adults This article discusses the effectiveness of certain therapies for aging adults with various illnesses and later life transitioning. Some of the therapies included are group therapy, life review therapy, and reality orientation. http://www.healthcare.uiowa.edu/icmh/evidence/documents/EBPOlderAdults.pdf	*Cycling Without Age* This is a program in which young people give rickshaw rides to older adults so they can feel "the wind in their hair" even if they have little mobility. It is an environmentally friendly means of connecting generations beginning in Denmark and now available in other countries, including some cities in the USA. http://cyclingwithoutage.org	*Caregiver Action Network* This organization offers support to caregivers through education, peer support, and outlets to share their stories. http://caregiveraction.org/
Center for Music Therapy in End of Life Care This organization provides resources on the effectiveness of music therapy in bereavement and offers workshops to learn more. http://www.hospicemusictherapy.org/resources/published-research/	*Positive Aging Resource Center* This is a helpful website which offers practical tips for emotional, physical, and mental health pertinent to the aging community. It is mainly for patients but also has a section for caregivers. http://www.positiveaging.org/index.html	*Well Spouse Association* This foundation offers support to spousal caregivers through emotional support in local chapters and educational resources. It is specifically designed for caring for those who are the caretakers of their spouses at the end of life and helping them through the many transitions. http://www.wellspouse.org/
Dignity therapy This article by the Chicago Tribune describes Dignity Therapy in aging adults and how it can provide meaning and purpose in end of life stages. It tells the story of a few patients who benefited from this meaningful story writing therapy. http://articles.chicagotribune.com/2012-01-11/health/sc-health-0111-dignity-therapy-20120111_1_patients-training-sessions-technique	*Fierce With Age* This is Dr. Carol Osborn's blog, which offers recommended reading, inspirational videos, and even online retreats for the aging population with particular emphasis on spirituality and resilience. http://fiercewithage.com	*The emotional survival guide for caregivers by Barry J. Jacobs* This is an excellent book for caregivers struggling with role reversals and coping through struggles associated with caring for a loved one. Written by a clinical psychologist and family therapist specializing in counseling medical patients and families. This link takes you to his website, which features a book summary along with where you can purchase the book. http://www.emotionalsurvivalguide.com/book.htm

(continued)

Table 10.1 (continued)

Resources for healthcare professionals	Resources for patients	Resources for caregivers and families
Respecting Choices (RC) is an internationally recognized, evidence-based advance care planning (ACP) model of care. http://www.gundersenhealth.org/respecting-choices	*Exergame with Kinect* This game was developed as an affordable, simple means of exercise for older adults. Participation in the game has been associated with improved balance, strength, walking, and motor control. The article was featured in the journal *Games for Health*, a potential resource for the aging population	*Coping with the death of a loved one* This workbook provides an outlet for caregivers to learn about the different stages of grief, rituals that one can do to help the grieving process, differences among ages and genders, and even exercises to complete throughout their bereavement. http://www.counsellingconnection.com/wp-content/uploads/2011/04/COPING-WITH-THE-DEATH-OF-A-LOVED-ONE.pdf
		The Caregiver's Handbook—National Care Planning Council This handbook gives caregivers information on common problems in caregiving, caring for the caregiver themselves, and legal/financial affairs. https://www.longtermcarelink.net/eldercare/the_caregivers_handbook.htm
		The Caregiver's Survival Handbook: How to Care for Your Aging Parent Without Losing Yourself This handbook gives information on how to get started with the initial conversations necessary to have with your loved one. It provides resources on finances, legal affairs, healthcare, insurance, housing, staying active, and caring for the caregiver.

ideation and depression, primary care physicians are trained to recognize depression and suicide ideation in older patients. In addition, mental health specialists are included on the treatment team. PROSPECT studies show that patients who receive this intervention had decreased severity of depression and are less likely to report suicidal ideation [40]. A study also found that patients participating in this intervention had lower mortality rates [41].

10.7 Conclusion

A wide range of psychological therapies falls within the term psychological interventions, including self-help support groups, low-intensity psychosocial interventions and higher-intensity psychological interventions. These interventions should be considered as a therapy option alongside other possible options (e.g., social support, lifestyle interventions, pharmacological therapy) rather than a singular approach to assisting patients and their family members. Increasing the Internet availability raises the possibility of using web-based therapy to support the management of anxiety and depression in older life. A number of studies are providing evidence that age is not a barrier to successfully treating anxiety and depression online [30, 42–44]. The increased availability of effective psychological interventions should provide much hope for older adults and their family members.

References

1. Forsman AK, Nordmyr J, Wahlbeck K. Psychosocial interventions for the promotion of mental health and the prevention of depression among older adults. Health Promot Int. 2011;26:85–107.
2. Givens J, et al. Older patients' aversion to antidepressants: a qualitative study. J Gen Intern Med. 2006;21:146–51.
3. Wilkinson P. Psychological treatments. In: Oxford textbook of old age psychiatry. 2nd ed. New York: Oxford University Press; 2013.
4. Gallagher-Thompson D, Thompson L. Treating late-life depression: a cognitive-behavioural approach, therapist's guide. New York: Oxford University Press; 2010.
5. Beekman AT, Copeland JR, Prince MJ. Review of community prevalence of depression in later life. Br J Psychiatry. 1999;174:307–11.
6. Bryant C, Jackson H, Ames D. The prevalence of anxiety in older adults: methodological issues and a review of the literature. J Affect Disord. 2008;109:233–50.
7. Prina AM, et al. Prevalence of anxiety and its correlates among older adults in Latin America, India and China: cross-cultural study. Br J Psychiatry. 2011;199:485–91.
8. Lam TP, et al. Proposed new diagnoses of anxious depression and bodily stress syndrome in ICD-11-PHC: an international focus group study. Fam Pract. 2013;30:76–87.
9. Löwe B, et al. Depression, anxiety and somatization in primary care: syndrome overlap and functional impairment. Gen Hosp Psychiatry. 2008;30:191–9.
10. Andreescu C, Reynolds CF. Late-life depression: evidence-based treatment and promising new directions for research and clinical practice. Psychiatr Clin N Am. 2011;34:335–55.
11. Miller MD, Morse J. Psychotherapeutic approaches for depression, cognitive impairment, and personality disorders in late-life. In: Geriatric psychiatry. New York: Oxford University Press; 2013.
12. Ayers CR, et al. Evidence-based psychological treatments for late-life anxiety. Psychol Aging. 2007;22:8–17.
13. DeBerry S, Davis S, Reinhard KE. A comparison of meditation relaxation and cognitive/behavioural techniques for reducing anxiety and depression in a geriatric population. J Geriatr Psychiatry. 1989;22:231–47.
14. National Collaborating Centre for Mental Health. Depression. The NICE guideline on the treatment and management of depression in adults (updated edition), National clinical practice guideline 90. London: British Psychological Society/Royal College of Psychiatrists; 2010.
15. New Zealand Guidelines Group. Identification of common mental disorders and management of depression in primary care. Wellington: New Zealand Guidelines Group; 2008.
16. Dowell A, Morris C, Dodds T, McLoughlin B. Psychological interventions in primary care mental health. In: Companion to primary care mental health. London: Radcliffe Publishing; 2012.
17. National Collaborating Centre for Mental Health. Depression. The NICE guideline on the treatment and management of depression in adults (partial update of NICE clinical guideline 23), National clinical practice guideline 90. London: British Psychological Society/Royal College of Psychiatrists; 2009.
18. Bridle C. Effect of exercise on depression severity in older adults: systematic review and meta-analysis of randomised controlled trials. Br J Psychiatry. 2012;201:180–5.
19. Mead N, et al. Effects of befriending on depressive symptoms and distress: systematic review and meta-analysis. Br J Psychiatry. 2010;196:96–101.

20. Kerse N, et al. Home-based activity program for older people with depressive symptoms (DeLLITE), a randomized controlled trial. Ann Fam Med. 2010;8:214–23.
21. Grant RW, Casey DA. Adapting cognitive behavioural therapy for the frail elderly. Int Psychogeriatr. 1995;7:561–71.
22. Alexopoulos GS, et al. Problem solving therapy and supportive therapy in older adults with major depression and executive dysfunction. Arch Gen Psychiatry. 2011;68:32–41.
23. Dowell AC, et al. Evaluation of the primary mental health initiatives: summary report. Wellington: University of Otago and Ministry of Health; 2009.
24. Gould RL, Coulson MC, Howard RJ. Cognitive behavioral therapy for depression in older people: a meta-analysis and meta-regression of randomized controlled trials. J Am Geriatr Soc. 2012;60:1817–30.
25. Gould RL, Coulson MC, Howard RJ. Efficacy of cognitive behavioral therapy for anxiety disorders in older people: a meta-analysis and meta-regression of randomized controlled trials. J Am Geriatr Soc. 2012;60:218–29.
26. Weissman MM, Markowitz JC, Kierman GL. Comprehensive guide to interpersonal psychotherapy. New York: Basic Books; 2000.
27. Miller MD. Clinician's guide to interpersonal psychotherapy in late-life: helping cognitively impaired or depressed elders and their care-givers. New York: Oxford University Press; 2009.
28. Serrano JP, et al. Life review therapy using autobiographical retrieval practice for older adults with depressive symptomatology. Psychol Aging. 2004;19:272–7.
29. Arean PA. Comparative effectiveness of social problem-solving therapy and reminiscence therapy as treatments for depression in older adults. J Consult Clin Psychol. 1993;61:1003–10.
30. Lynch TR, Epstein DE, Smoski MJ. Individual and group psychotherapy. In: Clinical manual of geriatric psychiatry. Washington: American Psychiatric Publishing; 2014.
31. Hall GR, Buckwalker KC. Progressively lowered stress threshold: a conceptual model for care of adults with Alzheimer's disease. Arch Psychiatr Nurs. 1987;1:399–406.
32. Gerdner LA, Buckwalter KC, Reed D. Impact of a psycho-educational intervention on caregiver response to behavioural problems. Nurs Res. 2002;51:363–74.
33. Abrams RC. Personality disorders in the elderly. Int J Geriatr Psychiatry. 1996;11:759–63.
34. Torgersen S, Kringlen E, Cramer V. The prevalence of personality disorders in a community sample. Arch Gen Psychiatry. 2001;58:590–6.
35. Reiss D, Steinglass P, Howe G. The family's organization around the illness. In: How do families cope with chronic illness? Hillsdale, NJ: Lawrence Erlbaum; 1993.
36. Gawande A. Being mortal. New York: Metropolitan Books; 2014.
37. Qualls S, Williams A. Caregiver family therapy: empowering families to meet the challenges of aging. Washington, DC: American Psychological Association; 2013.
38. Gilbody S, et al. Collaborative care for depression: a cumulative meta-analysis and review of longer-term outcomes. Arch Intern Med. 2006;166:2314–21.
39. Unützer J, et al. Collaborative-care management of late-life depression in the primary care setting. J Am Med Assoc. 2002;288:2836–45.
40. Alexopoulos GS, et al. Reducing suicidal ideation and depression in older primary care patients: 24-month outcomes of the PROSPECT study. Am J Psychiatr. 2009;166:882–90.
41. Gallo JJ, et al. The effect of a primary care practice-based depression intervention on mortality in older adults: a randomized trial. Ann Intern Med. 2007;146:689–98.
42. Andrews G. http://www.australianageingagenda.com.au/2014/07/18/elderly-succeed-internet-depression-treatment/.
43. Dear BF, et al. Internet-delivered cognitive behavioural therapy for depression: a feasibility open trial for older adults. Aust N Z J Psychiatry. 2013;47:169–76.
44. Alexander CL, et al. Bringing psychotherapy to primary care: innovations and challenges. Clin Psychol Sci Pract. 2010;17:191–214.

Exercise for Older Adults with Mental Health Problems

11

Roger Hilfiker

Abstract

Exercise or physical activity is considered as medicine, and both have several positive effects, which outweigh largely the risks. For older adults with mental health issues, physical activity and exercise might be even more important than for healthy people: exercise and physical activity can prevent or at least delay the onset of some mental disorders; they have therapeutic effects, either as the sole intervention or as an adjunct treatment for mental disorders. Patients are more likely to recover from a mental illness if they are regularly physically active. It is recommended for older adults to be physically active for at least 150 min per week at moderate intensity or for at least 75 min at vigorous intensity. Exercise adherence is quite low, and measures to improve exercise adherence should be implemented. Health-care providers should help older adults to find physical activities or exercise modalities that are perceived as pleasant. Caregivers of older adults with mental health issues should also be physically active, as this has a positive effect on the burden of carers of persons with mental health problems.

Key Points

- Although we do not have enough scientific evidence on how exactly to exercise with older adults with mental problems, we can be confident that physical activity and exercise have several positive effects.
- Physical activity or exercise should not add to the distress already present in older adults with mental health problems. Health professionals should help each older adult to find the physical activity that is fun to do or is at least not stressing.
- The history of exercises done should be taken into consideration. For someone who has been running his/her whole life, running in high age is no problem, but for someone who never regularly runs, other forms of exercise are probably better suited, at least to begin with.
- As some of the positive effects of exercise are due to the social component of it, group exercises should be offered.
- Before starting to exercise and from time to time, a risk screening by a medical doctor should be done.
- Physical activity does not have to be done in a gym; it can be part of everyday living such as household chores or walking.

R. Hilfiker (✉)
Physiotherapy, School of Health Sciences, HES-SO Valais-Wallis, Leukerbad, Switzerland

© Springer Nature Switzerland AG 2019
C. A. de Mendonça Lima, G. Ivbijaro (eds.), *Primary Care Mental Health in Older People*,
https://doi.org/10.1007/978-3-030-10814-4_11

11.1 Introduction

Exercise or physical activity is considered as medicine, and not a bad one [1–3]. Physical activities are activities where you move your body with your own energy. Activities can range from walking to the grocery store to walking the dog, taking the stairs instead of the elevator or gardening. Exercise is a subcategory of physical activity that is planned and structured. It includes activities such as strengthening, Tai Chi, yoga, running, cycling or stretching. Physical activity and exercise both have several positive effects, which outweigh largely the risks. For older adults with mental health issues, physical activity and exercise might be even more important; they can prevent or at least delay the onset of some mental disorders, and they have therapeutic effects, either as the sole intervention or as an adjunct treatment for mental disorders. Patients are more likely to recover from a mental illness if they are regularly physically active. Not only older adults with mental health issues should be physically active, but also their caregivers should be active: physical activity has a positive influence on the burden of carers of persons with mental health problems [4]. Exercise is medicine, but it should not be a bitter medicine. Because physical activity should be done the whole life, everybody should find a physical activity that is fun to do. Health professionals should help older adults to find physical activities and exercises that are fun for them. Exercise does not need to resemble a sporting activity such as weight lifting or running. It can be an activity such as dancing, walking or Tai Chi. Health professionals should know a large variety of exercises and physical activities. We all should do regularly physical activity and exercise every week, but exercises might be varied, and periods with frequent exercise sessions might be interrupted with periods with less.

11.2 Recommendations on Physical Activity and Exercise

Because of the positive effects, it is recommended for older adults to be physically active for at least 150 min per week at moderate intensity or for at least 75 min at vigorous intensity. These activities can be broken down to bouts of 10 min. If chronic conditions do not allow such an extensive physical activity volume, older adults should be physically active as much as tolerated and should avoid being sedentary [5]. Older adults living in long-term care facilities should exercise twice a week 35–45 min per session, and every resident who has no contraindication should have a personalized exercise programme [6].

The World Health Organization (WHO) recommends for older adults [7]:

1. Older adults should do at least 150 min of moderate-intensity aerobic physical activity throughout the week or do at least 75 min of vigorous-intensity aerobic physical activity throughout the week or an equivalent combination of moderate- and vigorous-intensity activity.
2. Aerobic activity should be performed in bouts of at least 10 min duration.
3. For additional health benefits, older adults should increase their moderate-intensity aerobic physical activity to 300 min per week or engage in 150 min of vigorous-intensity aerobic physical activity per week or an equivalent combination of moderate- and vigorous-intensity activity.
4. Older adults, with poor mobility, should perform physical activity to enhance balance and prevent falls on 3 or more days per week.
5. Muscle-strengthening activities, involving major muscle groups, should be done on 2 or more days a week.
6. When older adults cannot do the recommended amounts of physical activity due to

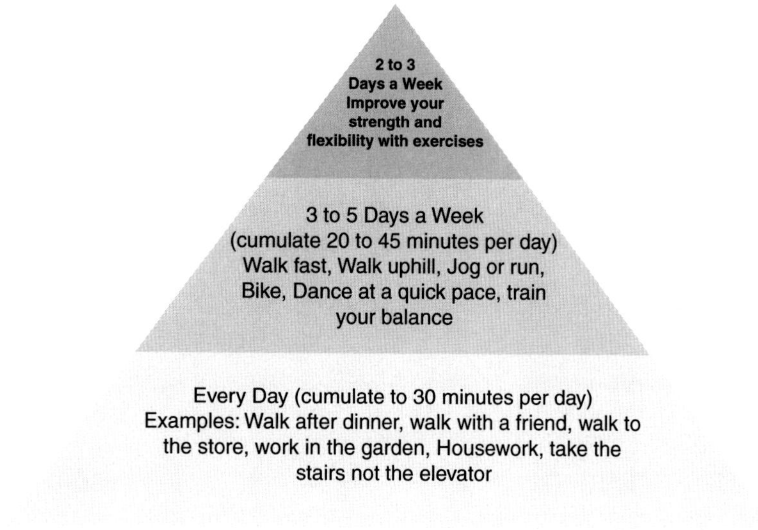

Fig. 11.1 Pyramid for recommendations of the weekly physical and exercise. See also https://www.cdc.gov/physicalactivity/basics/older_adults/ and http://www.who.int/dietphysicalactivity/factsheet_olderadults/en/

2 to 3
Days a Week
Improve your
strength and
flexibility with exercises

3 to 5 Days a Week
(cumulate 20 to 45 minutes per day)
Walk fast, Walk uphill, Jog or run,
Bike, Dance at a quick pace, train
your balance

Every Day (cumulate to 30 minutes per day)
Examples: Walk after dinner, walk with a friend, walk to
the store, work in the garden, Housework, take the
stairs not the elevator

health conditions, they should be as physically active as their abilities and conditions allow.

Figure 11.1 shows that older adults should be active every day for at least 30 min. The physical activity per day does not need to be done at once. Most recommendations say that one can break it up in smaller chunks of 10 min at least. Three to 5 days a week, older adults should add exercise at moderate or moderate to vigorous intensity to their daily physical activities, and they should exercise their balance. Balance exercises can be combined with activities of daily living, such as brushing teeth while standing in a tandem stand or even standing on one leg. Two to 3 days a week, they should add strengthening and flexibility exercises. There is evidence that more time being physically active, for example, 300 min per week, is even better. Most recommendations state that physical activity should be performed in bouts of at least 10 min. However, there is some evidence that even shorter bouts have positive effects [8]. This is important, for example, in frail older adults or older adults with dementia. Here, one can try to increase physical activity by, e.g.

standing up as often as possible, changing seats or rooms, walking short bouts, etc.

11.3 General Benefits and Risks of Exercise for Older Adults

Correctly performed regular physical activity, such as walking, or more vigorous exercises are not only safe but have several positive effects for older adults. The risk of developing major cardiovascular and metabolic diseases, osteoporosis, falls and fractures, muscular weakness or even cognitive impairments can be reduced [9]. Higher levels of physical activity were associated with lower all-cause mortality and cardiovascular-related mortality [10]. Aerobic exercise does not consistently improve cognitive function in older adults without cognitive impairments [11], but Tai Chi training improved processing speed and attention [12]. There is some evidence that lower levels of cardiorespiratory fitness are associated with the onset of dementia [13]; this would further the importance of aerobic exercise. Low-intensity activities, such as walking after dinner, seem protective for the onset of mild cognitive impairment [14].

11.3.1 Risks

There are some serious risks associated with exercise. During exercise, there is an increased risk for sudden cardiac death or myocardial infarction for individuals with a heart disease. Atherosclerotic coronary artery disease is most often the cause for an exercise-related death. The risk is highest for sedentary older adults when doing vigorous activities. This underlines the importance of screening for risk factors and a gradually progression of the activity intensity [15].

Physical activity and exercise also bear the risk for overuse problems and injuries of the musculoskeletal system. The best prevention for these overuse problems or injuries is a slow progression. With increased physical activity, the risk for falls might also increase, especially as the older adult will take more risk during physical activity. Persons at high risk for falls should probably first perform some exercises (i.e. balance and strengthening exercises), which reduce the risk for falls before engaging in activities with a high risk for falls (such as walking programmes). During a 2-year period of exercise in a large study of 631 participants in the intervention group and 629 in the control group, 5% of the participants had some musculoskeletal problems (versus only 1% in the control group) [16].

11.3.2 Pain and Physical Activity

Older adults with pain are less physically active than older adults without pain. This seems logical, as we all agree that pain is an unpleasant feeling and because physical activity might increase pain. Older adults with pain, e.g. due to osteoarthritis of the knee, often have doubts whether exercises are safe or beneficial for them [17]. Regrettably, health professionals often recommend a reduction in physical activity when older patients report painful joints, although a modifi-

cation of the activity would be a better choice in most of the cases. There is still a widespread belief that physical activity will increase the joint problems, which are attributed to wear and tear. In 2008, only about 60% of physiotherapists are convinced that exercise has positive effects for the symptoms of knee osteoarthritis [18], despite the strong scientific evidence that exercise is effective (and the evidence was already present at that time [19]). High-intensity sports, such as those that require rapid accelerations and instant decelerations, can increase the risk for osteoarthritis or its progression [20]. The same is true for continuous training with high impact on joints (e.g. downhill running, very-high-volume running, running with knee malalignment, running with overweight [21]). Running up to about 35 km per week is not associated with a higher risk for osteoarthritis; in contrary, it seems that running reduces the risk of osteoarthritis and reduces even more the risk for the need of a joint replacement [21–24]. Therefore, one can be confident that exercise at a moderate intensity and a moderate volume has positive effects on pain and function in patients with joint *problems* and is not a risk factor for osteoarthritis [25]. The best advice we can give is keep moving and, if overweight, lose weight. Pain can increase during exercise, or immediately after, but there is strong evidence that it has a positive effect on pain in the long term [26]. As a rule of thumb, pain should not persist for more than about an hour after stopping the physical activity. See Table 11.1 for pain symptoms that either allow to continue the exercise or should lead to a modification or a stop of the exercise. A common symptom is the delayed onset muscle soreness (DOMS) that can reach its highest pain level after 24–48 h. Health professionals should inform older adults about the meaning of different forms of pain during or after exercise and with what type of pain they can continue to exercise or when to stop.

11.3.3 Frailty and Physical Activity

Several definitions exist for frailty. Frailty can be defined as "a medical syndrome with multi-

Table 11.1 Pain types and when to continue or modify or even stop physical activity

Pain that allows to continue with exercise	Pain that needs modification of exercise
Mild to moderate pain at the beginning of exercise that decreases after some minutes	Moderate to severe pain. Change type of exercise (e.g. when severe knee pain during running change to walking uphill or cycling)
Mild to moderate muscle pain after the exercise that even gets worse the next day. Most probably delayed onset muscle soreness. This is not dangerous, and it will be less the next time you exercise	Stabbing or sharp pain during exercise. Change type of exercise, talk to a health professional
	Joint gets painful and hot and maybe swollen stop exercise. Restart adapted exercises when swelling and pain back to normal
	Chest pain: Contact a medical doctor

ple causes and contributors that is characterized by diminished strength, endurance, and reduced physiologic function that increases an individual's vulnerability for developing increased dependency and/or death" [27]. Frailty is not a contraindication for physical activity nor for exercise; in contrary, frailty is one of the most important reasons for an exercise prescription [28]. Exercise is the medicine that may reverse frailty or at least slow the increase of functional deficits [29]. The older and the frailer an older adult is, the more important it gets to add resistance and balance exercises to an aerobic training [30].

11.4 Benefits of Exercise for Older Adults with Mental Health Problems

Exercise has positive effects on muscle function, aerobic fitness, balance, quality of life and on mental health, but of course, mental health issues do not just disappear with exercise. Some of the beneficial effects of exercise are due to the social

interactions and social support during exercise interventions [31].

11.4.1 Exercise in Older Adults with Mild Cognitive Impairment

Aerobic exercise showed a small positive effect on global cognitive ability and on memory in older adults with mild cognitive impairments [32]. Combined physical and cognitive training induces neuroplastic changes in older adults [33].

Resistance training can delay the decline of, and may even increase cortical thickness in, older adults at risk for dementia [34]. This might protect from further cognitive decline. A resistance training, where six exercises were performed, each three times with eight repetitions, showed to improve global cognition, executive functions as well as verbal memory in older adults with mild cognitive impairments [35].

11.4.2 Exercise in Older Adults with Dementia

Aerobic exercise alone or combined with other exercises has positive effects on cognitive symptoms and on functioning in activities of daily life in older adults with dementia. Exercising without an aerobic component does probably have less positive influence on dementia [36]. One example of a successful approach shows that the implementation of a combined exercise programme is feasible and improves cognitive function [37]: The programme included aerobic, resistance, flexibility and balance exercises. To add cognitive components, participants were asked to say names of flowers, animals, fruits, etc. during exercises such as walking, bouncing a ball up and down a stair or exercising with weights. The programme was supervised and took place three times a week over 16 weeks.

What are the possible physiological mechanisms? It is most plausible that exercise increases brain vitality rather than acting on dementia-specific pathological mechanisms. Physical activity enhances neurotrophin levels, neurogenesis and vascularization, mediates neuroinflammation and inhibits neuronal integrity [36]. Sensorimotor exercises (i.e. exercises that challenge balance and muscle coordination) positively influence cognitive function, especially related to the visual-spatial network [38].

Exercise might also reduce the risk for falls by about 30% in older adults with dementia living in the community [39].

Because vascular- and lifestyle-related risk factors are associated with dementia risk, intervention that can modify these risk factors should also lead to a reduced risk of dementia. Combining interventions for diet, exercise, cognitive training and vascular risk monitoring showed a reduced cognitive decline when compared with a control group in a large Finnish study including 1190 older adults [16].

11.4.3 Exercise in Older Adults with Depression or Depressive Symptoms

Exercise, for example, a combination of endurance and strength training, has a positive effect on depressive symptoms in older adults [40, 41], and exercise also reduces depressive symptoms in adults with other psychiatric diagnoses [42]. The effects are comparable to the effects of pharmacological interventions and psychotherapy [43]. Exercise is not only effective for mild to moderate depression but also, as an add-on to other interventions, for older adults with severe depression [44]. The WHO [45] and the NICE [46] guidelines recommend that exercise is implemented in the standard treatment of depression. Although there is sound evidence that exercise at different intensities has positive effects on depressive symptoms, physical activity and exercise are not yet a priority in some of the guidelines on the treatment of depression. One reason for this slow integration of the positive evidence for exercise into the guidelines might be that there is still some uncertainty regarding the optimal dose response and the

type of exercise best suited for patients with depressive symptoms [47].

Because exercise has many other positive effects, it can be recommended that exercise should be an important part of the treatment in older adults with depression. Other forms of exercise, such as Tai Chi or Qigong, might also reduce depressive symptoms. Qigong, an ancient Chinese medical exercise form, seems better suited to reduce depressive symptoms than Tai Chi [48].

For all exercises, the amount of exercise should probably be more than 150 min per week to obtain a positive effect. Lower doses were often not successful [49]. Mixed aerobic and resistance exercises are probable best suited. Group sessions seem to have better effect than exercising alone, but this does not mean that every session must be in groups. For older adults with depression, exercise should probably be done with a moderate intensity instead of vigorous intensity. Effects seem to be larger when exercise is supervised by health professionals [50, 51].

Exercise might help by the means of biological factors such as increased turnover of neurotransmitters and endorphins or neurotrophic factors such as brain-derived neurotropic factor, the reduction of cortisol levels or the change in kynurenine metabolism. But also, psychological factors can lead to an improvement, for example, by an increase in self-efficacy [44].

Adverse events of physical activity and exercise in patients with depression are rare, but some older adults with depression may perceive exercise as stressful. Therefore, it is very important to customize exercise programmes and to find a physical activity or exercise modality that is enjoyable, but at least not stressful for the participant.

Exercise adherence is quite low, and measures to improve exercise adherence should be implemented. Motivation for exercise can be reduced because of the symptoms of depression, such as fatigue, indecisiveness, low self-esteem, loss of interest, loss of pleasure and poor sleep. Older adults with depression and a high level of anxiety and lower fitness are at the highest risk of not adhering to the exercise recommendations [52].

11.4.4 Exercise in Older Adults with Anxiety Disorders

Anxiety is treated with antidepressants and psychological treatments, and added exercise might improve the treatment. Exercise alone is better than a placebo but less effective than antidepressants. Therefore, exercise should be used in most cases combined with appropriate medication [53]. Tailored interventions are better suited than non-specific exercises, and the exercises should be performed for 3–4 sessions per week over at least 6 weeks. However, larger effects might be achieved when exercising over 15 weeks. One session should probably last at least 20 min, but stronger effects can be expected when session duration is over 30 min [54].

11.4.4.1 Exercise for Panic Disorders

Regular aerobic exercises can reduce the anxiety symptoms of patients with a panic disorder [55] but to a lesser amount than pharmacological treatments [56]. However, it seems that not every form of aerobic exercise has the same effect [57]. It seems that cognitive behavioural therapy might be better suited to reduce panic and agoraphobic symptoms [58], but given the positive effects of exercise and other outcomes, a combination of cognitive behavioural therapy and exercise might be better.

11.4.5 Exercise in Older Adults with Schizophrenia

Older adults with schizophrenia are less physically active than same-aged adults without schizophrenia. Cardiovascular mortality is increased in older adults with schizophrenia (and other psychiatric disorders, e.g. bipolar disorder); a large part of this increased mortality is attributed to smoking but also to reduced physical activity or lack of exercise [59]. This underlines the necessity to increase screening and treatment

for metabolic and cardiovascular risk factors. Hence, increased physical activity and exercise are important, and exercise can improve positive and negative symptoms [60].

11.4.6 Falls Risk and Exercise in Older Adults with Mental Health Problems

Falls risk increased with ageing and it is higher in older adults with mental health problems. For example, older adults with depression most often receive antidepressant medication that is associated with an increased falls risk [61]. Therefore, all older adults with mental health problems should be in a falls prevention programme including medication reviews, control of visual acuity, control of home hazards and the implementation of an exercise programme including strength and balance components [62]. Exercise programmes should be performed, if possible, for at least 3 h per week. Balance exercises should include highly challenging exercises for balance. Exercises should safely be made more challenging by reducing the base of support and by moving the centre of gravity and controlling body position during standing (i.e. reaching exercises, transferring body weight from one side to the other). If the participant needs to stabilize by touching something fix, then try to reduce this support (e.g. one finger instead of the whole hand; just touching, not grasping, etc.) [63].

Walking training can be included in addition to a balance exercise programme; however, high-risk patients should not perform walking programmes unsupervised. Strength training should be included in a falls prevention programme. If there is a pronounced weakness, there should be dedicated sessions for resistance training. See Fig. 11.2 for a progression of resistance training. If there is not a pronounced weakness, functional resistance trainings can be integrated in other exercise sessions, for example, after a short warm-up before a balance session, one can perform functional exercises such as squatting or simple standing up from a chair for several times.

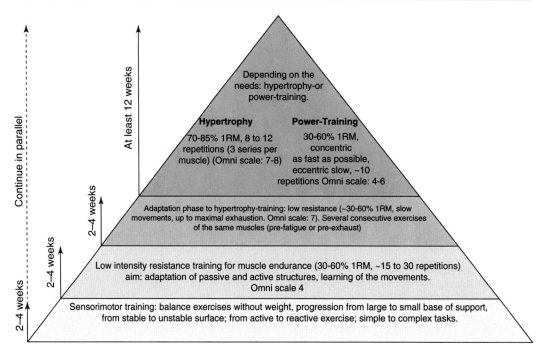

Fig. 11.2 Progression of resistance training. Physical activity readiness questionnaire

The more specific the weakness, the more specific the resistance training should be.

Dancing is an interesting approach for falls prevention as dancing has social, cognitive and physical aspects [64]. However, to prevent falls, dancing must be adapted to also include training elements such as stepping, reaction, strengthening and balance elements [65]. These elements can be easily implemented by a trained health professional. Dancing can so be used as a therapeutic approach.

11.4.7 Medical Clearance Before Exercise

The benefits of exercise clearly outweigh the risks, but there exist some health conditions that need attention. Most older adults will benefit from exercise, but diseases such as cardiovascular, pulmonary or metabolic disease may need some modifications or restrictions for their exercise programme. Older adults should see a medical doctor before starting exercise.

11.4.8 Exercise Modalities

For the prescription and monitoring of physical activity and exercise, we need to consider the intensity, the duration, the frequency and the progression of exercise training. The most important component is the intensity of the exercises.

In general, exercise intensity and volume should be low at the beginning of an exercise activity. A criterion-based progression is important. Criteria should consider the individual situation of the older adult as well as personal preferences.

11.4.8.1 Exercise Volume

To obtain positive effects on different age and inactivity-related problems, it is recommended to exercise for a weekly minimum of 150 min of moderate-intensity aerobic or 75 min of vigorous-intensity aerobic activity with additional muscle-strengthening exercises. Balance exercises should be added for all persons at risk for falls.

11.4.8.2   Exercise Intensity

Exercise intensity can be categorized in different zones (Table 11.2). There are no clear-cut boundaries between the zones. Exercising at the lower region of the light intensity zone can be used as regenerative training. The upper region of the light intensity zone is appropriate for beginners or for longer exercise sessions (i.e. longer than 1 h). The lower region of the moderate-intensity zone is ideal for an exercise duration of up to 45 min, whereas the higher region of the moderate-intensity zone is appropriate for shorter exercise durations. Exercising at the vigorous to very intensive training zone is appropriate for exercise durations up to 20 min. Exercise at high intensity should not be done too many times per week. Training above this zone should only be done interval training sessions.

The most appropriate measure to prescribe exercise intensity would be to use anchors such as metabolic or ventilatory thresholds (ventilator threshold, lactate threshold, maximal lactate

Table 11.2   Exercise intensity zones for aerobic (endurance) exercise

Zone	Description	% of VO2 max	Maximum heart rate	Heart rate reserve	RPE 6–20	Ability to talk comfortably
Very intensive	High-intensity interval training or other form of interval training should only be performed after medical clearance and under supervision of health professionals	>80%	>90	>80%	14–16–18	I can't speak comfortably; speaking a whole sentence fluently is not possible
Vigorous to very intensive intensity	Not necessary for health purposes Only possible over a short period Needs medical clearance	~80%	~90%	~80%	12–15 (mean 13.6 SD 1.8)[a]	I can speak but not entirely comfortably
Vigorous intensity	If you would do all your exercises at this intensity, you should do at least 150 min per week. But you can combine with lower intensities. For example, do 90 min at this intensity and 120 min at the lower intensity	60–80%	70–90%	60–80%	8–12	I can speak but I could not sing a song
Moderate intensity	If you would do all your exercises at this intensity, you should do at least 300 min per week. But you can combine with higher intensities. Remember: you can split the bouts of exercise; try to do some bouts of 10 min per day. But even shorter bouts are better than nothing	40–60%	55–75%	40–60%	6–8	Breathing is faster but speaking full sentences is possible and still comfortable
Light intensity	Could be done for hours (e.g. hiking). If done as warm-up: 5–10 min. Can be used as warm-up (5–10 min) or as regenerative training	<40%	<50%	<40%	<8	Breathing is just a little bit increased

[a]SD standard deviation; most older adults will rate the intensity in this zone as between 12 and 15 on the 6–20 scale. This illustrates that the interpersonal variability is high and the talk test provides more confidence for the monitoring of the exercise intensity. These values are from a large study [66]. All parameters have substantial interpersonal variability and, to be known exactly, should be determined by comprehensive exercise testing measuring ventilation, oxygen consumption, blood lactate levels, heart rate, etc. This would be important for maximizing performance gains. If exercise is mainly done for the improvement of health, these tests are not necessary. For the prescription of intensity, one probably best relies on the talk test, i.e. the different ability levels of speaking comfortably. In other words, if an older adult is exercising at an 80% of his heart rate reserve and is rating the perceived exertion at 15 on the 6–20 scale, you are not sure whether the intensity is too high. However, if the older adult is still able to speak a sentence fluently, but could not sing a song, you are sure that the intensity is not too high and not too low. If he is not able to speak a sentence fluently, you can be sure that he is exercising too hard

steady state, etc.) and to express the training intensity in a relative percentage of these anchors. However, this would need an exercise testing and a monitoring with heart frequency or blood lactate to determine the heart rate and the workload at each threshold. This is not feasible in most of the situations. Other parameters that are used for exercise prescription and monitoring are the percentage of maximum heart rate, percentage of heart rate reserve, percentage of maximum oxygen consumption, blood lactate and the rating of perceived exertion. Recommendations for the prescription and monitoring of the exercise intensity are often based on these parameters. However, the interpersonal variability is very large. If we take two randomly selected older adults and let them exercise at 70% of their heart rate reserve, the physiological responses may be very different. For person A 70% heart rate reserve might be a heart of 163 beats per minutes, and this intensity might be well below his individual anaerobic threshold. For Person B, a 70% of the heart rate reserve might be a heart rate of 154 beats per minute, and this person might be already above the individual anaerobic threshold, hence exercising too hard [67]. These differences may even be higher in older adults. This could lead to an overtraining and does increase the risk for cardiovascular events. Therefore, optimal tailored exercise intervention can only be determined based on comprehensive cardiopulmonary exercise testing that would provide sufficient information for the physiological responses at different exercise intensities. However, if physical activity or exercise is performed to improve health, this comprehensive testing is not always necessary nor always possible. The mentioned parameters can be used but should be regarded with caution. As we will explain below, the so-called talk test, or modified version of it, can be recommended for exercise prescription and monitoring when the aim is to improve health and functioning.

Exercise with the aim to improve general and mental health does not need to be intensive. However, the terms intensive or vigorous exercise are not always used with the same meaning or definition. This is not a problem, as we can give a simple recommendation: exercise for health in the older adult should allow a conversation, i.e. speaking in whole sentences should still be possible. For older adults who are already exercising for some time, the intensity can be increased: "talking in whole sentences is still possible, but singing a song would be difficult".

The intensity of aerobic exercise can be expressed in relation to the resting energy consumption or with the metabolic equivalent of task (MET, where 1 MET corresponds to the energy consumption during sitting) to the VO2 max or in relation to the individual anaerobic threshold.

Moderate-intensity: the heart rate and breathing are raised. Speaking is still comfortable. This corresponds to 4–6 METs. Brisk walking is classified as moderate intensity.

Vigorous-intensity activities: the heart rate and breathing are even higher. As a rule of thumb, talking is still possible, but singing a song would be too difficult. This corresponds to 6–8 METs.

Therefore, exercise prescription can also be done with the rating of the perceived exertion or even simpler methods, such as the talk test [68]. For the rating of the perceived exertion, the best-known scales are the 6–20, the 1–10 or the CR10 Borg scales. The different rating of perceived exertion scales can be obtained from http://www.borgperception.se; however, they are not free. The amount of the license fee depends on the use of the scale. It might be difficult to use these scales in patients with cognitive impairments [69, 70].

11.4.8.3   The Modified Talk Test

With the formal talk test, the person who exercises is asked to speak some sentences and to tell whether this talking was comfortable ("can you speak comfortably?"). If he responds yes, the exercise intensity is still mostly aerobic; if he gives somewhat equivocally, the exercise intensity is in the aerobic-anaerobic transition zone; if the answer is no, the exercise intensity is mainly anaerobic. The person who exercises should be on the same intensity level for about 2 min before doing the talk test [71]. However, the information on how comfortable talking is can also be used in a slightly different form: If one can speak comfortably, but there is already a slight increase in heart rate and breathing, then one is in the moderate-intensity zone. If one can speak but singing a song would not be possible anymore, one is exercising at a moderate to vigorous intensity level. If speaking full sentences is not possible anymore, one is exercising around or above the anaerobic threshold (something that is not necessary when performing continuous exercise for health but could be done in an intermittent form, such as high-intensity intermittent training). For interval or high-intensity intermittent training, the talk test is not feasible, because the exercise intervals are too short [72]. See also Table 11.2.

11.4.9 Resistance Training

The older a person gets, the more important is, as rule of thumb, resistance training. Ageing reduces not only the muscle mass (sarcopenia) but also the capacity of neural control, muscle activation and muscle coordination, resulting in lower muscle strength (dynapenia).

As a rule, we should first do large muscle exercises and second the smaller muscle exercises. Exercises involving multiple joints (e.g. squats) should be done before single-joint exercises (e.g. knee extension).

Exercise intensity is best monitored with a rating of the perceived exertion. The OMNI-RES scale is widely used for resistance training. The participant rated the intensity of effort, strain, discomfort or fatigue that he or she feels during the exercise. The OMNI-RES scale ranges from 0 to 10. 0 represents the absolute rest, i.e. sitting, and 10 reports a too high intensity or a load that could not be lifted. The anchors for the exercise levels are 1 "extremely light" and 9, the intensity of a weight that could just be lifted one time. The scale can also be used on older adults [73]. Furthermore, the scale can also be used to choose the optimal load during resistance training. The best method to define the exercise load during resistance training is the 1-repetition maximum test. However, the use of only the OMNI-RES is sufficient for a resistance training; if not, the

absolute maximal performance gain is necessary [73]. The OMNI-RES scale and its instructions can easily be found via Google.

Figure 11.2 shows a possible progression from sensorimotor exercises to muscle hypertrophy or power training. If an older person is not accommodated to resistance training or when starting a new period of training after a longer period of not performing resistance trainings (i.e. more than 1 months), an adaptation phase should be performed where first sensorimotor exercises improve coordination and reactivity. These exercises can be continued in parallel to all other resistance training periods, for example, during the warm-up. After a 2- to 4-week period, low-intensity resistance training at 30–60% of the 1-repetition maximum can be performed to improve local muscle endurance and an adaptation of passive and active structures, as well as to learn the correct performance of the exercises. For each exercise, 2–3 series should be performed with rest periods between the series of about 1 min. If the exercises for different muscles are alternated, such as in a circuit training, the rest periods can even be shorter than 1 min.

After a period of 2–4 weeks of local muscle endurance, one can progress to the phase of adaptation to hypertrophy training. The resistance (i.e. load) is still low (30–60% of 1RM), and the speed of the movements is slow, and one exercise is performed for about 40 seconds. Several exercises of the same muscle group can be performed with relative low rest periods, to achieve a fatigue that is rated with about a 7 on the 0–10 OMNI-RES scale.

Again, after a period of 2–4 weeks of the adaptation phase, the intensity can be increased depending on the needs of the older adult. If the main problem is sarcopenia (loss of muscle mass), a hypertrophy training is best suited. If the main problem is power or strength, a power training can be introduced. Some health professionals are reluctant to perform power training with older adults because they believe that the exercises performed at a relatively high speed for the concentric phase of the exercise are dangerous. However, there is evidence that power training is feasible and as safe as other exercise forms for older adults. Furthermore, the perceived exertion during power training is lower compared to hypertrophy training. During power training the emphasis is put on a fast concentric phase of the exercise movement and less on fatigue. The exercise is stopped when the participant cannot reproduce the same high speed as at the beginning. For safety reasons, the eccentric phase of the exercise is performed slowly.

For the hypertrophy training, intensities of about 70–85% of the 1-RM lead to the greatest increase in muscle mass. However, also lower intensities, e.g. 30–60% can lead to muscle mass increases. This is interesting for the training of older adults, where high-intensity loads are not always possible because of different comorbidities [74].

11.4.10 Balance Training

Balance training is important for most older adults, even more for older adults with mental health problems. Mental health problems can lead to a reduced balance [75–77].

Balance can be divided into the components "biomechanical constraints" (influenced, e.g. by postural alignment, strength and range of motion in joints), "stability limits/verticality" (influenced by limits of stability and the internal perception of postural vertical), "anticipatory postural adjustments" (important in tasks that require active moments of the body's centre of mass in anticipation of a change of position), "postural responses" (reactions, such as stepping, to an external perturbation), "sensory orientation" (body sway when visual or somatosensory information are changed) and "stability of gait" (stability during gait, i.e. reactions to internal and external perturbations) [78]. In older adults, these components are altered, depending on which body system is most reduced. For example, persons with osteoarthritis will have most limitations in the component "biomechanical constraints" [79], and persons with visual problems or those with polyneuropathies will have problems in the "sensory orientation" component.

Balance training should include activities that include progressively difficult postures that gradually reduce the base of support (e.g. from two-legged stand, semi-tandem stand, tandem stand to one-legged stand) and progressively reduce sensory input (e.g. standing with eyes closed); and the training should include dynamic movements that perturb the centre of gravity (e.g. tandem walk, circle turns), and it should include exercises that stress postural muscle groups (e.g. heel stands, toe stands).

11.4.11 Functional Exercises

Functional exercises consist of tasks that are similar to activities of daily living, such as standing up from a chair, climbing stairs, stepping, walking backwards, etc. These exercises aim to improve strength, balance and mobility. These functional exercises can be performed with older adults with dementia. In one study, the functional exercises, performed over 4 months, did delay the decline of functioning in activities of daily living in patients with dementia not related to Alzheimer's disease. In patients with Alzheimer's disease, the functional exercise programme was feasible, but did not postpone the decline in the functioning [80].

11.4.12 Combination of Cognitive and Physical Exercise

There are some good arguments of combining cognitive and physical exercise. However, there is conflicting evidence of whether the combination is better than using only one of both. In healthy older adults, combined exercises seem to be better than physical exercise only; however, for cognitive aspects, there is not yet enough evidence for an advantage of combined exercises compared to cognitive exercise only [81].

11.4.13 Computerized Cognitive Training

Computerized cognitive training can improve cognitive function in healthy older adults. Verbal memory, nonverbal memory, working memory, processing speed and visuospatial skills were the outcomes that could be improved. The expected effects are small but might still be relevant. The executive functions and attention seem to be more difficult to improve with computerized cognitive training. Furthermore, it seems that home-based computerized cognitive training is not effective. Group sessions seem to be the better approach [82].

Older adults with cognitive deficits can also benefit from computerized cognitive training; effects were found for attention, executive functions and memory. The effects are still observable after a follow-up period [83].

The best effects for computerized cognitive training were seen in group-based sessions with a duration per session of more than 30 min and not more than three sessions per week [83].

11.4.14 Exercise Adherence in Older Adults with Mental Health Problems

Only about half of adults with a mental health problem exercise because of an enjoyment of exercise. The most important effects of exercise are the following: improved physical health, increased fitness and energy, weight loss, improved appearance and the positive psychological effects, such as reduced stress, improved sleep and enhanced mood. However, stress, depression and low energy can limit exercise uptake or exercise adherence [84]. Most patients perceive a support from health professionals as a motivating factor.

11.4.15 Assessments for the Detection of Specific Needs that Could Be Addressed by Exercise

Although the increased use of assessments in older adults is a positive development, an assessment without a consequence is not recommended. Each assessment should have a clear aim and should be only done if its results might lead to a change or a decision. One of the simplest and

most relevant assessments is the simple measure of the walking speed, measured during a very short distance. Changes in walking speed seem to predict cognitive decline several years before the cognitive decline is noticed. Slow gait predicts decline in executive functions and in other cognitive domains, and changes in gait precede clinical symptoms of dementia. Walking speed is a sensitive measure and is indicative of subclinical cognitive decline. Testing walking speed is cheap and needs not a lot of resources and time [85]. Gait characteristics seem to better predict vascular dementia or other non-Alzheimer's dementia compared to dementia in patients with Alzheimer's disease [86]. Walking speed can be measured at normal pace or at fastest pace ("walks as fast as is safe, without running). Furthermore, walking speed can be measured with a start from standing still or time can be started when an older adult already is walking. Adding a second task, either a cognitive or a neuromuscular task might even be a more sensitive predictor of cognitive decline [87]. An example of the inability to perform multiple tasks is when an older adult stops walking while talking [88]. An increase of gait variability is also associated with cognitive impairments, especially during walking at a fast walking speed [89]. A variability of the stride length of more than 3% can be an indicator of cognitive problems.

Another simple test to screen basic mobility is the Timed Up and Go (TUG) test [90] in which a person is asked to stand up from a standard chair, walk 3 meters, turning around, walk back and sit down again. The TUG test has good reliability in older adults and in adults with cognitive impairments, but because of its relatively high absolute measurement error, results need to be interpreted with caution in older adults. The measurement error increases with the time needed to perform the task, but even with a time of 10 s, the expected true value could be within a range of 7–14 s [91]. The TUG test is also recommended and widely used for the screening of falls risk but, given the mentioned measurement error and the limited predictive value, should not be used alone [92].

One of the most widely used assessments in older adults is the short physical performance battery [93], consisting of a 4 m walk test for measuring gait speed, a timed five-chair stand test as well as a balance tests with feet held in different positions (feet together, semi-tandem, full tandem) for 10 s. The test takes about 10 min to complete and needs only a short course of training for the assessors.

11.4.16 Exercise with Older Adults with Dementia

Older adults who did not regularly exercise for some time should seek a medical doctor before starting with exercise. They should always seek a medical doctor if they have heart problems, high blood pressure, unexplained chest pain, breathing problems, dizziness or fainting episodes. A health professional should also be contacted if they have bone, joint or muscular problems, balance problems or fall frequently. These conditions will most probably not prohibit exercise but need medical clearance and might need supervision during exercise.

Exercise in the early to middle stages of dementia: most often older adults with mild dementia will have no problem in engaging in physical activity or exercise. All kind of activities and exercise can be considered, from gardening, walking to dancing or Qigong and Tai Chi.

In the later stage of dementia, physical activity remains important, and it may reduce the need for constant supervision from caregivers and may reduce the need for adaption such as walk-in bathtubs or stairlifts. Exercise at this stage often can be activities such as changing position from sitting to standing, walking into another room or moving to sit in different chairs from time to time. At this stage, it might be more difficult to achieve the recommended time-bouts of 10 min. But older adults with later-stage dementia should be encouraged to change positions as often as possible and to sit some time unsupported, if possible. Daily routines of moving around the house or block will help to maintain muscle strength and aerobic condition. Here are some exercises recommended from the British Alzheimer's Society [94]: (a) When standing up from bed or when going to bed,

shuffle along the edge of the bed in the sitting position, from one end of the bed to the other. (b) Stand with different feet positions or even on a single leg, supervised, with support if necessary. (c) Sit unsupported for a few minutes each day (i.e. do not lean the back against a support). (d) Stand up and move about as often and regularly as possible.

11.5 Conclusion

Physical activity and exercise have several positive effects in older adults, which outweigh the risks. They might be even more important for older adults with mental health issues by preventing or at least delaying the onset of some mental disorders. In addition, they have therapeutic effects, either as the sole intervention or in addition to other treatments. Patients are more likely to recover from a mental illness if they are regularly physically active. Caregivers of older adults with mental health issues should be also physically active, as physical activity has a positive effect on the burden of carers of persons with mental health problems.

References

1. Fortier M, Guerin E, Segar ML. Words matter: reframing exercise is medicine for the general population to optimize motivation and create sustainable behaviour change. Appl Physiol Nutr Metab. 2016;41:1212–5.
2. Naci H, Ioannidis JP. Comparative effectiveness of exercise and drug interventions on mortality outcomes: metaepidemiological study. BMJ. 2013;347:f5577.
3. Vina J, et al. Exercise acts as a drug; the pharmacological benefits of exercise. Br J Pharmacol. 2012;167(1):1–12.
4. Orgeta V, Miranda-Castillo C. Does physical activity reduce burden in carers of people with dementia? A literature review. Int J Geriatr Psychiatry. 2014;29(8):771–83.
5. American College of Sports Medicine, et al. American College of Sports Medicine position stand. Exercise and physical activity for older adults. Med Sci Sports Exerc. 2009;41(7):1510–30.
6. de Souto Barreto P, et al. Recommendations on physical activity and exercise for older adults living in long-term care facilities: a taskforce report. J Am Med Dir Assoc. 2016;17(5):381–92.

7. WHO. Physical activity and older adults recommended levels of physical activity for adults aged 65 and above. 2016. http://www.who.int/dietphysicalactivity/factsheet_olderadults/en/.

8. Glazer NL, et al. Sustained and shorter bouts of physical activity are related to cardiovascular health. Med Sci Sports Exerc. 2013;45(1):109–15.

9. McPhee JS, et al. Physical activity in older age: perspectives for healthy ageing and frailty. Biogerontology. 2016;17(3):567–80.

10. Evenson KR, Wen F, Herring AH. Associations of accelerometry-assessed and self-reported physical activity and sedentary behavior with all-cause and cardiovascular mortality among US adults. Am J Epidemiol. 2016;184(9):621–32.

11. Young J, Angevaren M, Rusted J, Tabet N. Aerobic exercise to improve cognitive function in older people without known cognitive impairment. Cochrane Database Syst Rev. 2015;(4):CD005381. https://www.cochranelibrary.com/cdsr/doi/10.1002/14651858.CD005381.pub4/abstract.

12. Kelly ME, et al. The impact of exercise on the cognitive functioning of healthy older adults: a systematic review and meta-analysis. Ageing Res Rev. 2014;16:12–31.

13. Schuch FB, et al. Are lower levels of cardiorespiratory fitness associated with incident depression? A systematic review of prospective cohort studies. Prev Med. 2016;93:159–65.

14. Krell-Roesch J, et al. Timing of physical activity, apolipoprotein E epsilon4 genotype, and risk of incident mild cognitive impairment. J Am Geriatr Soc. 2016;64:2479.

15. Jonas S, Phillips EM. ACSM's exercise is medicine™: a clinician's guide to exercise prescription. Philadelphia: Lippincott Williams & Wilkins; 2012.

16. Ngandu T, et al. A 2 year multidomain intervention of diet, exercise, cognitive training, and vascular risk monitoring versus control to prevent cognitive decline in at-risk elderly people (FINGER): a randomised controlled trial. Lancet. 2015;385(9984):2255–63.

17. Holden MA, et al. Role of exercise for knee pain: what do older adults in the community think? Arthritis Care Res (Hoboken). 2012;64(10):1554–64.

18. Holden MA, et al. UK-based physical therapists' attitudes and beliefs regarding exercise and knee osteoarthritis: findings from a mixed-methods study. Arthritis Care Res. 2009;61(11):1511–21.

19. Fransen M, McConnell S, Bell M. Exercise for osteoarthritis of the hip or knee. Physiotherapy. 2003;89(9):516.

20. Vannini F, et al. Sport and early osteoarthritis: the role of sport in aetiology, progression and treatment of knee osteoarthritis. Knee Surg Sports Traumatol Arthrosc. 2016;24(6):1786–96.

21. Ni GX. Development and prevention of running-related osteoarthritis. Curr Sports Med Rep. 2016;15(5):342–9.

22. Williams PT. Effects of running and walking on osteoarthritis and hip replacement risk. Med Sci Sports Exerc. 2013;45(7):1292–7.

23. Timmins KA, et al. Running and knee osteoarthritis: a systematic review and meta-analysis. Am J Sports Med. 2017;45:1447.

24. Chakravarty EF, et al. Long distance running and knee osteoarthritis. A prospective study. Am J Prev Med. 2008;35(2):133–8.

25. Lefèvre-Colau M-M, et al. Is physical activity, practiced as recommended for health benefit, a risk factor for osteoarthritis? Ann Phys Rehabil Med. 2016;59:196.

26. Anwer S, Alghadir A, Brismée J-M. Effect of home exercise program in patients with knee osteoarthritis: a systematic review and meta-analysis. J Geriatr Phys Ther. 2016;39(1):38–48.

27. Morley JE, et al. Frailty consensus: a call to action. J Am Med Dir Assoc. 2013;14(6):392–7.

28. Bauman A, et al. Updating the evidence for physical activity: summative reviews of the epidemiological evidence, prevalence, and interventions to promote "active aging". Gerontologist. 2016;56(Suppl 2):S268–80.

29. Bray NW, et al. Exercise prescription to reverse frailty. Appl Physiol Nutr Metab. 2016;41(10):1112–6.

30. de Labra C, et al. Effects of physical exercise interventions in frail older adults: a systematic review of randomized controlled trials. BMC Geriatr. 2015;15:154.

31. Zschucke E, Gaudlitz K, Ströhle A. Exercise and physical activity in mental disorders: clinical and experimental evidence. J Prev Med Public Health. 2013;46(Suppl 1):S12–21.

32. Zheng G, et al. Aerobic exercise ameliorates cognitive function in older adults with mild cognitive impairment: a systematic review and meta-analysis of randomised controlled trials. Br J Sports Med. 2016;50:1443.

33. Styliadis C, et al. Neuroplastic effects of combined computerized physical and cognitive training in elderly individuals at risk for dementia: an eLORETA controlled study on resting states. Neural Plast. 2015;2015:172192.

34. Suo C, et al. Therapeutically relevant structural and functional mechanisms triggered by physical and cognitive exercise. Mol Psychiatry. 2016;21:1645.

35. Fiatarone Singh MA, et al. The Study of Mental and Resistance Training (SMART) study-resistance training and/or cognitive training in mild cognitive impairment: a randomized, double-blind, double-sham controlled trial. J Am Med Dir Assoc. 2014;15(12):873–80.

36. Groot C, et al. The effect of physical activity on cognitive function in patients with dementia: a meta-analysis of randomized control trials. Ageing Res Rev. 2016;25:13–23.

37. de Andrade LP, et al. Benefits of multimodal exercise intervention for postural control and frontal cognitive functions in individuals with Alzheimer's disease: a controlled trial. J Am Geriatr Soc. 2013;61(11):1919–26.

38. Paillard T. Preventive effects of regular physical exercise against cognitive decline and the risk of

dementia with age advancement. Sports Med Open. 2015;1(1):4.

39. Burton E, et al. Effectiveness of exercise programs to reduce falls in older people with dementia living in the community: a systematic review and meta-analysis. Clin Interv Aging. 2015;10:421–34.

40. Catalan-Matamoros D, et al. Exercise improves depressive symptoms in older adults: an umbrella review of systematic reviews and meta-analyses. Psychiatry Res. 2016;244:202–9.

41. Adamson BC, Ensari I, Motl RW. Effect of exercise on depressive symptoms in adults with neurologic disorders: a systematic review and meta-analysis. Arch Phys Med Rehabil. 2015;96(7):1329–38.

42. Rosenbaum S, et al. Physical activity interventions for people with mental illness: a systematic review and meta-analysis. J Clin Psychiatry. 2014;75(9):964–74.

43. Bridle C, et al. Effect of exercise on depression severity in older people: systematic review and meta-analysis of randomised controlled trials. Br J Psychiatry. 2012;201(3):180–5.

44. Ravindran AV, et al. Canadian Network for Mood and Anxiety Treatments (CANMAT) 2016 clinical guidelines for the management of adults with major depressive disorder: section 5. Complementary and alternative medicine treatments. Can J Psychiatry. 2016;61(9):576–87.

45. WHO Mental Health. Physical activity. 2012. https://www.who.int/mental_health/mhgap/evidence/depression/q6/en/. Last accessed 22 March 2019.

46. NICE. Depression in adults: recognition and management. Published 2009, updated 2016. 2016 [cited 13.11.2016]. https://www.nice.org.uk/guidance/cg90/ifp/chapter/treatments-for-mild-to-moderate-depression.

47. Hallgren M, et al. Treatment guidelines for depression: greater emphasis on physical activity is needed. Eur Psychiatry. 2016;40:1–3.

48. Liu X, et al. A systematic review and meta-analysis of the effects of Qigong and Tai Chi for depressive symptoms. Complement Ther Med. 2015;23(4):516–34.

49. Dunn AL, et al. Exercise treatment for depression: efficacy and dose response. Am J Prev Med. 2005;28(1):1–8.

50. Schuch FB, et al. Exercise as a treatment for depression: a meta-analysis adjusting for publication bias. J Psychiatr Res. 2016;77:42–51.

51. Heinzel S, et al. Using exercise to fight depression in older adults: a systematic review and meta-analysis. GeroPsych. 2015;28(4):149.

52. Blumenthal JA, Smith PJ, Hoffman BM. Is exercise a viable treatment for depression? ACSMs Health Fit J. 2012;16(4):14.

53. Jayakody K, Gunadasa S, Hosker C. Exercise for anxiety disorders: systematic review. Br J Sports Med. 2014;48(3):187–96.

54. Wegner M, et al. Effects of exercise on anxiety and depression disorders: review of meta-analyses and neurobiological mechanisms. CNS Neurol Disord Drug Targets. 2014;13(6):1002–14.

55. Lamego MK, et al. Aerobic exercise reduces anxiety symptoms and improves fitness in patients with panic disorder. MedicalExpress. 2016;3(3). https://doi.org/10.5935/medicalexpress.2016.03.06.

56. Baldwin DS, et al. Evidence-based pharmacological treatment of anxiety disorders, post-traumatic stress disorder and obsessive-compulsive disorder: a revision of the 2005 guidelines from the British Association for Psychopharmacology. J Psychopharmacol. 2014;28(5):403–39.

57. Bartley CA, Hay M, Bloch MH. Meta-analysis: aerobic exercise for the treatment of anxiety disorders. Prog Neuro-Psychopharmacol Biol Psychiatry. 2013;45:34–9.

58. Hovland A, et al. Comparing physical exercise in groups to group cognitive behaviour therapy for the treatment of panic disorder in a randomized controlled trial. Behav Cogn Psychother. 2013;41(4):408–32.

59. Brown S, et al. Twenty-five year mortality of a community cohort with schizophrenia. Br J Psychiatry. 2010;196(2):116–21.

60. Rosa Rimes R, et al. Effects of exercise on physical and mental health, and cognitive and brain functions in schizophrenia: clinical and experimental evidence. CNS Neurol Disord Drug Targets. 2015;14(10):1244–54.

61. Stubbs B, et al. Falls in older adults with major depressive disorder (MDD): a systematic review and exploratory meta-analysis of prospective studies. Int Psychogeriatr. 2016;28(1):23–9.

62. Bunn F, et al. Preventing falls among older people with mental health problems: a systematic review. BMC Nurs. 2014;13(1):4.

63. Sherrington C, et al. Exercise to prevent falls in older adults: an updated systematic review and meta-analysis. Br J Sports Med. 2017;51:1750.

64. Kosmat H, Vranic A. The efficacy of dance intervention as a cognitive training for old-old. J Aging Phys Act. 2017;25:32.

65. Merom D, et al. Social dancing and incidence of falls in older adults: a cluster randomised controlled trial. PLoS Med. 2016;13(8):e1002112.

66. Scherr J, et al. Associations between Borg's rating of perceived exertion and physiological measures of exercise intensity. Eur J Appl Physiol. 2013;113(1):147–55.

67. Hofmann P, Tschakert G. Special needs to prescribe exercise intensity for scientific studies. Cardiol Res Pract. 2010;2011:209302.

68. Woltmann ML, et al. Evidence that the talk test can be used to regulate exercise intensity. J Strength Cond Res. 2015;29(5):1248–54.

69. Yu F, Demorest SL, Vock DM. Testing a modified perceived exertion scale for Alzheimer's disease. Psych J. 2015;4(1):38–46.

70. Yu F, Bil K. Correlating heart rate and perceived exertion during aerobic exercise in Alzheimer's disease. Nurs Health Sci. 2010;12(3):375–80.

71. Reed JL, Pipe AL. The talk test: a useful tool for prescribing and monitoring exercise intensity. Curr Opin Cardiol. 2014;29(5):475–80.

72. Reed JL, Pipe AL. Practical approaches to prescribing physical activity and monitoring exercise intensity. Can J Cardiol. 2016;32(4):514–22.

73. Gearhart RF Jr, et al. Strength tracking using the OMNI resistance exercise scale in older men and women. J Strength Cond Res. 2009;23(3):1011–5.

74. Csapo R, Alegre LM. Effects of resistance training with moderate vs heavy loads on muscle mass and strength in the elderly: a meta-analysis. Scand J Med Sci Sports. 2016;26(9):995–1006.

75. Bolmont B, et al. Mood states and anxiety influence abilities to maintain balance control in healthy human subjects. Neurosci Lett. 2002;329(1):96–100.

76. Nitz JC, Choy NL, Ogilvie M. The effect of depression on balance decline in mature women. Hong Kong Physiother J. 2005;23(1):27–35.

77. Bolbecker AR, et al. Postural control in bipolar disorder: increased sway area and decreased dynamical complexity. PLoS One. 2011;6(5):e19824.

78. Horak FB, Wrisley DM, Frank J. The balance evaluation systems test (BESTest) to differentiate balance deficits. Phys Ther. 2009;89(5):484–98.

79. Tamura T, et al. The impaired balance systems identified by the BESTest in older patients with knee osteoarthritis. PM R. 2016;8(9):869–75.

80. Toots A, et al. Effects of a high-intensity functional exercise program on dependence in activities of daily living and balance in older adults with dementia. J Am Geriatr Soc. 2016;64(1):55–64.

81. Zhu X, et al. The more the better? A meta-analysis on effects of combined cognitive and physical intervention on cognition in healthy older adults. Ageing Res Rev. 2016;31:67–79.

82. Lampit A, Hallock H, Valenzuela M. Computerized cognitive training in cognitively healthy older adults: a systematic review and meta-analysis of effect modifiers. PLoS Med. 2014;11(11):e1001756.

83. Lampit A, Valenzuela M, Gates NJ. Computerized cognitive training is beneficial for older adults. J Am Geriatr Soc. 2015;63(12):2610–2.

84. Firth J, et al. Motivating factors and barriers towards exercise in severe mental illness: a systematic review and meta-analysis. Psychol Med. 2016;46(14):2869–81.

85. Mielke MM, et al. Assessing the temporal relationship between cognition and gait: slow gait predicts cognitive decline in the Mayo Clinic Study of Aging. J Gerontol Ser A Biol Med Sci. 2013;68(8):929–37.

86. Beauchet O, et al. Poor gait performance and prediction of dementia: results from a meta-analysis. J Am Med Dir Assoc. 2016;17(6):482–90.

87. Deshpande N, et al. Gait speed under varied challenges and cognitive decline in older persons: a prospective study. Age Ageing. 2009;38:509.

88. Lundin-Olsson L, Nyberg L, Gustafson Y. Stops walking when talking as a predictor of falls in elderly people. Lancet. 1997;349(9052):617.

89. Montero-Odasso M, et al. Gait variability is associated with frailty in community-dwelling older adults. J Gerontol Ser A Biol Med Sci. 2011;66(5):568–76.

90. Podsiadlo D, Richardson S. The timed "Up & Go": a test of basic functional mobility for frail elderly persons. J Am Geriatr Soc. 1991;39(2):142–8.

91. Nordin E, Rosendahl E, Lundin-Olsson L. Timed "Up & Go" test: reliability in older people dependent in activities of daily living—focus on cognitive state. Phys Ther. 2006;86(5):646–55.

92. Barry E, et al. Is the Timed Up and Go test a useful predictor of risk of falls in community dwelling older adults: a systematic review and meta-analysis. BMC Geriatr. 2014;14(1):1.

93. Guralnik JM, et al. A short physical performance battery assessing lower extremity function: association with self-reported disability and prediction of mortality and nursing home admission. J Gerontol. 1994;49(2):M85–94.

94. Alzheimer's Society Factsheet: exercise and physical activity. 2015. https://www.alzheimers.org.uk/sites/default/files/migrate/downloads/factsheet_exercise_and_physical_activity.pdf. Last accessed 22 March 2019.

Advocating for Better Mental Health Care for Older Adults

12

Carlos Augusto de Mendonça Lima,
Gabriel Ivbijaro, Sudhir Kumar, and Jacob Roy

Abstract

A possible negative consequence of the rapid aging of the world population is the increase of the number of older adults with mental disorders. More than 20% of people aged 55 and more may suffer from mental health problems. Mental health problems have a significant impact on an older adult's ability to carry out the basic activities of everyday life and reduce the person's independence, autonomy, and quality of life. Despite the already significant and increasing number of well-prepared professionals, a well-developed body of knowledge, and a large number of caregivers, it is becoming more and more difficult to persuade the authorities to invest in the overall older adults' mental health. It is the responsibility of all mental health professionals, together with those involved, to advocate and to act to ensure that the distribution of available mental health resources is done in an equitable manner to adequately meet the needs of all. One of the ways to bring about a real change in the older adults' mental health care is to rely on the local, national, and international associations and organizations of the persons concerned by this theme. This chapter reviews some of these international organizations and their current projects.

C. A. de Mendonça Lima (✉)
Unity of Old Age Psychiatry, Centre Les Toises, Lausanne, Switzerland

G. Ivbijaro
NOVA University, Lisbon, Portugal

Waltham Forest Community and Family Health Services, London, UK

S. Kumar
Alzheimer's and Related Disorders Society of India, Ernakulam, Kerala, India

J. Roy
Alzheimer's and Related Disorders Society of India, Ernakulam, Kerala, India

Alzheimer's Disease International, London, UK

Key Points
- One of the consequences of the rapid aging of the world's population is the increase in the number of older adults with mental disorders who may overwhelm mental health systems.
- It is becoming increasingly difficult to convince the authorities to invest in the overall mental health of the elderly.
- One way to ensure an equitable distribution of available resources and to provoke a real change is to rely on local, national, and international societies, associations, and organizations to ensure a credible defense of interests.

© Springer Nature Switzerland AG 2019
C. A. de Mendonça Lima, G. Ivbijaro (eds.), *Primary Care Mental Health in Older People*,
https://doi.org/10.1007/978-3-030-10814-4_12

• This chapter presents some of these organizations active in Europe and in the world, as well as some of their strategies, projects, and actions.

12.1 Mental Health of Older Adults: An Important Public Health Subject

The world population aged over 60 is estimated to become 2 billion by 2050 [1]. In the same year, 30% of the population residing in the European Community area will be over 65 years of age, and 10% will be over 80 years of age. The growth of the older adults' number will be rapid in middle- and low-income countries, with enormous consequences for these vulnerable economies [2]. In the less developed regions, by 2050, older persons are expected to account for a fifth of the population. Many people live a long and happy life without any mental health problems, and, despite the widespread image that older people are sad, slow, and forgetful, mental disorders are not an inevitable consequence of aging. Nevertheless, one of the possible negative consequences of the rapid aging of the world population is the increase of the number of older adults with mental disorders, which is likely to overwhelm mental health systems in all countries [2] as they are now already doing.

More than 20% of people aged 55 and more may suffer from mental health problems. Biological changes can interfere with the functioning of the brain. Social change can lead to personal isolation or devaluation. Somatic diseases are also important factors in breaking an already fragile psychic balance. Mental disorders can exacerbate the symptoms and functional disabilities associated with medical illnesses and increase the overall cost of care [3].

Mental health problems can have a significant impact on an older adult's ability to carry out the basic activities of everyday life and reduce the person's independence, autonomy, and quality of life. The first step to reduce these negative consequences is simply by making a proper diagnosis. Unfortunately, mental health problems are not

often diagnosed and treated. Many older adults struggle without proper help—or simply without any help at all [4].

There are many prejudices about the meaning of mental illness. Many older adults today still see mental illness as a sign of weakness and are unlikely to admit their difficulties. In addition, symptoms of dementia and depression are too often considered as part of normal aging.

Despite the significant and increasing number of well-prepared professionals, a well-developed body of knowledge, and a large number of caregivers, it is becoming more and more difficult to persuade the authorities to invest in the overall older adults' mental health. This is not consistent with the growing demographic position of this age group in the population. The distribution of skilled mental health resources for caring older adults among the different regions of the world and income groups is significantly uneven, and in many countries, they are even scarce.

In this context, the absence of a comprehensive policy and targeted programs for the older adults' mental health is not surprising. Despite the improvement in educational programs, the recruitment of new human resources to work in favor of the older adults' mental health is becoming increasingly difficult. Even in Europe, where services are considered to be better developed, between 2011 and 2014, there were a 3% reduction in the median number of total psychiatrists per 100,000 inhabitants and an increase of only 1% in the median number of nurses per 100,000 inhabitants: Europe is the WHO region with the most skilled human resources in mental health and the region of the world with the highest rate of older adults [5].

Other health professions working with older adults are also affected. The lack of psychologists specialized in older adults' mental health severely reduces training opportunities for psychologists and is an obstacle to the development of positive attitudes toward the choice of a career with the older adults. The low availability of specialized psychologists also reduces the availability of supervision of nonspecialized psychologists providing support to older adults. However, the lack of adequate resources is not the only factor limiting the recruitment of adequate health personnel. Negative prejudices among the general public, decision-makers, and health-care providers, including doctors, have long contributed to making careers related to care of older adults less attractive than other specialties.

While in some parts of the world professionals interested in this area of care argue for designing specific services catering to the older adults, in some countries, there is a movement to close specific mental health services for older adults, considering that this exclusivity reinforces segregation within the health system. This specificity was originally recognized as being necessary to treat patients with multiple comorbidities and special needs and for which there was a natural tendency not to consider them as a priority adult population. Developing services should be closely matched with the resources available, existing heath systems, and prioritization. While developing specialist services at a national level may be appropriate for some health systems and countries, integration of old-age care and old-age mental health care into primary health services may be more appropriate in others.

The organization of services for older adults suffering from mental disorders needs vast improvement. There has been little attention on the needs of older adults suffering from anxiety and affective disorders, with suicidal ideation or with psychotic disorders.

It is the responsibility of all mental health professionals, together with those involved, to advocate and to act to ensure that the distribution of available mental health resources is done in an equitable manner to adequately meet the needs of all. The Declaration of Alma-Ata on Primary Health Care [6] states in Paragraph IV that every human being has the right and the duty to participate individually and collectively in the planning and implementation of health care. One of the ways to bring about a real change in the older adults' mental health care is to rely on the local, national, and international associations and organizations of the persons concerned by this theme. Putting together their energy, competences, and representativeness, it becomes more efficient to produce a significant change in all area concerned by mental health care for older adults: to produce better policies and more efficient programs and to develop more and better facilities to deliver care and education for all.

We will review some of these international organizations and their current projects.

12.2 The Nongovernmental Organizations

12.2.1 The European Association of Geriatric Psychiatry (EAGP: http://www.eagp.com)

The EAGP, the oldest association of the specialty (founded in 1972), has a very important role in bringing together old-age psychiatrists from European countries, creating opportunities for teaching, and promoting research. It is an association of professionals, which also encourages the development and promotion of national organizations of old-age psychiatry to join it. The objectives of the EAGP are to promote research, pre- and postgraduate training, and the development of old-age psychiatry and to cooperate with national and international organizations involved in the field. In addition to its congress, the association has participated at national and international congresses and as well to consensus meetings and has collaborated to significant consensus statements in the field.

Since 2013, the association organizes every 2 years in Lausanne the 1-week course in old-age psychiatry. This course offers a forum for bringing together European old-age psychiatrists with an academic or institutional potential. Participants have the opportunity to improve their knowledge on old-age psychiatry, to develop new ideas, and to share experiences about mental health programs and organizations. The course includes workshops, group discussions, and lectures by European experts in the field of geriatric psychiatry. The association also offers every year a 3-day refresher course for postgraduate training.

12.2.2 The International Psychogeriatric Association (IPA: http://www.ipa-online.org)

For more than 30 years, the International Psychogeriatric Association (IPA) has symbolized the entire mental health of the older adults. For the IPA, the spirit of connection, collaboration, and community is fundamental. The IPA facilitates the bringing together of professionals and their collaboration to interact and work together in research, to improve care practices, and to promote mental health improvement for all older adults around the world. The IPA promotes this spirit of community within the association but also seeks to work with other organizations that share its commitment, such as those included in its *IPA Affiliate Organizations* program (involving 27 associations from 24 countries), the World Health Organization, the United Nations, the World Psychiatric Association, the Alzheimer's Disease International, and many others.

Some activities of the IPA in addition to the organization of its congresses:

IPA Junior Research Awards in Psychogeriatrics: presented every 2 years at the International Congress, the IPA recognizes the best original research yet unpublished in the field of old-age psychiatry carried out by young professionals who are initiating in the specialty.

IPA Member Forums: these are the communities of IPA members who can connect and collaborate online as well as at meetings and congresses. Based on disciplines, regions of the world, and common interests in old-age psychiatry, members collaborate in forums to share best practices, communicate current projects, write articles, research, develop programs, and produce publications.

Expert Consensus Meeting: beginning in the 1990s, with the first meeting on behavioral and psychological symptoms of dementia (BPSD), until the most recent meeting for a universal definition of care and criteria for research on agitation, the IPA has been at the forefront of older adults' mental health. Regularly, IPA brings together renowned experts to conduct these invitational meetings only to examine and to discuss an important and determined issue in an effort to reach consensus and to advance the field.

12.2.3 The European Psychiatric Association (http://www.europsy.net)

The association was founded in October 1983 with the name of Association Européenne de Psychiatres (AEP) with the aim of promoting European psychiatry in the fields of research, treatment, and education. Another objective was to establish an association that would act as a privileged mediator between practitioners and public authorities on issues related to mental health policies.

In order to achieve these objectives, the ASP has gradually set up the organization of the annual European Congress of Psychiatry, as well as other regular scientific meetings, the publication of an international scientific journal, the award of research grants, and the creation of sections corresponding to sub-disciplines of psychiatry.

Since its foundation, the number of AEP members has grown steadily, and its openness to all member countries of the Council of Europe has evolved rapidly. As a result, in February 1989, it was granted consultative status with the Council of Europe, followed by a participatory status in 2003. In 2008, the Extraordinary General Assembly changed the name of the organization to become the European Psychiatric Association (EPA). Since 2012, the EPA offers the possibility for national psychiatric associations to become full members while retaining the possibility of individual membership: 39 national psychiatric associations from 36 European countries are by now members of the EPA.

EPA is the most visible psychiatric association in Europe, basing its growth on developing collaborative projects with other major psychiatric organizations such as the European College of Neuropsychopharmacology (ECNP), the German Research Network on Schizophrenia (ECSR), the International Society of Neurobiology and Psychopharmacology, the European Brain Council (EBC), and the European Union of Specialist Physicians (UEMS).

12.2.3.1 The Section of Old Age Psychiatry

EPA has created sections that have their own steering committees. These sections organize their own symposia under the aegis of EPA and annual conferences in Europe. The mission of the Section of Old Age Psychiatry is to promote the discipline of old-age psychiatry within the framework of the EPA, through the following objectives:

- To ensure that the executive committee and the board are well informed about issues of geriatric psychiatry
- To organize symposia and workshops during the EPA congress
- To collaborate with other international organizations with similar interests and participate in major international meetings relevant to the discipline
- To develop and disseminate educational materials for practitioners in the field
- To provide technical support to national member organizations of EPA

The Section of Old Age Psychiatry has proposed an itinerant course on dementia which was first presented in Riga in October 2013 at the annual meeting of the Latvian Psychiatric Society and after at the Portuguese National Congress of Psychiatry and Mental Health in November 2015. The section has collaborated with the fifth EPA Academia Summer School held in Strasbourg from 10 to 13 July 2015, with the theme of comorbidity between mental and physical disorders, focusing on the health of the elderly.

As an example of advocacy action, the section supported the Royal College of Psychiatrists Faculty of Old Age Psychiatry. In December 2013 the section contacted the EPA president to ask for a response on the risk of closure of specialized mental health services for the older adults in the UK. An open letter was published in *The Times* in January 2014 [7], with the signatures of representatives from the Royal College, EPA members, and other global specialists. The

EPA directors and its National Psychiatric Associations (NPA) board discussed this issue in Munich in March 2014. The EPA sent a letter in March 2014 to the UK Secretary of State for Health. The British health authority issued the following statement in its 2014 annual report: "Mental health problems in the elderly are common, often undiagnosed, but are amenable to treatment as in other age groups. Helping people with physical, psychological and social difficulties combined in the context of aging and the end of life requires specialization. This could be compromised by switching to generic services that are not organized according to the age of the users."

Finally, this section was represented at the meeting held in Lausanne in July 2002, where a paper on skill-based objectives for the training of specialists in old-age psychiatry was proposed [12].

12.2.4 The World Psychiatric Association (http://www.wpanet.org)

WPA is an association of national psychiatric societies aimed at increasing the knowledge and skills needed to work in the field of mental health and care for the mentally ill. Its member societies currently are 135, covering 117 countries, representing more than 200,000 psychiatrists.

WPA organizes the World Congress of Psychiatry every 3 years. It also organizes international and regional congresses and meetings, as well as thematic conferences. It has 65 scientific sections, aimed at disseminating information and promoting collaboration in specific areas of psychiatry. WPA has produced several educational programs and books. Encouraged by years of complaints about the political abuse of psychiatry, the WPA General Assemblies have formulated ethical guidelines on psychiatric practice, including the Madrid Declaration of 1996, amended in 1999 in Hamburg. WPA works equally well with the United Nations and the

World Health Organization to protect the rights of the mentally ill.

More recently, WPA has paid more and more systematic attention to teaching activities, often in coordination with the World Health Organization. Curricula have been developed, targeting psychiatrists and other health professionals around the world, particularly those residing in developing countries.

The Sections: they are the scientific backbone of WPA. They cover virtually all aspects of psychiatry and enjoy a high degree of independence under the WPA regulations under the supervision and direction of the secretary for the sections. Specifically, the aims of the sections are the collection, analysis, presentation, and dissemination of information on services, research and training in the various areas of psychiatry and mental health, and advancing knowledge in these fields.

The sections will achieve these by:

- The establishment of relations with national and international organizations which share the objectives of WPA in the specific area of the section, with a view to achieve better coordination of the activities of the interests of the section and the WPA
- The organization of scientific meetings on subjects of interest to the section
- The organization of symposia dealing with the specialty of the section at the World Congress of Psychiatry and other scientific meetings organized under the auspices of WPA
- The development of curricula, guidelines, and publications
- The elaboration of proposals for adoption as consensus declarations and position statements
- The promotion and conduction of international collaborative research

The Section of Old Age Psychiatry: The Section of Old Age Psychiatry has proposed symposia and working groups for the last 2 years at World Congresses of Psychiatry, WPA Regional Congresses, and other relevant associations such as the EPA and IPA. The section co-authored three consensus declarations

[8–10], jointly with WHO, and sent representatives at two other consensus meetings that produced relevant statements [11–13]. In 2009, it was at the origin of a consensus statement on ethics and the assessment of the capacity of older persons with mental disorders [14]. Finally, in 2002, the section, in collaboration with the WPA section on affective disorders, published a reference book on depression in the elderly [15] and conducted a survey in 2003 on the state of education in geriatric psychiatry in the world [16].

12.2.5 The World Federation for Mental Health (http://wfmh.com)

The WFMH is an international organization founded in 1948 to promote the prevention, treatment, and care of mental disorders at the global level and to promote mental health. Through its members and contacts in more than 100 countries in 6 continents, the federation has responded to international crises in mental health through its role as the sole credible advocacy base and as organizer of public education in the field of mental health. Its members (organizations and individuals) include mental health workers from all disciplines, consumers of mental health services, family members, and concerned citizens. This organization makes possible collaboration between governments and nongovernmental organizations to advance the cause of mental health services and of research and advocacy around the world.

WFMH supports older adults with mental disorders through two projects:

- The World Mental Health Day, which is celebrated on 10 October each year, with the overall objective of raising awareness of mental health issues worldwide and mobilizing efforts for mental health. The Day provides an opportunity for all stakeholders working on mental health issues to talk about their work and on what remains to be done to make mental health care a reality for people around the world. The WFMH leadership has chosen "Mental Health and Older Adults" as the theme for the World Mental Health Day in 2013—and for the WFMH annual report. The theme highlighted the lengthening of life expectancy, which in many developed countries involves more years at work, more years of active retirement, and a cohort of "very old" people, over 80 years. This creates a new concept of "old age." In low-income countries, citizens often have a shorter life span and receive limited assistance as they get older (http://wfmh.com/wp-content/uploads/2013/11/2013_wmhday_english.pdf).

- The World Dignity Project (www.worlddignityproject.com): Every human interaction represents an opportunity for one person to treat another with dignity—it is a meeting in dignity. People and families affected by mental illness can often describe what dignity should look like. However, experience shows a completely different reality. The stigma of mental illness can no longer be tolerated. Stigma interferes with the full participation of people in society and deprives them of their dignity. Making dignity in mental health a reality requires that every member of society works with others and that mental health problems become more visible and no longer considered as shameful. The World Dignity Project aims to identify and invite a million people, organizations, countries, and states to become members of the foundation by adopting the project symbol to make it possible to form a global movement to combat stigma linked to mental health and launch it to the general public all around the world since 2016.

12.2.6 Alzheimer Europe (http://www.alzheimer-europe.org/)

Alzheimer Europe (AE) is a nongovernmental organization aiming to raise awareness about all forms of dementia. Formed in 1996, AE is based in Luxembourg and operates a common European platform through cooperation among its 36 members, all of which are active Alzheimer's organizations in Europe. AE is primarily a lobbying organization that fosters awareness of dementia and care and research in EU institutions. This effort includes the European Alzheimer's Alliance, a group of more than 100 deputies of the European Parliament which aims to make dementia a public health priority. In addition, AE is a source of information on all aspects of dementia, including through annual research publications. The AE also publishes the *Dementia in Europe* and delivers a monthly newsletter to more than 5800 subscribers. At the national level, AE member associations have always been at the forefront of efforts to establish strategies to combat dementia in their countries. The annual AE conferences attract people from diverse backgrounds around dementia.

Here are some recent actions of the association:

Paris Declaration 2006: In 2006, AE and its member organizations adopted a declaration on the political priorities of the European Alzheimer Movement at the AE conference in Paris in 2006. In this Paris Declaration, Alzheimer Europe called on European policy makers to give Alzheimer's disease and other forms of dementia the political priority they deserved.

European Dementia Ethics Network: At the 2008 French Presidency Conference on Alzheimer's Disease, the president stressed the need for EU Member States to include in the discussion agenda some of the ethical challenges posed by dementia and advocated the creation of a European network for this purpose. This acknowledgment of the importance of the ethical aspects of dementia was taken up in the European Commission's Alzheimer's Disease Initiative: the European Dementia Ethics Network was created and became operational in 2009. By now, several of its working groups addressed ethical issues related to dementia research, restriction of freedom, and perception and representation of dementia and are currently working on a guide to help caregivers and people with dementia to address the ethical dilemmas they may encounter as a result of life experience with a person with dementia.

Elections to the European Parliament 2014: AE identified the elections to the European Parliament in 2014 as a key opportunity to contact current members of the European Parliament and candidates in the election and asked them to support the campaign of the organization to make dementia a European priority. AE asked them about the essential progress for people with dementia and their caregivers in the current mandate of the European Parliament and asked them to adopt their priorities for political action in the years to come.

Glasgow Declaration 2014: The Glasgow Declaration was published in 2014. It calls for the creation of a European dementia strategy and national strategies in all countries in Europe. The signatories also call on world leaders to recognize dementia as a public health priority and to develop a global plan of action on dementia.

European Collaboration on Dementia (EuroCoDe): The aim of the project is to create an European network of all actors in the field of dementia to jointly develop consensual indicators, to establish a permanent dialogue between these actors to identify ways to highlight synergies and closer collaborations in dementia European level. To develop these guidelines and indicators, the network brought together a number of European organizations, European projects, and informal collaborations.

12.2.7 Alzheimer's Disease International (http://www.alz.co.uk/)

ADI believes that the key to winning the fight against dementia lies in a unique combination of global solutions and local knowledge. As such, it operates at the local level, empowering Alzheimer's associations to promote and deliver care and support for people with dementia and their caregivers while working globally to draw attention to dementia: ADI has formal relations with the World Health Organization.

The ADI has an Alzheimer University, a series of hands-on workshops to help Alzheimer's staff and volunteers to build and to strengthen their organizations. ADI organizes an annual international conference which is a unique multidisciplinary event aimed at uniting people who have an interest in dementia around the world. World Alzheimer's Day, celebrated annually on 21 September, is an opportunity to raise global public awareness about dementia and its impact on families and to showcase the important work of its members around the world.

The *World Alzheimer Reports* provide the most comprehensive and up-to-date dementia data worldwide, including prevalence and economic impact.

The *10/66 Dementia Research Group* is made up of researchers who are studying the epidemiology of dementia, modalities, and services for the support of patients and their families in developing countries. ADI and the Fondation Médéric Alzheimer are working together to award the *Alzheimer's Award for Psychosocial Interventions* to promote this type of research aimed at supporting and improving the quality of life for people with dementia and their caregivers. The *IMPACT* study was designed to assess the current beliefs and behaviors of Alzheimer's disease and dementia among stakeholder groups from five European countries. The *Stroud Symposia Series* is a collaborative effort between the Stroud Center, the ADI, and the The Institute of Psychiatry, Psychology and Neuroscience in London and has collected stories about the experiences of people with dementia and their caregivers. These stories provided insight into the improvement in the quality of life of people with dementia and their caregivers.

12.3 The Governmental Organizations

12.3.1 The European Commission

The *European Commission's Directorate for Health and Consumers* and the Ministry of Health and Social Affairs of Spain co-hosted in

2010 in Madrid, with the support of the Spanish Presidency of the European Union, the conference Mental Health and Well-Being in Older People—Making It Happen (http://ec.europa.eu/health/mental_health/events/ev_20100419_en.htm).

The organizers invited 182 representatives from 29 European countries, the European Commission, and the European Parliament, including members of the health and social services authorities, governmental and nongovernmental organizations of professionals, and consumers. The conference stressed the right of older Europeans to the highest level of health and well-being. It was stressed that it is the duty of all to give greater priority to the promotion of mental health and well-being and to fight mental health problems. Several horizontal themes have been identified and should be taken into consideration in the developing measures to improve the mental health and well-being of older persons. Some principles have also been considered for building action to improve the mental health and well-being of the elderly.

The following five priority areas were discussed:

- The promotion of mental health in old age
- The prevention of mental disorders and the promotion of autonomy
- The older adults in vulnerable situations
- Health systems for care and treatment
- Support for informal caregivers

The conference invited the organizers to communicate the results to the presidency of the conference on *active and healthy aging* and encouraged the initiation of actions to promote the mental health and well-being of the older adults. The European Commission and Member States were invited to collaborate with regional and local authorities in partnership with professionals, informal patients and informal caregivers, NGOs, the older adults themselves, and other health sectors and the social sector concerned, to develop several initiatives to ensure the best possible mental health and well-being of older persons in Europe.

12.3.2 The United Nations

Through a series of decisions, conventions, and resolutions, the United Nations has made a decisive contribution to protecting the rights of all patients with mental disorders and disabilities. Two of them are:

- The United Nations Resolution 46/119 of 17 December 1991: Principles for the Protection of Persons with Mental Disorders and for the Improvement of Mental Health Care (http://www.equalrightstrust.org/ertdocumentbank/UN_Resolution_on_protection_of_persons_with_mental_illness.pdf)
- The United Nations Convention on the Rights of Persons with Disabilities of 2006 (http://www.un.org/disabilities/convention/conventionfull.shtml)

The UN was also linked to the 2002 Political Declaration and Madrid International Plan of Action on Aging [17] and the follow-up to the Second World Assembly on Aging in 2010 [18]. The Political Declaration committed itself to provide seniors with universal and equal access to care and services, including physical and mental health services. The United Nations Plan of Action on Aging provides a very specific contribution to the promotion of mental health in old age. Most recently, the United Nations Economic Commission for Europe (UNECE) realized in cooperation with the Government of Portugal at Lisbon in September 2017 the Ministerial Conference on Ageing (A Sustainable Society for All Ages: Realizing the potential of living longer).

The conference completed the third review and appraisal cycle (2012–2017) of the Madrid International Plan of Action on Ageing and its Regional Implementation Strategy (MIPAA/RIS). The focus was on "Realizing the potential of living longer." Conference panels addressed this theme through the lens of:

1. Recognizing the potential of older persons
2. Encouraging longer working life and ability to work
3. Ensuring aging with dignity

The *United Nations Convention on Older People's Rights*: the protection of the human rights of older peoples is still considered insufficient. Human rights, and their protection, are an important determinant of basic social health [17]. The Universal Declaration of Human Rights [19] deals with the rights of all human beings, but the rights and needs of certain groups are not sufficiently covered by it. The General Assembly of the United Nations decided on 16 November 2010 to set up a working group to strengthen the protection of the human rights of the older persons (http://globalaging.org/agingwatch/convention/humanrights/Strengthening20Rights%%20 2%20-[update]%20Low20Res.pdf%). A Convention on the Rights of Older Persons is the most effective way to ensure that all people now and in the future can enjoy their human rights in their old age on an equal basis with others. This agreement is necessary to:

- Establish legal norms that challenge and replace attitudes and behaviors that stigmatize and discriminate older people.
- Clarify how human rights are applicable to older age.
- Ensure that states understand their human rights obligations for all in their older age.
- Better understand and assert the rights in old age.
- Improve the accountability of states for their human rights obligations toward the elderly.
- Provide a framework for policy development and decision-making.

12.3.3 The World Health Organization

WHO, through its Department of Mental Health and Substance Abuse, plays a very important role in policy making, suggests the development of specific programs, and provides decision-makers around the world with relevant information on mental disorders. It is impossible to describe here all his actions in favor of the mental health of the older adults, but here are some of the most significant and recent.

The *WHO Collaborating Center for Psychiatry of the Elderly*: In 1994, WHO decided to appoint a collaborating center for the specific aspects of mental health for people over 65, and the University Service for Old Age Psychiatry of Lausanne was chosen. A protocol for a first collaboration was signed for the participation of this service in the program *Quality Assurance in Mental Health Care*. Quality indicators and a glossary to assess a day hospital in old-age psychiatry were developed, tested, and published [20]. Other indicators and glossaries were also developed to assess an outpatient facility and a liaison consultation in old-age psychiatry. Thanks to this first successful collaboration, the University Service of Old Age Psychiatry of Lausanne was appointed in 1996 as WHO-CC for Psychiatry of the Elderly and since then has assumed a consultative role for WHO in mental health for older adults.

Initially, this collaborating center received the mandate to organize three consensus meetings and to prepare and publish consensus statements on a definition of psychiatry for the elderly [9], the organization of care in psychiatry of the elderly [10], and the training in the psychiatry of the elderly [11]. These three meetings and documents were jointly organized and published in collaboration with WPA.

WHO decided to devote the year 2001 to mental health and published the World Health Report 2001: Mental Health, New Understanding, New Hope, to which the WHO-CC, Lausanne, contributed [21]. The collaborating center also organized a new consensus meeting on the reduction of stigma and discrimination against older persons with mental disorders and published it in several languages [11].

In 2012, the center organized another meeting to propose skill-based objectives for training in old-age psychiatry [12]. After its publication, the final document was submitted to the European Union of Specialist Physicians.

The WHO-CC has also contributed to the creation of fact sheets of references circulated by WHO. The latest, published in 2013, refers to depression. The center participates in the effort to raise awareness and disseminate information on old-age psychiatry in countries where this specialty is still underdeveloped, for example, in Brazil, where a project is under way to create a training program for caregivers. In addition, the center was also mandated to organize a collaboration among international experts in the revision of the International Classification of Mental and Behavioral Disorders (ICD-11). These include identifying the diagnostic features of psychiatric illness in older adults.

The Mental Health Gap Action Programme (mhGAP): After the World Health Year 2001 on mental health and the publication of WHR 2001 [21], WHO developed the mhGAP (http://www.who.int/mental_health/mhgap/en/) program to strengthen care services for people with mental disorders, neurological disorders, and substance dependence, particularly for low- and middle-income countries. The program states that with appropriate care, psychosocial assistance, and medicines, tens of millions of patients could be treated for depression, schizophrenia, and epilepsy and freed from their suicidal ideation and could begin to lead a normal life—even when resources are scarce. This program published the *mhGAP Intervention Guide for Mental, Neurological and Substance Use Disorders in Non-Specialized Health Settings* [22]. The IMH-mhGAP is destinated for health-care providers in primary and secondary care settings. It is presented in a succinct form to facilitate interventions by nonspecialized and already very busy staff. It details what to do, but does not attempt to explain how to do it. It is important that nonspecialized care providers be trained, supervised, and assisted in using the IMH-MhGAP in the assessment and management of people with mental, neurological, or psychoactive substance-related disorders. Although not specific to older adults with these disorders, it nevertheless presents a very useful chapter on dementia.

WHO and Dementia: In 2006, WHO published the document *Neurological Disorders: Public Health Challenges* [23]. It presents the public health perspective for neurological disorders and presents estimates and forecasts of the global burden of these disorders. Separate sections deal with some of the most important disorders in detail, dementia in particular. This chapter on dementia provides comprehensive information to decision-makers and can also be used as an awareness tool.

A major turning point, however, was the publication in 2012 of the report *Dementia: A Public Health Priority*, which was developed jointly by WHO and ADI [24]. The aim of this report is to raise awareness of dementia as a public health priority, to articulate a public health approach, and to advocate for action at national and international levels. Indeed, there is a lack of awareness and understanding of dementia in most countries, leading to stigma, barriers to diagnosis and care, impacting caregivers, families, and societies physically, psychologically, and economically. The report should enable governments, policy makers, and other stakeholders to address the impact of dementia as a growing threat to global health.

This hope has not been in vain. In March 2015, WHO organized its first Ministerial Conference on Global Action Against Dementia. Ministers [25] from several countries around the world, as well as experts from research, clinical communities, and NGOs, met in Geneva for the first time to discuss the global problems of dementia. The aim of the conference was to raise awareness of the socioeconomic burden created by dementia and to stress that this burden can be reduced if the world collectively commits dementia to a global public health priority.

12.4 Conclusion

It is clear that developing services catering to the mental health needs of older adults would be much easier in age-friendly cultures and societies and hence the importance of building and working toward them cannot be overemphasized. Awareness creation about the impact of mental health conditions on the older adults should be done among the general public, policy makers, funding bodies, as well as health-care and social care professionals.

We already count with two specific associations on old-age psychiatry (EAGP, IPA), sections of old-age psychiatry in international psychiatric associations (WPA, EPA), an association that plays a major role in defending the rights of the mentally ill (WHMH), and major associations involved in the debate on dementia (AE, ADI), plus official organizations such as the UN, WHO, and European Commission. National organizations including old-age mental health sections of psychiatric associations do play a role at the national level in several countries, some big and some small. With several of these organizations in existence, we would hope that the mental health of older adults would be fairly protected, but in reality there is a long journey before we reach this objective. There should be a concerted effort by all stakeholders involved including governmental and nongovernmental organizations, health and social sectors, and above all caregivers, service users, and general public.

It is extremely necessary to recognize the difficulties existing in the articulation of interests and in the provision of resources between these various actors. On the other hand, it is also necessary to accept the role of many other associations and medical organizations (World Federation of Neurology, International Association of Gerontology and Geriatrics, World Organization of National Colleges, Academies and Academic Associations of General Practitioners/Family Physicians, etc.) and nonmedical organizations (the International Council of Nurses, the International Federation of Occupational Therapists, many associations of psychologists, etc.) in their contribution to improving the mental health and well-being of the older adults and difficulties in articulating with the previous institutions. Finally, it should also be recognized the valuable role of national, regional, and local institutions in their efforts to collaborate with international institutions and who share the harsh reality of the older adults with their multiple health problems and with their material and social difficulties.

Many older adults do not yet receive the care they need. While in low- and middle-income countries this is mainly due to inadequate resources, in settings where care and assistance services are available, the reasons are lack of information, prejudice, and discrimination. Many professionals do not recognize the alarming severity of the problem and do not receive adequate mental health training in old age. The means to develop programs and services are too insufficient overall. But we must not deny that progress has been made. It is our responsibility to continue to develop them.

References

1. United Nations. World population ageing 2009. New York: UN; 2009.
2. World Health Organization, Alzheimer's Disease International. Dementia: a health public priority. Geneva: WHO; 2012.
3. American Association for Geriatric Psychiatry. Geriatrics and mental health—the facts. http://www.aagponline.org/prof/facts_mh.asp.
4. United States. Public Health Service. Office of the surgeon general. Mental health. A report of the surgeon general. Washington, D.C.: NIMH; 1999. http://profiles.nlm.nih.gov/ps/retrieve/ResourceMetadata/NNBBHS. Accessed 26 May 2013.
5. World Health Organization. Mental Health Atlas. Geneva: WHO; 2014. p. 2015.
6. Organisation Mondiale de la Santé. Déclaration d'Alma-Ata sur les soins de santé primaires. 12 September 1978. http://www.who.int/topics/primary_health_care/alma_ata_declaration/fr/.
7. Warner J, Graham N, de Mendonça Lima CA, Broadaty H, et al. Mental health — and how the other half lives. Letter to the editor. The Times, 24th January 2014.
8. World Psychiatric Association/World Health Organization. Psychiatry of the elderly: a consensus statement. (Doc: WHO/MNH/MND/96.7). Geneva: WHO; 1996. p. 11.
9. World Psychiatric Association/World Health Organization. Organization of care in psychiatry of the elderly: A technical consensus statement. (DOC: WHO/MSA/MNH/MND/97.3). Geneva: WHO; 1997. p. 15.
10. World Psychiatric Association/World Health Organization. Education in psychiatry of the elderly: a technical consensus statement. (DOC: WHO/MSA/MNH/MND/98.4). Geneva: WHO; 1998. p. 9.
11. Graham N, Lindesay J, Katona C, Bertolote JM, Camus V, Copeland JRM, de Mendonça Lima CA, Gaillard M, Nargeot MCG, Gray J, Jacobsson L, Kingma M, Kühne N, O'Loughlin A, Saracenon B, Taintor Z, Wancata J. Reducing stigma and discrimination against older people with mental disorders: a technical consensus statement. Int J Geriatr Psychiatry. 2003;18:670–8.
12. Gustafson L, Burns A, Katona C, Bertolote JM, Camus V, Copeland JRM, Dufey AF, Graham N, Ihl R, Kanowski S, Kühne N, de Mendonça Lima CA, Alvarez M, Rutz W, Tataru NL, Tudose C. Skill-based

objectives for specialist training in old age psychiatry. Int J Geriatr Psychiatry. 2003;18:686–93.

13. Katona C, Livingstone G, Cooper C, Ames D, Brodaty H, Chiu E. International Psychogeriatric Association consensus statement on defining and measuring treatment benefits in dementia. Int Psychogeriatr. 2007;19(3):345–54.

14. Katona C, Chiu E, Adelman S, Baloyannis S, Camus V, Firmino H, Gove D, Graham N, Ghebrehiwet T, Icelli I, Ihl R, Kalasic A, Leszek L, Kim S, de Mendonça Lima CA, Peisah C, Tataru N, Warner J. World psychiatric association section of old age psychiatry consensus statement on ethics and capacity in older people with mental disorders. Int J Geriatr Psychiatry. 2009;24(12):1319–24.

15. Baldwin RC, Chiu E, Katona C, Graham N. Guidelines on depression in older people. Practising the evidence. London: Martin Dunitz; 2002. Prepared under the auspices of the WPA Sections of Old Age Psychiatry and Affective Disorder.

16. Camus V, Katona C, de Mendonça Lima CA, Hakam AMA, Graham N, Baldwin R, Chiu E. on behalf of the WPA section on old age psychiatry. Teaching and training in old age psychiatry: a general survey of the World Psychiatric Association member societies. Int J Geriatr Psychiatry. 2003;18:694–9.

17. United Nations. Report of the second world assembly on ageing. Madrid 8–12 April 2002. New York: United Nations; 2002.

18. United Nations. Follow-up to the second world assembly on ageing. New York: United Nations; 2010.

19. United Nations. Universal declaration of human rights. New York: United Nations; 1948.

20. World Health Organization. Day-hospitals for the elderly. In: WHO. Quality assurance in mental health care. Check-lists & glossaries. Geneva: WHO; 2007. WHO/MSA/MNH/MND/97.2.

21. Organisation Mondiale de la Santé. Rapport sur la santé dans le monde 2001. La santé mentale : nouvelle conception, nouveaux espoirs. Genève: OMS; 2001. http://www.who.int/whr/2001/en/.

22. Organisation Mondiale de la Santé. Guide d'intervention mhGAP pour lutter contre les troubles mentaux, neurologiques et liés à l'utilisation de substances psychoactives dans les structures de soins non spécialisées: Programme d'action Combler les lacunes en santé mentale. Genève: OMS; 2011.

23. World Health Organization. Neurological disorders: public health challenges. Geneva: WHO; 2006.

24. World Health Organization. Dementia: a public health priority. Geneva: WHO; 2012.

25. World Health Organization. First WHO ministerial conference on global action against dementia: meeting report, WHO Headquarters, Geneva, Switzerland, 16–17 March 2015. http://apps.who.int/iris/bitstream/10665/179537/1/9789241509114_eng.pdf?ua=1&ua=1.

Part V

Mental and Behavioural Disorders (and Problems) in Older Adults in Primary Care

Anxiety Disorder in Older Adults

13

Valeska Marinho, Bruno Gherman,
and Sergio Luís Blay

Abstract

This chapter addresses anxiety disorders in late life, especially generalized anxiety disorder, which is highly prevalent and overloads health services. In addition, anxious patients usually have cognitive and social functioning decline, leading to a poorer quality of life. Despite this, it is a less studied topic than geriatric depression. Neurobiological research shows the involvement of the HPA axis, and basal cortisol levels are higher in those patients. The presentation of the symptoms is usually different in comparison with younger adults, and it is frequently comorbid with other psychiatric and physical diseases, complicating its management. The treatment should involve medicines, such as SSRIs and psychotherapy, especially cognitive behavioral therapy.

Key Points

- Anxiety disorders in late life have elevated prevalence and are frequently comorbid but not always chronic.
- GAD may not directly increase mortality in depressed elderly people but leads to increased use of health services, decreased cognitive and social functioning, and poor quality of life.
- Neurobiological markers could offer new insights into treatment, especially linking HPA axis and anxiety/depression.
- Treatment is usually less effective than in younger populations.
- Still less studied than geriatric depression and needs more studies with combined treatment strategies, such as pharmacotherapy plus psychotherapy.

13.1 Introduction

A wide variety of well-known mental health disorders are classified by DSM-5 criteria as anxiety disorders, including agoraphobia, panic disorder, generalized anxiety disorder (GAD), anxiety disorder due to a general medical condition, social phobia, and specific phobia. Obsessive compulsive disorder (OCD) and post-traumatic stress disorder (PTSD), which were

V. Marinho · B. Gherman
Center for Alzheimer's Disease and Related Disorders, Institute of Psychiatry, Universidade Federal do Rio de Janeiro, Rio de Janeiro, Brazil
e-mail: vm@valeskamarinho.med.br

S. L. Blay (✉)
Department of Psychiatry, Universidade Federal de São Paulo, São Paulo, Brazil

formerly classified as anxiety disorders in the DSM-IV, are now separate categories in the new edition of the DSM. Anxiety disorder is not the same as everyday anxiety, stress, and worry; they are persistent conditions that may interfere with daily life and lead to serious physical and mental discomfort [1].

Anxiety in late life was frequently neglected and unrecognized, but new data has shown that we are improving our ability in its recognition and diagnosis [2]. Anxiety disorders are prevalent in later life and are associated with increased risk for disability, increased use of health services, decreased cognitive and social functioning, and poor quality of life [3].

This chapter presents the recent literature focusing on anxiety disorders in older adults.

13.2 Epidemiology

Anxiety in older adults has been reported with lower rates than in younger adults, but data has shown that it may be underestimated [4].

Accurately assessing anxiety disorders is very challenging in all age groups. In the elderly, differences in presentation, content, and severity of anxiety symptoms make it more difficult to assess than in younger adults. In community samples, recent evidence reveals that anxiety in older adults is more common than depression, often preceding depressive disorders, and when co-occurring, they provide a worst outcome than either condition alone [5].

In a nationally representative US sample age of at least 65 years old, the National Comorbidity Survey Replication found an overall prevalence of DSM-IV criteria anxiety disorders, GAD, and any phobia of 7.0, 1.2, and 4.7%, respectively, whereas among participants of 55 years old and older, rates were 11.6, 2.0, and 6.5%, respectively [6]. Phobias and specific phobias were the most prevalent disorders in the older age group. In Australia, however, 2.8% of a representative sample aged 55–85 years old was diagnosed with GAD, approximately twice the US rate. The most significant predictors of a 12-month GAD were lifetime depression comorbidity, concerns about

having a serious illness despite doctor's reassurance, medication intake, and family history of anxiety or depression [7]. Studies in developing countries demonstrate substantial variation in the prevalence of anxiety, ranging from 0.1% in rural China to 9.6% in urban Peru. Estimates from the Latin America region, however, are similar to those from high-income European and North American countries [8].

Investigation of 70-year-olds showed that almost 14% of the women and 5% of the men met criteria for specific phobias. In most, fears were lifelong, although 8% had onset after age 50 [9].

Fear of falling, possibly because of changes in gait and balance, is the most common specific phobia in older people. It can be marked by excessive fear and avoidance; in more severe presentations, the consequences of this fear may be very complex, including avoiding everyday activities. One or more previous falls is the main risk factor for fear of falling. However, fear of falling is found in up to 50% of elderly who have had no previous falls [10].

Findings from previous studies suggested that anxiety is associated with an increased mortality rate in older men [11]. Recent investigations have shown that neither GAD nor mixed anxiety depression is associated with excess mortality [12]. Counter intuitively, GAD may even predict less mortality in depressive elderly people. The relation between GAD and its possibly protective effect on mortality merits further exploration.

13.3 Comorbidity

Anxiety disorders are frequently comorbid with other psychiatric and physical diseases, complicating its management in the elderly [13].

Similar to the general population, anxiety disorders in the late life frequently co-occur with depression [5]. In the National Comorbidity Survey Replication, 2.8% of adults 55 years of age and older had experienced co-occurring mood and anxiety disorders over the past year. Of those with a current anxiety disorder, 36.7% had comorbid major depressive disorder, while 51.8% of those with depression had a comorbid anxiety disorder. The rate of comorbidity with depression is higher for GAD compared to other anxiety disorders. The diagnosis of mixed anxiety/depression may be particularly relevant for older adults, whose symptoms may not meet strict diagnostic criteria for either disorder or may demonstrate a fluctuating symptom pattern [14]. Mixed anxiety and depression is a syndrome with a poorer prognosis, compared with anxiety or depression alone [15]. Also, anxiety disorders have consistently been found to have an adverse impact on cognitive functioning in older individuals, increasing the risk of cognitive decline [16].

Regarding physical comorbidity, a variety of medical conditions frequently coexist with anxiety disorders in older adults [17]. Cardiovascular disease, hyperthyroidism, diabetes, chronic pain, lung disease, and gastrointestinal problems have all been found to be significantly associated with anxiety disorders [18]. Diagnosing anxiety in the context of physical illness is a significant challenge in older adult. Given the deleterious consequences of mental disorders on the outcome of medical illnesses, detecting clinically significant anxiety in this context is crucial.

A growing body of research has focused on cardiac problems due to mutually adverse effect of cardiac problems and anxiety disorders. However, acute coronary syndrome patients meeting GAD criteria had a superior 5-year cardiac outcome. Possibly, they worry constructively and are more likely to seek help and be more adherent to cardiac rehabilitation programs [19].

13.4 Neurobiology of Anxiety in Older Adults

A relationship between polymorphism in the promoter region of the serotonin transporter gene, depression, and anxiety traits has been examined in many studies [20]. There is evidence to support the moderating effect of the serotonin transporter gene on the relationship between stressful life events and depression/anxiety. The effect is likely due to prolonged cortisol elevation in response to stress in carriers of the short allele [21].

Selective serotonin reuptake inhibitor (SSRI) efficacy has also been linked to genetic variation in the serotonin transporter gene. Further support comes from a recent treatment study that reported an association between serotonin transporter genotype and cortisol reductions after SSRI treatment in older adults with GAD [22].

High basal cortisol levels have been described in anxiety disorders (panic disorder and GAD). In the latter, studies suggest that such dysregulation may be state dependent, as higher cortisol levels can be found in patients with current anxiety disorder and lower cortisol levels for those in remission [23].

Also, hypothalamic-pituitary-adrenal (HPA) axis dysfunction in the elderly may influence cognitive performance in stress-related disorders. Elevated cortisol level is associated with poorer cognitive performance, which can partially be explained by the chronic effects of the hormone exposure on the hippocampus.

Findings from several studies suggest that, compared to older adults without GAD, those with GAD have poorer immediate and delayed episodic memory, as well as poorer set-shifting ability (a measure of executive function). Overall, anxiety treatment may improve cognitive ability in older adults [24].

13.5 Diagnosis and Assessment

The presentation of anxiety symptoms is usually different in older adults in comparison with younger patients, potentially making anxiety disorders more difficult to diagnose in the elderly [25]. Older adults tend to emphasize somatic rather than emotional symptoms of anxiety. They are also less likely to seek mental health services for their anxiety symptoms, with the consequence that the responsibility for diagnosing anxiety symptoms falls mainly on primary care physicians [26]. These issues pose a barrier to accurately diagnosing anxiety disorders in the elderly.

The phenomenon of anxiety can be divided into fear (as in phobias or panic disorder) or worry (as in GAD). Worry is a process of thoughts and images that are negatively affect-laden and, in severe forms such as GAD, relatively uncontrollable.

GAD is accompanied by somatic and psychological symptoms such as irritability, concentration problems, easy fatigability, sleep disturbances, muscle tension, and restlessness [27]. In older adults with GAD, about half experience their first onset after 50 years of age. Patients with late-onset GAD report more functional impairment and poorer health than those without GAD [28]. Furthermore, when GAD is comorbid with depression, risk for suicidal ideation increases [29]. Part of the challenge of diagnosing and treating GAD in the elderly is that worry content in older adults is different from that of younger adults. Older adults tend to worry regarding the health and welfare of loved ones instead of about work/school and relationships, the more common problems in younger adults [30]. Some scales have been developed to help the clinician in the assessment of anxiety symptoms specifically in older adults. The Geriatric Anxiety Inventory (GAI) has demonstrated adequate psychometric properties in this population and is currently validated in several languages [31].

Regarding specific phobias in older patients, the fear content typically involves situational fears, specifically fear of falling. The general definition for this condition is the loss of confidence in one's balance activities that ultimately impairs the performance of daily activities. Unfortunately, fear of falling is not specifically addressed in DSM-5. The prevalence of fear of falling increases with age and causes considerable impairment via decreases or avoidance of activity and social withdrawal. In community of older adults who do not have previous falls, the prevalence of fear of falling is estimated to be between 12% and 65% [32]. The prevalence increases up to 92% for those who have previous experience of falls [33]. The difficulty to diagnose fear of falling as a psychiatric disorder may come from the fact that the behavior is often considered normal and attributed to physical limitations due to comorbid medical disorders. Patients,

who have low objective fall risk but severe levels of fear of falling, as measured by a brief instrument such as the 7-item short form of the Falls Efficacy Scale, may warrant an intervention focused on excessive fear [34].

13.6 Treatment

Anxiety disorders in the elderly are frequently undetected and untreated. When treatment takes place, it usually involves benzodiazepines or other anxiolytic medications rather than antidepressants or psychotherapy. Unlike depression, little research has been conducted on treatment of anxiety in older adults.

Often the first step in medication management is discontinuation of harmful or inappropriate medication such as sedatives, anticholinergics, and antihistaminergics, including over-the-counter medications and herbal supplements.

Recent evidence suggests that SSRI pharmacotherapy is superior to psychotherapy as an acute treatment for geriatric anxiety [35]. Data from controlled trials support the use of escitalopram, duloxetine, pregabalin, venlafaxine, citalopram, and sertraline for late-life GAD [36].

Data are even scarcer with respect to treatment of other anxiety disorders, but evidence from controlled trials and open-label studies suggests the efficacy of sertraline, citalopram, and escitalopram, as well as of imipramine and alprazolam, for panic disorder in older adults. The SSRIs citalopram, escitalopram, and sertraline may be particularly effective treatments for anxiety in the elderly based on their low propensity for drug interactions and short half-lives [37].

Benzodiazepines are often the only treatment received by older adults with anxiety disorders, and they are prescribed more frequently to older adults than to younger adults. Although benzodiazepines are effective in reducing anxiety and may be useful as an adjunctive, as-needed, or short-term treatment strategy, long-term daily use is associated with falls, fractures, and cognitive decline in the elderly and is not recommended [38]. Among benzodiazepines, lorazepam has a relatively short half-life and no active metabolites and is therefore preferable to alprazolam or clonazepam, which are more likely to accumulate and achieve toxic levels in older adults.

In many cases, monotherapy may not be adequate. In that case, physicians should consider augmenting with other medications or with CBT that focuses on behavior intervention techniques such as relaxation therapy [39].

Research, mostly with older GAD patients, provides support for the effectiveness of cognitive behavioral therapy (CBT) relative to waiting list and active control conditions such as supportive therapy and attention placebo [39].

A recent RCT showed that CBT augmentation of SSRI treatment reduced peak cortisol levels for older adults with GAD. Since persistently high cortisol levels in aging are thought to increase age-related cognitive and medical problems, it suggests that there may be a benefit to health and cognition of CBT augmentation for late-life anxiety disorders [40]. Response to CBT for GAD in older adults may be compromised by memory impairment, executive dysfunction, or failure to complete at-home practice.

13.7 Conclusion

Given the seriousness of anxiety disorders in the elderly, further study of epidemiology, clinical features, comorbidity, neurobiology, disability, and treatment are needed to better understand this condition. It is also important to emphasize the importance of individual and coexisting mood and anxiety disorders in older adults as the treatment of this comorbid condition usually has poorer outcome. Further study of risk factors, course, and severity is needed in order to target intervention, prevention, and healthcare needs. Given the rapid aging of the world population, mostly in developing countries, the potential public health burden of late-life mental health disorders will likely grow as well, suggesting the importance of continued epidemiologic monitoring in the presence of anxiety disorders among elderly subjects both in clinical and community settings.

References

1. Blay SL, Marinho V. Anxiety disorders in old age. Curr Opin Psychiatry. 2012;25:462–7.
2. Bryant C, Mohlman J, Gum A, Stanley M, Beekman AT, Wetherell JL, Thorp SR, Flint AJ, Lenze EJ. Anxiety disorders in older adults: looking to DSM5 and beyond. Am J Geriatr Psychiatry. 2013;21(9):872–6.
3. Porensky EK, Dew MA, Karp JF, Skidmore E, Rollman BL, Shear MK, Lenze EJ. The burden of late-life generalized anxiety disorder: effects on disability, health-related quality of life, and healthcare utilization. Am J Geriatr Psychiatry. 2009;17(6):473–82.
4. Gum AM, King-Kallimanis B, Kohn R. Prevalence of mood, anxiety, and substance-abuse disorders for older Americans in the National Comorbidity Survey–Replication. Am J Geriatr Psychiatry. 2009;17:769–81.
5. King-Kallimanis B, Gum A, Kohn R. Comorbidity of depressive and anxiety disorders for older Americans in the National Comorbidity Survey—Replication. Am J Geriatr Psychiatry. 2009;17:782–92.
6. Byers AL, Yaffe K, Covinsky KE, Friedman MB, Bruce ML. High occurrence of mood and anxiety disorders among older adults: the National Comorbidity Survey Replication. Arch Gen Psychiatry. 2010;67(5):489–96.
7. Gonçalves DC, Pachana NA, Byrne GJ. Prevalence and correlates of generalized anxiety disorder among older adults in the Australian National Survey of Mental Health and Well Being. J Affect Disord. 2011;132:223–30.
8. Prina AM, Ferri CP, Guerra M, Brayne C, Prince M. Prevalence of anxiety and its correlates among older adults in Latin America, India and China: cross-cultural study. Br J Psychiatry. 2011;199(6):485–91.
9. Sigström R, Östling S, Karlsson B, Waern M, Gustafson D, Skoog I. A population-based study on phobic fears and DSM-IV specific phobia in 70-year olds. J Anxiety Disord. 2011;25(1):148–53.
10. Scheffer AC, Schuurmans MJ, van Dijk N, van der Hooft T, de Rooij SE. Fear of falling: measurement strategy, prevalence, risk factors and consequences among older persons. Age Ageing. 2008;37:19–24.
11. van Hout HP, Beekman AT, de Beurs E, Comijs H, van Marwijk H, de Haan M, van Tilburg W, Deeg DJ. Anxiety and the risk of death in older men and women. Br J Psychiatry. 2004;185:399–404.
12. Holwerda TJ, Schoevers RA, Dekker J, Deeg DJ, Jonker C, Beekman AT. The relationship between generalized anxiety disorder, depression and mortality in old age. Int J Geriatr Psychiatry. 2007;22(3):241–9.
13. Bower ES, Wetherell JL, Mon T, Lenze EJ. Treating anxiety disorders in older adults: current treatments and future directions. Harv Rev Psychiatry. 2015;23(5):329–42.
14. Jeste D, Blazer D, First M. Aging-related diagnostic variations: need for diagnostic criteria appropriate

for elderly psychiatric patients. Biol Psychiatry. 2005;58:265–71.

15. Almeida OP, Draper B, Pirkis J, Snowdon J, Lautenschlager NT, Byrne G, Sim M, Stocks N, Kerse N, Flicker L, Pfaff JJ. Anxiety, depression, and comorbid anxiety and depression: risk factors and outcome over two years. Int Psychogeriatr. 2012;24(10):1622–32.

16. Lenze EJ, Butters MA. Consequences of anxiety in aging and cognitive decline. Am J Geriatr Psychiatry. 2016;24(10):843–5.

17. El-Gabalawy R, Mackenzie CS, Shooshtari S, Sareen J. Comorbid physical health conditions and anxiety disorders: a population-based exploration of prevalence and health outcomes among older adults. Gen Hosp Psychiatry. 2011;33(6):556–64.

18. Garfield LD, Scherrer JF, Hauptman PJ, Freedland KE, Chrusciel T, Balasubramanian S, Carney RM, Newcomer JW, Owen R, Bucholz KK, Lustman PJ. Association of anxiety disorders and depression with incident heart failure. Psychosom Med. 2014;76(2):128–36.

19. Parker G, Hyett M, Hadzi-Pavlovic D, Brotchie H, Walsh W. GAD is good? Generalized anxiety disorder predicts a superior five-year outcome following an acute coronary syndrome. Psychiatry Res. 2011;188(3):383–9.

20. Karg K, Burmeister M, Shedden K, Sen S. The serotonin transporter promoter variant (5-HTTLPR), stress, and depression meta-analysis revisited: evidence of genetic moderation. Arch Gen Psychiatry. 2011;68(5):444–54.

21. Gotlib IH, Joormann J, Minor KL, Hallmayer J. HPA axis reactivity: a mechanism underlying the associations among 5-HTTLPR,stress, and depression. Biol Psychiatry. 2008;63:847–51.

22. Lenze EJ, Dixon D, Mantella RC, Dore PM, Andreescu C, Reynolds CF 3rd, Newcomer JW, Butters MA. Treatment-related alteration of cortisol predicts change in neuropsychological function during acute treatment of late-life anxiety disorder. Int J Geriatr Psychiatry. 2012;27(5):454–62.

23. Vreeburg SA, Zitman FG, van Pelt J, Derijk RH, Verhagen JC, van Dyck R, Hoogendijk WJ, Smit JH, Penninx BW. Salivary cortisol levels in persons with and without different anxiety disorders. Psychosom Med. 2010;72(4):340–7.

24. Butters MA, Bhalla RK, Andreescu C, Wetherell JL, Mantella R, Begley AE, Lenze EJ. Changes in neuropsychological functioning following treatment for late-life generalized anxiety disorder. Br J Psychiatry. 2011;199(3):211–8.

25. Wolitzky-Taylor KB, Castriotta N, Lenze EJ, Stanley MA, Craske MG. Anxiety disorders in older adults: a comprehensive review. Depress Anxiety. 2010;27(2):190–211.

26. Mackenzie CS, Reynolds K, Cairney J, Streiner DL, Sareen J. Disorder-specific mental health service use for mood and anxiety disorders: associations with age, sex, and psychiatric comorbidity. Depress Anxiety. 2012;29(3):234–42.

27. American Psychiatric Association. Diagnostic and statistical manual of mental disorders. 5th ed. Arlington: APA; 2013.

28. Chou KL. Age at onset of generalized anxiety disorder in older adults. Am J Geriatr Psychiatry. 2009;17:455–64.

29. Lenze EJ, Mulsant BH, Shear MK, Schulberg HC, Dew MA, Begley AE, Pollock BG, Reynolds CF 3rd. Comorbid anxiety disorders in depressed elderly patients. Am J Psychiatry. 2000;157(5):722–8.

30. Goncalves DC, Byrne GJ. Who worries most? Worry prevalence and patterns across the lifespan. Int J Geriatr Psychiatry. 2013;28:41–9.

31. Massena PN, de Araújo NB, Pachana N, Laks J, de Pádua AC. Validation of the Brazilian Portuguese version of geriatric anxiety inventory--GAI-BR. Int Psychogeriatr. 2015;27(7):1113–9.

32. Howland J, Lachman ME, Peterson EW, Cote J, Kasten L, Jette A. Covariates of fear of falling and associated activity curtailment. Gerontologist. 1998;38(5):549–55.

33. Gomez F, Curcio CL. The development of a fear of falling interdisciplinary intervention program. Clin Interv Aging. 2007;2(4):661–7.

34. Kempen GI, Yardley L, van Haastregt JC, Zijlstra GA, Beyer N, Hauer K, Todd C. The short FES-I: a shortened version of the falls efficacy scale-international to assess fear of falling. Age Ageing. 2008;37(1):45–50.

35. Gould RL, Coulson MC, Howard RJ. Efficacy of cognitive behavioral therapy for anxiety disorders in older people: a meta-analysis and meta-regression of randomized controlled trials. J Am Geriatr Soc. 2012;60(2):218–29.

36. Karaiskos D, Pappa D, Tzavellas E, Siarkos K, Katirtzoglou E, Papadimitriou GN, Politis A. Pregabalin augmentation of antidepressants in older patients with comorbid depression and generalized anxiety disorder-an open-label study. Int J Geriatr Psychiatry. 2013;28(1):100–5.

37. Gonçalves DC, Byrne GJ. Interventions for generalized anxiety disorder in older adults: systematic review and meta-analysis. J Anxiety Disord. 2012;26:1–11.

38. Ungar A, Rafanelli M, Iacomelli I, Brunetti MA, Ceccofiglio A, Tesi F, Marchionni N. Fall prevention in the elderly. Clin Cases Miner Bone Metab. 2013;10(2):91–5.

39. Wetherell JL, Petkus AJ, White KS, Nguyen H, Kornblith S, Andreescu C, Zisook S, Lenze EJ. Antidepressant medication augmented with cognitive-behavioral therapy for generalized anxiety disorder in older adults. Am J Psychiatry. 2013;170(7):782–9.

40. Rosnick CB, Wetherell JL, White KS, Andreescu C, Dixon D, Lenze EJ. Cognitive-behavioral therapy augmentation of SSRI reduces cortisol levels in older adults with generalized anxiety disorder: a randomized clinical trial. J Consult Clin Psychol. 2016;84(4):345–52.

Mercedes Fernández Cabana,
Alejandro García-Caballero, and Raimundo Mateos

Abstract

In this chapter, bereavement is defined as the response to the loss of a loved one, and the normal and pathological manifestations of that response are explained, as well as its expected progression, making reference to the mourning model as a process, proposed by Worden. The peculiarities of bereavement in old age are addressed, as well as the risk factors for the development of a complicated grief and the differential characteristics between a normal grief response and an episode of major depression or a psychotic disorder. Intervention guidelines are offered for the management of grief in the context of primary care and criteria that indicate the convenience of referral to specialised care and/or non-governmental resources, emphasising the importance of promoting instrumental and emotional support from the family and social environment of the mourners. The chapter also includes two clinical cases that illustrate the practical intervention with elderly people in grief.

M. Fernández Cabana
Servicio de Salud Mental, Hospital Virxe da
Xunqueira. Cee, A Coruña, Spain

A. García-Caballero
Department of Psychiatry, School of Medicine,
University of Santiago de Compostela (USC),
Santiago de Compostela, Spain

Department of Psychiatry, EOXI Ourense,
Ourense, Spain

South Galician Health Research Institute (IISGS),
Ourense, Spain

R. Mateos (✉)
Department of Psychiatry, School of Medicine,
University of Santiago de Compostela (USC),
Santiago de Compostela, Spain

Psychogeriatric Unit, CHUS University Hospital,
Santiago de Compostela, Spain
e-mail: raimundo.mateos@usc.es

Key Points
- Bereavement is defined as the response to the loss of a loved one.
- The normal response to bereavement is manifested by perceptual, cognitive and behavioural alterations, along with physical feelings and sensations related to the loss [1].
- In older adults, adjusting to life after a significant loss, such as the loss of a spouse, may be hindered by factors such as the existence of multiple losses, increased personal awareness of their own death and the interdependence that usually exists in the case of long-term partners [1].
- As the bereavement progresses, the intensity and frequency of the psychological distress should lessen [2].

© Springer Nature Switzerland AG 2019
C. A. de Mendonça Lima, G. Ivbijaro (eds.), *Primary Care Mental Health in Older People*,
https://doi.org/10.1007/978-3-030-10814-4_14

- Risk factors for the onset of complicated bereavement include a previous history of psychiatric disorders, a lack of perceived social support and cases in which the circumstances of the death are particularly distressing.
- The presence of frank psychotic symptomatology, depression or insuppressible suicidal thoughts is an indicator that the case should be referred to the mental health services.

14.1 Concepts and Expressions of Bereavement

Bereavement entails the series of psychological and psychosocial processes following the loss of someone with whom the person had a psychosocial connection [3]. In most cases, bereavement following the loss of a loved one is associated with an increased risk of suffering different psychological and physical disorders [4], which may result in an increased number of primary care visits. It is necessary to draw a distinction between those manifestations that are normal and expected and those that are not in order to offer appropriate and non-pathological support.

Feelings of loneliness, sadness, anger or impotence are common, along with sensations of yearning and anxiety (which may be manifested physically) with complaints of shortness of breath, chest tightness, anergy, etc. Responses of disbelief and shock may also emerge (particularly in the case of sudden deaths), as well as confusion and concern regarding the deceased and/or the circumstances of the death. There are often different perceptual alterations (which are gener-

ally temporary) such as feelings of presence and brief visual or audible hallucinations during which the mourner seems to perceive the deceased person.

On a behavioural level, sleep and eating disorders, distraction and a tendency towards isolation are frequent after the loss, with sobbing, whimpering and behaviours of searching for the deceased. Certain people try to avoid stimuli that remind them of the loss, while others constantly seek such stimuli, keeping the belongings of the deceased.

The aforementioned manifestations are normal [1] and must not be pathologised by those close to the mourner.

Although individual variability is the norm, certain researchers have attempted to classify this response into states [5] or stages [6–8], as can be observed at the Table 14.1:

On occasion, such attempts have been criticised, as it is thought that they transmit a vision of bereavement as a succession of stages through which people progress with certain passivity, while researchers such as Worden [1, 9] prefer to refer to bereavement as a process, which entails several different tasks in order to reach a satisfactory resolution. The first task to which he refers in his model is to *accept the reality of the loss*, in other words, the intellectual and emotional acceptance that the person has died and will not come back. This acceptance may take time, and behaviour such as keeping all of the belongings of the deceased for months or visiting psychics to "contact" the person indicate that this task is still unresolved.

The second task proposed by Worden [1] is to *process the pain of the grief*. This refers to the fact that, in general, it is necessary to recognise the suffering caused by the loss and work through the experience without denying its importance or

Table 14.1 Some proposals for classifying *the phases* of the grieving response

Author	States or stages of bereavement			
Kübler-Ross [5]	Denial	Anger/bargaining	Depression	Acceptance
Parkes [6]	Numbness	Yearning	Despair	Reorganisation
Bowlby [7]	Numbing	Yearning and searching	Despair	Reorganisation
Sanders [8]	Shock	Awareness of loss	Withdrawal	Healing/renewal

taking refuge in avoidance behaviours, such as sudden trips or the use of alcohol or drugs.

The third task proposed is *to adjust to a world without the deceased*. This may entail external adjustments (such as learning new skills or taking on roles that were once performed by the deceased), internal adjustments (confronting the effects of the death of a loved one on the mourner's own self-esteem, self-efficacy and on their definition of themselves) and spiritual adjustments, i.e. the way they see the world and their beliefs and values until that time. Those who find this task difficult will appear helpless and will not develop the new skills that they need, or they may isolate themselves so as not to confront the requirements of their environment.

Finally, the fourth task is to *find an enduring connection with the deceased in the midst of embarking on a new life*, in other words, finding ways to think about and remember the person that do not result in excessive emotional activation and that make it possible to engage with other people or activities and continue to experience life. However, in some cases people feel that their life ended with the death of their loved one and they are unable to relate to others or appreciate what life can still offer them.

The author [1] stresses that these tasks do not follow a strict order and that they do not have to be resolved sequentially, but rather they can be addressed simultaneously and at different times throughout the grieving process.

14.1.1 Bereavement in Later Life

At present, the population is progressively ageing, especially in developed countries. With age, there is an increased possibility of suffering multiple losses (and, therefore, multiple griefs) not only of loved ones but also in terms of status, physical and cognitive problems and, in some cases, awareness of the need to depend on others.

Over the years, people have increased awareness of their own vulnerability and mortality, and the death of their partner may precipitate their need to move house or enter an institution.

Furthermore, remaining in the house shared with their partner for so many years may lead to an intense sensation of loneliness, especially if the relationship was harmonious [1].

In later life, marriage has been associated with better mental health, possibly because it provides social support and increased self-esteem [10]. Thus, the loss of a partner after a long-term relationship entails the need for significant adjustments, both for men, who may need support to assume "feminised" tasks and to continue to feel a bond to their loved ones [10], and for women, who may require instrumental assistance or assistance of another kind [11].

Being widowed in later life has been linked to an increased risk of mortality related to heart problems [12] (this risk is greater in men [13]). The loss of a loved one may lead to worsening health in general, with symptoms such as weight loss and decreased functional capacity [14].

The loss of a partner is also associated with the onset of depressive symptoms, especially in the months following the death of the partner. A prior diagnosis of depression or anxiety disorders is a risk factor for complicated bereavement in older adults [14, 15]. It is also necessary to rule out psychotic disorders or dementia.

Deaths of friends and family also represent a progressive decrease of a person's social network, in other words, less possibility to receive support. Furthermore, cultural prejudice regarding old age may mean that older adults are neglected and do not receive accurate information in the event of the death of a loved one, with ideas such as "they do not understand", "they do not feel as much" or "better not to tell them".

However, research demonstrates that many older adults are able to work through grief in a satisfactory manner [16], especially those who have effective social support [17] and who are able to use positive coping strategies [18, 19].

It can be considered that the bereavement has been overcome when the person is able to remember the deceased with composure, without feeling overwhelmed by the memory, and is able to pay attention to the positive experiences shared [20].

14.2 Criteria for Detecting Abnormal Responses to Bereavement

There are certain risk factors that can hinder the grieving process. They are related to the relationship maintained with the deceased, the situation and characteristics of the patient and the cause and circumstances of the death.

The kind of connection that was held with the deceased is a factor that must be taken into account [21]. In this respect, when there was an ambivalent or excessively dependent relationship with the deceased, working through the bereavement may be more difficult. This is also the case when there is a certain uncertainty surrounding the death (when it is the result of an accident in a faraway place, deaths in which it is not possible to recover the body, etc.) or in the event of multiple losses. A previous history of difficulties to work through other situations of grief, a background of depressive episodes and certain personality characteristics related to an inability to tolerate emotional distress, as well as a tendency to respond with withdrawal or avoidance behaviour, are also personal risk factors.

With regards to the cause of death, death by suicide tends to be especially difficult for those left behind, as it is not usually interpreted as the final consequence of severe emotional suffering or mental illness but rather as a "choice" that could have been avoided, and mourners often think that *they should have done something to prevent the death* [22]. Therefore, feelings of guilt, suicidal thoughts, shame and stigma may emerge, given the social rejection that this cause of death provokes in the majority of cultures. There may also be a tendency to hide the cause of death [23], which reduces the possibility of receiving appropriate social support.

Sudden deaths, as a result of accidents, violence from others or physical problems (heart attacks, strokes, etc.), are usually more difficult to work through, as they entail more intense sensations of disbelief and unfairness, guilt and the need to blame others (e.g. medical staff) [1]. There may be unresolved issues after the sudden death of a loved one, and when this happens at an unexpected moment of the life cycle, it may jeopardise the grieving process.

The *Diagnostic and Statistical Manual of Mental Disorders* (fifth ed.; APA, 2013) has included "Persistent complex bereavement disorder" under the *conditions for further study* chapter, for cases in which there is an intense and sustained reaction to bereavement [24].

This diagnostic category would include common manifestations of grief, such as intense sorrow and emotional distress, yearning for the deceased and concern for the deceased or the circumstances of the death. Response to this distress would include symptoms such as difficulty accepting the death, with a sensation of numbness or disbelief regarding the loss, or bitterness or anger, and difficulties remembering the deceased in a positive manner, self-blame and excessive avoidance of stimuli associated with the loss.

Another of the proposed criteria would be social and/or identity alteration, with symptoms such as a desire to die to join the deceased, difficulty trusting other people, with disregard and a sensation of loneliness, difficulty keeping up with interests or making plans, a loss of the reason for living and a reduced feeling of individual identity.

Diagnosis will only be made in cases in which the grief is disproportionate or inconsistent with existing cultural or religious norms and when it results in clinically significant distress or impairment in social, occupational or other important areas, at least 12 months (in adults) after the death. Persistent complex bereavement disorder is associated with the onset of unhealthy behaviours such as the use of alcohol or tobacco, resulting in a lower quality of life and an increased risk of suffering medical conditions.

The manual [24] estimates that prevalence of persistent complex bereavement disorder is approximately 2.4–4.8%. It is more frequent in women, and there is a higher risk in cases of greater dependency on the deceased and when the deceased is a child. Other researchers estimate a prevalence of 10–25% of complicated bereavement among grieving older adults [25].

The DSM-5 also includes the specification "with traumatic bereavement" in cases of grief due to murder or suicide, in which distressing and persistent concerns may emerge regarding the traumatic nature of the death and the final moments of the deceased, their suffering and injuries or the malicious or intentional nature of the death.

Older adults who have lost a loved one (especially in the case of a long-term partner) may suffer high levels of depressive symptoms [26], and this response can be found in both men and women [27]. A distinction should be made between a depressive episode and bereavement (and the possible presence of both must be taken into account). Table 14.2 (modified from DSM-5 [24], 2013) shows the difference between the two.

Finally, perceptual alterations consisting of audible or visual illusions or hallucinations should be temporary and be followed by the criticism of the mourner. Such characteristics differentiate them from those that may appear in a psychotic disorder.

14.3 Possible Interventions and Recommendations for Specific Primary Care Management

Primary care services represent a privileged environment in which to care for people who are grieving and to offer them the monitoring that they need. In developed countries there are an

increasing number of requests for professional support to cope with grief and other psychological difficulties. In the past, this role was carried out by the community, the family or religious institutions, but as a result of the progressive secularisation of society, along with the scattering of the family and the progressive isolation of individuals, family doctors now receive many of these requests for help.

On occasion, long-term contact with patients in a primary care setting means that doctors have prior knowledge of the background of the mourner and information regarding the social support available to them [28, 29].

In the case of recurrent visits with physical complaints, it is important to explore if there has been a recent change in the person's life such as the loss of someone important. Such losses may be communicated directly by the patient or the patient's family and must not be ignored but rather addressed to the extent that the situation allows. Below we will describe some possible interventions:

- Dedicate a few minutes to investigate how the death occurred and the specific circumstances, enabling the mourner to express emotions. Avoid replying with clichés or trying to prematurely soothe the person.
- Ask how the person is and reassure them about expected symptoms of bereavement. Explain

Table 14.2 Criteria of normal grief response and major depressive episode

	Normal response to bereavement	Major depressive episode
Predominant affect	Emptiness and loss	Sadness, inability to experience happiness or pleasure
Mood	Dysphoria that gradually decreases in intensity and that appears in waves faced with certain stimuli	Persistent depressed mood that is not associated with specific thoughts or worries
Range of emotions	The pain may be accompanied by moments of humour and positive emotions	Intense unhappiness with less variability
Thoughts	Worry linked to thoughts and memories of the deceased	Self-criticism, pessimistic rumination
Self-esteem	Preserved	Feelings of worthlessness and self-hate are frequent
Thoughts of death	Typically passive, at times related to the idea of "joining" the deceased	There may be active suicidal thoughts, related to the feeling of worthlessness, indignity or inability to cope with the distress

to patients and their families that the grieving process is long and usually has ups and downs, especially on specific dates (such as celebrations and anniversaries of the death) and also 3–6 months after the death, when external support tends to decline.

- In the case of intense distress, openly explore as to whether there are possible suicidal thoughts, for example, by asking if the patient has considered the idea that it is not worth living. If the answer is yes, explore how structured the idea is and if they have thought how they would do it (the greater the level of intent and planning, the greater the risk).
- The use of psychiatric medications for acute bereavement is not recommended, except in cases of major depression or other mental disorders. Despite this, the prescription of such medications has increased in recent years [30]. The use of anxiolytics is contemplated for the first weeks after the death, to facilitate coping with the presence of intense anxiety or insomnia. They could be taken under the supervision of a carer, to prevent the mourner from taking potentially lethal doses.
- Explore the circumstances of the older adult, if they live alone and their perception of the availability of family support or a social network. Pay particular attention to older adults who have lost their partners and who feel that they have no valid social support.
- Ask if they are able to maintain their self-care (hygiene, diet, medications in the event of illness, etc.), and respectfully enquire if they are resorting to drugs or alcohol to cope with the distress that they feel and if the loss has also resulted in a significant decline in their economic resources.
- Encourage the instrumental and emotional support of family members and that of their social environment.
- If consulted on the matter, encourage the older adult to see the deceased to say goodbye and express their pain, which will facilitate acceptance of the death [31]. Advise against taking important decisions during the acute grieving period.

14.3.1 Referral Criteria

In order to decide whether it is necessary to refer the patient to specialised treatment, it is advisable to abide by clinical criteria and take the person's previous history into account, as well as cultural norms for the expression of distress.

The decision should also be based on the criteria of the actual patient, placing importance on their subjective interpretation of the death and their self-perception as to whether they are able to cope.

It will be useful to assess the contact held with nursing staff and the social services in cases in which there are self-care and economic difficulties.

General criteria to be taken into account for referral include the excessive duration of the distress (over 1 year according to certain authors), impaired health or self-care difficulties, the onset of frank psychotic symptomatology, insuppressible suicidal thoughts or clinical depression [32, 33].

14.4 Clinical Cases

Below we will examine two clinical cases in order to illustrate the different responses to the loss of a loved one.

14.4.1 Case 1

Healthcare Context: Interdisciplinary team at a community psychogeriatric unit (PGU). The patient is referred from his community mental health unit after assessment.

Mr. García is 83 years old, he is a widower and he is accompanied by his daughter. Level of Studies: Primary. He emigrated to Venezuela when he was 17, where he worked as a builder, married and had a daughter. He returned to his home country with his family when he was 63. He lives with his daughter, son-in-law and 19-year-old grandson.

According to his daughter, he looked after his wife, who had Parkinson's disease, for many years. When she died, 18 months ago, the patient suffered a significant physical and psychological depression. He was sad, restless and could not sleep. He started to suffer several falls (he was taking benzodiazepines).

Six months ago his daughter became alarmed after an extremely serious incident involving a pair of scissors, and she took him to the emergency department where they prescribed 50 mg/day of sertraline and 25 mg/day of quetiapine, and they referred him to the mental health unit. There he was diagnosed with a depressive adjustment disorder with behavioural disorders and mild cognitive impairment, and he was referred to the psychogeriatric unit for follow-up.

His daughter states that his mood has improved in recent months, but his memory is greatly impaired. One day he lost his keys in a park (they were later handed back to him), and on occasion he has lost money, so she withdraws his pension money from the bank for him.

The patient says that he is losing his memory and he finds it difficult to remember the name of people that he knows but that he is not too concerned about this because he knows that it is due to his age. Speaking in a fluent, coherent and orderly manner, he provides an alternative account to that of his daughter regarding the incident with the scissors. He says that he has been finding it very hard since the death of his wife with whom he had lived happily for over 60 years. He says that he was cutting up some cartons when his daughter challenged him and this angered him, but it was a misunderstanding, and it never occurred to him to attack her. He also appears upset because his family does not trust him (his daughter goes to the bank to withdraw money for him).

The patient gets up at 9:00, he visits a coffee shop on a regular basis, he gathers with other older adults in the park and he attends a memory workshop. He watches the television for 2 h. He drinks one glass of wine at a bar and half a glass with his main meal (1/4 of a litre per day). He has never been an excessive drinker or smoker.

With regards to his history of mental illness, he visited a general practitioner when he was around 40, at a time when he was stressed at work

and barely slept. The daughter confirms that he was prescribed Valium for a time and that he had subsequently took it again on occasions, but she has never seen him so depressed for large periods of time. When he was 50, he tried to return to Spain, but he found it very difficult and returned to Venezuela.

Mental Status Examination: His appearance is excellent, he is clean and he is willing to collaborate. Affective contact is good. There is no evidence of psychotic symptomatology. He is euthymic and there are hardly any symptoms of anxiety. He now eats and sleeps well. MMSE = 24/30 points, which for his age and low level of studies is considered as high performance in our environment.

Prior Personality: Mister García describes himself as a "methodical and responsible" person.

Based on his recent positive evolution, his psychopharmacological treatment is continued, and he is advised to increase his social relations.

At a revision held 9 months later, he is cheerful and he states "I'm alone, because my wife has died, but I have my daughter... we might fight at times but we're happy (he laughs at his joke)... although I am losing my memory".

His daughter confirms his positive evolution and plays down his memory losses, which are now minor.

Final Diagnosis: Complicated bereavement with a moderate depressive episode and a psychomotor agitation crisis. It is assessed that the grieving process is progressing in a satisfactory manner, thus reversing cognitive impairment (although there are still subjective complaints).

Follow-up Plan: His pharmacological treatment is continued, and he is still advised to increase his social interaction. A follow-up appointment is scheduled after a year, and he can call if necessary. A written report is submitted to his primary care physician.

Discussion: Case 1

This case is an example of complicated bereavement in a person with a good prior level of mental balance. The good relationship with the deceased and the high level of family and social support were factors in his positive prognosis. The cognitive impairment which is frequently associated with depression has not progressed, so the onset of dementia has been ruled out, despite the emphasis placed on this matter initially by the patient and his daughter. Despite the positive evolution of the case, it should be followed up conjointly by the primary care centre and on the specialised mental health level, in this case, the community psychogeriatric unit [34].

14.4.2 Case 2

Healthcare Context: A medium-sized nursing home, with an in-house medical and nursing service. The psychogeriatric unit collaborates through a referral and liaison programme, with monthly visits from the psychologist and psychiatrist. The case has been addressed in conjunction with both professionals and in direct collaboration with the residential centre's doctor, social worker and nurse.

Mr. Martínez is 88 years old and he was widowed 6 months ago.

Level of Studies: Primary. He worked on fishing boats.

He is referred to our PGU by the doctor at the nursing home because one night he got out of bed saying that he wanted to jump out of the window.

The first interview is performed by the psychologist. At first, the patient denies any psychotic symptomatology, and he complains of foot pain because his shoe bothers him. When asked about his deceased wife, he says that he misses her, despite the fact that it was quite difficult for him when she was ill. He says that he dreams a lot and he admits that he is sad and has a "fear of living". He is worried about everything. He says that he is waiting to be transferred to another home that is closer to where his niece lives, who they raised as a daughter. He says that he does not care about dying and, if he had the strength, he would take his own life.

The psychiatrist visits him the following week. He states that he has head pain and is depressed, "I feel hopeless... I remember my wife and sometimes it feels like I can see her and that she is with me". He accepts that "for her it was better to die, she was in a lot of pain, she wanted to die".

He has delusional ideas of bankruptcy: "I'm worried about my bank book, and if they're going to trick me, when I signed I realised that it was like I was signing my death sentence, I signed so many times... there are six thousand euros... I became obsessed with the idea... I don't know if it's true or not... I think about it a lot... yesterday I went to the bank to complain but I don't know what I said..."

He has persistent suicidal thoughts: "...I thought about jumping off somewhere, I don't belong here".

Good cognitive status according to his level of studies: MMSE = 21/30. He has been taking a benzodiazepine to sleep for several years.

He is diagnosed with complicated bereavement with major depression, with suicidal thoughts and delusional ideas of wrong being done to him. He is prescribed 75 mg/day of venlafaxine.

After 6 weeks a clear improvement is observed and he is calmer.

After 4 months he is well, calm and coherent. He refers to the possible transfer to another home with less anxiety, "I'm not as bothered now". He eagerly recounts how yesterday "I ate a cake and I smoked a cigar, I thought it would harm me, but it didn't".

After 6 months he is admitted to hospital with lower gastrointestinal bleeding due to diverticulosis. He suffered an episode of delirium while he was in the hospital, and in his discharge report, a diagnosis of dementia was made.

A short time after his discharge from hospital, at the home he is serene and euthymic. His cognitive status is similar to the last time (MMSE = 21/30). It is verified that he does not have dementia, and as the hospital reduced the pharmacopoeia, eliminating the antidepressant, it is decided that no psychiatric drugs will be prescribed.

Two months later, he suddenly expresses a fear that his bank books will be altered, "I become obsessed with strange things like this". "I always felt hopeless about everything in life". Although he appears euthymic, the recurrence of delusional ideas renders it advisable for him to resume taking 75 mg/day of venlafaxine. Based on his positive evolution and after several months, the venlafaxine was reduced to 37.5 mg/day.

At his 18-month follow-up, he was euthymic. He was advised to go for walks outside of the centre, accompanied by a volunteer. After 30 months he was stable. The patient died 4 years after becoming widowed.

Discussion: Case 2

In this case we have a person with complicated bereavement and a major depressive episode, with suicidal thoughts and delusional ideas of wrong being done to him. His depressive personality was a predisposing factor, and the fact that he had certain family support was a factor in his positive prognosis.

He demonstrated a positive and quick response to pharmacological treatment and psychotherapeutic support. The positive evolution of the case highlights the diagnostic error made during his time at the hospital: his delirium was confused with dementia.

Mr. García was never transferred to another home, and despite this his evolution was positive. He died 4 years later (at the age of 92) without ever having developed dementia.

14.5 Conclusion

Cognitive, perceptual and behavioural alterations, along with physical feelings and sensations, are normal responses to bereavement. However, the bereavement process can be exacerbated by risk factors related to the relationship maintained with the deceased, the situation and characteristics of the patient and the cause and circumstances of the death. Support for bereaved individuals used to be provided by the family, community or religious institutions. Due to increasing secularisation of society, changing family structures and isolation of older adults, people may turn to family doctors for help. Primary care practitioners should have structures in place to be able to help directly or at least refer to appropriate services, sometimes within the non-governmental sector.

This chapter has provided some case studies and very practical ways of supporting bereaved individuals.

References

1. Worden JW. Grief counseling and grief therapy. A handbook for the mental health practitioner. 4th ed. New York: Springer; 2009.
2. Payás A. Las tareas del duelo. Madrid: Paidós; 2010.
3. Tizón JL. Pérdida, pena y duelo: vivencias, investigación y asistencia. Paidós Ibérica: Barcelona; 2004.
4. Stroebe M, van Son M, Stroebe W, Kleber R, Schut H, van den Bout J. On the classification and diagnosis of pathological grief. Clin Psychol Rev. 2000;20(1):57–75.
5. Kübler-Ross E. On death and dying. New York: Macmillan; 1969.
6. Parkes CM. Bereavement: Studies of grief in adult life. New York: International Universities Press; 1972.
7. Bowlby J. Attachment and loss: Vol. 3. Loss, sadness, and depression. New York: Basic Books; 1980.
8. Sanders C. Grief: the mourning after. New York: Wiley; 1989.
9. Worden JW. Grief counseling and grief therapy. A handbook for the mental health practitioner. New York: Springer; 1982.
10. McLaren S, Gomez R, Gill P, Chesler J. Marital status and suicidal ideation among Australian older adults: the mediating role of sense of belonging. Int Psychogeriatr. 2015;27(1):145–54.
11. DiGiacomo M, Lewis J, Phillips J, Nolan M, Davidson PM. The business of death: a qualitative study of financial concerns of widowed older women. BMC Womens Health. 2015;15:36.
12. Carey IM, Shah SM, DeWilde S, Harris T, Victor CR, Cook DG. Increased risk of acute cardiovascular events after partner bereavement: a matched cohort study. JAMA. 2014;174(4):598–605.
13. Stahl ST, Arnold AM, Chen JY, Anderson S, Schulz R. Mortality after bereavement: the role of cardiovascular disease and depression. Psychosom Med. 2016;78(6):697–703.
14. Shear MK, Ghesquiere A, Glickman K. Bereavement and complicated grief. Current Psychiatry Report. 2013;15(11):406.
15. Bruinsma SM, Tiemeier HW, Verkroost-van Heemst J, van der Heide A, Rietjens JA. Risk factors for complicated grief in older adults. J Palliat Med. 2015;18(5):438–46.
16. Burns RA, Browning CJ, Kendig HL. Examining the 16-year trajectories of mental health and well-being through the transition into widowhood. Int Psychogeriatr. 2015;27(12):1979–86.
17. Powers SM, Bisconti TL, Bergeman CS. Trajectories of social support and well-being across the first two years of widowhood. Death Stud. 2014;38(6–10):499–509.

18. Ong AD, Bergeman CS, Bisconti TL, Wallace KA. Psychological resilience, positive emotions, and successful adaptation to stress in later life. J Pers Soc Psychol. 2006;91(4):730–49.

19. Ong AD, Bergeman CS, Bisconti TL. The role of daily positive emotions during conjugal bereavement. J Gerontol B Psychol Sci Soc Sci. 2004;59(4):P168–76.

20. Latiegi A. Prevención y tratamiento del duelo patológico. In: Astudillo W, Arrieta C, Mendinueta C, Vega de Seonae I, editors. La familia en la terminalidad. Bilbao: Sociedad vasca de cuidados paliativos; 1999.

21. Kho Y, Kane RT, Priddis L, Hudson J. The nature of attachment relationships and grief responses in older adults: an attachment path model of grief. PLoS One. 2015;10(10):e0133703.

22. Tal I, Mauro C, Reynolds CF, et al. Complicated grief after suicide bereavement and other causes of death. Death Stud. 2016;41(5):1–9.

23. Sveen CA, Walby FA. Suicide survivors' mental health and grief reactions: a systematic review of controlled studies. Suicide Life Threat Behav. 2008;38(1):13–29.

24. American Psychiatric Association. Diagnostic and statistical manual of mental disorders. 5th ed. Washington, DC: Author; 2013.

25. Nam I. Complicated Grief Treatment for older adults: The critical role of a supportive person. Psychiatry Res. 2016;244:97–102.

26. Sikorski C, Luppa M, Heser K, et al. The role of spousal loss in the development of depressive symptoms in the elderly - implications for diagnostic systems. J Affect Disord. 2014;161:97–103.

27. Lee HJ, Lee SG, Chun SY, Park EC. Sex differences in depressive effects of experiencing spousal bereavement. Geriatr Gerontol Int. 2017;17(2):322–9.

28. Ferreiro JA, Mateos R. International commentaries: Spain. In: Chew-Graham CA, Baldwin R, Burns A, editors. Integrated management of depression in the elderly. Cambridge: Cambridge University Press; 2008. p. 171–5.

29. Cerecedo-Pérez MJ, Tovar-Bobo M, Rozadilla Arias A. Medicalization I. 'Disease labeling: all business'. Atención Primaria. 2013;45(8):434–8.

30. Shah SM, Carey IM, Harris T, DeWilde S, Victor CR, Cook DG. Initiation of psychotropic medication after partner bereavement: a matched cohort study. PLoS One. 2013;8(11):e77734.

31. Núñez MA, Carballo N, Fernández-Cabana M, Pérez MA. Cuidados Paliativos en Oncología. Algoritmo de actuación ante el duelo y manejo psicológico del paciente terminal y su familia. In: CHUOU, editor. Diagnóstico y tratamiento en medicina hospitalaria: Enfoque práctico. Libro do Peto. Ourense: Complexo Hospitalario Universitario de Ourense; 2014.

32. Richardson R, Lowenstein S, Weissberg M. Coping with the suicidal elderly: a physician's guide. Geriatrics. 1989;44(9):43–47, 51.

33. Pérez-Sales P. Trauma, guilt, grief. Towards an integrative psychotherapy. Bilbao: Desclee de Brower Ed.; 2006.

34. Mateos R. Asistencia en Psiquiatría Geriátrica. De la Teoría a la Praxis. In: Agüera L, Cervilla J, Martín M, editors. Psiquiatría Geriátrica. 2nd ed. Madrid: Masson; 2006. p. 909–45.

Bodily Distress Syndrome (BDS), Bodily Stress Syndrome (BSS) and Health Anxiety in Older Adults

15

Gabriel Ivbijaro, David Goldberg,
Lucja Kolkiewicz, Todd M. Edwards,
Clifton McReynolds, and Igor Svab

Abstract

Disorders of bodily distress or bodily experience occur across all age groups including older adults. Understanding this condition in older adults particularly in primary care is very important because over 25% of primary care consultations are accounted for by people who are aged 65 years and older and it significantly impacts caregivers. Treatment of BDS requires professionals from multiple disciplines who can effectively collaborate to optimize care.

G. Ivbijaro (✉)
NOVA University, Lisbon, Portugal

Waltham Forest Community & Family Health Services, London, UK

D. Goldberg
King's College, London, UK

L. Kolkiewicz
NOVA University, Lisbon, Portugal

East London NHS Foundation Trust, London, UK
e-mail: lucja.kolkiewicz@nhs.net

T. M. Edwards
Marital and Family Therapy Program, University of San Diego, San Diego, CA, USA
e-mail: tedwards@sandiego.edu

C. McReynolds
Chicago, IL, USA

I. Svab
Medical Faculty, University of Ljubljana, Ljubljana, Slovenia
e-mail: igor.svab@mf.uni-lj.si

Key Points

- Disorders of bodily distress or bodily experience occur across all age groups, including older adults.
- Despite the difficulties with agreeing shared terminology, the available research shows that treatment is possible for people with disorders of bodily distress and there is hope for patients, their carers and health-care professionals.
- The key requirements for making a diagnosis and developing a care package include history, co-occuring illnesses, investigations to rule out somatic illness and, when necessary, additional tests.
- There is positive evidence to support the use of pharmacological interventions and a range of non-pharmacological interventions, including problem-solving therapy, mindfulness and family interventions.
- Collaborative or integrated care provides the best opportunity for success and maintenance of recovery.

15.1 Introduction

There have been many terms used to describe psychosomatic conditions associated with multiple physical symptoms for which physi-

© Springer Nature Switzerland AG 2019
C. A. de Mendonça Lima, G. Ivbijaro (eds.), *Primary Care Mental Health in Older People*,
https://doi.org/10.1007/978-3-030-10814-4_15

cians are unable to find an immediate explanation of the aetiology.

Some of the terms used to describe these disorders have been considered unacceptable by patients who experience these conditions and by the doctors that treat these conditions because they are ambiguous and negative [1–4]. Terms have included MUS (medically unexplained symptoms) [5], SSD (somatic symptom disorder) [6] and BDS (bodily distress syndrome) [4, 7, 8]. Other terminology used includes fibromyalgia syndrome and somatoform disorder [9, 10].

Henningsen et al. [2] proposed that any terminology adopted to describe these disorders should be acceptable to patients, be acceptable and useable by doctors and health-care professionals, not reinforce dualistic thinking, be able to be readily used in patients who also have pathologically established disease, be adequate as a standalone diagnosis, have a clear core theoretical concept, facilitate the possibility of multidisciplinary medical and psychological treatment, have similar meaning in different cultures, be neutral with regard to aetiology and pathology and have a satisfactory acronym [2].

In addition to these criteria, it is important that terminology used should not result in stigma and should not take away the hope of recovery from either the patient or the therapist. It should provide an opportunity for the severity of illness to be described or measured and enable the opportunity for care packages to be designed in collaboration with the patients so that there can be a shared outcome.

More recently, with the introduction of ICD-11 WHO [11], new terminology has been proposed under a parent heading of 'Disorders of bodily distress or bodily experience', and subcategories include bodily distress disorder (BDD) described as:

- Characterised by the presence of bodily symptoms that are distressing to the individual and excessive attention directed toward the symptoms, which may be manifested by repeated contact with health-care providers. If another health condition is causing or contributing to the symptoms, the degree of attention is clearly excessive in relation to its nature and progres-

sion. Excessive attention is not alleviated by appropriate clinical examination and investigations and appropriate reassurance. Bodily symptoms are persistent, being present on most days for at least several months. Typically, bodily distress disorder involves multiple bodily symptoms that may vary over time. Occasionally there is a single symptom—usually pain or fatigue—that is associated with the other features of the disorder [11].

15.1.1 Finding a Suitable Definition for Clinicians in Primary Care

The concept of BDD contained in the main ICD-11 is suitable for mental health professionals, since, although patients typically have many symptoms, it includes patients who may have only a single somatic symptom. The version of the ICD-11 intended for use in primary health care (ICD-11 PHC) has modified this definition, in view of the many patients with only one or two somatic symptoms. Patients who have *three or more somatic symptoms* without any physical explanation are said to have bodily stress syndrome (BSS).

Bodily stress syndrome has been adapted for the needs of primary care and is clearly a more conservative concept than BDD. Extensive research in both primary care and general hospital care has been conducted in Denmark by Fink et al. [7, 12, 13].

They used a definition of this common disorder as patients with at least three persistent symptoms over time attributable to autonomic overarousal (cardiorespiratory, gastrointestinal, musculoskeletal) or as general symptoms of tiredness and exhaustion. The patient's concern over health expresses itself as excessive time and energy devoted to these symptoms. The symptoms are distressing and/or result in significant disability. This is an important advance in classification, as it drops the previous concept of 'unexplained'.

Another important concept in primary care is health anxiety, which appears to overlap considerably with BSS. It replaces the previous concept of 'hypochondriasis'. Like BSS, it is a better concept to share with the patient and may lead to a therapeutic dialogue. Although patients often also have somatic symptoms, it is not a requirement that they should have any.

15.2 Diagnostic Criteria

15.2.1 Bodily Stress Syndrome (BSS)

15.2.1.1 BSS: Presenting Symptoms/ Complaints

The patient presents with multiple somatic symptoms over time in association with high distress and accompanied by disability. The symptoms may be influenced by culture and change over time.

15.2.1.2 BSS: Clinical Description

The patient suffers from multiple persistent bodily symptoms, which are present at the same time. In order to diagnose BSS, the symptoms must at some stage present as autonomic arousal symptoms, musculoskeletal tension or general/ neurological and cognitive symptoms and result in significant disruption in daily life. Symptoms are distressing and/or result in significant disruption in daily life, as well as persistent concerns about the medical seriousness of the symptoms.

15.2.1.3 BSS: Required Symptoms

The patient *must have*:

- At least three persistent symptoms over time attributable to autonomic overarousal (cardio-respiratory, gastrointestinal, musculoskeletal) or as general symptoms of tiredness and exhaustion. The patient's concern over health expresses itself as excessive time and energy devoted to these symptoms.
- The symptoms are distressing and result in significant disability.

Symptom patterns *may include*:

- Examples of cardiopulmonary arousal: palpitations, precordial discomfort, breathlessness without exertion, hyperventilation, hot or cold sweats, trembling or shaking and dry mouth
- Examples of gastrointestinal arousal: abdominal pains, frequent loose bowel movements, feeling bloated, regurgitations, constipation, diarrhoea, nausea, vomiting and burning sensation in chest or epigastrium
- Examples of musculoskeletal tension: pains in arms or legs, muscular aches or pains, pains in the joints, feelings of paresis or localised weakness, back ache, pain moving from one place to another and unpleasant numbness or tingling sensations
- Examples of general unspecific symptoms: concentration difficulties, impairment of memory, excessive fatigue, headache and dizziness

15.2.1.4 BSS: Severity

Mild: The patient complains of symptoms or problems in only one bodily system, and while there is some disability, most activities can be managed, with increased difficulty.

Moderate: There are multiple problems in one or two bodily systems, and there is marked distress or disability associated with the symptoms.

Severe: There are symptoms in multiple bodily systems and disability/distress is severe.

15.2.1.5 BSS: Childhood Variations

Bodily distress in children may be mono-symptomatic, and the type of symptoms varies with age, with abdominal pain and headache common in smaller children, whereas the prevalence of fatigue and neurological symptoms seems to increase with age. Bodily distress in children may continue into adult life.

15.2.1.6 BSS in Older Patients

Disorders of bodily distress or bodily experience occur across all age groups including older adults [12]. Understanding this condition in older adults particularly in primary care is very important because over 25% of primary care consultations are accounted for by people who are aged 65 years and older [13, 14].

15.2.2 Health Anxiety

15.2.2.1 Health Anxiety: Presenting Symptoms

The patient may present with any physical symptom and symptoms may change over time. The main problem is not the symptom itself but *persistent worry about potential health problems.*

15.2.2.2 Health Anxiety: Clinical Description

Health preoccupation is a disorder of the awareness of one's body with a high degree of illness worry.

15.2.2.3 Health Anxiety: Required Symptoms

One (or more) of the following three phenomena:

- The patient may have obsessive rumination with intrusive thoughts, ideas or fears of harbouring illness that cannot be stopped or can only be stopped with great difficulty.
- Either worrying about or preoccupation with fears of harbouring a severe physical disease or the idea that disease will be contracted one in the future or preoccupation with other health concerns.
- Attention and intense awareness on bodily functions, physical sensations, physiological reactions or minor bodily problems that are misinterpreted as serious disease.

15.2.2.4 Health Anxiety: Childhood Variations

Children may be subject to parent's health preoccupation. In young children with health preoccupation, the specific cognitive distortions may be difficult to verify directly, but their presence might be based on observations of the child's behaviour such as being hard to calm down or divert when having physical symptoms or a tendency to complain a lot about pain and physical symptoms when there seems not to be much wrong.

15.3 Assessment and Treatment

Despite the difficulties with agreeing shared terminology, the available research shows that treatment is possible for people with disorders of bodily distress or bodily experience and there is hope for patients, their carers and health-care professionals [4, 15–18].

Many of these patients will be managed in primary care, so there is a need for primary care to be innovate, able to collaborate with secondary and social care and capable of shared decision-making with patients, just as in all other conditions [19–22].

15.3.1 History Taking and Investigations

There are many clinical guidelines available to support clinicians who treat disorders of bodily distress [23, 24].

The key requirements for making a diagnosis and developing a care package include:

(a) *History* that looks for presence of pain, parts of the body that are affected, whether anatomical pathways are followed, other physical symptoms, what organs are affected other psychological symptoms including sleep disturbance, fatigue, concentration and memory.
(b) *Co-occuring physical or mental illness* to account for some of the symptoms.
(c) *Investigations* to rule out somatic illness including physical examination: blood tests including full blood count (FBC); liver function tests (LFTs); renal function tests; creatinine phosphokinase (CPK), antinuclear antibodies (ANA), C-reactive protein (CRP), and erythrocyte sedimentation rate (ESR); vitamin D levels, folic acid levels, rheumatoid factor (RF), and thyroid function tests including thyroid-stimulating hormone (TSH).
(d) *Additional tests.* These are possible, but the clinician must be clear in their mind about what they are looking for and what this test

will achieve because it is essential to avoid over investigation especially as we know that there are high health-care utilisation costs associated with these conditions [25].

Once the history, examination and investigations are complete, it is essential to share the outcome with the patient in order for the clinician and patient to jointly develop a care package following a biopsychosocial approach.

15.3.2 Monitoring Progress

Direct involvement in assessing their symptoms and the impact of interventions provided as part of their individualised care package by using visual analogue scales has been shown to be useful [26]:

- *Symptom intensity* has been measured using a numeric analogue scale that asks the question 'during the last 7 days, the overall intensity of my bodily symptoms was…'.
- The patient is then asked to rate themselves on a Likert scale with 0 described as 'no symptoms at all' and 10 described as 'worst possible symptoms'.
- *Symptom interference* has been measured using a numeric analogue scale that asks the question 'during the last seven days my bodily symptoms interfered with daily life activities'.

The patient is then asked to rate themselves on a Likert scale with 0 described as 'not at all' and 10 described as 'interfered completely'.

This two numeric analogue scale has been translated into more than 20 languages [26].

15.3.3 Non-pharmacological Interventions

There is positive evidence to support the use of a range of non-pharmacological interventions in patients who present with bodily distress disorders. A 2014 Cochrane Review looking at interventions for somatisation disorder, undifferentiated somatoform disorder, somatoform disorders unspecified, somatoform autonomic dysfunction, pain disorder, alternative somatoform diagnoses proposed in the literature and medically unexplained physical symptoms (MUPS) concluded that psychological therapies were superior to usual care or waiting list in terms of reduction of symptom severity. They specifically found that cognitive behaviour therapy (CBT) reduces somatic symptoms and that the effect of this lasts beyond a year at the conclusion of therapy [15].

Being Patient Centred The patient must be at the centre of all decisions about the treatment plan, and trust needs to be built between the patient and the caregiver. The caregiver must recognise their own feelings of frustration and know how to manage them so that they do not have a negative influence on the therapeutic relationship [4, 27, 28].

Cognitive Behaviour Therapy (CBT) Cognitive behaviour therapy (CBT) has been by far the most extensively researched psychological intervention for bodily distress disorders, and, as a single treatment, only CBT has been adequately studied to allow tentative conclusions for practice to be drawn [15]. CBT focuses on addressing or changing cognitions and behaviours that people have in interaction with their symptoms, and combining CBT with graded exercise has also been shown to be of significant benefit, although concordance to this combination of therapy is low [29].

Mindfulness Therapy There is evidence to support the use of mindfulness-based therapies in the treatment of bodily distress disorders based on the treatment outcomes in somatisation disorder, functional somatic syndromes such as fibromyalgia, irritable bowel syndrome (IBS) and chronic fatigue syndrome (CFS) [30–32].

Use of the Consultation Liaison Model The usefulness of the psychiatric liaison-consultation model where psychiatrists see the patient in the presence of the other treating physician has been reviewed. Although the other treating physician finds this useful, there is limited evidence that this approach significantly improves the patient's symptoms [33].

Body Mind Approach™ Separating the mind and body for patients with bodily distress is unhelpful. Body-based psychotherapy that uses mindful, kinetic practice derived from dance movement therapy can be useful for adults including the older adult population. This type of therapy connects the person's inner feelings of distress with their bodily feelings of movement during the therapy to promote healing and recovery [34, 35].

Couple Therapy and Family Interventions As with most health problems, family members are on the front lines of caring for patients with BDS/BSS, particularly when the patient is in later life. Family members are affected by the illness and, in turn, have an effect on the patient and the illness. In a study of adults with somatisation disorder, patients reported significantly higher levels of family conflict and significantly lower levels of family cohesion, which is characterised by frequent arguments, emotional distance and poor support [36]. In a couple or marital relationship, conflict and distance likely exist in a demand-withdraw interactional pattern: patient attention-seeking behaviour is associated with partner withdrawal, and partner attention-providing is associated with patient withdrawal [37]. A common theme in this pattern is the avoidance of emotional pain. An avoidance of emotional pain may be linked to emotional and/or physical trauma, which is discussed elsewhere in this chapter.

When family members are present in treatment, doctors can directly observe a significant context for the illness—organisational patterns (e.g. roles, rules), communication and illness beliefs in the family [38]. For example, family members frequently have strong beliefs about the cause of BDS/BSS and the role of health professionals in treating BDS/BSS. A common trap that family members encounter is blaming the patient with BDS/BSS for faking symptoms or being weak, which may create significant tension in the relationship. Family members may also worry that something is significantly wrong with their loved one and look for reassurance and a clear treatment plan. Education for family members that link psychological, relational and physical processes will help family members better understand the patient and potentially decrease misunderstanding and conflict [39, 40]. If family involvement is not possible, it is still helpful to inquire about the family, both currently and historically.

15.3.4 Pharmacological Interventions

In some cases pharmacological treatments are useful.

Antidepressant Medication Antidepressant medication, particularly tricyclic antidepressants (TCAs) and serotonin-noradrenaline reuptake inhibitors (SNRIs), has been found to be useful, particularly in pain relief resulting in a 35–50% improvement in pain in some patients. However there is no advantage in treating with a combination of antidepressants from the same or different classes because the side effects outweigh any clinical benefits gained [17].

Antipsychotic Medication Some people have advocated for the use of antipsychotic medication in bodily distress specifically to treat pain, sleep disturbance, depression and anxiety in patients with fibromyalgia; however this is not supported as a clinical intervention or as part of the care package because the side effects outweigh any benefits [41]. In people with a proven comorbid psychosis, antipsychotic medication will have an important part to play.

15.4 Collaborative Care

There are many reasons that people present with bodily distress. Some are biological, some are social, and some are psychological and can include early- and late-onset trauma and exposure to parental illness. There may be precipitating factors for bodily distress that the patient is unable to recognise such as recent infection, accidents, physical and emotional trauma and loss events.

This complexity means that it is difficult for a single individual practitioner to possess all the skills necessary to manage a patient presenting with bodily distress, so a collaborative or integrated approach to care provides the best opportunity for success and maintenance of recovery [19, 42].

The ICD11 PHC produced some draft management guidelines for both BSS and HA, and they are given below.

15.4.1 Management Guidelines: Bodily Stress Syndrome (BSS)

[There are as yet no official guidelines on the management of BSS. These guidelines are based on the considerable research which has already been done on 'patients with unexplained somatic symptoms'].

15.4.1.1 BSS: Essential Information for the Patient and the Family

Bodily stress syndrome is a common disorder in primary medical care and consists of three or more somatic symptoms in a particular group (musculoskeletal, cardiovascular, gastrointestinal, neurocognitive) which used to be referred to by separate terms such as fibromyalgia, effort syndrome or irritable bowel syndrome. However, these should not be thought of as independent clinical entities and can usefully be thought of as symptoms that are fairly common and are related to stress. Our bodily organs are controlled by a part of our nervous system called the autonomic nervous system. When we are stressed, this can lead to overarousal of this system, leading to common symptoms like palpitations, abdominal pain, shortness of breath, diarrhoea and backache. These symptoms are very real and can cause pain and discomfort [1].

15.4.1.2 BSS: General Management and Advice to Patient and Family

Primary care staff should take a comprehensive history from the patient, covering the somatic, cognitive, emotional, behavioural and social dimensions. For example, are there one or several patterns of symptoms, how long do they last, and does the patient take medication for pain? What does the patient think about the origin of these symptoms—and does the family agree with this? Is there any avoidance behaviour, and does sick leave have to be taken? Aim for a shared definition of the problem, with education and explanation, and a clear explanation of factors that will inhibit recovery, for example, repeated negative somatic investigations. It is important to be optimistic about the symptoms and stress that they are reversible, even when they have lasted a long time [2].

Patients with BSS need to be treated with attention to how disabled they are by their symptoms and how long the symptoms have lasted. Those with only *minor disability*, or of less than 3 months duration, should be treated entirely by the GP. Giving firm assurance and being positive about the prognosis can be therapeutic in patients with mild BDS/BSS, as symptoms will decrease in 50–75% of the patients over a period of 6–15 months [3].

Those with *moderate disability* can be offered sessions with other attached workers within primary care.

15.4.1.3 BSS: Management Interventions

If *stress is related to a particular life problem*, then 'problem-solving', by a nurse or other attached worker, can also be useful, and such skills can be readily taught to health-care workers and given in primary care.

15.4.1.4 BSS: Medication Advice

For those with depression of at least moderate severity, antidepressants have also been shown to be effective, but some other studies have shown no difference between antidepressant and a placebo, nor was there difference between the various antidepressants [4].

Patients with predominant bowel symptoms ('irritable bowel syndrome') may benefit from diet low in indigestible fibres or low in fermentable oligosaccharides, disaccharides, monosaccharides and polyols (FODMAP diet). Diarrhoea or constipation may be treated with antispasmodics or laxatives as appropriate. Loperamide may also be helpful with diarrhoea (but note that side effects can include stomach cramps and bloating, dizziness, drowsiness and rashes). Regular exercise is also helpful.

Those with backache or headache may benefit from painkillers, but addictive medication should be avoided.

15.4.1.5 BSS: Liaison and Referral

If assistance from psychologists is available, *cognitive behaviour therapy* may be beneficial to these patients. It has been shown to be superior to treatment as usual in primary care [5], and individual CBT is better than either group CBT or usual treatment [6].

Meditation using mindfulness techniques has also been shown to be superior to usual treatment [7] and has also been shown to be cost-effective in primary care [8].

Those with *long histories* and *severe disability* may be referred to specialist *mental health services*—either to a clinical psychologist or to a psychiatrist. When this is not practicable, long-term patients should be seen from time to time by the primary care clinician, to check whether new symptoms suggestive of new physical disease have appeared and to investigate these symptoms only if they sound typical of such diseases. Continuity of care is important: patients should be offered regular planned follow-up appointments and treated with sympathy and concern.

15.4.2 Management Guidelines: Health Anxiety

[There are as yet no official guidelines on the management of health anxiety. This guideline takes account of recent research on this disorder].

15.4.2.1 Health Anxiety: Essential Information for the Patient and the Family

When people suffer from health anxiety, they worry excessively about their health and monitor it repeatedly. Typically, they ruminate about illness, so that when they start thinking about a potential disease, this thought recurs persistently. The constant fear of disease creates considerable distress. Health anxiety is common in the community and medical settings [1, 2]. Most of those with health anxiety consult health professionals repeatedly, but are helped only briefly by the reassurance that usually follows, and a cycle of recurring consultations and investigations is set up. This reinforces health anxiety and the condition persists.

15.4.2.2 Health Anxiety: General Management and Advice to Patient and Family

The most important initial intervention is to help these patients *feel understood*; using a collaborative strategic approach, you need to build up an understanding that what they are suffering from is fear of disease rather than having the disease they fear. One of the common mistakes in management is to say that the symptoms are imagined. The symptoms of the health anxious patient are not imagined; they are often very troubling and profound, but they are interpreted wrongly as symptoms of a physical disease instead of mental discomfort and associated bodily sensations.

The second message to be delivered is that reassurance, no matter how provided, does not solve the problem. Reassurance provides short-term temporary relief, which can become addictive, but doubt always sets in and the benefit of reassurance is lost. Such 'safety-seeking behaviours' have been shown to greatly exacerbate health anxiety [3].

The third important message is to avoid what is now recognised as cyberchondria, the frequent information seeking from the Internet or from other media outlets. This only tends to exacerbate fears of illness as the patient tends to ignore the high frequency of common disorders and focus on the rare and potentially fatal ones. Part of therapy is to use the Internet in a sensible and informed way.

Once the negative effects of these behaviours are understood, the problem of health anxiety becomes more accessible to management. Once worry has been identified as the major component of the problem, therapeutic intervention becomes focused on this.

15.4.2.3 Health Anxiety: Psychological Interventions

Stress management, cognitive behaviour therapy adapted for health anxiety, computerised cognitive behaviour therapy (CCBT), acceptance and commitment therapy and mindfulness-based cognitive therapy are effective in the treatment of health anxiety [4–8]. The beneficial effects can last for many years [9]. Patients with high scores on health anxiety scales at baseline show the greatest improvement, and those with high depression ratings initially have lower levels of response [10]. The presence of health anxiety with co-existing disease does not impair the success of treatment [11].

15.4.2.4 Health Anxiety: Medication Advice

There is no specific drug treatment for health anxiety, but some slight evidence that the SSRI drug, fluoxetine, may be of value [43]. Most people with health anxiety are concerned about adverse effects of drugs and are generally averse to this mode of treatment.

15.4.2.5 Health Anxiety: Management Advice Regarding Special Issues that are Specific to the Diagnostic Category that Merit Separate Consideration

The important difference between health anxiety and other anxiety disorders is that patients rarely complain of health anxiety; indeed they are more likely to regard it as a necessary condition to ward off disease rather than a disorder. Enabling patients to realise that they have an anxiety disorder is the most important first step in management, but it must be done in such a way that the patient appreciates that the therapist understands their concerns and can empathise with them

instead of making comments such as 'its all your imagination'. Most people with health anxiety know they worry but do not consult practitioners with special knowledge of mental health, preferring to see doctors in general medicine.

At present there are very few services available in most countries for the treatment of health anxiety. Nonetheless, if the simple and straightforward advice is given as above, it can have at least some effect on the outcome of the problem.

15.4.2.6 Health Anxiety: Liaison and Referral

In many people these fears of illness and consequent beliefs are entrenched, and skilled management is often necessary to effect a lasting change. Referral to a clinical psychologist may be appropriate. General nurses may also be trained in psychological treatments and have been shown to be more acceptable and more effective as therapists than psychologists in medical settings [44], possibly because they are perceived as more acceptable to patients who still wish to have treatment given by someone who has a sound background in medical practice.

15.5 Research Opportunities and Recommendations

(a) Organisation of health care should enhance the possibilities for collaborative care for these patients.

(b) Primary care should be given enough support to manage these patients, minimising the unnecessary referrals and medicalisation of these patients.

(c) Teaching about BDS/BSS should be included into curricula at undergraduate level so that all future doctors understand the nature of this disease.

(d) At postgraduate level, future specialists, especially in primary care, should gain knowledge and skills how to manage these patients.

(e) Research about BDS/BSS should become a greater priority in allocation of research funds.

References

1. Creed F, Guthrie E, Fink P, Henningsen R, Reif W, Sharpe M, White P. Is there a better term than 'medically unexplained symptoms'? J Psychosom Res. 2010;68:5–8. https://doi.org/10.1016/j.jpsychores.2009.09.004.
2. Henningsen P, Fink P, Hausteiner-Wiehle C, Reif W. Terminology, classification and concepts. In: Creed F, Henningsen P, Fink P, editors. Medically unexplained symptoms, somatisation and bodily distress. Cambridge: Cambridge University Press; 2011.
3. Salmon S, Peters S, Stanley I. Patients' perceptions of medical explanations for somatisation disorders: qualitative analysis. Br Med J. 1999;318:372–6.
4. Ivbijaro G, Goldberg D. Bodily distress syndrome (BDS): the evolution from medically unexplained symptoms (MUS). Ment Health Fam Med. 2013;10:63–4.
5. Edwards TM, Stern A, Clarke DD, Ivbijaro G, Kasney LM. The treatment of patients with medically unexplained symptoms in primary care: a review of the literature. Ment Health Fam Med. 2010;7:209–21.
6. American Psychiatric Association. Somatic symptom and related disorders. In: Diagnostic and statistical manual of mental disorders. 5th ed. Washington DC: APA; 2013.
7. Fink P, Toft T, Hansen MS, Ørnbøl E, Olesen F. Symptoms and syndromes of bodily distress: an exploratory study of 978 internal medical, neurological, and primary care patients. Psychosom Med. 2007;69:30–9.
8. Fink P, Schröder A. One single diagnosis, bodily distress syndrome, succeeded to capture 10 diagnostic categories of functional somatic syndromes and somatoform disorders. J Psychosom Res. 2010;68:415–26.
9. Häuser W, Henningsen P. Fibromyalgia syndrome: a somatoform disorder? Eur J Pain. 2014;18(8):1052–9. https://doi.org/10.1002/j.1532-2149.2014.00453.x.
10. Haller H, Cramer H, Lauche R, Dobos G. Somatoform disorders and medically unexplained symptoms in primary care- a systematic review and meta-analysis of prevalence. Dtsch Arztebl Int. 2015;112:279–87. https://doi.org/10.3238/arztebl.2015.0297.
11. World Health Organization. International classification of diseases 11th revision. Geneva: WHO; 2018. https://icd.who.int/browse11/l-m/en#/http%3a%2f%2fid.who.int%2ficd%2fentity%2f794195577.
12. Wijeratne C, Hickie I. Somatic distress syndromes in later life: the need for paradigm change. Psychol Med. 2001;31:571–6.
13. Commonwealth Department of Health and Family Services, General Practice Branch. General practice in Australia. Canberra: Commonwealth of Australia; 1996.
14. Budtz-Lilly A, Vestergaard M, Fink M, Carlsen AH, Rosendal M. Patient characteristics and frequency of bodily distress syndrome in primary care: a cross-sectional study. Br J Gen Pract. 2015;65(638):e617–22. https://doi.org/10.3399/bjgp15X686545.
15. Van Dessel N, den Boeft M, van der Wouden JC, Kleinstäuber M, Leone SS, Terluin B, Numans ME, van der Horst HE, van Matwijk H. Non-pharmacological interventions for somatoform disorders and medically unexplained physical symptoms (MUPS) in adults. Cochrane Database Syst Rev. 2014;11:CD011142. https://doi.org/10.1002/14651858.CD011142.pub2.
16. Walitt B, Klose P, Üçeyler N, Phillips T, Häuser W. Antipsychtics for fibromyalgia in adults. Cochrane Database Syst Rev. 2016;6:CD011804. https://doi.org/10.1002/14651858.CD011804.pub2.
17. Thorpe J, Shum B, Moore RA, Wiffen PJ, Gilron I. Combined pharmacotherapy for the treatment of fibromyalgia in adults. Cochrane Database Syst Rev. 2018;2:CD010585. https://doi.org/10.1002/14651858.CD010585.pub2.
18. Welsch P, Üçeyler N, Klose P, Walitt B, Häuser W. Serotonin and noradrenaline reuptake inhibitors (SNRI's) for fibromyalgia. Cochrane Database Syst Rev. 2018;2:CD010292. https://doi.org/10.1002/14651858.CD010292.pub.2.
19. Funk M, Ivbijaro G (eds). Integrating mental health into primary care: a global perspective. WHO/Wonca: 2008.
20. Ivbijaro GO, Enum Y, Khan AA, Lam SS-K, Gabzdyl A. Collaborative care: models for treatment of patients with complex medical-psychiatric conditions. Curr Psychiatry Rep. 2014;16:506.
21. Ivbijaro G. Mental health: a resilience factor against both NCDs and CDs. In: Commonwealth health partnerships 2012. Cambridge: Nexus Strategic Partnerships; 2012. p. 17–20.
22. Rosendal M, Blankenstein AH, Morriss R, Fink P, Sharpe M, Burton C. Enhanced care by generalists for functional somatic symptoms and disorders in primary care. Cochrane Database Syst Rev. 2013;10:CD008142. https://doi.org/10.1002/14651858.CD008142.pub2.
23. Häuser W, Ablin J, Perrot S, Fitzcharles M-A. Management of fibromyalgia: key messages from recent evidence-based guidelines. Pol Arch Intern Med. 2017;127(1):47–56. https://doi.org/10.20452/pamw.3877.
24. Petzke F, Brückle W, Eidmann U, Heldmann P, Köllner V, Kühn T, Kühn-Becker H, Strunk-Richter M, Schiltenwolf M, Settan M, von Wachter M, Weigl M, Häuser W. General treatment principles, coordination of care and patient education in fibromyalgia syndrome: updated guidelines 2017 and overview of systematic review articles. Schmerz. 2017;31(3):246–54. https://doi.org/10.1007/s00482-017-0201-6.
25. McAndrew LM, Phillips LA, Helmer DA, Maesto K, Engel CC, Greenberg LM, Anastasides N, Quigley KS. High healthcare utilization near the onset of medically unexplained symptoms. J Psychosom Res. 2017;98:98–105. https://doi.org/10.1016/jpsychores.2017.05.001.

26. Rief W, Burton C, Frostholm L, Henningsen P, Kleinstäuber M, Kop WJ, Löwe B, Martin A, Malt U, Rosmalen J, Schröder A, Sheddon-Mora M, Toussaint A, van der Feltz-Cornelis C, on behalf of the EURONET-SOMA Group. Core outcome domains for clinical trials on somatic symptom disorder, bodily distress disorder, and functional somatic syndromes: European Network on Somatic Symptom Disorders Recommendations. Psychosom Med. 2017;17(9):1008–15. https://doi.org/10.1097/PSY.0000000000000502.

27. Trimbos Instituut /Netherlands Institute of mental Health and Addiction. *Multidisciplinaire Richtlijn SOLK en Somatoforme Stoornissen.* [multidisciplinary guideline medically unexplained symptoms and somatoform disorders]. Houten: Ladenius Communicatie BV; 2010.

28. Olde Hartman TC, Rosendal M, Aamland A, van der Horst HE, Rosmalen JGM, Burton CD, Lucassen PLBJ. What do guidelines and systematic reviews tell us about the management of medically unexplained symptoms in primary care? BJGP Open. 2017;1(3):BJGP-2016-0868. https://doi.org/10.3399/bjgpopen17X101061.

29. Busch AJ, Schachter CL, Overend TJ, Peloso PM, Barber KA. Exercise for fibromyalgia: a systematic review. J Rheumatol. 2008;35(6):1130–44.

30. Henningsen P, Zipfel S, Herzog W. Management of functional somatic syndromes. Lancet. 2007;369(9565):946–55.

31. Fink P, Rosendal M. Recent developments in the understanding and management of functional somatic symptoms in primary care. Curr Opin Psychiatry. 2008;21(2):182–8.

32. Fjorback LO, Arendt M, Ørnbøl WH, rehfeld E. Mindfulness therapy for somatization disorder and functional somatic syndromes – randomized trial with one-year follow-up. J Psychosom Res. 2013;74:31–40. https://doi.org/10.1016/j.jpsychores.2012.09.006.

33. Hoedeman R, Blankenstein AH, van der Feltz-Cornelis CM, Ktol B, Stewart R, Groothoff JW. Consultation letters for medically unexplained physical symptoms in primary care. Cochrane Database Syst Rev. 2010;12:CD006524. https://doi.org/10.1002/14651858.CD006524.pub2.

34. Payne H. The body speaks its mind: the BodyMind ApproachTM for patients with medically unexplained symptoms in primary care in England. Arts Psychother. 2015;42:19–27. https://doi.org/10.1016/j.aip.2014012.011.

35. Payne H. The BodyMind approach™: supporting people with medically unexplained symptoms/somatic symptom disorder. J Psychother Couns Psychol. Reflect. 2017;2(2):5–7.

36. Brown RJ, Schrag A, Trimble MR. Dissociation, childhood interpersonal trauma, and family functioning in patients with somatization disorder. Am J Psychiatr. 2005;162:899–905.

37. Hilbert A, Martin A, Zech T, et al. Patients with medically unexplained symptoms and their significant others: illness attributions and behaviors as predictors of patient functioning over time. J Psychosom Res. 2010;68:253–62.

38. Families RJ. Illness, and disability: an integrative treatment model. New York: Basic Books; 1994.

39. Watson WH, McDaniel SH. Relational therapy in medical settings: working with somatizing patients and their families. J Clin Psychol. 2000;56:1065–82.

40. McDaniel H, Doherty WJ, Hepworth J. Medical family therapy and integrated care. In: 2nd edition. Washington, D.C.: American Psychological Association; 2014.

41. Walitt B, Klose P, Üçeyler N, Phillips T, Häuser W. Antipsychotics for fibromyalgia in adults. Cochrane Database Syst Rev. 2016;6:CD011804. https://doi.org/10.1002/14651858.CD011804.pub2.

42. Budtz-Lilly A, Schröder RMT, Fink P, Vestergaard M, Rosendal M. Bodily distress syndrome: a new diagnosis for functional disorders in primary care? BMC Fam Pract. 2015;16:180. https://doi.org/10.1186/s12875-015-0393-8.

43. Fink P, Rosendal M, Olesen F. Classification of somatization and functional somatic symptoms in primary care. Aust N Z J Psychiatry. 2005;39:772–81.

44. Budtz-Lilly A, Fink P, Ørnbøl E, Vestergaard M, Moth G, Christensen KS, Rosendal M. A new questionnaire to identify bodily distress in primary care: the 'BDS checklist. J Psychosom Res. 2015;78:536–45.

Biopsychosocial Approaches to Depression in the Older Adults

16

David Baron and Jessica Uno

Abstract

There is no health without mental health. This commonly cited phrase is particularly true in the elderly. Depression can be challenging to diagnose and treat in older adults patients and has a significant negative impact on the overall quality of physical and emotional well-being. A comprehensive biopsychosocial approach to assessment and management of depression is necessary to ensure maximal quality of life. Assessment of mood must take into account current life stressors, such as chronic and acute health problems, social isolation, age-related cognitive decline, prior history of depressions, recent losses (family, friends), drug and alcohol use, and financial challenges. Treatment interventions should address issues identified in the biopsychosocial assessment, with an emphasis on psychosocial treatment (such as enjoyable exercise and increased social interactions). Pharmacotherapy should be used cautiously and conservatively, as side effects and drug-drug interactions are a common problem in this population. Keeping the *Golden Years* truly golden requires attention to the overall mood state of older adult patient, not a sole focus on physical functioning.

Key Points

- Depression is a common, and potentially life-threatening, diagnosis in older adults patients treated in a primary care setting.
- The diagnosis of depression in this population can be challenging given its symptom presentation and co-occurring psychosocial stressors and chronic medical abnormalities associated with aging.
- A regular, enjoyable, medically sound exercise program should be considered in the treatment of all depressed older adults patients.

16.1 Introduction

Diagnosing depression in the older adult can be challenging. The differential diagnosis of the classic symptoms of a major mood disorder, including altered sleep, appetite, energy levels, sad mood, hopelessness, poor concentration, and suicidal ideation, may result from life events. However, major life events such as the death of a friend or spouse, new disabilities, and financial instability are more frequent in old age. Primary depression must also be distinguished from organic causes secondary to

D. Baron (✉) · J. Uno
Keck School of Medicine, University of Southern California, Los Angeles, CA, USA
e-mail: dave.baron@usc.edu

© Springer Nature Switzerland AG 2019
C. A. de Mendonça Lima, G. Ivbijaro (eds.), *Primary Care Mental Health in Older People*,
https://doi.org/10.1007/978-3-030-10814-4_16

comorbid medical conditions or medications. This can be a daunting task when 92% of older Americans have at least one chronic condition, with 77% of seniors enduring at least two. It follows that as of 2015, the average geriatric patient takes 14–18 prescriptions per year. This creates an extremely challenging situation when it comes to understanding potential drug-drug interactions and the effect on mood and behavior.

As complicated as this problem seems, the solution is within reach. Depression is approached differently in adolescents and middle-aged adults. Logically, late-life depression also requires its own detection and management strategies. With increased knowledge of its unique symptoms, geriatric depression becomes less insidious. Additionally, primary care providers (PCPs) should become familiar with the full continuum of appropriate biopsychosocial interventions. While late-life depression treatment may create challenges when attempting pharmacologic management, psychosocial interventions hold great potential as primary and adjunctive treatment strategies. Behavioral and lifestyle changes, especially enjoyable exercise, can make a significant and lasting impact on clinical management of depression.

All symptoms of depression in the older adults should be evaluated from a context-dependent perspective. Mislabeling a presenting symptom as being caused by an underlying mood disorder, when it is actually the result of a medical abnormality or current life stressor, will negatively impact creation of effective treatment. Conversely, subjecting a patient to unnecessary medical treatments and diagnostic tests for "medical" symptoms, which are the results of a depressive disorder, is costly and could increase morbidity. Thorough evaluation of the etiology of every presenting symptom will result in a more accurate diagnosis and better serve the biopsychosocial needs of depressed older adult patients.

This chapter builds on previous chapters discussing history taking strategies and the wider determinants of mental health in older patients.

16.2 Differences in Late-Life Depression

The presentation of depression in the geriatric population may differ significantly from depression seen in middle-aged adults and young people. Relying on the classic adult presentation of depression when diagnosing geriatric patients is problematic. Misidentifying depression among the older adult is especially dangerous because it is associated with an increased suicide risk, especially among older white men. Additionally, late-life depression has a high association with increased healthcare costs, family stress, and an impaired quality of life that hinders enjoyment of one's golden years. Other obstacles that complicate late-life depression are the cultural infantilization of older patients and ageist beliefs about their diminished abilities. Depression is *not* a normal feature of aging, but it is a highly treatable condition, meriting vigilance from the PCP. It is important for the clinician to understand that discussing mood and emotional symptoms may be difficult for the older adult patient. Discussions of mood and emotional stress are often viewed as inappropriate topics for discussion with their medical doctor. As a result, somatic symptoms may be the presenting complaint, as these *are* appropriate to tell their doctor. Differentiating mood symptoms presenting as somatic complaints from purely physical complaints is important to ensure an effective treatment intervention.

One confusing feature of geriatric depression is cognitive impairment. Executive dysfunction is often the initial complaint that brings older adult patients in for evaluation. While "slow thinking" or "brain fog" is a common experience of younger people with depression, it may be especially pronounced in depressed older adult patients who are already concerned about developing dementia. At the same time, depressive symptoms confound the workup of neurodegenerative diseases and age-related memory impairment. However, careful questioning of the patient can assist in differentiating between depression and dementia. A sense of apathy is more prominent in geriatric depression and often translates into features such as reduced short-term recall, poor concentration, and disorganization. Depressed, non-demented patients are not necessarily experiencing memory impairment; they just may not *care* anymore as a result of being depressed.

In addition to apathy, the interview with a depressed patient may express different key phrases regarding mood. Sad mood may present in older patients as disinterested behavior and statements of *hopelessness, helplessness, being a burden*, or *worthlessness*.

> Statements implying the patient has nothing to live for:
>
> "I have nothing to look forward to."
> "All my friends are dead."

> Statements implying that the patient believes himself or herself to be better off dead:
>
> "I'm just a burden on my family."
> "They don't need me around anymore."

Other signs of depression manifest as subtle behavior changes. Sleeping difficulties are commonly reported. A depressed older adult patient may report poor sleep but is not aware he or she is napping excessively during the day or falling asleep while watching television in the early evening. Another important confounding variable is the lack of any exercise or activity during the day. These symptoms are often overlooked in depressed older adult patients because popular culture tends to portray these behaviors as typical of old age.

Occasionally, the cognitive symptoms of geriatric depressions can be taken to extremes in a phenomenon formerly labeled "pseudodementia." Now referred to as "depression with reversible dementia," this syndrome consists of cognitive impairment, reaching a level of severity resembling dementia. As its name suggests, this "dementia" will resolve when the underlying depression is treated. While this may sound like an alarming challenge for the PCP, depression with reversible dementia differs from depression in Alzheimer's patients. Reversible dementia patients exhibit more symptoms of anxiety. Additionally, they often feature early-morning awakening and loss of interest in past pleasurable activities.

> **Interview Strategies for Diagnosis**
> Several aspects of a patient's history are especially helpful in diagnosing late-life depression. A few questions to focus on include:
>
> • Have they had prior depressive episodes earlier in life?
> • What prior treatments for depression have the patient tried?
> • Which worked well? Which did not work well, and why?
> • What current life stresses is the patient experiencing?
>   – Financial insecurity?
>   – Health insurance issues?
>   – Family?
>   – New disability or loss of mobility?
>   – Recent retirement?

For late-life depression, the interviewer should place extra emphasis on past psychiatric history, in addition to current social stressors. It can provide clues for making an accurate diagnosis. Past history of depression should include any side effects of prior pharmacologic treatment. Patients frequently discontinue their depression medications because of adverse side effects, lack of efficacy, or expense. These negative experiences play a large role in discouraging the older adult patient from seeking treatment for subsequent episodes. On the contrary, a positive experience in the past may help ensure compliance with another course of medications.

Finally, it is important to remind geriatric patients that just because they are old, it does not mean they should be depressed. Rather, they should enjoy life and all it has to offer.

16.3 Case Studies

16.3.1 Case 1

Mrs. F is 78 years old and recently widowed. She was in good health and led an active life until 8 months ago, when her husband of 55 years suffered a stroke. He died of medical complications 2 months ago. Mrs. F refused to leave her home and move in with her daughter after her husband's death. She did not want to attend a medical evaluation, but her daughter insisted. Ms. F has no past history of depression and has enjoyed good health throughout her senior years. She developed breast cancer when she was 42, but she is a cancer survivor with no relapse. Her only medication is a multivitamin. Her physical exam is unremarkable and age-appropriate, and her routine labs are all within the normal range. Her daughter is concerned that her mother is becoming depressed because she is sleeping more than usual, has lost weight, and only eats two meals a day. Mrs. F denies persistent sadness, but her daughter has noticed her becoming tearful on occasion. The daughter is requesting her mother be put on antidepressants and forced to move in with her, despite Mrs. F denying being depressed or needing assistance with activities of daily living.

16.3.1.1 Discussion

Although depression is common in older adults, it is important to conduct a comprehensive assessment of all presenting symptoms. Loss of loved ones is inevitable with advancing age but does not always result in an episode of depression and the need for a trial of antidepressants.

In this case, when the doctor asked the patient about her daughter's concerns, she provided the following explanations. She did not want to leave her home until she was no longer able to care for herself. She appreciated her daughter's concern

but did not want to conform her life to fit her daughter and give up her personal space. She also did not invite her daughter to move in, as they disagree on housekeeping. She admitted to only eating two meals a day but claimed she did not like cooking for one and always ate when she was hungry. She kept cans of Ensure in her refrigerator, and drank at least one can a day. She denied sleeping more, but explained that when her daughter called numerous times a day, she would often not answer and claim she had been sleeping, rather than saying she did not want to speak with her daughter for the third time that day. Mrs. F did admit to missing her husband, but she was happy he was out of his misery.

"It was very tough to watch him slowly wither away," she said, with tears in her eyes. When asked about suicidal thoughts, she denied them, claiming, "When God is ready, we'll be together again. We talk every day, and I know he is always by my side."

Mrs. F's remark about talking with her husband every day is a common long-term coping method among those who have lost a spouse. It is a way they maintain a connection with deceased loved ones and keep them alive in their hearts. Such statements are not necessarily symptoms of psychosis. Unlike the aforementioned stereotypes of older adults, this habit is appropriate among geriatric patients. It is often referenced in popular films such as *Forrest Gump* and Pixar's *Up*.

If concerned, PCPs should request a psychiatric consult. The guidelines for distinguishing the normal grief response from psychosis apply. Ask the patient if the deceased person talks back to them or tells them to do things like join them in the grave. If the response is something like "No, but I know he's always listening," then psychosis is less of a concern. In this case, Mrs. F's response is not concerning for suicidal ideation or overt hallucinations. She says she will rejoin her husband "when God is ready." Her attitude is that his spirit is watching over her, not commanding her. Remember, psychosis is not just defined by hearing voices but by losing touch with reality. Providers should ask themselves, "Is this truly a thought process that is out of touch with reality?

Or is it part of the patient's coping style?" As long as this behavior isn't interfering with the patient's health, it can be considered benign and a potential coping strategy.

Preserving Autonomy and Dignity Mrs. F's case counters the assumption that older adult patients are senile or poor historians. It highlights the need to speak directly with the patient, rather than relying on depression-screening tools or collateral information. Presuming that a patient cannot speak for herself is disempowering and denies the patient's autonomy. Providers should try to maintain a sense of independence for the individual. Acknowledge that depression treatment is a team effort. Respecting an individual's autonomy over her body, her health, and her safety can facilitate recovery from depression. Since feelings of helplessness or worthlessness often pervade late-life depression, the last thing the patient needs is to be undermined or patronized.

The most important intervention would be to listen to the patient and ask what she feels she needs to move on with her life. Ongoing assessment is necessary, as denial of underlying mood symptoms is not uncommon. It is critical to work *with* the patient, as opposed to forcing her into a living situation she does want. In this case, the patient was willing to call her daughter daily and to come over for dinner at her daughter's at least twice a week. She also agreed to go food shopping with the daughter twice a month and join an AARP exercise class. No medications were prescribed, and the patient agreed to speak with her doctor if she experienced any physical symptoms. A diagnosis of grief reaction was made.

Living Situation The lifestyle interventions employed in Mrs. F's case resulted from productive negotiation that respected Mrs. F's dignity. With respect to living situation, it is ideal to allow the patient to stay in her own home and environment as long as possible. Always ask the patient, "Where would you feel happiest?" If a patient has the capacity to understand her situation and the competence to make her own decisions, going against her wishes is unethical. First, do no harm. Forcing someone out of her home prematurely

may be harmful, psychologically and possibly physically. As long as the home is made safe for its senior resident, it is a positive setting for depression recovery.

Enjoyable Exercise A critical component of Mrs. F's treatment plan is her exercise class. Enjoyable exercise should be a core component in any geriatric depression intervention. Not only does enjoyable exercise benefit the body, it also creates purpose in life. Giving older adult patients something to look forward to each day can ameliorate feelings of hopelessness. Enjoyable exercise reminds them that they still have something to live for. The neurocognitive benefits of enjoyable exercise include improved mood, better sleep, and increased energy levels. Oftentimes, enjoyable exercise has a ripple effect that promotes a healthy lifestyle in general. Patients are inspired to pursue additional ways to stay active and engaged.

Enjoyable exercise also has a valuable social aspect. Mrs. F's isolation was detrimental to her mental wellness. Taking an exercise class will introduce her to peers who may share her experiences. If a patient complains of things like, "All my friends are dead," then enjoyable group exercise is one way to build a new support network.

Recommendations of exercise may initially be met with reluctance. Patients may believe their arthritis, back pain, etc. will worsen or get in the way. However, providers can help alter the patient's desired exercise activity to accommodate her physical limitations. For instance, a patient may have enjoyed modern dance earlier in life. She might try a comparable activity like tai chi, an activity that emphasizes graceful movement and balance but spares the joints. If the patient previously enjoyed gymnastics, she could consider yoga and other sports involving flexibility. Physicians should also educate patients to "listen to their bodies" when engaging in enjoyable exercise. Teach them which signs may indicate that an exercise is too strenuous, such as chest pain or shoulder pain. By knowing what to look for, patients are empowered to supervise their own health and prevent injuries. When in doubt, customize the intervention to whatever is best for the patient.

Takeaway Points
- Exercise should be considered as a therapeutic modality for all depressed patients.
- Exercise should be fun for the patient and medically cleared to initiate.
- The social aspects of an exercise program should be considered for elderly patients.

- Medications, prescription or over-the-counter
- Occult disease presenting with organic depression
- Alcohol abuse
- Mild head trauma (concussion) the patient doesn't remember (i.e., occurred while amnesic from alcohol or medications)

16.3.2 Case 2

Mr. D is a 74-year-old man referred for evaluation of progressive cognitive decline and memory deficits. On initial exam, he admits to lacking interest in previously pleasurable activities and feeling like a burden to his family. His wife reports that he suffered an episode of depression in his 40s, and he has always drank too much alcohol. He was never diagnosed or treated for either of these problems. Since retiring from his job 2 years ago, Mr. D has put on 15 pounds and developed type 2 diabetes and hypertension. He takes a diuretic and an ACE inhibitor and a statin. He has stopped playing golf, a game he loved all of his life, claiming he gets too tired and no longer enjoys playing. His days are spent watching TV and napping. Mr. D screens positive on the Geriatric Depression Scale, but denies being depressed, claiming, "I'm not crazy." Given his past history of depression combined with his current symptoms, Mr. D is prescribed an SSRI for his depression. One week after seeing his doctor, Mr. D attempts suicide with a handgun but survives.

16.3.2.1 Discussion

Chief complaints of cognitive decline and memory deficits require a rigorous workup, because many different sources can be to blame.

Causes of Apparent Cognitive Decline

- Age-related memory (normal)
- Primary depression

From the start, Mr. D used one of the key phrases expressing feelings of worthlessness. Providers should follow up statements like these with "What do you mean by that?" and start exploring for suicidal ideation, plans, and means to attempt. Depressed white older males are at the highest risk for completed suicide. Although not being the demographic with the highest number of attempts, their efforts are more often lethal, compared to other groups such as women and teenagers. Sad mood may not be a presenting symptom in this age group, but a history of prior depression (especially prior suicide attempts), substance abuse, poor physical health, and low self-esteem are all significant risk factors for suicide.

Inquiring about patient access to firearms is an essential precaution. Once someone has said life isn't worth living, you *must* assess suicide risk.

- If your patient has a gun, ask why he keeps a gun.
  - Recreational purposes?
  - Self-defense?
- How many firearms does he own?
- Where do they keep it?
  - Is it locked in a closet or gun safe?
  - Is it in an unsecured cabinet?
  - Is it in his car?
  - Where is ammunition stored?
- Discuss family precautions to monitor or restrict gun access to a suicidal patient.

- If a patient is reluctant, it's helpful to remind him, "you might not feel suicidal now, but you've said you feel down sometimes. You might feel worse later, so to be safe, let's lock up the gun."

Despite making a diagnosis of depression in this patient, prescribing an antidepressant was not sufficient. Mr. D would have benefitted from a more comprehensive, biopsychosocial intervention, including a referral for an initial psychiatric evaluation to rule out other causes, given the potential lethality of the case. The appropriate strategy would have been to refer to a psychiatrist for consultation. Initially, the patient may feel the PCP is dismissing or abandoning him by referring him to a psychiatrist, especially if the patient insisted he was "not crazy" or denied feeling depressed. The PCP should reassure the patient that psychiatric referral is part of a thorough medical approach for their overall health. Do not rush the patient in telling their story. It is very important to take this additional time to explain your logic and get feedback from the patient.

Sample Explanation
"There are some things I am worried about that are affecting your quality of life. There might be reasons for these symptoms that require a specialist, so I want to refer you. If you had a cough that wouldn't go away or chest pain, I would refer you to a cardiologist to better treat your problem. In this case, it is important you see a psychiatrist so that we can provide the best possible care for you."

Medications and Substance Use While evaluating Mr. D, one should consider how other factors such as medications and alcohol affect depression. Mr. D's social history includes frequent alcohol use which merits a thorough investigation. Alcohol consumption could be either the main cause of his cognitive impairment and depressed mood, or it could be exacerbating his primary depression.

When approaching Mr. D's alcohol use, several aspects should be clarified. First, ask *why* he drinks. Problematic alcohol consumption is not always caused by an addiction disorder. Does he drink to forget or to enjoy himself? Is he self-medicating with alcohol, such as in PTSD? Are his drinking patterns the result of tolerance changes as he aged? Does he drink because it helps him fall asleep? Also clarify how much alcohol intake occurs over a discrete length of time. Nursing one beer over an hour is different from consuming a bottle of wine each night before bed. A useful question to ask is, "When you buy a 6-pack of beer, how long does it last you?" Some may say it lasts them a few days, but for others it may last them a few months. Exploring these questions help characterize the patient's alcohol profile and identify the best approach strategies. Because patients may be embarrassed to discuss their alcohol use with their PCP, attempts should be made to corroborate drinking behavior with family or caregiver reports.

After better understanding a patient's alcohol use, it is important to discuss benefits of cutting back on alcohol consumption. To avoid sounding judgmental, PCPs can emphasize their concerns about alcohol's negative impact on two major symptoms: sleep disturbances and cognitive impairment. Alcohol may help the patient get to sleep initially but ultimately interferes with sleep quality. Alcohol changes the architecture of sleep, leading to increased awakenings and decreased restorative, restful sleep. If the patient is actually engaging in light or moderate alcohol use, such as enjoying one glass of wine after dinner, recommend he drink his wine at least 2 h before bedtime.

Alcohol can contribute to cognitive impairment even when the patient is sober. As patients age, their alcohol tolerance decreases. While drinking, they experience increased disturbances of coordination and balance, leading to increased risk of falling. Consequently, older patients are more prone to suffering mild concussions that they later don't remember. These subclinical concussions may present during sober periods with symptoms of memory impairment, mood changes, and neurocognitive slowing.

Equally important to consider are concurrent over-the-counter and prescription medication use. Given Mr. D's recent diagnoses of hypertension and type 2 diabetes, he likely takes prescription medications. Recall that numerous medications, especially antihypertensives, are known to carry a risk for inducing psychosis and mood symptoms. The 2012 Beer's Criteria published by the American Geriatrics Society is a useful list to reference. In the setting of multiple comorbid conditions, the onset of mood symptoms is clinically relevant. Major depressive disorder has a gradual onset. If a patient presents with acute-onset symptoms of depression, medications, substance use, or occult disease should be considered as the underlying etiology. Depression can be one of the first symptoms of certain cancers, such as non-small cell lung cancer and pancreatic cancer.

Treatment Pharmacologic interventions may play a role in Mr. D's treatment, but they should not be the sole intervention, especially with recurrent depressive episodes. For this patient, the key issues to address are his feeling out of control of his life and fearful of his future. Recommended ways to address these components of the patient's depression include listening to his concerns and fears, addressing any automatic negative thoughts or beliefs, and exploring social stressors. In addition to enjoyable exercise, various modes of therapy and counseling can help Mr. D achieve sustainable remission of his depression.

Options to offer Mr. D include talk therapy, peer support groups, pet therapy, family counseling, and cultural or spiritual resources, such as church, temple, mosque, or meditation.

Takeaway Points
- Medications may play a role in treating depression but should be used wisely.
- Non-medication interventions should be recommended for every depressed patient, especially elderly patients.

- Do not rush the intake process; take time to listen to the elderly patient's "story."

16.3.3 Case 3

Mr. T, a 78-year-old man, comes into the office after being referred for treatment of recurring depression. He has a prior history of two major depressive episodes. The last one was 12 years ago. He denies ever feeling life was not worth living, but he is reporting poor sleep, poor appetite, decreased energy, and little enjoyment in his life. He reports being active prior to retiring from work 6 years ago. He has a supportive marriage of 40 years but feels little motivation to join his wife on daily activities, such as grocery shopping or going for a walk. His wife is concerned he is becoming more withdrawn and irritable over time. He is very reluctant to take antidepressant medications, as he has had issues with side effects in the past. In discussing non-medication treatment options with him, he is resistant to attending talk therapy but says he would consider an exercise program. After discussing the basics of an effective exercise program with his family physician, elevating his heart rate to a safe level, as determined by baseline cardiac status, and maintaining it for 15–20 minutes, he asks what form of exercise is best. He reports becoming bored with brisk walking, and he does not like going to the gym or swimming. When asked about activities he used to enjoy, he mentions playing tennis. "I watch the kids playing these days, and I would not be able to get a single shot back," he reports. After a discussion with his wife, she calls a local tennis club and discovers an over-75 league. Despite never playing tennis herself, she joins the league with her husband after they are both medically cleared to play. After 3 months they report playing 3 days a week, and they join their new tennis friends for lunch after playing at least weekly. The patient reports much improved sleep and increased energy. He looks forward to playing, and he is planning to take his wife to attend a major pro tennis tournament. His wife reports he has not seemed this engaged in life since retiring from work and reports how involvement with him has also improved her life.

16.3.3.1 Discussion

The role of regular exercise in improving mood is well documented. One fact that is not always addressed is the "enjoyment factor." Exercise that is not fun for the patient is not likely to be continued. It should be of no surprise that successful diets do not focus on giving up all the foods that one enjoys. None of the positive effects of regular exercise will be experienced if the activity is not continued on a consistent basis.

When prescribing exercise for treating depression, an initial assessment of cardiac status and orthopedic issues should be completed. It is important to assure the patient that they are healthy enough to engage in regular physical activity. This assessment is useful to determine how to adjust desired exercise activities to fit the patient's physical condition. Once the initial screen is completed (this can be part of an annual physical), the patient should be instructed on how to "listen to their body." As previously mentioned in Case 1, chest pain or joint pain should be reported to their doctor, not merely self-treated with over-the-counter analgesics.

Once the initial screen is completed, focus on finding an enjoyable form of exercise/activity. As was this case in this patient, discussing past enjoyable activities is an excellent starting point. Providing a list of potential activities to the patient is helpful rather than just telling the patient to "go exercise." Make this an integral component of all treatment recommendations. Discussion of the social component is also helpful. An exercise program is more effective when social support systems are involved. Even solo activities, like jogging or swimming, are more effective when done in a group setting or with a friend. This will enhance the enjoyment factor and positively enhance long-term adherence. Another strategy to improve outcomes is to inform significant others to comment on observed improvement in mood, physical appearance, and activity tolerance.

Exercise should be a part of every treatment intervention. The human body is meant to move. Even a patient with significant health issues can be encouraged to engage in medically monitored exercise.

16.4 Conclusion

An effective treatment plan for geriatric depression integrates components across the biopsychosocial spectrum. This is not unique to psychiatric conditions. For example, successful treatment of diabetes would never include only insulin administration. Adequate treatment would require dietary changes, stress reduction, weight management, and exercise to achieve optimal, sustainable results.

There are a number of medications approved for the treatment of depression. Always keep in mind the side effect profiles of each medication and be prepared to offer alternatives should the patient find the adverse effects intolerable. When prescribing antidepressants, use a lower dose than for younger individual, and carefully monitor the response. Outpatient therapies like electroconvulsive therapy (ECT) are available for severe, refractory cases. In moderate depression, pharmacotherapy should be initiated after more conservative treatment strategies, such as talk therapy or lifestyle modifications, have failed.

Additionally, keeping one's brain active in the later years has been found to improve neurocognitive function and psychological wellness in seniors. This doesn't mean using gimmicky programs like "brain improving games," which have recently become popular on the consumer market. Research has shown these "brain games" do little to maintain or improve mental function. However, activities that involve learning, critical thinking, or strategy have been linked to improved performance on cognitive evaluations. These activities can range from solving sudoku puzzles to taking a class at the community college. Synthesizing and integrating new mental skills during retirement is highly recommended alongside enjoyable exercise. The role that the individual plays is therefore very important.

Non-governmental organizations (NGOs) can also play an important role in assisting older adults at risk of depression. These NGOs provide practical support with day-to-day tasks and companionship to older adults who may otherwise become isolated. In the UK, some general practitioners work in partnership with such organizations. A scheme called "social prescribing" or community referral allows GPs to "prescribe" social activity and other nonclinical services for a patient whose primary problem is not medical. These services incorporate many of the factors that make enjoyable exercise an effective tool for improving the quality of life in older adults.

In conclusion, the depressed elderly patient best benefits from a biopsychosocial approach structured around each individual's needs and concerns. By combining enjoyable exercise, social engagement, and appropriate pharmacologic treatment, PCPs can effectively guide their geriatric patients toward a happier and healthier life.

Suggested Reading

1. Almeida OP, McCaul K, Hankey GJ, Yeap BB, Golledge J, Norman PE, Flicker L. Duration of diabetes and its association with depression in later life: the health in men study (HIMS). Maturitas. 2016;86:3–9.
2. ASCP Fact Sheet. Administration on Aging, 2012; Center for disease control and prevention, 2012; National Council on Aging, 2014. https://www.ascp.com/articles/about-ascp/ascp-fact-sheet.
3. Conradsson M, Rosendahl E, Littbrand H, Gustafson Y, Olofsson B, Lövheim H. Usefulness of the geriatric depression scale 15-item version among very old people with and without cognitive impairment. Aging Ment Health. 2013;17(5):638–45.
4. D'ath P, Katona P, Mullan E, Evans S, Katona C. Screening, detection and management of depression in elderly primary care attenders. I: the acceptability and performance of the 15 item geriatric depression scale (GDS15) and the development of short versions. Fam Pract. 1994;11(3):260–6.
5. Hoeft TJ, Hinton L, Liu J, Unützer J. Directions for effectiveness research to improve health services for late-life depression in the United States. Am J Geriatr Psychiatry. 2016;24(1):18–30.
6. Kapp MB. Geriatric depression. Elder Law Rev. 2016;10:1.
7. Kwak YT, Song SH, Yang Y. The relationship between geriatric depression scale structure and cognitive-

8. behavioral aspects in patients with Alzheimer's disease. Dementia and Neurocognitive Disorders. 2015;14(1):24–30.
8. Lavretsky H, Reinlieb M, St. Cyr N, Siddarth P, Ercoli LM, Senturk D. Citalopram, methylphenidate, or their combination in geriatric depression: a randomized, double-blind, placebo-controlled trial. Am J Psychiatr. 2015;172(6):561–9.
9. Li Z, Jeon YH, Low LF, Chenoweth L, O'Connor DW, Beattie E, Brodaty H. Validity of the geriatric depression scale and the collateral source version of the geriatric depression scale in nursing homes. Int Psychogeriatr. 2015;27(9):1–10.
10. Lockwood KA, Alexopoulos GS, van Gorp WG. Executive dysfunction in geriatric depression. Am J Psychiatr. 2014;159(7):1119–26.
11. Lyness JM, Noel TK, Cox C, King DA, Conwell Y, Caine ED. Screening for depression in elderly primary care patients: a comparison of the Center for Epidemiologic Studies—Depression Scale and the geriatric depression scale. Arch Intern Med. 1997;157(4):449–54.
12. Morimoto SS, Kanellopoulos D, Manning KJ, Alexopoulos GS. Diagnosis and treatment of depression and cognitive impairment in late life. Ann N Y Acad Sci. 2015;1345(1):36–46.
13. Poelke G, Ventura MI, Byers AL, Yaffe K, Sudore R, Barnes DE. Leisure activities and depressive symptoms in older adults with cognitive complaints. Int Psychogeriatr. 2016;28(01):63–9.
14. Rapp MA, Dahlman K, Sano M, Grossman HT, Haroutunian V, Gorman JM. Neuropsychological differences between late-onset and recurrent geriatric major depression. Am J Psychiatr. 2014;162(4):691–8.
15. Riepe MW. Clinical preference for factors in treatment of geriatric depression. Neuropsychiatr Dis Treat. 2015;11:25.
16. Roose SP, Sackeim HA, Krishnan KRR, Pollock BG, Alexopoulos G, Lavretsky H, Old-Old Depression Study Group. Antidepressant pharmacotherapy in the treatment of depression in the very old: a randomized, placebo-controlled trial. Am J Psychiatr. 2015;161(11):2050–9.
17. Spyrou IM, Frantzidis C, Bratsas C, Antoniou I, Bamidis PD. Geriatric depression symptoms coexisting with cognitive decline: a comparison of classification methodologies. Biomedical Signal Processing and Control. 2016;25:118–29.
18. Thomas AJ, Davis S, Morris C, Jackson E, Harrison R, O'Brien JT. Increase in interleukin-1β in late-life depression. Am J Psychiatr. 2014;162(1):175–7.
19. Yesavage JA, Brink TL, Rose TL, Lum O, Huang V, Adey M, Leirer VO. Development and validation of a geriatric depression screening scale: a preliminary report. J Psychiatr Res. 1983;17(1):37–49.
20. Yesavage JA, Sheikh JI. Geriatric depression scale (GDS) recent evidence and development of a shorter violence. Clin Gerontol. 1986;5(1–2):165–73.

Suicidal Behaviour in Older Adults

17

Diego De Leo and Urska Arnautovska

Abstract

Suicide rates among older adults are the highest in nearly every part of the world. Also in late life, suicide is a multifactorial problem with several interrelated factors that vary with age, gender and culture. Depression is one of the main risk factors for suicide in older adults; however, cultural variations do exist that change the hierarchy of importance of risk factors. In the oldest olds, men appear to be more vulnerable than women to adverse life circumstances. Thus, suicide prevention in older adults should pay particular attention to the many socio-environmental conditions that may be relevant in this age, especially social isolation, loneliness, financial insecurity and physical illnesses. Early detection and treatment of affective disorders are key interventions to reduce the risk of suicide in this late part of life. Ageistic perspectives are still very present also among health professionals and should be counteracted with great determination. Promoting a culture of adaptation to the changes imposed by the advancing of age should form the essential part of a process central to suicide prevention.

Key Points
- Suicide rates among individuals aged 65 years and older are the highest for both men and women in almost all regions of the world.
- Suicide methods among older adults vary across the world.
- Depression tends to be considered as a normal part of ageing and may often be missed by primary care doctors.
- Risk factors for suicide among older adults include mental disorder, physical illness and social factors.
- Protective factors include engagement in valuable activities, high levels of education and socioeconomic status and religious or spiritual involvement.

D. De Leo (✉)
Australian Institute for Suicide Research and Prevention, Griffith University,
Mount Gravatt, QLD, Australia

Slovene Centre for Suicide Research, University of Primorska, Koper, Slovenia
e-mail: d.deleo@griffith.edu.au

U. Arnautovska
School of Applied Psychology and Mental Health Institute Queensland, Griffith University,
Mount Gravatt, QLD, Australia

17.1 Epidemiology

Although declining in many parts of the world for the past 30 years [1], suicide rates among individuals aged 65 years and older are still the

© Springer Nature Switzerland AG 2019
C. A. de Mendonça Lima, G. Ivbijaro (eds.), *Primary Care Mental Health in Older People*,
https://doi.org/10.1007/978-3-030-10814-4_17

highest for both men and women in almost all regions of the world, as indicated by the World Health Organization report, *Preventing Suicide: A Global Imperative* [2]. In addition, increase in life expectancy and decrease in mortality due to causes of death other than suicide created expectations that the absolute number of older adults' suicide might be growing further. Using data from 17 countries, Shah and colleagues [3] have identified that suicide rates continue to grow up to extreme ages (i.e. in centenarians), with a curve of the trend line steeper in men than in women. However, older adults seem to have benefitted more than other age groups from the improvements in general health assistance and quality of life which have been witnessed in many countries in recent years [2], as testified by the fact that their rates have declined more than in younger individuals [1, 2].

Compared to suicide rates, nonfatal suicidal behaviour (including suicide attempts) decreases proportionally with increasing age [4]. This has been clearly shown by the results of the WHO/EURO Multicentre Study on Suicidal Behaviour (a very large cooperative effort), which found that only 9% of 22,665 episodes of 'parasuicide' (hospital treated) were made by older adults (65+ years) compared to 50% of the episodes made by individuals in the 15–34 years age group [5]. Compared to younger individuals (especially youth), where the number of nonfatal behaviours is exceedingly high, the ratio between fatal and nonfatal suicidal behaviour can become very small in old age, varying from 1–2 [5] to 1–4 [6] (in youth, if we consider non-suicidal self-injury episodes, it can reach 1–5000 [7]). While nonfatal behaviour is particularly frequent in women of younger age groups, the prevalence tends to be equal in advanced age [8]. The gender paradox in suicide rates (the difference between sexes, with rates of male subjects much higher than those of their female counterparts) is often explained by the more frequent help-seeking behaviour in females and the use of more violent methods in males (such as firearms or hanging) [9–11].

Contrarily to common beliefs, approaching the natural end of life is not accompanied by an increased frequency of suicide ideation or death

wishes: both types of thoughts are more prevalent in youth and young adults, as shown by the community survey performed in Australia in the context of the WHO/SUPRE-MISS Study [12].

A note of caution should be expressed in relation to the validity of suicide mortality data in old age as well as in the general population [13, 14]. In fact, mortality data for suicide in older adults are often under-reported; 'accidents' (e.g. falls, drowning, etc.), refusal to take life-sustaining medication or overdosing with drugs such as insulin or opioids can all be recorded as non-suicide cases. In a recent book chapter, De Leo and Arnautovska examined in detail many of these conditions [15].

17.2 Is Suicide in Old Age Different?

Suicide in old age is often considered to be the result of a rational decision. Lack of positive expectations, frailty, dependency from others, loss of spouse and solitude are frequently considered motivations that could 'explain' cases of suicide. Aggregation of different factors, for example, bereaving the death of partner in a dependent and frail individual, may reinforce the paradigm of rational choices. Similarly, suicide can be interpreted as a 'legitimate exit' from life when loss of reputation, dignity or dramatic change in social status is experienced.

Ageistic views tend to consider depression as a normal feature of ageing [16]. However, depression is not an obvious response to any particular stressor such as, for example, deteriorated physical health, loss of a spouse or financial difficulties. 'Depression' should indicate a pathological alteration and not a normal reaction to stressors of various nature. There are several different forms of depression, possibly involving also different and complex aetiologies; all these forms are strongly associated to suicide [17]. Although depression is an important risk factor for suicidal behaviour also in old age, it is possible that its role has been overemphasized. Sadness, disillusionment, disappointment, disengagement and lack of positive expectations are frequent travel mates in the life journey of every individual and not necessarily symptoms of depression. As such, there should be no need for a medical dictionary to describe and understand these common feelings. But when does sadness become depression (i.e. a mental disorder)? In the words of Maj [18], this happens essentially in three main situations: (1) when the reaction is unrelated to a life event or disproportionate to it, (2) when there is a qualitative difference (e.g. a *gestalt*, an entity that goes beyond the sum of symptoms) and (3) on pragmatic grounds, assuming there is a continuum of severity from ordinary sadness to clinical depression [18]. Many psychiatrists today tend to privilege this latter interpretation to qualify a condition as 'depressive' in psychiatric terms. However, from a suicide prevention perspective, there could be both pros and cons in a similar attitude. In theory, approaching a patient with attention and prudence is always to be preferred to a predisposition that considers life stressors as inevitable and all reactions to them as normal. This may bring to underestimating and undertreating depression, especially in old age where life stressors may easily aggregate [17]. On the other hand, adopting a very limited medical vocabulary (where everything is defined as 'depression') may induce a too narrow attitude to treatment, often limited to prescribing an antidepressant drug. In this way, the appreciation of the multifactorial nature of suicidality also becomes too limited and the possibilities of counteracting the complexities of a suicidal progression too modest. Given there are no 'magic bullets' for depression, there is no 'quick fix' for suicidal behaviour, and very seldom a drug prescription can make a positive difference.

Also in old age suicide methods vary from country to country and gender. For example, in the United States, the most common method for older men is gunshot, while for older women it is poisoning, mostly by overdosing medications [9]. In England and Wales, hanging is the most common method for older men, while for women poisoning with medications [19]. In places with many high-rise buildings, like Hong Kong and Singapore, jumping from a height represents the most common method [20]. Despite cultural and gender differences, the increased lethality of methods chosen by older adults is seen around the world and reflects the fact that the ratio suicide/suicide attempts is much lower in older adults than in other age groups [5, 21]. Greater determination to die and more attention to avoid being rescued by third parties concur with this phenomenon [22].

17.3 Risk Factors

17.3.1 Mental Disorders

In literature, a psychiatric diagnosis has been reported as present between 71% and 95% of suicide cases of older adults. The most common diagnosis is affective disorder, which is present from 54% to 87% of these cases [23, 24], and is associated with the highest population attributable risk for suicide in late life [25]. Although depressive disorder occurs only in 8–16% of the general older adult population [26], suicide among older adults is likely to happen in the context of a depressive episode. In fact, depression—both as chronic depressive symptoms and as first episode in old age—has been identified as the most powerful independent risk factor for suicide in old age [27]. More recent studies on subjects of 60 years of age and more, based on the method of psychological autopsy, have however shown that depression is less frequently present in these patients than in those of younger age: in fact, among older adults, the prevalence of the disorder did not reach 50% of cases, while for subjects under 60 years of age, it was close to 60% [28].

Even if depression may appear as the most prominent clinical picture, several age-related medical conditions (e.g. cardiovascular disorders, stroke, chronic pain, etc.) are often concomitant to it [29]. These comorbidities sometimes make the identification of depression difficult or delay its recognition and treatment; thus, depression might end by being regarded as irrelevant or secondary to a somatic condition.

Also, depression in older adults is often accompanied by symptoms of anxiety or a full-blown anxiety disorder. These conditions may frequently increase the risk of suicide [30, 31]. For example, in a historical series of suicide cases in older adults in a general hospital, a common factor was the presence of severe anxiety, poorly responsive to treatments, with the majority of suicide cases occurring in the first hours of morning, when anxiety symptoms are often stronger and supervision probably less tight [32].

Although alcohol abuse represents a less common risk factor for suicide in older adults compared to what is found in young adults [33], it remains an important indicator of risk for both sexes. Usually, alcohol abuse increases the risk of suicide through its interaction with other factors that are particularly prevalent among older adults, such as depressive symptoms, medical conditions, a negatively perceived health status and poor control of social environment. These factors are then capable to stimulate further intake of alcohol, and the vicious circle that is thus established can easily become lethal. The association between alcohol abuse and suicide has been noted in many countries, western and non-western, but is particularly marked in the Baltic republics and other countries of the former Soviet bloc [34]. In any case, either alcohol abuse or any other substance abuse appears as less prevalent among older adults than among younger subjects [28]. Similar considerations apply to the association between suicide and psychotic disorders, which are much less represented in suicide cases of people of advanced age than in those of younger individuals [28, 35].

Even personality disorders appear to be less frequently associated with cases of suicide in older adults compared to younger persons [36]. As for the presence of specific personality traits in suicidal older adults, cognitive rigidity (particularly lack of openness to new experiences), apprehensiveness and anankastic traits seem to be particularly common among suicides in older adults [25, 37].

Despite the high prevalence of dementia diagnosis in advanced age, this condition does not seem to be significantly associated with an increased risk of suicide [38]. The few cases reported in the literature relate to subjects with preserved insight, who are aware of the seriousness of the diagnosis, with evidence of depressive symptoms, of younger age and not showing any positive response to anti-dementia drug treatment [39].

17.3.2 Psychosocial Factors

There are several reasons why research in suicide prevention in older adults has tended to focus on depression as a risk factor. One obvious reason is the presence of many psychosocial factors (such as impoverishment, isolation, relocation to a nursing home and bereavement) that may increase susceptibility to depression [40]. However, even in the absence of an affective disorder, these factors can markedly upset the life of an individual, often creating living conditions too poor to be accepted and increasing the risk of suicide at very advanced age too. Men, particularly when single, widowed or divorced, are often reported to be at increased risk of suicide [41]. Financial problems, low level of education, lack of social and/or religious support networks [42] and feelings of loneliness [43] may increase the risk of suicide. In particular, isolation and a lack of social interactions are important risk factors for suicide in older adults, even after accounting for the influence of mood disorders. The existence of relationship problems in the family or the presence of a very tense climate or discord may also represent important stressors by increasing the sense of emotional isolation and then being associated with suicidal behaviours [22]. In fact, loneliness may result from the loss of an important intimate relationship or a social role that previously helped to preserve a person's sense of self-esteem and dignity. Also early traumatic experiences (e.g. history of abuse during childhood, loss of a parent, etc.) can have consequences in later life and be associated with increased likelihood of suicidal behaviour [37, 44].

Usually, a death represents a significantly stressful event, especially if it involves the loss of a child or close relative [45]. For the older old (80+ years), the loss of a partner increases the risk of suicide in particular during the first year after the death, with men being affected more strongly by this stressful life event than women [42]. Consequently, widowhood can significantly increase the risk of suicide and attempted suicide in older adults [5]. Loneliness is also reflected in the solitary nature of suicides among older adults, which are more often performed at home [35]. Even the loss of a pet can be a significant trigger for a suicidal crisis [45].

Retirement is an event related to the ageing process with potentially negative effects on the mental health of an older adult. The risk of suicide is particularly high in the first 2–3 years after the termination of the employment [17]. Of particular relevance in this context are changes in income, social status, and social and family role interactions. These changes can lead to feelings of worthlessness and loss of self-esteem and purpose in life [22].

Geographic areas with large proportions of house tenants are characterised by higher suicide rates for older people, in particular for older males. These observations are consistent with the results of studies from English-speaking countries, suggesting that housing is one of the most important needs in people's lives [46–48]. Those who cannot afford a private retreat are more likely to suffer from social unrest, have low incomes and experience inability to work, which are all factors that are linked to a higher risk of suicide in English-speaking countries [49]. Precipitating factors for suicidal behaviour among older adults are also represented by forced relocation (such as when the landlord wants back the unit), a recent placement in a nursing home or the anticipation of such an event [50, 51].

One particular situation that older adult individuals are frequently involved in is murder-suicide [52]. Although this is a relatively rare phenomenon, older adults are disproportionately represented among both perpetrators and victims of domestic homicide-suicide [53, 54]. The existing evidence shows that the vast majority of cases of murder-suicide are committed by men against a female spouse with a firearm [54, 55]. As many as 40% of the actors were involved in providing assistance to a spouse with a long-term illness or with a disability [54]. It has been suggested that over 70% of the murder-suicide cases in senior citizens might recognize suicide as a primary motivation [56].

17.3.3 Physical Illness

Somatic and functional-impairment conditions significantly increase the risk of suicide during the entire life span [57]. Studies comparing suicides of subjects aged 65+ years with living controls found that serious physical illnesses (particularly visual impairment and neurological and malignant diseases) were independently associated with suicide among males [58, 59].

Hospitalisation can be a risk factor for suicide in older adults [52]. In Finland, for example, approximately 30% of suicides in older adults between 1988 and 2003 occurred within 1 month of discharge from hospital [60]. Interestingly, approximately 80% of diagnoses given during the hospitalization were nonpsychiatric. In Denmark, men over 80 years hospitalized with medical illnesses had the highest suicide rate of all age groups, while the risk of suicide in men over 80 years with three or more medical illnesses requiring hospitalization was also three times higher than that of those with no comorbidities [61].

Abuse or inappropriate use of prescription medications, particularly painkillers and those used to treat psychiatric disorders, can also place older adults at increased risk of suicide. Research from Canada has found that the risk is heightened by multiple prescriptions and increases with medication strength [62, 63].

In a case-control study, Conwell and colleagues [64] compared 86 people over age 50 who died by suicide with the same number of matched living controls. They found that suicide cases had more DSM-IV Axis I disorders, worse physical health and greater functional impairments compared to controls. Cases of suicide had a history of psychiatric treatment, admission to medical or surgical hospital in the previous year and more frequent home visits than controls. In a multivariate model, the presence of any active psychiatric disorder and any loss in instrumental activities of daily living (e.g. food preparation, shopping, ability to use the phone, etc.) contributed independently to the risk of suicide [64].

Comorbidity of psychiatric disorders with physical disabilities appears to particularly increase the risk of suicide in older adults [65], with loneliness adding to that risk [42].

17.4 Protective Factors

Unfortunately, the study of protective factors for suicide in old age is still in its infancy. Factors identified as potentially protective include high levels of education and socioeconomic status, engagement in valuable activities and religious involvement [66]. For example, involvement in Catholic practices has been associated with lower rates of suicide compared to non-Catholics [67, 68]. Intensity of faith and participation in social activities connected to the religious practice seem to be the most important explanations for this effect [68]. Furthermore, the presence of significant levels of social support, either represented by intimate friends or relatives, can constitute an important protective factor. A recent psychological autopsy study has evidenced that individuals who died by suicide were particularly missing the help (or receiving less than needed) from both relatives and friends [28]. Marriage seems to constitute a protective factor, particularly for older adult males [10, 69].

In any case, in the words of Conwell, '…none of the risk factors that are known to us has predictive power sufficient to permit the identification of a person at risk of suicide. Very few studies have included large-size samples enough to allow multivariate models of risk and protective factors. Therefore, our understanding of the role of each single factor remains very limited. We know very little of the impact of the combination of several factors' (p. 249) [25].

17.5 Treatment of Suicidality in Older Adults

As already mentioned, suicidal behaviour in old age is generally characterized by close association with depression, strong intention to die and high lethality [25]. Interventions need to balance risk and protective factors, bearing in mind that these will be of different significance depending on the cultural and social context [70]. For exam-

ple, depression may have a strong association with suicidality in the United States but much less so in countries like India and China [71].

Risk of suicide is often not recognized in older patients [22]. In fact, many older adults who take their life have consulted their (general practitioner) GP shortly before their death. In a study that examined contacts with different health professionals in the 3 months prior to death [suicide cases ($n = 261$) compared to sudden death controls ($n = 182$)], 76.9% of suicide cases and 81.9% of sudden death cases visited their GP. Persons who died by suicide had significantly more frequently contacts with mental health professionals than sudden death controls. People with a diagnosable mental health disorder at the time of suicide attended GP surgeries approximately with the same frequency of people without a mental health diagnosis. Overall, in the 3 months prior to death, approximately 90% of people who died by suicide and by sudden death sought help from the health-care system, mainly from GPs. With reference to health-care contacts, people who had or did not have a diagnosable psychiatric disorder did not appear as distinguishable at the GP surgery level [72]. In 8% of suicide cases, contact happened within 2 days from death, in 22% of cases between 3 and 7 days, in 30% of cases between 1 and 4 weeks and in 27% of cases between 1 and 3 months [37].

An investigation from the United States showed that primary care physicians would be less willing to treat suicidal older adults compared to younger patients and would be more likely to believe that suicidal ideation in an older individual is frequently 'rational' [73].

As a matter of fact, communication of suicidal thoughts tends to be less common among men and older adults who die by suicide than it is among women and younger people who do it [74]. In addition, older people tend to minimize their psychological problems and consider them to be related to physical illness. As a result, family and friends can be the first to note that an older adult is at risk of suicide [75, 76].

In addition to considering the acute stress factors described above, risk assessment of suicide in older adults should not overlook the impact of chronic stress factors such as loneliness, complicated pain and severe disability. These might trigger suicidal tendencies, especially in the absence of social support [22].

As noted earlier, an older person may present a greater determination to die than their younger counterparts [6]. Indeed, the presence of previous attempts of suicide in older adults strongly indicates the risk of repeated suicide attempts and fatal suicidal behaviour [77]. The results of the WHO/EURO Multicentre Study on Suicidal Behaviour largely confirmed this. In fact, during a period of 12 months following the index episode of attempted suicide, 11% of participants aged 65+ years repeated their nonfatal behaviour, but 13% died by suicide [41].

In most countries, males have higher rates of suicide [78], while females have higher rates of nonfatal suicidal behaviour [79]. In adults, depression is about twice as common in women than in men [80]. In theory, this should make women the most exposed to the risk of suicide. However, females seem to be able to better address life stressors than their male counterparts and possess particularly resilient attitudes even in very advanced age [81]. Disparities in resilience could be explained by the different coping strategies used by older men and women in times of stress [81]. Men are generally less likely than women to seek treatment for psychological problems [82, 83] and also to adhere to this treatment once initiated, compared to women [84]. In patriarchal societies, cultural script for masculinity has promoted the suppression of emotions in men, by discouraging them from showing sadness, grief or crying or seeking interpersonal support in times of trouble [81, 82].

With these characteristics in mind, and considering that the systematic treatment of depression in the older adult is also expected to reduce suicidal ideation [85, 86], the PROSPECT study (Prevention of Suicide in Primary Care Elderly: Collaborative Trial) assessed whether interventions at primary care level reduced main risk factors for suicide in an older adult population [85]. Treatment management was shared among social workers, nurses and psychologists. The intervention group consisted of 598 patients recruited from 20 primary care practices in New York. Within a 12-month period, three follow-ups were set up to evaluate changes in suicide ideation and severity of depression. At 4 months, patients showed a remarkable decrease in suicidal thoughts compared with the usual level of care (12.9% vs 3.0%, respectively). In addition, patients in the intervention group had a more favourable course of depression both in terms of symptom severity and reduction speed. These results are consistent with those of the IMPACT study (Improve Mood-Promoting Access to Collaborative Care) [86]. The latter study included 1801 adults aged 60+ years, who suffered from major depression or dysthymia. Randomized participants had access to a depression care manager who offered problem-solving treatment for 12 months in addition to antidepressants prescribed by primary care physicians. The control group received care as usual. Participants in the intervention group showed significantly lower rates of suicide ideation than participants receiving usual care at all follow-ups.

Regardless of the specific type of mental disorder, hopelessness was identified as the most important psychological condition that may be seen in patients with a variety of different psychiatric conditions. Hopelessness has been associated with suicide ideation and behaviour. It was also identified as a moderator between cognitive functioning in dementia and suicidal behaviour in the few cases of suicide observed in patients diagnosed with dementia. In fact, the preservation of a certain level of insight (as mentioned above) can lead to depression and despair, which in turn can lead to suicide ideation [39]. Detecting hopelessness may be particularly relevant in the field of primary care, where older patients may feel hopeless about their experience of illness.

There is currently no evidence of effectiveness of any specific therapy for older adults with a personality disorder who are at risk of suicide. Future research could, therefore, need to identify appropriate treatments for such conditions and examine how these therapies could help to prevent suicide in people with these disorders.

A group of international experts belonging to the International Association for Suicide Prevention Interest Group on Suicide in Old Age [87] has reviewed 19 studies with an empirical assessment of a suicide prevention program for adults aged between 60 years and older. The review concluded that most of the studies focused on reducing risk factors (particularly depression and isolation) and seemed to reduce the risk of suicide more successfully in women than in men. Most of the studies showed a reduction of suicide ideation in patients or in suicide rates of the communities targeted by the study. The same group of experts proposed a set of recommendations to address senior citizens at risk of suicide [88]. The recommendations stressed the need for multi-component approaches, to be based on available scientific evidence and having an organized system of distribution of resources while monitoring the effectiveness of each intervention that could support the efforts through various levels.

A similar approach could be identified in a community-based suicide prevention program, carried out in 1995–2002 in Yuri, Japan, involving 6819 older adults (65+ years). This program suggested that a combination of group activities (including social activities, voluntary work and recreation), psycho-education (focusing on depression and suicide risk factors) and self-assessment of depression were effective in reducing suicide in women, but not in men [89].

At the level of general prevention, limiting access to means of suicide is one of the most effective universal strategies to reduce suicide rates in the world [90]. However, there is no convincing evidence yet that access restriction may be effective with populations of older adults.

At selective/indicated level, there are experiences that have mostly used limited samples, samples of convenience or specific communities. The Tele-Help/Tele-Check program, established in the Veneto region of northern Italy, represents a form of assistance and support to a special community. This assistance uses an approach essentially based on providing support through the phone. In case of special needs or emergencies, a pre-established network of people may intervene to meet the needs. The articles describing the impact of this system presented results of the assistance to some 20,000 older adults selected for the presence of somatic chronic diseases and/or mental problems and physical or emotional isolation [91]. A staff member trained to offer emotional and psychosocial support and, at the same time, to monitor the conditions of the customer contacted each client at least twice a week. Ten years after its introduction, the number of suicides among older adults in the region was much lower than expected, with a statistically significant impact among female users [92].

Older adults seem more likely to approach their GP for help, rather than specialist mental health services [23]. Social services (e.g. senior centres, public transport companies, peer support groups) and communities (e.g. banks, utility companies, pharmacists and mailmen) can represent potential gatekeepers [25]. In the United States, a program based on these gatekeepers was able to reach socially and economically disadvantaged seniors at risk of suicide. Employees of community businesses, specially trained to recognize people in need of help and to refer them to geriatric and mental health services, were remarkably successful in identifying people at risk. Thus, in this project, those gatekeepers were responsible for 40% of all referrals to local services for older adults [93]. Given this promising evidence, the training of gatekeepers at community level was proposed as a potentially useful method to identify older individuals at risk for suicide [25]. It is clear, however, that every effort needs to be done to promote the integration of older people in social groups and communities (religious and non-religious). By providing a social support network, connectedness can help to moderate isolation and loneliness and to promote feelings of belonging and self-esteem [94].

Overall, however, the evidence on the effectiveness of suicide prevention interventions for older adults remains limited. There is consensus that a multifactorial approach and multiple levels of suicide prevention could reduce suicide in older adults [88]. On the other hand, elements of national prevention strategies that could be of relevance also for late-life suicide are (1) awareness of suicide and its public health dimension,

(2) recognizing suicide risk factors and controlling those that are modifiable, (3) coordination of mental health and substance abuse control programs, (4) development and implementation of strategies to reduce the stigma associated with mental illness and suicidal behaviour and (5) creating programs to improve help-seeking behaviour, particularly among males [2].

Most national suicide prevention strategies recognize the high risk of suicidal behaviour in individuals aged 65 years and over [2]. Strategies aimed at this age group generally promote mental health, with particular emphasis on the early recognition and treatment of depression. To achieve these objectives, access to integrated mental health services and adequate treatment and support for older adults and their carers are often provided [15]. Studies on the effectiveness of mental health services for older adults provide encouraging evidence, in particular for those services involving community multidisciplinary teams [95].

17.6 Conclusions

Even if they remain the highest, suicide rates among older adults are falling in most western countries [1, 2]. At the basis of suicide reduction, it is possible that older adults have particularly benefitted from improvements in overall levels of health care and quality of life, more than any other age group. Having been (and still being) the most disadvantaged demographic segment, improvements in older adults have shown a proportionately greater size compared to the others [1]. Hopefully, this phenomenon might continue with the same pace, but targeted action would be required to achieve a steeper decrease in the trend line.

The improvement of social support and the detection and early treatment of affective disorders are key interventions to reduce risk of suicide in old age [87]. Prevention based on community actions and training of gatekeepers seems to be an important strategy. In particular, community programs that promote a sense of usefulness and belonging and preserve social integration and social status should be pushed vigorously. Governments must continue to pay attention to improving retirement programs, facilitating access to general health and mental health services and developing support systems. To actually test the validity of actions undertaken and verify their applicability to different cultural contexts remain imperative.

Combating stigma and ageistic perspectives—still deeply rooted in both laymen and professionals—must be done with great determination. Meanwhile, actively promoting a culture of adaptation to different stages of life and to the changes imposed by the advancing of age should form the essential part of a process, bringing to better successful ageing avenues.

Suicide among older adults is a multifactorial problem with several interrelated factors involved. These factors vary with age, gender and culture. Depression is only one of the risk factors for suicide in older adults and not necessarily the most important one, especially in some cultures. Suicide prevention in older adults should broaden its focus and pay attention to the many socio-environmental conditions that may be relevant in older age, especially social isolation, financial security and physical health. This would certainly help to better counteract suicide ideation and behaviours in this difficult part of life.

Acknowledgments Thanks are due to colleagues that have helped in growing our interest towards the theme of suicide in old age, particularly Prof José' Bertolote, Dr. Karolina Krysinska and Prof Brian Draper.

References

1. Bertolote J, De Leo D. Global suicide mortality rates – a light at the end of the tunnel? Crisis. 2012;33:249–53.
2. WHO. *Preventing suicide: a global imperative.* Geneva: World Health Organization; 2014.
3. Shah A, Zarate-Escudero S, Bhat R, De Leo D, Erlangsen A. Suicide in centenarians: the international landscape. Int Psychogeriatr. 2014;26:1703–8.
4. De Leo D, Scocco P. Treatment and prevention of suicidal behaviour in the elderly. In: Hawton K, van Heeringen K, editors. The international handbook of suicide and attempted suicide. Chichester: Wiley; 2000. p. 555––570.

5. De Leo D, Padoani W, Scocco P, et al. Attempted and completed suicide in older subjects: results from the WHO/EURO multicentre study of suicidal behaviour. Int J Geriatr Psychiatry. 2001;16:300–10.

6. McIntosh JL, Santos JF, Hubbard RW, et al. Elderly suicide research, theory and treatment. Washington, DC: American Psychological Association; 1994.

7. Shaffer D, Jacobson C. Proposal to the DSM-V childhood disorder and mood disorder work groups to include non-suicidal self-injury (NSSI) as a DSM-V disorder. Arlington: American Psychiatric Association; 2009. Retrieved from http://www.dsm5.org/Proposed%20Revision%20Attachments/APA%20DSM-5%20NSSI%20Proposal.pdf.

8. Shah A, Bhat R, Mac Kenzie S, et al. Elderly suicide rates: cross/national comparison of trends over a 10-year period. Int Psychogeriatr. 2008;20:673–86.

9. Karch D. Sex differences in suicide incident characteristics and circumstances among older adults: surveillance data from the National Violent Death Reporting System – 17 US states, 2007-2009. Int J Environ Res Public Health. 2011;8:3479–96.

10. Kolves K, Potts B, De Leo D. Ten year of suicide mortality in Australia: socio-economic and psychiatric factors in Queensland. J Forensic Legal Med. 2015;36:136–43.

11. Schriivers DL, Bollen J, Sabbe BG. The gender paradox in suicidal behavior and its impact on the suicidal process. J Affect Disord. 2012;138:19–26.

12. De Leo D, Cerin E, Spathonis K, Burgis S. Lifetime risk of suicide ideation and attempts in an Australian community: prevalence, suicidal process, and help-seeking behaviour. J Affect Disord. 2005;86:215–25.

13. De Leo D. Can we rely on suicide mortality data? Crisis. 2015;36:1–3.

14. Williams RF, Doessel DP, Sveticic J, De Leo D. Accuracy of official suicide mortality data in Queensland. Aust N Z J Psychiatry. 2010;44:815–22.

15. De Leo D, Arnautovska U. Prevention and treatment of suicidality in older adults. In: O'Connor R, Pirkis J, editors. International handbook of suicide prevention. Research, policy and practice. Chichester: Wiley-Blackwell; 2016.

16. Rabheru K. Special issues in the management of depression in older patients. Can J Psychiatr. 2004;49:41–50.

17. De Leo D, Diekstra RFW. Depression and suicide in late life. Goettingen: Hogrefe & Huber; 1990.

18. Maj M. When does depression become a mental disorder? Br J Psychiatry. 2011;199:85–6.

19. Shah A, Buckley L. The current status of methods used by the elderly for suicides in England and Wales. J Inj Violence Res. 2011;3:68–73.

20. Chia B-H, Chia A, Ng W-Y, Tai B-C. Suicide methods in Singapore (2000–2004): type and associations. Suicide Life Threat Behav. 2011;41:574–83.

21. Dombrovski AY, Szanto K, Duberstein P, Conner KR, Houck PR, Conwell Y. Sex differences in correlates of suicide attempt lethality in late life. Am J Geriatr Psychiatr. 2008;16:905–13.

22. De Leo D, Draper B, Krysinska K. Suicidal elderly people in clinical and community settings. In: Wasserman D, Wasserman C, editors. Oxford textbook of suicidology and suicide prevention. New York: Oxford University Press; 2009. p. 703–19.

23. Conwell Y, Thomson C. Suicidal behaviour in elders. Psychiatr Clin North Am. 2008;31:333–56.

24. Shah AK, De T. Suicide and the elderly. Int J Psychiatry Clin Pract. 1998;2:3–17.

25. Conwell Y. Suicide later in life. Challenges and priorities for prevention. Am J Prev Med. 2014;47:S244–50.

26. Blazer DG. Depression in late life: review and commentary. J Gerontol Series A. 2003;58:249–65.

27. Reynolds CF III, Kupfer DJ. Depression and aging: a look to the future. Psychiatr Serv. 1999;50:1167–72.

28. De Leo D, Draper B, Snowdon J, Kolves K. Suicides in older adults: a case-control psychological autopsy study in Australia. J Psychiatr Res. 2013;47:980–8.

29. Montano CB. Primary care issues related to the treatment of depression in elderly patients. J Clin Psychiatry. 1999;60:45–51.

30. Diefenbach GJ, Woolley SB, Goethe JV. The association between self-reported anxiety-symptoms and suicidality. J Nerv Ment Dis. 2009;197:92–9.

31. Fawcett J. Severe anxiety and agitation as treatment modifiable risk factors for suicide. In: Wasserman D, Wasserman C, editors. Oxford textbook of suicidology and suicide prevention. New York: Oxford University Press; 2009. p. 407–11.

32. De Leo D. Suicide in a general hospital: the case of the elderly. Crisis. 1997;18:5–7.

33. Krysinska K, Heller TS, De Leo D. Suicide and deliberate self-harm in personality disorders. Curr Opin Psychiatry. 2006;18:95–101.

34. Kolves K, Varnik A, Tooding LM, et al. The role of alcohol in suicide: a case-control psychological autopsy study. Psychol Med. 2006;36:923–30.

35. Harwood D, Jacoby R. Suicidal behaviour among the elderly. In: Hawton K, van Heeringen K, editors. The international handbook of suicide and attempted suicide. Chichester: Wiley; 2000. p. 275--292.

36. Neulinger K, De Leo D. Suicide in elderly and youth population: how do they differ? In: De Leo D, editor. Suicide and euthanasia in older adults. Göttingen: Hogrefe & Huber Publishers; 2001. p. 137–54.

37. Draper B, Kõlves K, De Leo D, Snowdon J. A controlled study of suicide in middle-aged and older people: personality traits, age, and psychiatric disorders. Suicide Life Threat Behav. 2014;44:130–8.

38. Schneider B, Maurer K, Frolich L. Dementia and suicide. Fortschr Neurol Psychiatr. 2001;69:164–73.

39. Haw C, Harwood D, Hawton K. Dementia and suicidal behaviour: a review of the literature. Int Psychogeriatr. 2009;21:440–53.

40. Capurso A, Capurso C, Solfrizzi V, et al. Depression in old age: a diagnostic and therapeutic challenge. Recenti Prog Med. 2007;98:43–52.

41. Erlangsen A, Jeune B, Bille-Brahe U, Vaupel J. Loss of a partner and suicide risk among oldest

old: a population-based register study. Age Ageing. 2004;33:378–83.

42. Turvey CL, Conwell Y, Jones MP, et al. Risk factors for late-life suicide: a prospective, community-based study. Am J Geriatr Psychiatr. 2002;10:398–407.

43. Rubenowitz E, Waern M, Wilhelmson K, et al. Life events and psychosocial factors in elderly suicides – a case-control study. Psychol Med. 2001;31:1193–202.

44. De Leo D, Padoani W, Lonnqvist J, et al. Repetition of suicidal behaviour in elderly Europeans: a prospective longitudinal study. J Affect Disord. 2002;72:291–5.

45. De Leo D, Cimitan A, Dyregrov K, Grad O, Andriessen K. Bereavement after traumatic death: helping the survivors. Göttingen: Hogrefe; 2013.

46. Navarro C, Ayala L, Labeaga JM. Housing deprivation and health status: evidence from Spain. Empir Econ. 2010;38:555–82.

47. Burrows S, Laflamme L. Living circumstances of suicide mortality in a south African City: an ecological study of differences across race groups and sexes. Suicide Life Threat Behav. 2005;35:592–603.

48. Law CK, Kolves K, De Leo D. Influences of population-level factors on suicides in older adults: a national ecological study from Australia. Int J Geriatr Psychiatry. 2016;31:384–91.

49. Baum F. The new public health. 3rd ed. Melbourne: Oxford University Press; 2008.

50. Loebel JP, Loebel JS, Dager SR, et al. Anticipation of nursing home placement may be a precipitant of suicide among the elderly. J Am Geriatr Soc. 1991;91:407–15.

51. Torresani S, Toffol E, Scocco P, Fanolla A. Suicide in elderly South Tyroleans in various residential settings at the time of death: a psychological autopsy study. Psychogeriatrics. 2014;14:101–9.

52. O'Dwyer S, De Leo D. Older adults and suicide. In: Wasserman D, editor. Suicide: an unnecessary death. 2nd ed. Cambridge: Cambridge University Press; 2016. p. 215–27.

53. Bell CC, McBride DF. Commentary: homicide-suicide in older adults—cultural and contextual perspectives. J Am Acad Psychiatry Law. 2010;38:312–7.

54. Malphurs JE, Cohen D. A statewide case-control study of spousal homicide-suicide in older persons. Am J Geriatr Psychiatr. 2005;13:211–7.

55. Bourget D, Gagne P, Whitehurst L. Domestic homicide and homicide-suicide: the older offender. J Am Acad Psychiatry Law. 2010;38:305–11.

56. Salari S. Patterns of intimate partner homicide suicide in later life: strategies for prevention. Clin Interv Aging. 2007;2:441–52.

57. Conwell Y, Duberstein PR, Cox C, et al. Risk factors for suicide in later life. Biol Psychiatry. 2002;52:193–204.

58. De Leo D, Hickey P, Meneghel G, et al. Blindness, fear of sight loss, and suicide. Psychosomatics. 1999;40:339–44.

59. Waern M, Rubenowitz E, Runeson B, et al. Burden of illness and suicide in elderly people: case-control study. Br Med J. 2002;324:1355.

60. Karvonen K, Hakko H, Koponen H, Meyer-Rochow VB, Rasanen P. Suicides among older persons in Finland and time since hospitalization discharge. Psychiatr Serv. 2009;60:390–3.

61. Erlangsen A, Vach W, Jeune B. The effect of hospitalization with medical illnesses on the suicide risk in the oldest old: a population-based register study. J Am Geriatr Soc. 2005;53:771–6.

62. Juurlink DN, Herrmann N, Szalai JP, Kopp A, Redelmeier DA. Medical illness and the risk of suicide in the elderly. Arch Intern Med. 2004;164:1179–84.

63. Voaklander DC, Rowe BH, Dryden DM, Pahal J, Saar P, Kelly KD. Medical illness, medication use and suicide in seniors: a population-based case-control study. J Epidemiol Community Health. 2008;62:138–46.

64. Conwell Y, Duberstein PR, Hirsch JK, et al. Health status and suicide in the second half of life. Int J Geriatr Psychiatry. 2009;6:147–8.

65. Kaplan MS, McFarland BH, Huguet N, et al. Physical illness, functional limitations, and suicide risk: a population-based study. Am J Orthopsychiatry. 2007;77:56–60.

66. Fiske A, Wetherell JL, Gatz M. Depression in older adults. Annu Rev Clin Psychol. 2009;5:369–89.

67. Durkheim E. Suicide: a study in sociology. Illinois: Free Press; 1951. (First published in 1897).

68. De Leo D. Struggling against suicide. Crisis. 2002;23:23–31.

69. Harwood DMJ, Hawton K, Hope T, et al. Suicide in older people: mode of death, demographic factors, and medical contact before death. Int J Geriatr Psychiatry. 2000;15:736–43.

70. De Leo D. Cultural issues in suicide and old age. Crisis. 1999;20:53–5.

71. Fleischmann A, De Leo D. The World Health Organization's report on suicide: a fundamental step in worldwide suicide prevention. Crisis. 2014;35:289–91.

72. De Leo D, Draper BM, Snowdon J, et al. Contacts with health professionals before suicide: missed opportunities for prevention? Compr Psychiatry. 2013;54:1117–23.

73. Uncapher H, Arean PA. Physicians are less willing to treat suicidal ideation in older patients. J Am Geriatr Soc. 2000;48:188–92.

74. Conwell Y, Duberstein PR, Cox C, et al. Age differences in behaviours leading to completed suicide. Am J Geriatr Psychiatr. 1998;6:122–6.

75. Dombrovski AY, Szanto K. Prevention of suicide in the elderly. Ann Long-Term Care. 2005;13:52–32.

76. Waern M, Beskow J, Runeson B, et al. Suicidal feelings in the last year of life in elderly people who commit suicide. Br Med J. 1999;354:917–8.

77. Hawton K, Harriss L. Deliberate self-harm in people aged 60 and over: characteristics and outcome of a 20-year cohort. Int J Geriatr Psychiatry. 2006;21:572–81.

78. Bertolote J, Fleischmann A. A global perspective on the magnitude of suicide mortality. In: Wasserman D, Wasserman C, editors. Oxford textbook of suici-

dology and suicide prevention. New York: Oxford University press; 2009. p. 91–8.

79. Hawton K, Harriss L. The changing gender ratio in occurrence of deliberate self-harm across the lifecycle. Crisis. 2008;29:4–10.

80. Accortt EE, Freeman MP, Allen JJ. Women and major depressive disorder: clinical perspectives on causal pathways. J Women's Health. 2008;17:1583–90.

81. Canetto SS. Elderly women and suicidal behavior. In: Canetto SS, Lester D, editors. Women and suicidal behaviour. New York: Springer; 1995.

82. Cochran SV, Rabinowitz FE. Gender-sensitive recommendations for assessment and treatment of depression in men. Prof Psychol. 2003;2:132–40.

83. Galdas PM, Cheater F, Marshall P. Men and help-seeking behaviour: literature review. J Adv Nurs. 2005;49:616–23.

84. Vörös V, Osváth P, Fekete S. Gender differences in suicidal behaviour. Neuropsychopharmacol Hung. 2004;6:65–71.

85. Bruce ML, Ten Have TR, Reynolds CF III, et al. Reducing suicidal ideation and depressive symptoms in depressed older primary care patients: a randomized controlled trial. J Am Med Assoc. 2004;291:1081–91.

86. Unützer J, Tang L, Oishi S, et al. Reducing suicidal ideation in depressed older primary care patients. Am Geriatr Soc. 2006;54:1550–6.

87. Lapierre S, Erlangsen A, Waern M, et al. A systematic review of elderly suicide prevention programs. Crisis. 2011;32:88–98.

88. Erlangsen A, Nordentoft M, Conwell Y, et al. Key considerations for preventing suicide in older adults. Crisis. 2011;32:106–9.

89. Oyama H, Watanabe N, Ono Y, et al. Community-based suicide prevention through group activity for the elderly successfully reduced the high suicide rate for females. Psychiatry Clin Neurosci. 2005;59:337–44.

90. Mann JJ, Apter A, Bertolote J, et al. Suicide prevention strategies: a systematic review. J Am Med Assoc. 2005;294:2064––2074.

91. De Leo D, Carollo G, Dello Buono M. Lower suicide rates associated with a Tele-help/Tele-check service for the elderly at home. Am J Psychiatr. 1995;152:632–4.

92. De Leo D, Dello Buono M, Dwyer J. Suicide among the elderly: the long-term impact of a telephone support and assessment intervention in northern Italy. Br J Psychiatry. 2002;181:226–9.

93. Florio ER, Hendryx M, Jensen JE, et al. A comparison of suicidal and nonsuicidal elders referred to a community mental health program. Suicide Life Threat Behav. 1997;27:182–93.

94. Krause N. Church-based social support and mortality. J Gerontol. 2006;61B:140–6.

95. Draper, B. & Low, L. (2004). What is the effectiveness of old-age mental health services? Retrieved March 24, 2015, from WHO Regional Office for Europe Web site: http://www.euro.who.int/document/E83685.pdf.

Psychosis in Older Adults

18

Carlos Augusto de Mendonça Lima,
Emanuela Sofia Teixeira Lopes,
and Aleksandra Milicevic Kalasic

Abstract

There is an increase of the prevalence of psychotic symptoms in older adults. The presence at this period of life of the highest comorbidity rate, the changes of the central nervous system with ageing, and the particular high frequency of life stressors during this period of life may all explain this. Psychotic symptoms are present in an important number of medical and psychiatric conditions and they make part of psychotic disorders in late life too. The same classification of disorders with psychotic symptoms in adults may be used for older adults. Primary psychotic symptoms exist in persistent psychotic disorders (schizophrenia, delusional disorder, and schizoaffective disorder), acute psychotic disorder, and personality disorders (paranoid, schizoid, and schizotypal personality disorders). Secondary psychotic symptoms include major and minor neurocognitive disorders, delirium, organic mental disorders, disorders due to psychoactive substance use, bipolar disorders, and depressive episode. Somatic disorders, comorbidities and iatrogenic causes are included at this cluster. Assessment and management of psychosis in older adults at primary care require an organization of the mental health-care system. The management of psychosis in older adults implies the proper use of multidisciplinary therapeutic interventions: pharmacotherapy and psychological, social, and occupational therapy. All forms of stigma and discrimination against older adults with psychosis and their carers should be eliminated.

C. A. de Mendonça Lima (✉)
Unity of Old Age Psychiatry, Centre Les Toises,
Lausanne, Switzerland

E. S. T. Lopes
Unity of Health and Clinical Psychology, Hospital da
Senhora da Oliveira - Guimarães, EPE,
Creixomil, Portugal

A. M. Kalasic
Department for Social Work, Faculty for Media and
Communication, Singidunum University,
Belgrade, Serbia

Municipal Institute of Gerontology and Palliative
Care, Singidunum University, Belgrade, Serbia

Key Points
- There is an increase of the prevalence of psychotic symptoms in older adults.
- The presence at this period of life of the highest comorbidity rate, the changes of the central nervous system with ageing, and the particular high frequency of life stressors during this period of life may all explain this.
- Psychotic symptoms are present in an important number of medical and psychiatric conditions and they make part of psychotic disorders in late life too.

© Springer Nature Switzerland AG 2019
C. A. de Mendonça Lima, G. Ivbijaro (eds.), *Primary Care Mental Health in Older People*,
https://doi.org/10.1007/978-3-030-10814-4_18

- The same classification of disorders with psychotic symptoms in adults may be used for older adults.
- Primary psychotic symptoms exist in persistent psychotic disorders (schizophrenia, delusional disorder, and schizoaffective disorder), acute psychotic disorder, and personality disorders (paranoid, schizoid, and schizotypal personality disorders).
- Secondary psychotic symptoms include major and minor neurocognitive disorders, delirium, organic mental disorders, and disorders due to psychoactive substance use, bipolar disorders, and depressive episode. Somatic disorders, comorbidities and iatrogenic causes are included at this cluster.
- Assessment and management at primary care require an organization of the mental health-care system.
- The management of psychosis in older adults implies the proper use of multidisciplinary therapeutic interventions: pharmacotherapy and psychological, social, and occupational therapy
- All forms of stigma and discrimination against older adults with psychosis and their carers should be eliminated.

Clinical Case

Mrs. M. L., 72-year-old-patient, is a retired economist, married without children living in Belgrade, Serbia. She describes a difficult relationship with her husband. She has previously experienced episodes of anxiety treated with serotonin reuptake inhibitors in the past.

She presented a fear that she was being stalked by someone and was suspicious of being robbed. Her husband didn't understand her behavior and believed that she was inventing and exaggerating everything as usual so she was seen at her sister in law's house by the psychiatrist.

Mrs. M. L. was noted to be wide eyed and frightened and was looking around the room suspiciously, she had little spontaneous speech but eventually said that she was being "attacked by an armature." Her sister-in-law reported that Mrs. M. L. was refusing to eat or to sleep because she believed that she was being watched by someone and was drinking small amounts of water. She denied hallucinations in any modality but her behavior suggested that hallucinations may be present and she described delusions of persecution and robbery. She was well orientated and had no insight into her condition.

A working diagnosis of late-onset psychosis in an older adult was made.

18.1 Introduction

"Wisdom comes with old age," we use to say. This statement forgets that the two most important threatens to "wisdom" are highly prevalent at this period of life: dementia and psychosis.

Psychosis is characterized by thought and perception distortions associated to emotional (sadness, anxiety), behavioral symptoms (apathy, aimlessness, self-absorbed attitude, excitement, posturing, stupor), vegetative changes (loss of energy, sleep, appetite), and neurocognitive impairments (executive functioning: planning, reasoning, problem solving, cognitive flexibility; attention; memory; verbal and visual learning; processing speed and social cognition) [1]. Patients often don't realize the pathological character of these symptoms. They represent a source of distress for patients, families, and the community. Interestingly, psychotic symptoms such as being spied by a neighbor, cheated by family members, and facing to intruders at home were just considered until some decades ago as eccentric behaviors of older adults [2, 3]. With the development of different classifications of mental disorders it became easier to make the proper diagnostic. But this illustrates how older adults with psychotic symptoms were—and still are—victims of prejudices, stigma, and discrimination.

One of the consequences of this is the few number of studies on psychosis in older adults besides considerable efforts to change this like the joint meeting of the European Association of

Geriatric Psychiatry and the Section for the Psychiatry of Old Age of the Royal College of Psychiatrists at London in 1992 [4], the International Late-Onset Schizophrenia Group Consensus Conference met in July 1998 [5], and the Potsdam Conference on Late-Onset Mental Disorders in 1999 [6].

There is an increase of the prevalence of psychotic symptoms in older adults. This may be explained by the presence at this period of life of the highest comorbidity rate, by the changes of the central nervous system with ageing, and finally also because of the particular high frequency of life stressors during this period of life (retirement, financial difficulties, bereavement, deaths of peers, physical disability) [7].

Thought and perception distortions are frequently found in primary care (PC) context. At low and middle income countries, primary care professionals may often be the only available resource to identify and manage the psychotic symptoms of older adults [8]. As part of these symptoms may belong to an ancient chronic psychosis, patients often are already very well known by PC: not only the professionals have followed the disorder onset and its evolution but they also know which personal and community resources are available. In the case of late-onset psychotic symptoms, PC has the patient's medical history, can quickly identify potential somatic disorders at the origin of the psychotic symptoms or recognize potential negative effects of drugs being used, and estimate the potential risk of drugs interactions. Independently of the economical country level, PC is an important resource to help in the management of treatments.

18.2 Epidemiology

Psychotic symptoms are present in an important number of medical and psychiatric conditions. In order to determine the frequency of a clinical phenomenon we need to precisely know to which condition we want to refer. In the case of psychotic symptoms we just can have a very approximate estimation: in fact we can say that besides the efforts to estimate the frequency of psychosis

in older adults, results tend to underestimate the true prevalence.

The prevalence of all range of psychotic disorders in older adults with more than 65 years is 4–6% [9–13] and for those with more than 85 years as high than 10% [13]. The majority of these cases are related to psychotic symptoms in dementia. More than 23% of older adults will experience psychotic symptoms at some time and dementia is the main cause [14]. The proportion of older adults with schizophrenia whose onset was later than 40 years is 23.5% [15]. The annual incidence of schizophrenia-like psychosis increases by 11% every 5 years since the age of 60 years [15]. Paranoid schizophrenia occurs in 60% of cases and 30% is delusional disorder. The other form of psychosis occurs in 10% of cases. Paranoid and systematic delusions tend to increase with age in patients with schizophrenia, while symptoms of disorganization tend to decrease [16]. The diagnosis of a nonorganic psychosis first manifesting in older adults is not rare in tertiary care (about 30% of admissions at an old age psychiatric hospital) [17]. The most common etiology of psychosis in older adults is presented in Fig. 18.1 [18].

The prevalence of schizophrenia and delusional disorders for older adults is 0.5–1%, 5 times more frequent in women than in men

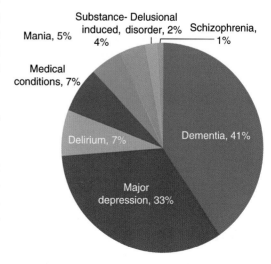

Fig. 18.1 Distribution of most common causes of psychosis in older adults [18]

(possibly because the onset of schizophrenia in women is later) [13]. Relatives of patients with very-late-onset schizophrenia have a lower morbid risk than the relatives of patients with early-onset schizophrenia [19, 20]. Older adults with good premorbid educational level, occupational, and psychosocial functioning are less impaired in case of late-onset schizophrenia than in those with early-onset schizophrenia [21–23].

The main risk factors for psychotic symptoms include female gender, brain degeneration with cognitive decline, brain neurochemical changes associated to the ageing process (which have relevant consequences on pharmacokinetics and pharmacodynamics for all drugs), comorbid medical conditions, medications (such as dopaminergic and anticholinergic), substance abuse, social isolation, adequate stimulation deprivation, sensory deficits, and premorbid personality (paranoid) [15, 24].

18.3 Classification of Psychosis in Older Adults

The same classification of disorders with psychotic symptoms in adults may be used for older adults. The proposed classification here presented, with the respective diagnostic criteria, may quickly change next year with the publication of the International Classification of Diseases, 11th revision, to which a working group of old age psychiatrists was invited to review the classification of psychotic disorders. Table 18.1 presents the classification of the disorders where psychotic symptoms may be present.

Traditionally psychotic symptoms can be related to two main groups of disorders. The primary psychotic group includes functional disorders with no detectable physiological and anatomical change, an influence of substances, or iatrogenic causes. Psychotic symptoms constitute the core group of the diagnostic criteria. This group includes the persistent psychotic disorders, the acute psychotic disorder, other psychotic disorders, and the personality disorders. The secondary psychotic group includes some functional disorders (the psychotic symptoms are not the main symptoms) and the organic disorders where

Table 18.1 Classification of disorders presenting psychotic symptoms

Primary psychotic symptoms	Secondary psychotic symptoms
Psychiatric disorders *Persistent psychotic disorders* • Schizophrenia • Delusional disorder • Schizoaffective disorder *Acute psychotic disorder* • Acute and transient psychotic disorder *Other psychotic disorders*	*Psychiatric disorders* • Major and minor neurocognitive disorders (dementia) with psychotic symptoms • Delirium • Organic mental disorders (hallucinosis, catatonic, delusional) • Mental and behavioral disorders due to psychoactive substance use • Bipolar affective disorder with psychotic symptoms • Depressive episode/recurrent depressive disorder with psychotic symptoms
Personality disorders • Paranoid personality disorder • Schizoid personality disorder • Schizotypal disorder	*Somatic disorders and comorbidities* *Iatrogenic causes of psychosis*

a disturbance of normal functioning may be explained by a biological detectable cause.

18.3.1 Primary Psychotic Symptoms

18.3.1.1 Psychiatric Disorders

Persistent Psychotic Disorders

• *Schizophrenia*: is characterized by disturbances that involve the most basic functions which give the normal person a sense of individuality, uniqueness, and self-direction. Multiple mental functions are affected including thinking (e.g., delusions, formal thought disorders), perception (e.g., hallucinations), self-experience (loss of the sense of agency or feeling of ownership of the experience), cognition (impaired attention, verbal memory, and social cognition), volition (e.g., loss of motivation), affect (blunted emotional expression), and psychomotor behavior (catatonia). Persistent delusions, persistent hallucinations, thought disorders, and distortions of self-experience are considered core symptoms. At least one of these needs to be present for at least one month for the diagnosis. Other symptoms include negative symptoms (apathy and anhedonia, paucity of speech, and blunting of emotional expressions, not due to depression or to any medication), disorganized behavior (odd, eccentric, aimless, and agitated activity), and psychomotor disorders (excitement, posturing, or waxy flexibility, negativism, mutism, and stupor).

The diagnosis of schizophrenia should not be made when the symptoms exist less than one month, when they occur concurrently or within a few days of a diagnosable depressive or manic episode, and when it is possible to demonstrate the effects of a psychoactive substance or the presence of a general medical condition.

Schizophrenia can arise at any time in life—from childhood to very late age: the expression of symptoms shows a great variation when its onset is at the extremes of life. Understanding these variations can help to identify the causes of the disorder and its risk factors. A consensus statement was published in 1998 proposing, in an arbitrary way, cut-offs with potential clinical and research utility. Schizophrenia diagnosed before 40 years is classified as having an early onset; schizophrenia diagnosed between 40 and 60 years is recognized as having a late onset; schizophrenia diagnosed by the first time after 60 years is recognized as having a very late onset [5, 25].

There are several arguments to justify this classification: there are three adult peaks of onset corresponding to adult life, middle age, and old age [26, 27]. Female gender is associated with late age onset. There are no important differences in terms of symptoms between early- and late-onset schizophrenia [17], but in very late-onset schizophrenia there are low prevalence of formal thought disorder and affective blunting, while visual hallucinations are more frequent [28, 29]. No differences in type or severity of neurocognitive impairments were found between early- and late-onset cases, besides late-onset schizophrenia presents milder cognitive impairments (cognitive flexi-

bility and abstraction) [30]. Familial schizophrenia (suggesting hereditary form of the disorder) is more common in earlier than in late-onset cases [20]. For other authors it was found that the following symptoms were more present and more severe in early-onset cases than in very late-onset cases: hallucinations, assiduity loss, grandiosity, reference and influence delusions, and friendship poverty. Very late-onset cases had more persecutory delusions and more vascular cerebral lesions/vulnerability [31].

- *Delusional disorder*: is characterized by the development either of a single delusion or of a set of related delusions that are unusually persistent (at least three months) and sometimes lifelong. Other defining symptoms of schizophrenia (persistent auditory hallucinations, disorganized thinking, negative symptoms) are not present, although various forms of perceptual disorders (hallucinations, illusions, misidentifications of persons) thematically related to the delusion are still consistent with the diagnosis. Apart from actions and attitudes directly related to the delusion or delusional system, affect, speech, and behavior are typically normal [32]. Clear and persistent auditory hallucinations and/or negative symptoms are incompatible with the diagnosis. The delusions are not due to the direct effects of a medical condition or substance on the CNS.

Delusional disorder is recognized as a frequent phenomenon in old age. This disorder is associated with premorbid personality (schizotypal, paranoid), hearing loss, low socio-economic status, and migration. Unfortunately, there are very few studies on this population but it seems that older adults are reluctant to seek treatment and they are more resistant to it. The delusional disorder is frequently more distressing to family members or neighbors than for the patient who frequently denies the existence of a problem [33]. It may be a part of several different types of nonorganic psychosis manifesting for the first time in the elderly and this may subsequently evolve into different diagnostic categories [34].

The classification according to the age of onset can contribute to a better understanding of their epidemiology, psychopathology, and outcome. It was also proposed to use the same cut-off ages than used for schizophrenia to separate the cases in three groups (early onset, late onset, and very late onset).

- *Schizoaffective disorder*: is an episodic disorder with both symptom criteria of schizophrenia and a major mood episode (either depressive, manic, or mixed) that are prominent within the same episode of illness, preferably simultaneously or at least within a few days of each other. There are prominent symptoms of schizophrenia (delusions, hallucinations, disorders of self-experience, formal thought disorders) which are accompanied by typical symptoms of a depressive episode (depressed mood, loss of interest, reduced energy), a manic episode (elevated mood, increase in the quality and speed of physical and mental activity), or a mixed affective episode [35].

Conditions that meet the above requirements, but with a duration of less than one month, should be diagnosed initially as acute transient psychotic disorders or as other psychotic disorder, depending on the clinical presentation. In cases where the symptoms of schizophrenia co-exist with an affective episode of mild severity, the individual should be diagnosed with schizophrenia with prominent depressive and/or manic symptoms.

Schizoaffective disorders with first onset later in life are extremely rare, and for instance, there is no reason to distinguish between late-onset and early-onset schizoaffective disorders [36].

Acute Psychotic Disorder

- *Acute and transient psychotic disorder*: is characterized by acute onset of psychotic symptoms which emerge without a prodrome and reach their maximal severity within two weeks. Symptoms include delusions, hallucinations, disorganization of thought processes, perplexity or confusion, and disturbances of affect and mood. Catatonia-like psychomotor disturbances may be present. In most cases there is marked fluctuation of symptoms, sometimes from day to day. The duration of

the disorder rarely exceeds three months. When the disorder recurs, periods of remission are typically longer and the outcome is generally better than in schizophrenia. The symptoms are not due to direct effects of a medical condition or psychotropic substance use.

Symptoms are often precipitated by stressors or unexpected situations (death of a loved one, including animals, sudden change of wealth or other social issues—including moving to another domicile, diagnosis of severe disorder). Commonly, the premorbid functional level returns once the stressors are identified and managed [37]. This condition can be considered as a particular reaction to severe stress and an adjustment disorder.

Other Primary Psychotic Disorders

This category includes disorders with primary psychotic symptomatology that do not meet the criteria for schizophrenia, delusional disorder, schizoaffective disorder, acute and transient psychotic disorder, schizotypal disorder, or for psychotic types of affective disorders. Psychotic conditions due to brain disorders, general medical conditions, or substance use/withdrawal need to be excluded.

Table 18.2 presents the diagnostic criteria for the above disorders, such as proposed to the ICD-11.

18.3.1.2   Personality Disorders

Three personality disorders were included in this chapter because (1) their importance as risk factor for some of the above psychiatric disorders, (2) their characteristics may represent just a step between an adjusted personality and a psychotic disorder, (3) some classifications include them as a full psychiatric disorder since they have many aspects in common with the other disorders that they are related, and (4) they represent an important source of suffering and are problems for social integration and performance.

There are few studies of personality in older adults. They are behavioral patterns with inflexible responses to diverse situations of life. These patterns are stable in time and older adults have lived with them all their lives: there is no late-onset

Table 18.2 Diagnostic criteria for psychosis proposed to WHO for the ICD-11

Psychotic disorder	Diagnostic guidelines
Schizophrenia	The symptoms can be divided into and often occur together such as: (a) persistent delusions of any kind (b) persistent hallucinations in any modality (c) thought disorder resulting in severe cases in incoherence or irrelevant speech, or neologisms (d) distortions of self-experience (e) negative symptoms such as apathy and anhedonia, paucity of speech, and blunting of emotional expressions; it must be clear that these are not due to depression or to medication (f) disorganized behavior, including odd, eccentric, aimless, and agitated activity (g) psychomotor disorders such as excitement, posturing, or waxy flexibility, negativism, mutism, and stupor At least two of the symptom categories [at least one of them should include symptoms from the core symptoms (a) to (d)] should have been clearly present for most of the time during a period of 1 month or more The diagnosis of schizophrenia should not be made: (1) For conditions that meet the above requirements but with a duration of less than 1 month (2) If the symptoms of schizophrenia occur concurrently or within a few days of a diagnosable depressive or manic episode (3) If the disturbance is due to demonstrable effects of a psychoactive substance or to a general medical condition
Delusional disorder	• Development of a delusion or set of related delusions persisting for at least 3 months • Delusions are variable in content across individuals while showing remarkable stability within individuals over time. They may evolve over time. Common forms of delusions: persecutory, hypochondriac/somatic, grandiose, delusional jealousy, and erotomania • Delusions may be accompanied by actions, which may be extreme, directly related to the content of the delusions • Clear and persistent auditory hallucinations and/or negative symptoms are incompatible with the diagnosis • Apart from the actions and attitudes directly related to the delusional system, affect, speech, and behavior are unaffected • Anxiety and/or depression may be present intermittently, but do not persist over time. Delusions must be present at times when there is no disturbance of mood • The definitional criteria for schizophrenia or any other psychotic disorder have never been fulfilled at any time • The delusions are not due to the direct effects of a medical condition or substance on the CNS
Schizoaffective disorder	A diagnosis of schizoaffective disorder should be made only when the symptom criteria of schizophrenia and of a depressive, manic, or mixed episode of moderate or severe degree are present simultaneously or within a few days of each other • The disorder is characterized by episodes in which delusions, hallucinations, or other symptoms of schizophrenia co-occur with a depressive, manic, or mixed affective episode • The duration of symptomatic episodes is at least four weeks for both psychotic and affective symptoms • The psychotic and mood symptoms are not due to the direct physiological effects of a substance, a general medical condition or its treatment • The disturbance is not better accounted for by a diagnosis of schizophrenia, an episode of a mood disorder with psychotic features, a mental disorder due to a general medical condition or its treatment, or a substance-induced disorder

(continued)

Table 18.2 (continued)

Psychotic disorder	Diagnostic guidelines
Acute and transient psychotic disorder	Acute onset of psychotic symptoms, with or without other symptoms, that emerge without a prodrome, progressing from a non-psychotic state to a clearly psychotic state within 2 weeks • Symptoms typically change rapidly, both in nature and intensity. Such changes may occur from day to day, or even within a single day • In addition, there are often other symptoms such as disturbances of affect, transient states of perplexity, or impairment of attention and concentration. Importantly, if present, these symptoms do not meet the criteria for mood disorders or delirium, respectively • The disorder is transient with duration usually not exceeding 3 months • The onset of this disorder is usually associated with a rapid deterioration in social and occupational functioning. Following remission, the person is generally able to retain the premorbid level of functioning. The symptoms of this disorder are not due to direct effects of a medical condition or psychotropic substance use
Other primary psychotic disorders	"Other primary psychotic disorder" should be coded if the number or duration of psychotic symptoms (i.e., delusions, hallucinations, formal thought disorder, grossly disorganized, or catatonic behavior) do not fulfill the criteria for any specific psychotic disorder or to justify any other specific diagnosis. Psychotic conditions due to brain disorders, general medical conditions, or substance use/withdrawal need to be excluded

or very late-onset personality disorder, at least not in absence of brain damage or deterioration. Their presence may significantly limit the capacity of the older adult to cope with the several stressors common at these period of life and be, in some cases, a premorbid state of late- and very late- onset psychotic disorders.

Three conditions can be here listed. All of them may be a premorbid condition for schizophrenia and delusional disorder. They represent at the DSM-5 the Cluster A Personality Disorder [38]:

(a) Paranoid personality disorder: It is characterized by a pervasive distrust and suspiciousness of others such that their motives are interpreted as malevolent.
(b) Schizoid personality disorder: It is a pervasive pattern of detachment from social relationships and a restricted range of expression of emotions in interpersonal settings.
(c) Schizotypal personality disorder: It is also a pervasive pattern of social deficits marked by acute discomfort with, and reduced capacity for, close relationships as well as by cognitive or perceptual distortions and eccentricities of behavior.

18.3.2 Secondary Psychotic Symptoms

18.3.2.1 Psychiatric Disorders

Psychotic symptoms may be present during the course of some psychiatric disorders which may be divided into three clusters:

• Organic disorders at directly affecting the central nervous system:
  – Major and minor neurocognitive disorders (dementia) with psychotic symptoms
  – Delirium
  – Organic mental disorders (hallucinosis, catatonic, delusional)
• Mental and behavioral disorders due to psychoactive substance use
• Mood disorders
  – Bipolar affective disorder with psychotic symptoms
  – Depressive episode/recurrent depressive disorder with psychotic symptoms
• *Major and minor neurocognitive disorders (dementia) with psychotic symptoms*: Psychotic symptoms during the course of a neurocognitive disorder, such dementia, make part of what is

known as behavioral and psychological symptoms of dementia (BPSD). These symptoms are very well described in Chap. 21 of this book and will not be developed here. BPSD are frequent in dementia (2/3 of patients will present at least one of them at a given time), they are a sign of severity of the dementia and it contributes to increase the suffering of patients and the burden of their caregivers [39–41]. It may increase the risk of institutionalization, violence, abuse, and older adult neglect [15, 42].

- *Delirium*: the Chap. 20 of this book is dedicated to delirium. The definition used by the authors is: "Delirium is primarily a disturbance of consciousness, attention, cognition, and perception but can also affect sleep, psychomotor activity, and emotions. It is a common psychiatric illness among medically compromised patients and may be a harbinger of significant morbidity and mortality."

- *Organic mental disorders*: there are several conditions causally related to brain dysfunction because of trauma, a primary brain disease, to a systemic disease affecting the brain secondarily, to endocrine disorders, and to the use of toxic substances. What will differ them from delirium is the fact that they don't include necessarily the impairment of consciousness and attention as well of the cognitive disturbance. Among the several forms listed some include psychotic symptoms as main symptoms:

  - *Organic hallucinosis*—persistent or recurrent hallucinations occurring in clear consciousness (with or without delusional elaboration).

  - *Organic catatonic disorder*—diminished or increased psychomotor activity with catatonic symptoms like those observed in schizophrenia. It may be confounded with delirium as it may rarely occur without clear consciousness.

  - *Organic delusional disorder*—persistent or recurrent delusions (with or without hallucinations) dominating the clinical picture in the presence of an organic etiology.

- *Mental and behavioral disorders due to psychoactive substance use*: Acute intoxication, induced persistent psychotic disorders, and substance withdrawal must be considered. The most common drugs causing such problems in older adults are alcohol, tobacco, and caffeine. Prescribed drugs as sedatives or hypnotics, and opioids (for chronic pain) are at the origin of such difficulties too. The psychotic disorder related to the substance use may take different forms such schizophrenia-like, delusional, hallucinatory, polymorphic, depressive, manic, and mixed. In general, consciousness is clear but it may also be clouded.

- *Bipolar affective disorder with psychotic symptoms*: The presence of psychotic symptoms is a sign of higher severity of bipolar disorder. Besides most frequently the first episode of mania occurs early in life, and it can also occur later. Older adults with psychotic symptoms in mania usually have grandiose delusions, irritability, and sexual inappropriate behaviors. Patients usually don't recognize them as ill and they may have delusions of possessing great fortune, exceptional skills, and superpowers. Psychotic symptoms during the depressive phase of bipolar disorder don't differ of those of depressive episode and of recurrent depression.

- *Depressive episode/recurrent depressive disorder with psychotic symptoms*: Psychotic symptoms in depression also represent a sign of severity of the depressive episode. They are more common in late-onset depression than in earlier onset. The delusions concern more hypochondriac features, punishment for unforgivable acts, or of catastrophes affecting beloved ones. The majority of delusions are mood congruent [14].

18.3.2.2 Somatic Disorders and Comorbidities

These conditions are cited here because:

- They are at the origin of psychotic symptoms in two major conditions (delirium and organic mental disorders);
- Primary care is a good context to detect and manage them without being necessary to refer the patient to a secondary level.

They may include almost all internal medicine conditions. We should always have in mind the possibility of acute and chronic pain, water and electrolytic disturbances, and infections. Tumors, endocrine disorders, cardiovascular disorders, respiratory chronic conditions, urinary disturbances, intestine transit disturbances, and in particular, sensory impairments (hearing and sighting incapacities) can all be at the origin of persistent and/or acute psychotic symptoms.

18.3.2.3 Iatrogenic Causes of Psychosis

The use of prescribed and non-prescribed drugs may cause psychotic symptoms and also be at the origin of delirium and organic mental disorders. Again primary care teams are at the good place to detect any deviance in the use of these drugs. The medication potentially causing psychotic symptoms include: antihistamine, anti-Parkinson drugs, anti-arrhythmics, anti-inflammatory drugs, anticonvulsants, steroids, sedatives, and anticancer drugs.

Invasive procedures, referral to specialists/hospitals, and any other intervention perceived by an older person as threatening can be at origin of psychotic symptoms. It is important to spend the necessary time to explain the reason why these prescriptions are made and to check the person understanding, to execute them as friendly as possible, and to avoid unnecessary procedures.

18.4 Assessment and Management at Primary Care for an Older Adult with Psychotic Symptoms [1]

18.4.1 Organizing Mental Health Care for Older Adults

To assess and to manage psychotic disorders in older adults is complex. It often requires particular knowledge and skills but it also depends on how the health system is organized at local, regional, and national level. Clinical decisions on what to do, in which priority, when, and to whom to refer are all depend on how the health-care system is structured and how much easy the access to mental health care is. This is not specific only to psychosis but also to all mental health disorders in older adults.

WHO is working alongside governments, NGOs, national academic, and research teams to improve access to high quality mental health treatment and care for all in need. Key messages and actions that WHO is promoting are as follows [43]:

- Stop the human rights violations in mental health facilities;
- Develop mental health laws which respect human rights, promote adequate health care, and stop social exclusion;
- Put in place mental health policies and strategic plans that enable national authorities to prioritize and coordinate all mental health actions in the country so as to maximize positive outcomes for people with mental illness and the communities in which they live;
- Provide appropriate treatment, care, and support through better mental health services and the mobilization of untapped community resources; and
- Advocate for better recognition and action for mental health in national development agendas and programs.

As mentioned at the WHO/WPA consensus statement on organization of care in psychiatry of the elderly [44], all people have the right of access to a range of services that can respond to their health and social needs. These needs should be met appropriately for the cultural setting and in accordance with scientific knowledge and ethical requirements. Governments have a responsibility to improve and maintain the general and mental health of older people and to support their families and carers by the provision of health and social measures adapted to the specific needs of the local community.

The inclusion of topics related to the mental health of older adults in national mental health policies is mandatory. According to these policies, it is necessary to develop specific programs to address coordinated response to the mental health needs of this population. Another important step is to train professionals to recognize the symptoms and to develop their skills on how to manage them, offering appropriate response to the person and support for the carers. Therapeutic resources have to be available, not only the essential drugs but also psychological resources and opportunities for appropriate psychiatric rehabilitation. All these actions depend on the national economic development and Table 18.3 proposes a list of required actions for the care of older adults in case of psychosis, according to the national income level.

18.4.2 Managing Psychosis in Older Adults

18.4.2.1 General Principles

Any older adult should be routinely and specifically enquired about the presence of psychotic symptoms: check the presence of beliefs not shared by others and if he/she is hearing voices or seeing things that nobody else perceives. Co-lateral investigation may inform about any behavioral and activity changes. Assess always the neurocognitive functioning.

Be aware of possessing good skills on how to interview an older adult with psychosis. The first step for the assessment and the management of psychosis is to build supportive and empathic relationship with the person [45]. This can be particularly challenging in patients with paranoid symptoms. Treat patient with respect and offer care in the least restrictive environment as possible [46]. Be optimist and encourage hope. The person with psychosis should be provided with a diagnosis and be informed about it in a language easy to be understood [46]. Explain the nature of the symptoms and that they are related to a mental disorder that can be treated [1]. Assess the risk of self-harm and the risk for the others.

Take into account cultural and religious aspects, particularly in case of older adults from different origins than yours. If necessary, seek advice and supervision of an experienced professional on transcultural aspects of psychiatry, if available [45].

Health needs of older adults are diverse. At primary care it is easier to manage the prevention, early detection, and treatment of the majority of somatic health problems. Older adults with psychosis are at risk to develop several health disorders in particular in the case of those carrying for a long time their mental disorder. Routinely monitor weight, cardiovascular, and metabolic indicators. Promote good healthy behavior (avoid alcohol and other non-prescribed drugs, physical activity, regular sleep, good personal hygiene, avoid stressors), check the diet habits, detect excessive weight gain, abnormal lipid, and glucose levels, offer help to stop smoking [45]. Note carefully all the drugs being used (even those not prescribed). Assess the consumption of any other substance potentially dangerous (including alcohol and caffeine).

Offer to those who take care of older adults with psychosis the possibility to express their own needs, feelings, and questions. This could reduce the level of expressed emotions inside the relationship context. With the person's consent, inform them about the diagnosis, prognosis, available supports (including social support), and how to lead with crisis situations. Include them in the decision-making care plan. Educate carers to avoid to convince the person that his/her beliefs are false and tell how to assume a neutral and supportive attitude [1, 46].

Explain to the person and the carers about the therapeutic elements, the necessity to take regularly some drugs, and the need for regular controls. Tell about the possibility of relapse of symptoms and how to lead with this.

Identify potential stressors and try to propose strategies to reduce them. Propose help to reduce isolation: encourage the person to improve social activities, to contact prior old friends, and to establish new relationships. Use the resources of the community: make the person to contact his/her religious community, identify the leisure and cultural activities groups, and promote the participation to physical activities with other persons. Group occupational therapy may be necessary for same persons. This may reduce

Table 18.3 Required actions for the care of older adults with psychosis

Actions	Low income countries	Middle income countries	High income countries
Providing care in primary care	Recognize psychosis care as a component of PC Include the recognition and treatment of psychosis in training curricula of all health personnel, including refresher training to PC physicians	Develop locally relevant training materials Provide refresher training to PC physicians	Improve effectiveness of management of psychosis in PC Improve referral patterns
Making appropriate treatments available	Increase availability of essential antipsychotics Develop and evaluate basic educational and training interventions for caregivers	Ensure availability of essential antipsychotics in all health-care settings Make effective caregiver interventions generally available	Provide easier access to newer antipychotics Provide access to psychological interventions both for older adults as for their caregivers
Giving care in the community	Older adult people with psychosis are best assessed and treated in the place where they are living Develop and promote standard needs assessments for use in primary and secondary care Initiate pilot projects on development of multidisciplinary community care teams, day care, and short-term respite care Move people with psychosis out of inappropriate institutional settings	Initiate pilot projects on integration of psychosis care with general health care Provide community care facilities (with multidisciplinary community teams, day care, respite, and inpatient units for acute assessment and treatment) Encourage the development of residential and nursing-home facilities	Develop alternative residential facilities Provide community care facilities Give individualized care in the community to people with psychosis
Educating the public	Promote public campaigns against stigma and discrimination Support nongovernmental organizations in public education	Use the mass media to promote awareness of mental health of older adults and foster positive attitudes	Launch public campaigns for early help-seeking, recognition, and appropriate management of mental health disorders in old age
Involving communities, families, and consumers	Support the formation of self-help groups Fund schemes for nongovernmental organizations	Ensure representation of communities, families, and consumers in policy-making, service development, and implementation	Foster advocacy initiatives
Developing human resources	Train primary health-care workers Initiate higher professional training programs for doctors and nurses in geriatric psychiatry and medicine Develop training and resource centers	Create a network of national training centers for physicians, psychiatrists, nurses, psychologists, and social workers	Train specialists in advanced treatment skills

Table 18.3 (continued)

Actions	Low income countries	Middle income countries	High income countries
Supporting more research	Conduct studies in primary health-care settings on the prevalence, course, outcome, and impact of psychosis in the community	Institute effectiveness and cost-effectiveness studies for community management of psychosis	Extend research on the causes of psychosis in older adults Carry out research on service delivery Investigate evidence on the prevention of psychosis in older adults

negative symptoms. This therapy combines psychotherapy strategies with activities aimed at creativity expression [1].

The improvement of the person's autonomy and independence is one of the main goals of the treatment. Offer to the person support to improve his/her life skills and to enhance independent living skills. Even if the older adult lives in a context of restriction of his/her liberty (nursing homes) all efforts should be made to improve his/her skills to make choices (dressing, menus).

18.4.2.2 Therapeutic Resources

The offer of the therapeutic resources will depend on the diagnosis at the base of the psychotic symptoms: we don't treat psychotic symptoms in affective disorders, major neurocognitive disorders, delirium, or other organic mental disorder in the same way that those present in persistent and acute psychotic disorders. Here we will essentially discuss the treatment for these last conditions. Two main therapeutic interventions should be easily available: pharmacotherapy and psychotherapy. The use of both together increases the chance of the best recovery. Antipsychotics should be used routinely but psychotherapy will be used according to some conditions described below.

Pharmacotherapy

The main rules to be followed are [1, 46]:

- As soon as the proper diagnosis is made, initiate an antipsychotic medication;
- Weigh the risks and benefits with the patient, their family members, or their surrogate decision maker;
- Prescribe one antipsychotic at a time. Avoid regular combined antipsychotic medication (except for short periods);

- Start with the lowest dose and titrate up slowly to reduce side effects;
- Monitor before use of an antipsychotic: weight, blood pressure, fasting sugar, cholesterol, ECG, assess any movement disorder, nutritional status, and level of physical activity.
- Monitor regularly during the treatment, the therapeutic response, the side effects (some of them can be both provoked by the antipsychotic or by the psychosis), the emergence of movements disorders, weight, pulse, and blood pressure, fasting blood glucose and lipid levels, adherence, and any change in other health condition.

The choice of the antipsychotic should be based upon the side effects and how it is supposed to affect the person's life. Antipsychotics in older adults have shown to increase the risk of mortality, stroke, neurocognitive decline, extrapyramidal symptoms, sedation, and a serious but rare condition called neuroleptic malignant syndrome [47]. Atypical and conventional antipsychotics have also shown to have an increased risk of falls but they have been preferred than conventional antipsychotics because they have less severe side effects.

Psychotherapy

There are few studies of psychotherapy for older adults with psychosis. Nevertheless, NICE [45] proposes some recommendations that can be used for this population. Essentially there are two possible psychological interventions: cognitive behavior therapy (CBT) and family therapy. Healthcare professionals taking in charge one of these two interventions should have particular skills in delivering this therapy to older adults with psychosis and be regularly supervised. It could be very difficult to deliver this kind of care at primary care level and the majority of times these healthcare professionals work at a secondary level facility.

CBT may help older adults to establish links between their thoughts, feelings, and actions and their symptoms and functioning level as well help these persons to re-evaluate their perceptions, beliefs, and thoughts to their symptoms. Other goals may be to help people to learn how to monitor their own thoughts, feelings, or behaviors, to promote alternative ways of coping with their symptoms, to reduce distress, and to improve functioning [45].

Family intervention in the presence of the person (if possible) should take account of the relationship between the main carer and the person with psychosis, and have a specific supportive, educational, or treatment function, including negotiated problem solving and crisis management [45].

18.4.2.3 Preventing Psychosis in Older Adults

Psychotic symptoms in older adults related to somatic disorders and/or because of iatrogenic causes can be prevented by the good control of somatic conditions: the prevention for them should also prevent the psychotic symptoms. Avoiding the use of drugs for persons at risk to develop psychosis, regularly monitoring the use of all substances, and encouraging older adults to stop smoking, to use alcohol very moderately, and to reduce caffeine consumption may all contribute to reduce risks. An attention has to be paid to prevent drug interactions as well as to the impact of pharmacokinetics and pharmacodynamic changes related to ageing and to existing conditions.

Delirium can be prevented by the control of the main predisposing factors: age >65 years old (because of the higher number of comorbid pathology and polypharmacy, increasing the risk of noxious drug interactions and side effects), the use of physical restraints, malnutrition, more than three medications added, use of bladder catheter, any iatrogenic event, and finally acute insults (acute bacterial/viral infection, fractures,

metabolic alterations, intense uncontrolled pain, hypoxia and ischemia, and sleep deprivation) [48–50].

Psychotic symptoms in case of major neurocognitive disorders make part of the conditions and are relatively difficult to prevent. Psychotic symptoms, as one of the major symptoms of BPSD, may occur in particular such physical discomfort, as a drug side effect, psychological ill-being, environmental or caregiver inadequacy, or any combination of the former. The premobid personality may contribute to its onset.

There is no possible prevention for personality disorders: the possible therapeutic interventions should be used years before. But CBT may have an impact to increase the acceptance of own self and help to promote alternative ways of coping with life's difficulties, to reduce distress, and to improve functioning. There is no indication to administration of antipsychotics in this case.

Psychotic symptoms in the course of an affective disorder (bipolar, depressive disorder, or recurrent depression) are a sign of severity. The prevention consists on earlier interventions in life to treat them (psychological and/or pharmacological) as rarely they start later in life. Antidepressants may prevent depressive relapse and mood stabilizers may prevent both bipolar and depressive episodes relapse but their use have to be very well monitored.

In the case of any distressed older adult with social functioning decline and with psychotic symptoms it should be assessed without delay by a specialist. This may be difficult in lower income countries without specialists easily available but in the presence of these symptoms the evaluation of any medical condition is mandatory. History, physical examination, laboratory examination, and brain image if available should respond if there are medical conditions or side effect of drugs. Don't offer antipsychotics to reduce the risk of or preventing psychosis.

18.4.2.4 Managing Early-Onset Psychosis in Older Adults [45]

An older adult with a history of psychosis started early in life is someone who should know enough well his mental disorder and probably is already known by the primary care professionals. If the history points for good results of previous treatments start to use them. Offer crisis intervention resolution. Assess the risks for the person's and career's security. Consider all available resources to help the person in the community and refer him/her to an inpatient unit only if there is no other better solution. Referral to a specialized mental health service will depend upon local availability of such a service. Consider in this case the possibility of the person to refuse this solution: lead with the medical and legal aspects of an involuntary hospitalization according to the local rules.

The treatment options include oral antipsychotic medication with psychological intervention. Review existing medication and adapt the doses or replace it by another antipsychotic if necessary. CBT and family intervention may start during the acute phase or later. Consider occupational therapy. The treatment should be continuously be monitored and be offered as long as necessary to prevent relapse. After discharge of the inpatient unit, the follow-up may be assured by a specialized outpatient unit or by primary care team if clear orientations are available.

Other situations where an older adult with psychosis should be referred by primary care to a specialized unit are a poor response to treatment, a non-adherence to medication, intolerable side effects, comorbid substance misuse, and the risk to self and others security [45].

18.4.2.5 Managing Late or Very Late-Onset Psychosis in Older Adults

There is a higher risk of organic mental disorders or of major neurocognitive disorders in the case of late or very late-onset psychosis and all efforts should be made in order to make an early diagnosis of these conditions. Monitor for other possible conditions such as affective disorders, anxiety, substance misuse, and somatic health problems. Otherwise, the psychotic condition should be treated as any first psychotic episode.

A complete and multidisciplinary assessment should be made, if possible in a specialized board. Psychiatrist, neurocognitive psychologist,

and trained nurse and social work should work together to address the following points [45]:

– Medical assessment including medical history, physical examination, identification of all drugs being used;
– Psychiatric assessment with identification of risk factors, personality profile, past mental health problems, use of substances (alcohol, caffeine, etc.);
– Identification of social determinants of health and disease (accommodation, social network, financial conditions, leisure activities, family constellation, spiritual and cultural needs, etc.);
– Identification of past and present stressors (in particular with recent and past losses) and trauma. Assess the possibility of a post-traumatic stress disorder;
– Satisfaction with own life.

If possible, avoid using antipsychotics for a first episode at primary care level unless a specialist recommends it. Otherwise, offer antipsychotic medication as mentioned before. CBT and family interventions should make part of the care plan. Occupational therapy should be offered if available.

18.4.2.6 Recovery and Follow-Up

Once the acute psychotic episode is under control, continuous treatment should be provided involving multidisciplinary approach. Pharmacology, psychological, social, and occupational interventions should be available. Promote autonomy and independence; fight all forms of possible stigma and discrimination against the persons and the carers.

General practitioners and other primary health-care professionals can manage the residual symptoms, if they exist. These professionals should monitor the physical health of older adult with psychosis under treatment as frequently as possible. Attention should focus not only on any sign of psychotic relapse but also on cardiovascular disease risk assessment, lipid modification, and of fasten glucose levels.

In case of older adults whose illness has not responded enough to treatment, diagnosis should be reviewed; the adherence to treatment has to be assured, with drug monitoring when possible. Other causes of non-response should be considered as comorbidity, drug interaction, and the use of other substances.

18.5　Conclusion and Future Developments

Psychotic symptoms in older adults are still today object of little interest of researchers. Psychopathological understanding of late and very late-onset disorders may help to define new therapeutic strategies. Older adults with psychotic symptoms are very vulnerable to stigma and discrimination: it is necessary to develop specific topics to protect them at the national mental health policy. Integration with other sectors of the society may be necessary to promote their protection: educational sector, justice, and security forces all together should collaborate together for a better result. In case of loss of autonomy because of the mental disorder, legal protection should be offered and regularly reviewed. For that it is necessary to assess the capacity to consent. How to lead with a growing older adult population with a long history of psychosis is a challenge: the majority of protocols of care, rehabilitation procedures, and goals were developed for younger adults, very often with the intention to insert them at the working market. This is not possible for older adults at the age of retirement and solutions will have to be found. Structures to support these persons and their families to live in the community are still missing and residential facilities are not prepared in their majority to cope with chronic psychotic older adults. To achieve the highest possible level of quality of life for older adults with psychosis, two complementary dimensions must be taken into account: the psychological well-being and individual resilience besides their deficiencies.

References

1. WHO. mhGAP intervention guide version 2.0. Geneva: WHO; 2016. p. 33.
2. Seeman MV, Jeste DV. Historical perspective. In: Hasset A, Ames D, Chiu E, editors. Psychosis in the elderly. London: Taylor & Francis; 2005. p. 1–9.
3. Hassett A. In: Hasset A, Ames D, Chiu E, editors. Defining psychotic disorders in an aging population. London: Taylor & Francis; 2005. p. 11–22.
4. Katona C, Levy R. Delusions and hallucinations in old age. London: Gaskell; 1992.
5. Howard R, Rabins PV, Seeman MV, Jeste DV, The International Late-Onset Schizophrenia Group. Late-onset schizophrenia and very-late-onset schizophrenia-like psychosis: an international consensus. Am J Psychiatry. 2000;157:172–8.
6. Marneros A. Late-onset mental disorders: the potsdam conference. London: Gaskell; 1999.
7. Berrios GE. Psychotic symptoms in the elderly. In: Katona C, Levy R, editors. Delusions and hallucinations in old age. London: Gaskell; 1992. p. 3–14.
8. WHO and WONCA. Integrating mental health into primary care. A global perspective. Geneva: WHO; 2008.
9. Christenson R, Blazer D. Epidemiology of persecutory ideation in an elderly population in the community. Am J Psychiatry. 1984;141:1088–9.
10. Henderson AS, Korten AE, Levings C, Jorm AF, Christensen H, Jacomb PA, Rodgers B. Psychotic symptoms in the elderly: a prospective study in a population sample. Int J Geriatr Psychiatry. 1998;13:484–92.
11. Forsell Y, Henderson AS. Epidemiology of paranoid symptoms in an elderly population. Br J Psychiatry. 1998;172:429–32.
12. Keith SJ, Regier DA, Rae DS. Schizophrenic disorders. In: Robins LN, Regier DA, editors. Psychiatric disorders in America: the Epidemiological Catchment Area Study. New York: Free Press; 1991. p. 33–52.
13. Subramaniam M, Abdin E, Vaingankar J, Picco L. Prevalence of psychotic symptoms among older adults in an Asian population. Int Psychogeriatr. 2016;28(7):1211–20.
14. Khouzam HR, Battista MA, Emes R, Ahles S. Psychoses in late life. Evaluation and management of disorders seen in primary care. Geriatrics. 2005;60(3):26–33.
15. Karim S, Harrison K. Psychosis in the elderly. In: Chew-Graham CA, Ray M, editors. Mental health and older people. Cham: Springer; 2016. p. 181–94.
16. Harris MJ, Jeste DV. Late-onset schizophrenia: an overview. Schizophr Bull. 1988;14:39–45.
17. Häfner H, Löffler W, Riecher-Rössler A, Häfner-Ranabauer W. Schizophrenia and delusions in middle aged and elderly patients. Epidemiology and etiological hypothesis. Nervenarzt. 2001;72(5):347–57.
18. Barak Y, Levy D, Szor H, Aizenberg D. First-onset functional brief psychoses in the elderly. Can Ger J. 2011;14(2):30–3.
19. Webster J, et al. Late-life onset of psychotic symptoms. Am J Geriatr Psychiatry. 1998;6:196–202.
20. Pearlson GD, Kreger L, Rabins PV, Chase GA, Cohen B, Wirth JB, Schlaepfer TB, Tune LE. A chart review

study of late-onset and early-onset schizophrenia. Am J Psychiatry. 1989;146:1568–74.

21. Howard R, Graham C, Sham P, Dennehey J, Castle DJ, Levy R, Murray R. A controlled family study of late-onset non-affective psychosis (late paraphrenia). Br J Psychiatry. 1997;170:511–4.

22. Kay DWK, Roth M. Environmental and hereditary factors in the schizophrenias of old age ("late paraphrenia") and their bearing on the general problem of causation in schizophrenia. J Ment Sci. 1961;107:649–86.

23. Post F. Persistent persecutory states. Oxford: Pergamon Press; 1966.

24. Tune LE, et al. Schizophrenia in late life. Psychiatr Clin N Am. 2003;26:103–13.

25. Howard R, Rabins PV, Castle DJ. Late onset schizophrenia. Petersfield: Wrightson Biomedical; 1999.

26. Van Os J, Howard R, Takei N, Murray RM. Increasing age is risk factor for psychosis in the elderly. Soc Psychiatry Psychiatr Epidemiol. 1995;30:161–4.

27. Sham P, Castle D, Wessely S, Farmer AE, Murray RM. Further exploration of a latent class typology of schizophrenia. Schizophr Res. 1996;20:105–15.

28. Rabins PV, Pauker S, Thomas J. Can schizophrenia begin after age 44? Compr Psychiatry. 1984;25:290–4.

29. Almeida O, Howard R, Levy R, David AS. Psychotic states arising in late life (late paraphrenia): psychopathology and nosology. Br J Psychiatry. 1995;166:205–14.

30. Jeste DV, Symonds LL, Harris MJ, Paulsen JS, Palmer BW, Heaton RK. Nondementia nonpraecox dementia praecox? Late-onset schizophrenia. Am J Psychiatry. 1997;5:302–17.

31. Girard C, Simard M. Elderly patients with very late-onset schizophrenia-like psychosis and early-onset schizophrenia: cross-sectional and respective clinical findings. Open J Psychiatry. 2012;2:305–16.

32. Gabriel E. Delusional disorders (of earlier onset) in old age. In: Katona C, Levy R, editors. Delusions and hallucinations in old age. London: Gaskell; 1992. p. 171–6.

33. Targum SD. Treating psychotic symptoms in the elderly patients. Primary Care Companion J Clin Psychiatry. 2001;3(4):156–63.

34. Broadway J, Mintzer J. The many faces of psychosis in the elderly. Curr Opin Psychiatry. 2007;20(6):551–8.

35. Marneros A, Deister A, Rohde A. Schizophrenic, schizoaffective and affective disorders in the elderly: a comparison. In: Katona C, Levy R, editors. Delusions and hallucinations in old age. London: Gaskell; 1992. p. 136–52.

36. Marneros A. Late-onset schizoaffective disorders. In: Marneros A, editor. Late-onset mental disorders. London: Gaskell; 1999. p. 98–106.

37. Pillman F, Balzuweit S, Haring A, Bleink R, Marneros A. Suicidal behavior in acute and transient psychotic disorders. Psychiatry Res. 2003;117(3):199–209.

38. American Psychiatric Association. Desk reference to the diagnostic criteria from DSM-5. Washington: APA; 2013.

39. Waldö ML, Gustafson L, Passant U, Englund E. Psychotic symptoms in frontotemporal dementia: a diagnostic dilemma. Int Psychogeriatrics. 2015;27(4):531–9.

40. Sweet RA, Hamilton RL, Lopez OL, Klunk WE. Psychotic symptoms in Alzheimer's disease are note associated with more severe neuropathologic features. Int Psychogeriatr. 2000;12(4):547–58.

41. Ballard C, O'Brien J, Coope B, Fairbairn A. A prospective study of psychotic symptoms in dementia sufferers: psychosis in dementia. Int Psychogeriatr. 1997;9(1):57–64.

42. Tran M, Bédard M, Molloy DW, Dubois S. Associations between psychotic symptoms and dependence in activities of daily living among older adults with Alzheimer's disease. Int Psychogeriatr. 2003;15(2):171–9.

43. WHO. Mental health action plan 2013-2020. Geneva: WHO; 2013.

44. WHO/WPA. Organization of care in psychiatry of the elderly: a technical consensus statement. Geneva: WHO; 1997.

45. National Institute for Health and Care Excellence. Guidelines (CG178), psychosis and schizophrenia in adults: treatment and management. Feb 2014.

46. Golberg D, Ivbijaro G, Kolkiewicz L, Ohene S. Schizophrenia in primary care mental health. In: Ivbijaro G, editor. Companion to primary care mental health. London: WONCA and Radcliffe; 2012. p. 353–62.

47. Masand PS. Side effects of antipsychotics in the elderly. J Clin Psychiatry. 2000;61(Suppl 8):43–9.

48. Inouye SK, Charpentier PA. Precipitating factors for delirium in hospitalized elderly persons: predictive model and interrelationship with baseline vulnerability. JAMA. 1996;275(11):852–7.

49. Cerejeira J, et al. The cholinergic system and inflammation: common pathways in delirium pathophysiology. J Am Geriatr Soc. 2012;60(4):669–75.

50. Nogueira V, et al. Improving quality of care: focus on liaison old age psychiatry. Ment Health Fam Med. 2013;10(3):153.

Sexuality in Older Adults

19

António Pacheco Palha

Abstract

The author presents some reflexions on sexuality in older adults having in mind that advanced age is not an undifferentiated experience. It is pointed out that some stereotypes are associated with ageing like social isolation, pain problems, difficulties to manage one's own life and inability for sexual life.

Some comments related with the body are done, and it is suggested a concept of timeless body, considering the importance of nonverbal communication in the recreation of sex interest. So, the satisfaction in personal relationship and satisfaction in sexual performance can be achieved in this age. It was concluded that is fundamental for the promotion of sexual health, an active role of the primary care physicians that should be prepared to understand the sexuality of older adults.

Key Points

- Advanced age is not an undifferentiated experience. It is important to know that the idea of successful ageing includes longevity and quality of life, namely, in affective life.
- Some stereotypes associated with ageing are social isolation, health problems/pain, disinterest and the inability to perform sexually and manage one's own life.
- No age body and timeless body. All these new ideas are very important to consider a new time for the sexuality of older people.
- Affection helps in recreating sex, and nonverbal communication takes on new dimensions and becomes a necessity in older adults.
- Although ageing is significantly linked to a decrease in various aspects of sexual activity, satisfaction in personal relationships and satisfaction in sexual performance do not decline with age.
- In overview it is fundamental for the promotion of sexual health in older adults to have the primary care physicians prepared to understand the sexuality context of the ageing woman and man.

A. P. Palha (✉)
Department of Psychiatry, School of Medicine, University of Oporto (Jubilee), Porto, Portugal

World Psychiatry Association (WPA), Geneva, Switzerland

European Federation of Sexology, Tilburg, The Netherlands

© Springer Nature Switzerland AG 2019
C. A. de Mendonça Lima, G. Ivbijaro (eds.), *Primary Care Mental Health in Older People*,
https://doi.org/10.1007/978-3-030-10814-4_19

Mental health is an important dimension of each person's general health, namely, when we are faced with sexuality in older adults. It is therefore important to consider sexual difficulties in older adults.

The concept of mental health comprises welfare, self-confidence, autonomy, competence, intergenerational dependence and self-actualisation of the individual's emotional and intellectual potential. From an intercultural viewpoint, it is virtually impossible to define mental health. However, it is generally agreed that mental health is more than the absence of mental illness [1], and from that definition I intend to emphasise not only the importance of the sense of autonomy and competence, but also the need for self-actualisation of emotional and intellectual potential of older women or men. In 1975, over 30 years ago, the WHO [2] defined sexual health as the "harmonious integration of the somatic, emotional, intellectual and social aspects of sexual being, with the goal of enriching personality, communication and love" [2]. It is appropriate to refer to a definition of sexual health in a sense, like love, that is part of the definition itself. We can raise the question – can older people fall in love for another person?

More recently (2001), the WPA (World Psychiatry Association) Section of Psychiatry and Human Sexuality, supported by its president Juan Mezzich and by an expert group in which I participated, published the book *Psychiatry and Sexual Health* [3], where sexual health was defined as a "dynamic and harmonious state involving erotic and reproductive experiences in the physical and spiritual fields, based on an informed, ethical, free and responsible chosen culture and not only on the absence of sexual dysfunction" [4].

Sexuality is a global reality that involves the entire human personality throughout life with an energy that motivates us to seek contact, affection, pleasure and well-being and that influences feelings, thoughts, actions and interactions. This magic process begins at birth and ends only with death. Thus, it can be said that sexuality is a very personal thing that is not limited to the genitalia.

We consider the following integral dimensions: biological, psycho-emotional, communicative, ethical, sociocultural and political. These are very important when dealing with sexuality issues in older adults and in gerontopsychiatry. Mental illness affects all aforementioned dimensions, where most affected ones depend on each disease.

In 1962, renowned gerontologist Strehler [5] proposed five criteria for normal ageing:

1. Cumulative: Ageing effects increase with time.
2. Universal: All members of a species display ageing signs.
3. Progressive: Ageing is a series of gradual changes.
4. Intrinsic: Changes take place even in a "perfect" environment.
5. Deleterious: All changes comprise normal biological functions.

He also stated that ageing is a set of changes that occur in post-reproductive life and that cause a decrease in the body's ability to maintain homeostasis—the regulation of biological processes for efficiency and survival. Older people show some typical ageing signs—wrinkles, grey hair, etc. These depend on the ageing process or the individual's lifestyle (environmental and social factors) and their possible prevention.

Advanced age is not an undifferentiated experience. It is important to know that the idea of successful ageing includes longevity and quality of life [6]. The following aspects are considered important for interaction: social involvement and participation, disease reduction and promoting of physical and mental activity.

The word "old" no longer has a positive meaning. Nowadays, it is taken as explicit repudiation, unkindness or as sign of disrespect. Almost nobody likes to be treated as sir or madam. It is a sign that ageing is happening and it is visible to others [7].

New expressions such as "third age", "senior citizens" or "middle aged" appear as an attempt to extend the boundaries of age, leaving them undefined.

"It leads to the anguish of age and wrinkles, obsessions such as health, eating, hygiene, controlling (check-up) and maintenance (sauna massage, sports, diets) rituals, solar cults and therapeutics (over-consumption of medical and pharmaceutical products)" [8].

For the first time in history, most people in societies like ours can make plans about their future ageing, namely, in its affective life.

Third age and ageing are currently associated to a set of negative stereotypes, with adverse consequences for individuals belonging to this age group and the society in which they live.

A new report from the United Nations Population Fund (UNFPA) [9] in 2012 estimated that the number of people over 60 years old on the planet will increase by almost 200 million in the next 10 years. Data shows that the older adult population will surpass the milestone of one billion people. In 2050, they will reach two billion people, or 20% of the world population, and by 2025 about 10.4% of the older adult population in the world will have more than 65 years old. It is estimated that in Europe alone, it will be about 21%, which is expected to happen between 2000 and 2025, showing an increase of about 3.5% worldwide [10]. According to UNFPA [9], the ageing population will be more visible in emerging countries. Nowadays, two in every three people with the age of 60 or more live in developing countries. In 2050, this number will rise to about four in every five people. The report shows that 47% of older adult men and 24% of older women still participate actively in the labour market. However, data shows that many older adults around the world are victims of abuse, discrimination and violence. The report calls on governments, civil society and the general public to work together in order to stop these destructive practices and invest in older people. "In economic terms, contrary to popular belief, a large number of older people contribute to their families, supporting financially younger generations and national and local economies, by paying taxes", the report states.

The evolutionary psychology clinic believed that evolutionary changes that occurred in humans during childhood/adolescence up to old age were universal, unidimensional, unidirectional and irreversible.

Stable capabilities in adulthood were followed by a "fatal" mental deterioration of old age!

Nowadays, it claims that there are different mental capacities/intellectuals with different evolutions, leaving the idea of being a single whole. It is for the affective life of each person (and its dimension).

Traditionally it has been said that men and women experience ageing in a different manner. Women are associated to an earlier age; masculinity is associated with qualities such as competence, autonomy and self-control, being these qualities more "resistant" to ageing. In women, qualities such as beauty and the ability to procreate are more valued, being these qualities most affected by premature ageing. There are all kinds of stereotypes associated with ageing, being the association between ageing and dementia too wide that even forgetfulness/memory impairment and the lack of learning ability are factors that are considered normal in the process of ageing older adults. When retirement age arrives, it is a time of decisions for them older adults, and it becomes a void impossible to fill. It comes with the fear of passivity and depending on third parties is an almost inevitable factor. Other negative stereotypes associated with ageing are social isolation, health problems/pain, disinterest and the inability to perform sexually and manage one's own life.

The secret for a successful ageing: traditionally, it is one in which the bodies have developed the ability to camouflage any sign or trace that shows the sense of time. The ideal body in our time is not the longevity body nor the curvilinear one, but the body that transgresses the boundaries of time: no age body and timeless body. All these new ideas are very important to consider a new time for the sexuality of older people.

Longevity is something relatively new in human history, and it still does not know much about the dynamics between the older adult and one's environment, particularly regarding issues related with sexuality.

There is a set of biopsychosocial influences that allow women to maintain the lifestyle they had before menopause: the level of professional fulfilment, their positive body image (they feel that they still retain some of their youth, being attractive without the apparent fear of ageing), a tight gratifying sexual behaviour and a responsible role in the family by being active and involved in decisions related to the organisation of domestic life, especially in guiding children [11].

Culture in its broadest sense can alter the physiology of women. Studies around the world show that the prevalence of heat in menopausal women ranges from 0% in women of Mayan culture up to 80% in women of German culture [12].

When we talk about clinical sex, we cannot forget to mention the pioneering work of Masters and Johnson [13], a pair of American therapists who unwrapped the model of defining the sexual response cycle, which comprises four phases—excitement, orgasm, plateau and resolution. This, some years later, was modified by Ellen Kaplan [14] with the inclusion of the initial phase of the triphasic desire model of sexual response—desire (excitement), orgasm and resolution. This consideration for desire is important in many psychiatric conditions [15]. On the other hand, studies performed by Masters and Johnson [16] reported that sexuality in older people is seen as a reduction in sexual response—progressively with age, in which the factors to consider are annoyance with partner (a), fatigue, physical or mental illness or the fear of failing.

In recent years, there have been several criticisms made upon these concepts, which are at the basis of sexual dysfunction classifications, embodied in DSM-III (1980) [17], since such classifications do not seem to fit in certain multicultural populations.

Menopause has some symptoms that are usually transient and harmless, yet they are unpleasant and sometimes disabling. Estimates are that by the year 2030, 1200 million women will be menopausal. For women in menopause, sexual intercourse is debilitating and advances ageing and death. Satisfaction with sexual intercourse after menopause decreases considerably, and older women still enjoy sex, even when they were probably sexually disturbed when they were young. Older people with chronic illnesses or disabilities should refrain from sexual relations [12].

In some classic books on Sex of famous sexologist, like Kraft-Ebing at the end of XIX century and H. Ellis in the second third of XX century,

it's a possibility to meet some prejudices in relation to old people sexuality reflecting the social and cultural values of each social era.

H. Ellis wrote (1933) "There is a frequent and well-marked tendency in women for a rush of sexual desire in menopause - the last flame of a dying fire that can easily cover some morbid aspects. Similarly, in humans, when years start to take their toll, sex drive can suddenly become urgent and this last exacerbation of sexuality is even more dangerous when translated into an attraction for young girls and acts of indecent familiarity with children" [18].

Krafft-Ebing [19] describes sexuality in older people as perverse as Ellis [18] have decades later, mentioning that there is a frequent and well-marked tendency in women for a rush of sexual desire in menopause – the last flame of a dying fire that can easily cover some morbid aspects. Similarly, in humans, when years start to take their toll, sex drive can suddenly become urgent, and this last exacerbation of sexuality is even more dangerous when translated into an attraction for young girls and acts of indecent familiarity with children.

A study performed by Kinsey et al. [20, 21] and presented in their important books on sexual behaviour of american male and female showed that in a total of 12,000 interviews, only 186 individuals were over 65 years old, and in a total of 1646 pages only 7 were aimed at sexuality in seniors.

At this point, it becomes essential to advise and show some techniques that can help in improving performance and ageing. Some of them are the changing of sexual techniques (caresses, kisses, etc.), a greater relaxation and genital stimulation, via manual or oral appeal and with medication, if necessary [22]. It has been said that "All dysfunctions increase with age, except for lubrication, which reaches its maximum at the onset of menopause" [23] and the possibility that "Older men might experience more pleasure and intimacy during coitus than younger ones" [24].

Parenting is one of the most important periods of adult life transition for both men and women and even for homosexual couples [25].

The role of physicians (including psychiatrists and gynaecologists) regarding sexuality in the climacteric and old age should consider the effective treatment of menopausal problems, particularly sexual changes in women and ageing in men, oral treatment for erectile dysfunction and detection of side effects caused by psychotropic medication in sexual performance. Certainly, endocrine support might be necessary.

Sexuality is necessary for the physical and mental well-being of older adults. Sexual practices are the same in all ages and might be satisfactory for the couple.

The second half of the twentieth century produced a series of changes in social morality that founded the so-called sexual revolution. Eroticism in old age was subsequently caused for deep reflexion—the "modernization of old age".

In 1969, American gerontologist Butler [26] defined a form of discrimination against old age as "ageism", which comprised grouped prejudices similar to those related to race, religion and ethnicity. Butler underlined the stereotypes about the relationship between age and fatigue, sexual disinterest, intellectual slowness, the inability to learn, unproductiveness and moodiness.

As it happens in other ages of life, it has the overall aim of promoting the development and optimisation of the best human possibilities in the field of interpersonal relations in general and sex in particular.

In the counselling of older adults there are some mistakes that should be avoided:

1. Transmitting a young and coital model about sexuality that causes anxiety.
2. Conveying a vision of things that disqualifies all one's past life and makes one feel frustrated or finished.
3. Forgetting that all people, even older adults, are in need of emotional ties, especially to dispose of attachment figures, and of a network of social relationships.
4. Advising practices contrary to the wishes of religious or cultural beliefs of the older adults themselves.

Affection helps in recreating sex, and nonverbal communication takes on new dimensions and becomes a necessity, as in another phase of mere instinctual discharge. Somehow, the tryst helps to recreate the meaning of life; it gives us another taste and harmony. In 1990, Vega [27] said that older adults had a 46.3% need for affection, 43% need for medical care, 26.6% need for less isolation and 11.5% need for more family affection.

After 60 and 70 years of age, being happy is not necessarily a race against time, against oneself, in order to succeed in professional careers and to test the physical and intellectual abilities, often close to the limit of individual resistance. The emotional needs of an individual above 60 years old are more important that all that. Older adults, after this age, want to live in serenity in order to have a mutual understanding with their life partner, and patience and tolerance to guide their interpersonal relationships within the family through tenderness and friendship, while having an active sex life.

By the end of the twentieth century, the prospect became more optimistic, with a new attitude about sexuality in old age, a line of postmodern discourse, relativizing certain moral parameters and discourses of power that establish a temporal perspective with strict limits. So Moody [28] proposes the course of postmodern life as being an extension of adult age (adulthood in two directions—backwards with the disappearance of childhood and forth with the disappearance of old age).

So, humans will live especially at an age dictated by adult age that incorporates the ideas of responsibility, autonomy and diversified consumption [29].

Although ageing is significantly linked to a decrease in various aspects of male sexual activity, satisfaction in personal relationships and satisfaction in sexual performance do not decline with age. Even some people who have a reduced number of erections during sleep and penile rigidity report, as well as their partners, that they are in regular and satisfying relationships.

To be in a healthy and active ageing process, it is essential to discover new things that have not yet been taught. Living the new, the unexpected, doing what has been done before but differently, seeing what has been seen before but differently, discarding what has been learned (old) and embracing the unknown (new).

The nonverbal communication takes on new dimensions and becomes a necessity, as another phase of mere instinctual discharge. Somehow, the romantic encounter helps to recreate the meaning of life; it gives you another taste.

Middle-aged sexuality and "greater age" lead us to a sense of harmony and tenderness, with the progressive removal of biological turbulence (hormonal, but not only) and conflict within an harmonious relationship with the environment, profession and family.

Predictors of sexual interest and sexual activity in older people include the couple's previous level of sexual activity, physical and psychological health, availability, interest and health. These factors are similar in both heterosexual and homosexual people [30]. Older people residing in institutions are less sexually active than older people living in communities. Only 10% are sexually active, while 20% showed interest in sex [31].

In this line of thought, it is consistent to introduce the concept of self-realisation, understood as the personal dynamics and ability that each human body has of upgrading its own capabilities, keeping true to the more fundamental individual references. We dare to say, as Patterson [32] states, that "self-realization is the only basic motivation of all human beings". Nowadays, most seniors have a satisfying and more frequent sex life. There is a new concept of "sexual maturity" for older adults.

Some things to take into account: sexual pleasure in the older adult is not just a matter of genital erection or orgasm; it is also what is provided by touch or oral contact. The level of pleasure is probably the best index of sexual activity in older people. It is important to remember that it is possible to have orgasms without an erection and that orgasms change greatly in their features.

There is few data on homosexuality in older people; an article published by Berger [33] in 1984 that focuses on levels of global adjustment in older adult homosexuals but does not deal with their sexuality [22]. It is necessary to have more research in this area of sexuality.

"You know that, as age advances, prejudice in all sectors of life is also present, particularly in sexual ones (myths and taboos). We can say that these prejudices are some of the worst and cruellest ones to the human person. It is said that older people have no more interest in sex that they do not need sex and it is ugly when they think or do it. However, if we look at the biology of these people, they would present ample capacity for sexual fulfilment" [34].

19.1 Conclusion

In overview it is fundamental for the promotion of sexual health in older adults to have the primary care physicians prepared to understand the sexuality context of the ageing woman and man. At the same time, that should deal of specific problems of sexual dysfunctions.

To finish this general overview on sexuality in the process of ageing, it is important to consider thinking that "sex" is a gift for the young is beyond unfair; it is absurd. Age is no barrier for having an active sex life! And that sexuality should contribute for the discovery of experiences and emotions that are timeless and should last until the heat disappears from the body.

As last comment in a world where the pharmaceutic means use to be prescribed frequently as a frequent solution in sexual medicine for older adults, we should have in mind that "Tenderness is the best emotional growth and enabling co-existence of human beings" [35].

Sexual difficulties should form part of general health assessment of older adults. Family doctors should not assume that there are no problems. The assessment should be sensitive to the patient's cultural beliefs and respect their dignity.

References

1. WHO. The world health report 2001. Mental health: new understanding, new hope. Geneva: World Health Organization; 2001.
2. WHO. The world health report 1975. Education and treatment in human sexuality: the training of health professionals. Geneva: WHO; 1975. Technical Report Series No. 572.

3. Mezzich J, Hernandez-Serrano R. Psychiatry and sexual health: an integrative approach. Edwardsville: RLP Group, Inc; 2006.
4. WPA. Programa educacional de saúde sexual. N.Y. 2001.
5. Strehler B. Time, cells and aging. New York/London: Academic; 1962.
6. Rowe JW, Kahn RL. Successful aging. New York: Pantheon/Random House; 1998.
7. Magalhães CS. A importância do domicílio para o idoso – O contributo do Serviço de Apoio Domiciliário. Dissertação de Mestrado. Polo Braga: Universidade Católica Portuguesa. 2012.
8. Lypovetsky G. A era do vazio – ensaio sobre o individualismo contemporâneo. Lisboa: Relógio D'Agua; 1997.
9. UNFPA. United Nations Population Fund. 2012. ISBN: 978-0-89714-007-2.
10. World Population Prospects: The 1998 Revision. Volume 3. United Nations Publications. 2000.
11. Hilditch JR, Lewis J, Peter A, et al. A menopause-specific quality of life questionnaire: development and psychometric properties. Maturitas. 1996;24:161–75.
12. Payer L. The menopause in various cultures. In: Burger H, Bullet M, editors. A portrait of menopause. Park Ridge: Parthenon; 1991. Portuguese Society of Menopause (2006). Portugal.
13. Masters W, Johnson V. Human sexual response. Boston: Brown and Company; 1966.
14. Kaplan HS. The new sex therapy. London: Baillière-Tindall; 1974.
15. Kaplan HS. Hypoactive sexual desire. J Sex Marital Ther. 1977;3:3–9.
16. Masters W, Johnson V. Human sexual incompatibility. Buenos Aires: Inter Médica; 1976.
17. American Psychiatric Association (APA). Diagnostic and statistical manual of mental disorders. 3rd ed. Washington, DC: American Psychiatric Association; 1980.
18. Ellis H. Psychology of sex. 2nd ed. London: Heineman Publisher; 1933.
19. Kraft-Ebing. Psychopathia sexualis. 1st ed. Stuttgart: Verlag von Ferdiand Enke; 1886.
20. Kinsey A, Pomeroy W, Martin C. Sexual behavior in the human male. Philadelphia: Saunders; 1948.
21. Kinsey A, Pomeroy W, Martin C, et al. Sexual behavior in the human female. Philadelphia: Saunders; 1953.
22. Dominguez A. La Sexualidade en un adulto mayor. 2005.
23. Osborn M, Hawton K, Gath D. Sexual dysfunction among middle aged women in the community. Br Med J. 1988;296:959–62.
24. Janus S, Janus C. The Janus report on sexual behaviour. New York: Wiley; 1993.
25. Palha AP, Lourenço MF. Psychological and cross-cultural aspects of infertility and human sexuality, vol. 31. Basel: Karger Publishers; 2011. p. 164–83.
26. Butler R. Age-ism: another form of bigotry. The Gerontologist. 1969;9:243–6.
27. Vega W. Hisparüc families in the 1980s: a decade of research. J Marriage Fam. 1990;52:1015.
28. Moody H. Ethics in aging society. Baltimore: John Hopkins University. Press; 1993.
29. Iacub R. Proyetar la Vida: El desafio de los Mayores. Buenos Aires: Ediciones Manantial; 2001.
30. Klingman EW. Office evaluation of sexual function and complaints. Clin Geriatr Med. 1991;7(1):15–39.
31. Spector IP, Fremeth SM. Sexual behaviors and attitudes of geriatric residents in long-term care facilities. J Sex Marital Ther. 1996;22:235–46.
32. Patterson CH. The therapeutic relationship. Monterey. 1985
33. Berger RM. Realities of gay and lesbian aging. Soc Work. 1984;29(1):57–62.
34. Lopes G. Sexualidade Humana. 2ª edição ed. Rio de Janeiro: Medsi; 1993. p. 77–81. ISBN: 85-7199-058-1.
35. Pasini W. O Amor e Tempo. Livraria Civilização Editora. 2000.

Part VI

Neurocognitive Disorders (and Problems) in Older Adults in Primary Care

Manuel Coroa, Horácio Firmino, Vasco Nogueira, and Luiz Miguel Santiago

Abstract

Delirium is a common and serious acute neuropsychiatric syndrome and is known to increase the risk for subsequent functional decline and mortality. The etiologies of delirium are diverse and multifactorial and often reflect the pathophysiological consequences of an acute medical illness, medical complication or drug intoxication. Delirium can have a widely variable presentation and is often missed and underdiagnosed as a result. At this chapter we discuss the prediction, etiology, prevention, diagnosis, subtypes and treatment (pharmacological and non-pharmacological) of delirium in the elderly population.

Key Points
- Delirium is a common, preventable condition and can be a medical emergency.
- Delirium amongst older adults is largely underdiagnosed and often leads to long, costly hospital admissions.
- There are validated, effective and easy-to-use screening and diagnostic tools.
- Due to the modifiable risk factors, prevention must be the way forward.

20.1 Introduction

Despite being a common and potentially reversible cause of behavioural disturbance, delirium has been largely ignored by health service planners and practitioners, which inadvertently aggravate and increase its incidence amongst older adults [1, 2], *leading to more expensive and longer hospitalization periods, as well as worse prognosis* [3].

The overwhelming lack of measures to prevent, manage and reduce its impact is bewildering, especially if we take the following aspects into consideration: the large amount of modifiable and non-modifiable risk factors and the potentially inducing drugs identified; the number of fast, simple, effective and validated tools for its screening and diagnostic; and the largely studied pharmacologic and non-pharmacologic interventions for its prevention and treatment.

M. Coroa · H. Firmino (✉)
Department of Psychiatry and Mental Health, Psychogeriatric Unit, Coimbra University Hospital Center, Coimbra, Portugal

V. Nogueira
Department of Psychological Medicine, Faculty of Medicine, University of Coimbra, Coimbra, Portugal

L. M. Santiago
Primary Health Care and General Practice of Faculty of Medicine of University of Coimbra, Coimbra, Portugal

© Springer Nature Switzerland AG 2019
C. A. de Mendonça Lima, G. Ivbijaro (eds.), *Primary Care Mental Health in Older People*,
https://doi.org/10.1007/978-3-030-10814-4_20

Delirium has been pointed as one of the top three conditions for which quality of care needs to improve [4].

20.2 Historical Background

Also known as "acute confusional state", "encephalitis" or "everyman's psychosis", delirium was first identified and described by Hippocrates and its peers (400–366 B.C). They have noticed the existence of an acute mental disorder accompanied by fever, behavioural alteration and sleep disruption with a severity degree directly linked to the severity of the fever and which was clearly different from those mental disorders with no apparent cause (dementia).

In the later 1880s, the discovery of the cause-effect connection between syphilis and the so-called general paralysis of the insane (GPI or paralytic dementia) has factually proven that some mental disorders might be caused by an identifiable organic cause and consequently be treated.

Recently, there are some prevalence studies placing delirium as one of the most common complications of hospital admission for older patients [5] and linking its development to higher mortality and morbidity rates during and after the hospitalization period [6, 7]. There are also reports of a significant impact on healthcare economics, with an increase *of the hospitalization per day average cost of about 2½ times* [5].

Despite this, delirium remains an *underdiagnosed* syndrome with non-diagnostic rates as high as 72% and also some poor 2.7% of correct informatics codification [6–9].

These impressive findings unveil the urgent need to implement aggressive measures to assure its prevention, early diagnostic and correct management amongst healthcare professionals, family and other caretakers.

20.3 Epidemiology

On its majority, delirium prevalence studies ran in hospitalized patient estimate that it occurs in up to 30% of all medically ill patients, being

Table 20.1 Incidence and prevalence of delirium [8, 9]

Setting	% with delirium
Prevalence in hospitalized medically ill patients[a]	10–30%
Prevalence in hospitalized elderly patients	10–40%
Prevalence in hospitalized cancer patients	25%
Prevalence in hospitalized AIDS patients	30–40%
Prevalence in terminally ill patients	80%
Prevalence in hospice	29%
Prevalence in intensive care unit	
With mechanical ventilation	60–80%
Without mechanical ventilation	20–50%
Prevalence in community	
Persons 85 years or older	14%
Regardless the age	1%
Prevalence at hospital admission	10–31%
Prevalence in long-term care facility and postacute care	1–60%
Incidence during hospital admission after hip fracture	28–61%
Incidence during hospital admission after surgery	15–53%

[a]High-risk conditions and procedures include cardiotomy, hip surgery, transplant surgery, burns, renal dialysis and lesions of central nervous system

especially common amongst the elder, postoperative patients and terminally ill patients, with prevalence rates of around 80% for the latter [8]. See Table 20.1.

A recent multicentric point prevalence study (*Delirium Day*), which involved 1867 older patients (aged 65 years or more) across 108 acute and 12 rehabilitation wards in Italian hospitals, concluded that delirium occurred in more than *one out of five patients* in acute and rehabilitation hospital wards, with higher prevalence in neurology wards (28.5%) and lower in rehabilitation wards (14.0%). Despite its inherent diagnosis difficulty degree, the commonest subtype of delirium was the hypoactive, followed by the mixed type, hyperactive and finally the nonmotoric [10].

Unfortunately, the epidemiology of this syndrome in primary health and community institutions is quite unknown and needs further work to be more accurately set. There is an estimated prevalence of 14% in persons above 85 years of age and around 1% regardless the age [9].

20.4   Etiology and Pathophysiology

Functional changes occur in a large number of neurotransmitters: the most frequent and best characterized are a reduction of cholinergic function and an increase in dopaminergic and gabaergic function, although alterations in almost all neurotransmitter systems (serotoninergic, noradrenergic, glutaminergic, histaminergic) have been found.

20.4.1 Microstructural Abnormalities and Delirium

A recent study has proved that microstructural abnormalities in the cerebellum, hippocampus, thalamus and basal forebrain are directly linked to increased delirium incidence and severity when controlling for age, vascular comorbidities, gender and baseline cognitive performance [11].

20.4.2 Acetylcholinesterase Activity Levels as Predictor

In a cohort study, low preoperative acetylcholinesterase activity levels correlated positively with the postoperative development of delirium [12].

20.4.3 The Neuroinflammatory Hypothesis of Delirium

There is consistent evidence that the liberation of inflammatory mediators to the blood stream caused by acute peripheral stimulation may also induce an acute inflammatory response in the central nervous system. This inflammatory stress subsequently generates neurobehavioural and cognitive symptoms due to neuronal and synaptic dysfunction.

The reflex central response produces a complex multifactorial inflammatory axis characterized by dysfunction of the brain-blood barrier, neurochemical disturbances with decrease of the acetylcholine activity and an increase of dopamine and norepinephrine and consequent disconnection of brain areas.

Also, some identified risk factors (e.g. age and neurodegenerative disorders) work as response amplifiers, exaggerating the microglial activation following systemic inflammatory events.

This mutual influence is the result of multiple communication pathways that allow the brain to be continuously monitoring the immune state of the body and promptly react through the hypothalamic-pituitary-adrenal (HPA) axis whenever there is an activation of the innate immune system [13].

20.5   Clinical Aspects: What Is It?

"Delirium is primarily a disturbance of consciousness, attention, cognition, and perception but can also affect sleep, psychomotor activity, and emotions. It is a common psychiatric illness among medically compromised patients and may be a harbinger of significant morbidity and mortality" [14].

The *global disorder of cognitive functions and attention with altered awareness and consciousness constitute the cardinal features of this syndrome.* Sleep-wake cycle disruption, abnormal activity status and responsiveness are considered additional. Delirium is also characterized by having an acute onset and a tendency to fluctuate along the day, being usually worse at night. Prodromal symptoms such as insomnia, anxiety, drowsiness and nightmares may precede the fully developed syndrome [15].

These symptoms must constitute a significant difference from the patient's usual status and must not be better explained by any other subjacent mental disorder. In addition, there should be supportive evidence linking them to an undergoing physiological event, medical disease, trauma, drug intoxication/abstinence, etc. Also, they usually *revert* (completely or partially) with the resolution of the causing event. Unfortunately it is still considered an innocuous and inevitable consequence of hospitalized patients.

The constellation of signs and symptoms presented is no more than the manifestation of the neurophysiological alterations directly or indirectly induced by one of the underlying processes previously mentioned.

20.6   Clinical Subtypes

According to its clinical presentation, it may be divided in three main subtypes: *hyperactive, mixed and hypoactive*.

20.6.1 Hyperactive Subtype

It is the least common and the most frequently diagnosed subtype of delirium [16]. Patients with hyperactive delirium are restless and demanding an extraordinary amount of attention from staff, inclusively during the night, and might as well interact negatively with other patients, which usually are unable to share the room with these other.

Mydriasis, tachycardia, profuse sweating, flushed face, tremors, hypertension, fear and rage may appear as a result of the increased sympathetic activity found in this patients [15].

20.6.2 Hypoactive Subtype

This hypoactive subtype of delirium, unlike the hyperactive, is the most difficult to diagnose, and, unfortunately, it is positively linked to increased mortality rate, advanced age, palliative care, number of comorbidities and severity [17]. It is clinically characterized by sedation, psychomotor and consciousness impairment and low-debt speech [18].

20.6.3 Mixed Subtype

This clinical subtype of delirium combines characteristics from both hypoactive and hyperactive phenotypes, as patients usually present a cyclic agitation-sedation alternation along the day, being the hypoactive phase more frequent at night [16]. Its prevalence is usually reported as the highest, accounting for approximately half of the cases. However, there are prevalence studies and authors that report a higher prevalence for the hypoactive subtype, which is explained by its higher probability of escaping diagnosis. These prevalence variations might also be influenced by the sample dimension, the kind of nursery ward and hospital or even by the assessment methods used and the subjective nature of the scoring.

20.7   Predisposing and Precipitating Factors

In elder people, delirium is rarely caused by one single factor, and is commonly associated with medical and surgical illness, intoxication, withdrawal states and central nervous system disease [16].

Checking the patient's socio-demographic information, lifestyle habits, medical and surgical antecedents as well as the chronic medication list (including the self-prescript and alternative medicine ones) should be enough to the delirium's predisposing and precipitating factors, as well as the potentially inducing drugs (e.g. tricyclic antidepressants, high-potency anti-histaminic drugs, etc.) (Table 20.2).

There are numerous predisposing factors for delirium. Age > 65 year's old is surely the most important, not only by normal ageing physiologic alterations (e.g. brain-blood barrier vulnerability, lower functional reserve, sleep quality loss, tendency to fall, etc.) but also by the higher number of comorbid pathology associated (e.g. dementia, diabetes, renal insufficiency, cancer, etc.) [9]. As expected, the higher number of comorbid pathology is linked with polypharmacy, increasing the risk of noxious drug interactions and side effects.

Epidemiologic data places patients with terminal illness as the most vulnerable for developing delirium, justifying special attention.

The use of physical restraints, malnutrition, more than three medications added, use of bladder catheter and any iatrogenic event may be considered independent delirium precipitating factors in hospital environment, being all modifiable and having a cumulative effect with each other and with the predisposing factors [19].

Table 20.2 Predisposing and precipitating factors for delirium

Predisposing factors	Precipitating factors	Delirium-inducing medications
Demographic factors Age > 65 years Male sex	*Acute insults* Dehydration Fracture Hypoxia/ischemia Infection Medications Metabolic derangement Severe illness Shock Surgery Uncontrolled pain Urinary or stool retention	*Avoid on patients with high risk of developing delirium** Anticholinergics Antipsychotics Benzodiazepines Chlorpromazine Corticosteroids H2-receptor antagonists Cimetidine Famotidine Nizatidine Ranitidine Meperidine Sedative hypnotics
Comorbidities/conditions/events Dementia Depression Elder abuse Falls History of delirium Malnutrition Polypharmacy Pressure ulcers Sensory impairment Premorbid state Inactivity Poor functional status Social isolation Alcoholism Chronic pain History of baseline lung, liver, kidney, heart, or brain disease Terminal illness	*Environmental exposures* Intensive care unit Sleep deprivation Tethers	

Adapted from Kalish et al. [9]
*Evaluate risk/benefit ratio

Acute insults such as acute bacterial/viral infection, fractures, metabolic alterations, intense uncontrolled pain, hypoxia and ischemia and sleep deprivation are also consistently appointed as precipitating factors [20, 21].

20.8   Diagnostic

The diagnostic is essentially based on clinical skills, depending on the healthcare professionals concern and ability to recognize the core signs and symptoms.

Obtaining side information from family, friends and previous caretakers about the patient's baseline neurocognitive state also plays a crucial role in the diagnostic. This simple and so often forgotten step is often enough to determine the mode of the symptomatic onset (acute vs. chronic), which is essential for the distinction between delirium, dementia and depression.

The clinical evaluation of these patients must always include a scrupulous objective exam. *Vital sign measurement* and all the other basic procedures are usually enough to guide further complementary procedures or might even unveil the underlying cause.

Hydro-electrolytic alterations screening; renal and hepatic function assessment; complete blood count, blood cultures and arterial blood gas pressure; endocrinal function study; electrocardiography and electroencephalography; and drug abuse screening should be considered according to the presented symptoms and clinical suspicion. See Table 20.3.

Table 20.3 Evaluation of potential causes for delirium based on clinical suspicion

Suspicion	Evaluation
Cardiovascular disease	Electrocardiography
	Troponin and myoglobin serum levels
	d-Dimers and fibrinogen measurement
Hypovolemia	Assess dehydration or blood loss
	Complete blood count
	Urine-specific gravity test
	Blood urea/nitrogen ratio
Endocrine disease	Measurement of thyroid hormones
	Cortisol measurements
	Serum glucose levels
	ACTH stimulation test
Gastrointestinal disease	Liver function assessment
	Amylase and lipase serum levels
	Simple orthostatic (tangential) abdominal X-ray
	Abdominal CT
Infectious disease	Blood cultures
	Complete blood count
	Chest radiography
	Computed tomography
	Lumbar puncture
	Acute phase markers
	Urinalysis with culture
	Skin examination
Renal disease	Creatinine
	Blood urea/creatinine ratio
	Serum electrolyte measurement
Nutritional problems	Measurement Vit. B12 levels
	Folate measurement
	Albumin and pre-albumin measurement
Neurologic disease	Extended neurological examination
	Head-CT
	Electroencephalography
	Lumbar puncture
Respiratory difficulty	Pulse oximetry
	Arterial blood gas measurement
	Chest X-ray
	Oral obstruction inspection
Pain	Assess the severity
	Watch out for potential delirium-inducing analgesics

(continued)

Table 20.3 (continued)

Suspicion	Evaluation
Substance/drug abuse	Review of social, occupational and drug exposure history
	Urine drug screening
	Acetaminophen dosing
	Serum alcohol levels
	Serum salicylate levels
Medication-induced	Medication reconciliation
	Special attention to anticholinergic drugs
	History of previous adverse reactions

20.9 Diagnostic Tools

With a sensitivity range from 46 to 100%, the Confusion Assessment Method (CAM) scale is considered the *gold standard* tool to diagnose delirium [22]. It has been used on over 4000 published studies, and it's available in 12 different languages [23]. It allows the diagnostic and severity assessment of delirium and inclusively might be used for screening purposes.

Regarding the improvement of the home-care quality to patients with or in-risk of developing delirium, the Hospital Elder Life Program (HELP) has developed the *Family Assessment Method (FAM-CAM)*, which is based on a shortened version of CAM and can also be used by trained family members to early detect and evaluate delirium (http://hospitalelderlifeprogram.org/private/fam-cam-disclaimer.php?pageid=01.09.00). It has already been validated, and a study with 58 caretakers has reported *sensitivity up to 88% and a specificity of 98%*, with high correlation with CAM [11, 12, 22]. See Table 20.4.

As a matter of fact, delirium is far from being restricted to the geriatric population, as it also occurs within the paediatric patients, especially in intensive care units (ICU). This acknowledgement led to the development of the *Paediatrics CAM-ICU*, which actually represents a simplified adaptation from the original CAM to match the verbal and non-verbal expected development of a normal 5-year-old child [24].

Table 20.4   Delirium assessment scale summary

Scale	Average time taken	Applicable by	Screening	Diagnosis	Severity	Sensitivity (S) and specificity (Sp)
Confusion Assessment Method (CAM)	<5 min	Non-psychiatrist clinicians	V	V	V	S: 46–100%[a] Sp: 63–100%[b]
Family Assessment Method (FAM-CAM)	<5 min	Trained interviewer	V	V	V	S: 65–88% Sp: 98%
Nursing Delirium Screening Scale (NDSS)	1 min	Nurses	V	V		S: 85.7% Sp: 86.8%
NEECHAM confusion scale	10 min	Nurses	V			S: 95% Sp: 78%
Confusion State Evaluation	< 30 min	Nurses, physicians, psychologists		V	V	
Paediatrics CAM-ICU (pCAM-ICU)						S: 83% Sp: 99%
Delirium Observation Screening Scale (DOSS)	5–10 min	Research assistant		V		
Delirium Rating Scale-Revised-98 (DRS-R-98)	16 min	Psychiatrist				
4-AT	2 min	Trained interviewer	V	V		S: 89.7% Sp: 84.1%

Adapted Grover and Kate [24]

[a]Lower sensitivity ratings were reported when the scale was applied by nurses or research assistants

[b]Lower specificity ratings were reported when the evaluated patients had comorbid psychiatric pathology

Despite the existence of many specific delirium assessment scales, the use of general cognitive assessment tools such as the *Mini-Mental State Exam* (MMSE), the *Montreal Cognitive Assessment* (MoCA) and the *General Practitioner assessment of Cognition* (GPCOG) is highly recommended. Their results are invalid when applied in acute confusional states, but they can and should be used in clinical practice to assess the clinical features included in delirium screening/diagnostic "scales" like CAM. If available, recent pre-delirium performance scores on these tests may be used to document the acute nature of the deficits.

20.10   Delirium vs. Dementia

To distinguish these two neurocognitive disorders based on a single observation of an unknown patient may be extremely difficult, even impossible, due to the large symptomatic overlap between them. Awareness and attention impairment, memory deficits, hallucinations, delusions, sleep-wake cycle disruption, agitation, sedation or even symp-

tom fluctuation (etc.) might be present on both. However, they often coexist and interact in poorly understood ways, being dementia a known predisposing factor for delirium and vice versa [25].

Delirium differs from other neurocognitive disorders by having a *fast onset* (hours to days), *link to medical condition* (e.g. infection, trauma, etc.), *substance intoxication/withdrawal and medication, potential reversibility* and *symptom length* (usually acute on delirium vs. permanent on dementia).

20.11   Prevention

To reduce the risk of developing delirium is important to reduce the risks which are known to be modifiable: use of eyeglasses and eating aids, provision of orienting information (as calendars and clock), objects that people have in their home, early mobilization, correction of dehydration, modification of unnecessary noise and stimuli, promotion of a good sleep hygiene and prevent urinary catheters and physical restraint.

20.12 Treatment

The essential part of the treatment is to *identify and solve/treat* the culprit event(s) (e.g. infection, hydro-electrolytic disturb, sensory impairment, etc.). Delirium's severity normally follows the result of the implemented measures to treat the "original" cause(s).

Behavioural control is fundamental to ensure the quality of the provided care. Agitated patients often difficult the healthcare professional's action (e.g. self-removal of venous accesses, self-injury, accidents, etc.).

Drug-induced cases are usually easily reverted with the suspension of the causing one(s). In privation cases (e.g. BZD, alcohol, etc.), the reintroduction of the missing drug or its substitution for an equivalent one is often successful.

20.12.1 Non-pharmacologic Interventions

"Nonpharmacologic interventions were defined as including behavioural interventions, monitoring devices, rehabilitation, environmental adaptations, psychological and social supports, medication reductions, complementary and alternative medicine, and system and process changes" [26]. Also, the diagnostic of delirium *is not* a formal indication for pharmacological treatment.

Training and educating delirium-specialized multidisciplinary teams (including physicians, nurses and other healthcare professionals) are recommended for improving the care quality ministered to elder patients and for preventing delirium. These teams are known to be more efficient on the evaluation, diagnostic and application of pharmacological and non-pharmacological prevention and treatment. They also allow multicomponent interventions, which are highly recommended by experts, who also recommend its formal inclusion in hospital healthcare plans.

Also, the establishment of a solid and trustful relationship between the healthcare professionals, caretakers and the patient's family should be granted. Educating close family members and caretakers is crucial for the post-discharge period

outcome, preventing readmissions through the correction of the assessed modifiable risk factors and by increasing the early identification probability of an eventual relapse.

20.12.2 Multicomponent Interventions (MCI)

The latest NICE guidelines on this matter state that patients should be evaluated within the first 24 h (counting from hospital admission) and should benefit of a MCI comprehending a set of carefully designed individualized pharmacological and non-pharmacological interventions to be applied by a specialized team. This strategy reduces delirium incidence, and its duration and severity but has no apparent impact on mortality and institutionalization rate reduction [27].

Some examples of non-pharmacological interventions are time-space reorientation and cognitive stimulation, sensorial deficits correction (e.g. use of glasses and hearing aids), nasogastric and urinary probe removal (as soon as possible) and promotion of toileting routines, physical immobilization avoidance and early mobilization, to provide an environment with adequate levels of sensorial stimulation and adequate nutritional and hydric support and promote sleep hygiene routines. These interventions combined with a rational pharmacological use to control some of the predisposing/precipitating factors (e.g. effective pain control and *anticholinergic drug use avoidance*) are able to reduce delirium rates in one-third [26].

20.13 Pharmacological Measures

Delirium symptom-aimed pharmacologic measures (e.g. antipsychotic drugs for agitation or hallucinations) should only be considered when non-pharmacological interventions are not successful and if the patient's behaviour represents danger for himself and to third ones or creates an important obstacle to the assistance quality.

When controlling the exuberant agitation and other behavioural disruptions often found in delirium, which occurs mostly at night, inexperienced clinicians might use high doses of antipsychotic and other sedative drugs. A careless pharmacological intervention might perpetuate delirium and convert a hyperactive subtype into hypoactive one (with the associated increase in the morbidity and mortality rates), and, in severe cases, patients can be found almost comatose in the day after.

There is no consensus on the timing or the best drug to use in any of these situations; however, there is evidence supporting the benefits of the implementation of pharmacological therapy within the first 24 h (counting from the diagnostic) in ICU patients [28, 29].

- Behavioural control with low doses of haloperidol [0.25–0.5–3 mg per day, I.M. (I.V. formulations should be only used on ICU)] is the best option for treating hyperactive delirium symptoms due to its pharmacokinetic and pharmacodynamics properties (low anticholinergic and low sedative effects). Low doses of risperidone (0.5–1 mg per day) can be used as an alternative on haloperidol intolerance cases [30, 31].
- Kishi et al. [32] concluded that second-generation antipsychotics are more effective and safer than haloperidol for treating delirium, despite the lack of large sample comparative studies. Also, there were no significant effectiveness and outcome differences reported between risperidone and olanzapine and between amisulpride and quetiapine [32].

Some authors describe a "subclinical" type of delirium, a clinical situation where the diagnostic criteria are only partially fulfilled, and a single study points that risperidone was effective on reducing the probability of progression to a full-blown delirium [33].

However, due to the actual lack of evidence, the usage of antipsychotic drugs for preventing delirium in elder patients is not recommended [26].

Until this moment all cholinesterase inhibitors (e.g. rivastigmine) are contraindicated for preventing and treating delirium. However, a recent study shows that perioperative rivastigmine patch application could reduce the occurrence of postoperative delirium in older patients with low cognitive status, but it is necessary to obtain more evidence through further studies on a larger number of older patients with cognitive impairment [34].

Symptomatic control through benzodiazepines in single therapy should be avoided because of its known delirium precipitating and aggravating potential. Its usage is mainly reserved to specific types of delirium such as *delirium tremens* or benzodiazepine withdrawal syndrome. However, they might be helpful in the sleep-wake cycle regularization being lorazepam (0.5–1.5 mg per day) and oxazepam (7.5–15 mg per day) the best options [31].

Ondansetron, valproic acid, methylphenidate and gabapentin have also been tested, but the evidence of its benefit is very limited.

20.14 Special Types of Delirium

20.14.1 Delirium Tremens

Delirium tremens is caused by alcohol deprivation, and it has especially higher mortality rates (up to 35% if untreated). It is mostly characterized by the core clinical features of delirium plus exuberant and uncontrollable tremors, serious sense-perception alterations, including visual and tactile hallucinations, cardiac rhythm alterations and general autonomic dysfunction. The use of benzodiazepines qs has formal indication for preventing and treating *delirium tremens*. Oxazepam is the most frequently used because of its half-life and absence of hepatic metabolization. Gabapentin may also be used with the same purpose [35].

20.14.2 Benzodiazepine Withdrawal Syndrome

The *benzodiazepine withdrawal syndrome*, in severe cases, produces a spectrum of symptoms identic to those observed in *delirium tremens*, but, in spite of the latter, the first one develops slower (3–7 days after suspension). Benzodiazepine reintroduction (along with behavioural and symptomatic control) will often work [36].

20.15 Conclusions

- Delirium is underdiagnosed at old age population at primary care.
- Delirium is frequently appointed as the most frequent complication of hospital admission, leading to longer hospitalization periods, increased healthcare cost and higher morbidity and mortality rates.
- Delirium is an *underdiagnosed* syndrome, with non-diagnostic rates up to 72%, and also lacks the formal inclusion of effective prevention, detection, treatment and management strategies in health programmes.
- Prevention is the more important strategy to reduce the rate of delirium, with the known modifiable conditions.
- In most cases there is a secondary reason which can be resolved.
- "A LOAP (liaison old age psychiatry) service may play an important role for the early recognition of psychiatric conditions amongst elderly inpatients as well as the effective management and prevention of adverse outcomes, particularly for patients with delirium. The effective communication of these services with outpatient clinics, community mental health teams and day-care centers can be an important measure to reduce hospital readmissions and overutilization of health resources [21]".
- Further studies with larger samples and ingenious designs are needed to reduce the actual evidence limitation in some delirium-related features.

References

1. Inouye SK, Schlesinger MJ, Lydon TJ. Delirium: a symptom of how hospital care is failing older persons and a window to improve quality of hospital care. Am J Med. 1999;106(5):565–73.
2. McCusker J, et al. Environmental risk factors for delirium in hospitalized older people. J Am Geriatr Soc. 2001;49(10):1327–34.
3. Jorge-Ripper C, et al. Prognostic value of acute delirium recovery in older adults. Geriatr Gerontol Int. 2016;17(8):1161–7.
4. Fong TG, Tulebaev SR, Inouye SK. Delirium in elderly adults: diagnosis, prevention and treatment. Nat Rev Neurol. 2009;5(4):210–20.
5. Leslie DL, Inouye SK. The importance of delirium: economic and societal costs. J Am Geriatr Soc. 2011;5:S241–3.
6. Bellelli G, et al. Under-detection of delirium and impact of neurocognitive deficits on in-hospital mortality among acute geriatric and medical wards. Eur J Intern Med. 2015;26(9):696–704.
7. Gustafson Y, et al. Depression in old age in Austria, Ireland, Portugal and Sweden. Eur Geriatr Med. 2013;4(3):202–8.
8. Brown T, Boyle M. Delirium. Br Med J. 2002;325(7365):644.
9. Kalish VB, Gillham JE, Unwin BK. Delirium in older persons: evaluation and management. Am Fam Physician. 2014;90(3):150–8.
10. Bellelli G, et al. "Delirium Day": a nationwide point prevalence study of delirium in older hospitalized patients using an easy standardized diagnostic tool. BMC Med. 2016;14(1):106.
11. Cavallari M, et al. Neural substrates of vulnerability to postsurgical delirium as revealed by presurgical diffusion MRI. Brain. 2016;139(Pt 4):1282–94.
12. Cerejeira J, et al. Low preoperative plasma cholinesterase activity as a risk marker of postoperative delirium in elderly patients. Age Ageing. 2011;40(5):621–6.
13. Cerejeira J, Lagarto L, Mukaetova-Ladinska EB. The immunology of delirium. Neuroimmunomodulation. 2014;21(2–3):72–8.
14. Trzepacz P, et al. Treatment of patients with delirium. In: A.P. Association, editor. Practice Guidelines for the treatment of Psychatric Disorders. Arlington: American Psychiatric Association; 2006. p. 71.
15. Lipowski Z. Delirium (acute confusional states). JAMA. 1987;258(13):1789–92.
16. Hogg J. Delirium. In: Robert Jacoby CO, Dening T, Thomas A, editors. Oxford textbook of old age psychiatry. New York: Oxford University Press; 2008. p. 505–17.
17. Leonard M, et al. Phenomenological and neuropsychological profile across motor variants of delirium in a palliative-care unit. J Neuropsychiatry Clin Neurosci. 2011;23(2):180–8.
18. Diana Rafaela JC. Delirium. In: Horácio Firmino MRS, Cerejeira J, editors. Saude mental das pessoas mais velhas, vol. 291-304. Coimbra: LIDEL; 2016.
19. Inouye SK, Charpentier PA. Precipitating factors for delirium in hospitalized elderly persons: predictive model and interrelationship with baseline vulnerability. JAMA. 1996;275(11):852–7.
20. Cerejeira J, et al. The cholinergic system and inflammation: common pathways in delirium pathophysiology. J Am Geriatr Soc. 2012;60(4):669–75.

21. Nogueira V, et al. Improving quality of care: focus on liaison old age psychiatry. Ment Health Fam Med. 2013;10(3):153.

22. Inouye SK, et al. Clarifying confusion: the confusion assessment method: a new method for detection of delirium. Ann Intern Med. 1990;113(12):941–8.

23. Ely EW, et al. Evaluation of delirium in critically ill patients: validation of the Confusion Assessment Method for the Intensive Care Unit (CAM-ICU). Crit Care Med. 2001;29(7):1370–9.

24. Grover S, Kate N. Assessment scales for delirium: A review. WJP. 2012;2(4):58–70.

25. Fong TG, et al. The interface between delirium and dementia in elderly adults. Lancet Neurol. 2015;14(8):823–32.

26. Panel TAGSE. Postoperative delirium in older adults: best practice statement from the American Geriatrics Society. J Am Coll Surg. 2015;220(2):136–148. e1.

27. Holt R, Young J, Heseltine D. Effectiveness of a multi-component intervention to reduce delirium incidence in elderly care wards. Age Ageing. 2013;42(6):721–7.

28. Heymann A, et al. Delayed treatment of delirium increases mortality rate in intensive care unit patients. J Int Med Res. 2010;38(5):1584–95.

29. Michaud CJ, Thomas WL, McAllen KJ. early pharmacological treatment of delirium may reduce physical restraint use a retrospective study. Ann Pharmacother. 2013;48(3):328–34.

30. Morandi A, et al. Consensus and variations in opinions on delirium care: a survey of European delirium specialists. Int Psychogeriatr. 2013;25(12):2067–75.

31. Seitz DP, Gill SS, van Zyl LT. Antipsychotics in the treatment of delirium: a systematic review. J Clin Psychiatry. 2007;68(1):11–21.

32. Kishi T, et al. Antipsychotic medications for the treatment of delirium: a systematic review and meta-analysis of randomised controlled trials. J Neurol Neurosurg Psychiatry. 2015;87(7):767–74.

33. Hakim SM, Othman AI, Naoum DO. Early treatment with risperidone for subsyndromal delirium after on-pump cardiac surgery in the elderly a randomized trial. J Am Soc Anesthesiol. 2012;116(5):987–97.

34. Youn YC, et al. Rivastigmine patch reduces the incidence of postoperative delirium in older patients with cognitive impairment. Int J Geriatr Psychiatry. 2016;32(10):1079–84. https://doi.org/10.1002/gps.4569.

35. Myrick H, Malcolm R, Brady KT. Gabapentin treatment of alcohol withdrawal. Am J Psychiatr. 1998;155(11):1626j–1626.

36. Mackinnon GL, Parker WA. Benzodiazepine withdrawal syndrome: a literature review and evaluation. Am J Drug Alcohol Abuse. 1982;9(1):19–33.

Neurocognitive Disorders in Old Age: Alzheimer's Disease, Frontotemporal Dementia, Dementia with Lewy Bodies, and Prion and Infectious Diseases

21

Armin von Gunten, Eduardo Nogueira, Henk Parmentier, and Irênio Gomes

Abstract

Dementia is a clinical syndrome of cognitive decline resulting in impaired activities of daily living. It affects a person in their personhood, which, together with behavioural and psychological features, causes enormous suffering for both patient and caregiver.

Many diseases cause dementia, but neurodegenerative, vascular, and mixed disorders are most often involved. The type of dementia may influence the clinical presentation, its course, and the available therapeutic options. Thus, an aetiopathogenic assessment is crucial and includes somatic, cognitive, psychopathological, functional, and paraclinical investigations.

Most dementias have no cure although depression and substance-induced cognitive impairment are central differential diagnoses as they are potentially reversible when treated. Antidementia drugs have a limited indication. Psychosocial treatments, in particular of behavioural and psychological features, are paramount and often efficient. Medication, if required, complements psychosocial treatment. Treatment options must be evaluated dynamically as the patient and caregiver needs change over time.

Primary care is an essential component of the care provided to people with dementia, from early detection to treatment across all stages of the illness, to help alleviate patient and caregiver suffering.

A. von Gunten (✉)
Service de Psychiatrie de l'Age Avancé, Department of Psychiatry, University of Lausanne Medical Center (CHUV), Lausanne, Switzerland
e-mail: armin.von-gunten@chuv.ch

E. Nogueira · I. Gomes
Instituto de Gerontologia et Geriatria,
Pontifícia Universidade Católica do Rio Grande do Sul—PUCRS, Porto Alegre, Brazil

H. Parmentier
Woodstreet Medical Center, London, UK

Medical Faculty, Universidade NOVA de Lisboa, Lisbon, Portugal

Key Points
- Parallel to population ageing, the number of patients with dementia is increasing in nearly all countries of the world.
- While more than half of all the demented already live in low- and middle-income countries, this number is likely to rise to over 70% by 2050.
- Dementia is a syndrome caused by a variety of different diseases among which the mixed, neurodegenerative, and vascular disorders are the most common ones in the elderly.

© Springer Nature Switzerland AG 2019
C. A. de Mendonça Lima, G. Ivbijaro (eds.), *Primary Care Mental Health in Older People*,
https://doi.org/10.1007/978-3-030-10814-4_21

- Detecting cognitive impairment and diagnosing dementia are fundamentally important tasks for all general practitioners.
- Assessment is complex and multidimensional including somatic, cognitive, psychopathological, functional, and paraclinical investigations with the patient and their caregivers being the sources of information.
- Depression and substance-induced cognitive impairment are a central differential diagnosis as they may be treated causally and potentially be cured.
- Among, e.g. metabolic disorders, a number of infectious disorders must be looked for.
- For most dementias, however, there are no disease-modifying treatments.
- Enhancing the patient's quality of life is the central treatment aim.
- Treating the patients' comorbidities is paramount.
- Behavioural and psychological features of dementia must be looked for actively as they are usually accessible to efficient treatment. Treating behavioural and psychological symptoms is a crucial focus of treatment.
- Enhancing the patient's functional capacity is a further treatment aim.
- Antidementia drugs have a limited indication.
- Medication, if required, complements psychosocial treatment.
- Enhancing the caregivers' quality of life is a further aim to pursue.
- Treatment and care options have to be evaluated repeatedly over time as the patient and caregiver needs are likely to change constantly.

21.1 Introduction

Dementia has entered collective awareness as a major public health issue. As the occurrence of dementia is related to older age, its prevalence increases in parallel with the increase of human longevity. It has become one of the most frequent clinical conditions in the elderly in both high-income and middle- and low-income countries.

Dementia is in everybody's mouth not only as a result of its high frequency but also of the profound impact it has on a person. It affects a person in its intimacy and personhood and may cause enormous suffering and disability for those having the disease.

Dementia changes the lives not only for those who have it, but most of the time, it weighs heavily on family members and caregivers. Dementia comes with an enormous physical and psychological cost with many of the caregivers having excess morbidity and mortality as compared to those who do not have to care for a demented person [1].

The physical and psychological burden the caregivers are enduring cannot be estimated as easily as the economic costs of dementia which is thought to be as astronomic as 604 billion US$ worldwide in 2010 [2].

Dementia may be defined from a clinical perspective as a syndrome of cognitive or intellectual decline that is often progressive with the decline impacting by definition on activities of daily living. Dementia is caused by a number of diseases, more often than not neurodegenerative, vascular, and mixed disorders, but more rarely other conditions primarily or secondarily affecting the brain are involved. The type of dementia may influence the clinical presentation, its course, and the available therapeutic options. As dementia is often progressive, the needs are likely to change over the course of the disease.

Although most dementias have no cure and no disease-modifying treatments are available, much can be done to alleviate both the demented and their caregivers alike so as to improve their quality of life. An adequate response to the needs of people with dementia and their families usually requires a combination of medical, psychological, and social care interventions depending, among other factors, on the stage of the dementia. Primary care is an essential component of the care provided to people with dementia, from early primary prevention, early detection, and treatment in the most advanced stages of the illness [3].

21.2 The Dementia Syndrome

21.2.1 Epidemiology of Ageing and the Dementias

Over the twentieth century, a spectacular increase of the median longevity has occurred in humans with a further spurt during the second half of the century. This is primarily due to better living conditions and secondarily to medical progress. Thus, in less developed countries, the longevity increase is largely the result of much reduced mortality at younger ages, particularly in childhood, and from infectious disease [4]. In high-income countries, the continuing increase in life expectancy is now mainly due to the declining mortality at older ages [5].

The brunt of this increase is borne by the elderly segment of the population in high-income countries, but even in low-income countries, the proportion of the elderly is increasing rapidly. Thus, the proportion of persons 60 years or older currently exceeds 30% only in Japan, but by the middle of this century, many countries will have a similarly high proportion of older people [6]. Overall, there is evidence that the older the age segment the higher the relative increase. This evolution will go on for some time although limits are likely to be set by the vascular disease epidemics and, of course, maximal longevity in the human species. However, the evolution of the Swiss population is an example of the increasing proportion of the elderly in the general population. Thus, the number of those aged 20–64 years will be about 20% between 2010 and 2040, while the increase of those aged 80 years or more will be about 120% within the same time frame in the canton of Vaud (http://www.scris.vd.ch). Over the last 50 years or so, the number of nonagenarians increased by about 25 times and that of the centenarians by over 60 times. As mentioned, this development is not limited to high-income countries as it is also happening with some delay in most middle- but also low-

income countries. In the 1990s, the segment of those 60 or older took over those aged 12–24 years in terms of their total number. This phenomenon will be observed approximately by the fifth decade of this century in low- and middle-income countries, a major difference being the observation that the absolute number of the elderly in these countries will be much higher than that in high-income countries (http://www.imf.org/external/pubs/ft/fandd/2006/09/picture.htm).

Life expectancy has increased markedly, and this holds true for both life expectancy with or without incapacity. Some subjects may remain independent for long periods into older age, while others require help and care over extended periods of their lives. Older people are living longer, but the quality of these extra years is unclear [7]. It remains to be seen whether or not health at retirement and its evolution differ in the baby boomer generation compared to cohorts born before and during World War II.

The main risk factor for dementia is increasing age. Thus, the epidemiology of the dementia is likely to be similar to that of the general population with a substantial increase of those suffering from dementia in the older segments. Although the dementias are quite rare at the populational level at the age of 65 years—with perhaps 1–2% having dementia or 2–5% between 65 and 74 years—this prevalence rate is rocketing up exponentially in the older segments as it doubles every 5 years or so. Thus, 30–40% of those 85 years old or more and about half of the elderly aged 90 years, and more so beyond this age, have dementia [8, 9]. The syndrome affects approximately 5–8% of individuals over age 65, 15–20% of individuals over age 75, and 25–50% of individuals over age 85 [10]. How to define dementia in the oldest-old remain a challenge, and controversial and trustworthy prevalence and incidence data are still scarce in the oldest-old age group. However, recent preliminary results now indicate that dementia and Alzheimer's disease continue to rise also at very high ages with both incidence and prevalence of dementia being highest in the oldest-old [11, 12].

Worldwide, 35.6 million people have dementia, a number that will rise to 65.7 million in 2030 and 115.4 million in 2050 [13]. The average estimated prevalence of dementia for those aged 60 years or over, in all regions, is 4.7%. High-income countries still have a higher relative prevalence of dementia than low-income countries. However, while Europe and North America are expected to experience an increase of 40% and 63% respectively, a 117% growth in East Asia and a 134–146% growth in Latin America are forecast for the next 20 years. While more than half of all the demented (58%) currently live in low-income countries, this number is likely to rise to 71% by 2050 [14].

In high-income countries, where 35–50% of the people with dementia live in nursing homes [3], direct social care costs account for more than half of the total costs [15]. In low- and middle-income countries, where the large majority of people with dementia live at home and depend on care provided by their families, informal care costs represent two-thirds of the total costs. Overall, the costs of direct medical care represent a small part of all costs worldwide (around 16%), while the costs of informal care and the direct costs of social care amount to 42% of all costs worldwide. A large majority of the total global costs of dementia (89%) are incurred in high-income countries, 10% in middle-income countries, and less than 1% in low-income countries. However, less than half of the people with dementia live in high-income countries, 40% live in middle-income countries, and 14% live in low-income countries [14].

21.2.2 Clinics

21.2.2.1 Defining Dementia

Dementia is a syndrome rather than a disease characterized clinically by an acquired cognitive deficit sufficient enough to interfere negatively with the requirements of daily living. However, diagnosing dementia based on this definition is challenging as almost every term making up the description can be controversially defined. The debate will not be settled neither through DSM-V [16] nor the future ICD-11.

However, definitions evolve. Thus, the mandatory presence of a memory deficit to qualify for a diagnosis of dementia may favour the diagnosis of AD and discard what is more and more recognized as non-memory dementias such as those found, e.g. in vascular brain disorders. Although the requirement of a memory deficit is still part of the ICD-10 definition [17], this has already been changed in DSM-V and will been introduced in ICD-11.

The current tendency is to diagnose the underlying disease (AD, FTD, etc.), but this will not further the debate on when to consider someone as demented or as having a major neurocognitive impairment DSM-V denomination. For the time being, dementia is defined according to ICD-10 or DSM-V (Table 21.1) and the hopefully soon to come ICD-11.

Thus, dementia remains a syndrome and its diagnosis relies solely on history taking and clinical examination.

Despite much progress in the search of consensual definitions and clinical assessments, not all shadowy zones have been discarded. As an example, whether or not a dysexecutive syndrome leading to frontosubcortical memory impairment is to be considered a deficit of one or two cognitive domains, i.e. executive functioning and memory, remains speculative. This is of some importance as a diagnosis of dementia requires the presence of an impairment of at least two cognitive domains. The causal relationship between a cognitive deficit and a functional impairment, required to diagnose dementia, may be difficult in view of the presence of some other diseases handicapping the patient in their everyday activities. Although the diagnosis of dementia implies the presence of a threshold to be crossed how exactly this threshold is defined is still not entirely clear (cf. staging of dementia).

A patient's entry point into the clinical setting is often a memory or more generally a cognitive complaint either by the patient, a family member, or an informal caregiver. In these cases, an investigation of the complaint is warranted. However, the question of a systematic screening of cognitive disorders in the population remains ultimately unanswered despite the high prevalence of these disorders of perhaps 5% of those over 64 years of age [18] with increasing levels as age

Table 21.1 Defining dementia (ICD-10) and major neurocognitive disorder (DSM-V)

ICD-10 (abbreviated)
• G1. There is evidence for each of the following:
– A decline in memory, most evident in the learning of new information. The decline should be verified by a reliable history from an informant, supplemented, if possible, by neuropsychological tests or quantified cognitive assessments
– A decline in other cognitive abilities characterized by deterioration in judgement and thinking, such as planning and organizing, and in the general processing of information. Evidence should be obtained from an informant and supplemented, if possible, by neuropsychological tests or quantified objective assessments. Deterioration from a previously higher level of performance should be established
• G2. Awareness of the environment is preserved sufficiently long to allow the unequivocal demonstration of the symptoms in criterion G1
• There is decline in emotional control or motivation or a change in social behaviour manifested as at least one of:
– Emotional lability
– Irritability
– Apathy
– Coarsening of social behaviour
• Criterion G1 should have been present for at least 6 months
DSM-V (abbreviated)
• Evidence of significant cognitive decline from a previous level of performance in one or more cognitive domains (complex attention, executive function, learning and memory, language, perceptual-motor, or social cognition)
– Concern of the individual, a knowledgeable informant, or the clinician that there has been a significant decline in cognitive function
– A substantial impairment in cognitive performance, preferably documented by standardized neuropsychological testing or, in its absence, another quantified clinical assessment
• The cognitive deficits interfere with independence in everyday activities (i.e. at a minimum, requiring assistance with complex instrumental activities of daily living such as paying bills or managing medications)
• The cognitive deficits do not occur exclusively in the context of a delirium
• The cognitive deficits are not better explained by another mental disorder (e.g. major depressive disorder, schizophrenia)

advances. Although a population-based screening seems to be an unreasonable suggestion, such high prevalence rates may justify a more systematic screening of cognitive disorders from 75 years of age upwards [19].

21.2.2.2 Differential Diagnosis

The aetiological definition of dementia is vast, but some entities are particularly frequent in the elderly. This holds true for the neurodegenerative dementias, including AD and Lewy body (LB) disorders, various vascular brain disorders resulting in dementia such as multi-infarct dementia, or subcortical vascular encephalopathy as well as mixed cases. Some neurodegenerative and vascular disorders are less frequent in the elderly (Huntington's disease, CADASIL, etc.), but FTD remains an important differential diagnosis although it usually starts earlier than AD, mostly in the sixth decade of life.

A range of metabolic, infectious, or nutritional disorders are of importance in the differential diagnosis of dementia in the elderly (Table 21.2).

A number of anamnestic elements are helpful to orientate the differential diagnosis and include the type and evolution of the deficits (initial symptoms and signs and their evolution over time, neurological and psychiatric symptoms and signs, exaggerated use of alcohol or other psychoactive substances, sleep complaints and disorders, current medication status such as the use of multiple and/or psychotropic drugs, traumatisms, vascular diseases or coagulopathies, etc).

Primary psychiatric disorders including above all depression, substance use disorders, and to a minor degree psychosis can masquerade dementia and are among the most important differential diagnoses. These disorders are of particular importance as they have a potential of reversibility. About 10% of all patients investigated for dementia suffer from depression, often accompanied by cognitive impairment sometimes as profound as to respond to the criteria of dementia, but which is potentially treatable and curable. This is a high percentage that contrasts with a 1% prevalence of primary somatic disorders with a potential of curability including dementias secondary, e.g. to thyroid or metabolic disorders, infectious diseases, normal pressure hydrocephalus, and others [20].

A confusional state or delirium may be of subacute onset in the elderly and at times difficult to differentiate from dementia if its course is protracted. Of course, delirium occurs in dementia

Table 21.2 Differential diagnosis of dementia

Type	Examples	Testing
Degenerative	AD, FTLD, Lewy bodies, Parkinson, Huntington, multiple system atrophy, prion disorders, CBD, PSP, MND	Medical history, physical examination, lab tests, imaging, EEG, ENMG, LP, neuropsychological testing
Inflammatory/ autoimmune/ infectious	Systemic lupus erythematosus, Sjögren, Behçet, polyarteritis nodosa, sarcoidosis, celiac disease, Hashimoto's encephalitis, HSV, HIV, CMV, EBV, Lyme, syphilis, Whipple, tuberculosis, malaria, fungal meningitis	Lab tests, LP
Vascular	CNS vasculitis, macro-/micro-infarcts, microangiopathic diseases, thrombotic thrombocytopenic purpura, hyperviscosity syndromes, chronic subdural haematoma	Lab tests, neuroimaging, carotid duplex, ECG, skin biopsy (CADASIL), muscle biopsy (vasculitis)
Neoplastic	Primary and secondary malignancies, paraneoplastic syndromes	Lab tests, LP, imaging
Toxic/metabolic	Uraemia, hepatic encephalopathy, hypo-/ hyperthyroidism, hyperPTH, hypo-/hypercorticism, porphyria, vitamin deficiencies, alcohol, drugs, heavy metal poisoning, Wilson	Lab tests, liver biopsy
Neurological	Hydrocephalus, epilepsy, multiple sclerosis	EEG, imaging
Psychiatric	Depression, schizophrenia, bipolar disorder, obsessive-compulsive disorder, conversion, etc.	Clinical assessment

AD Alzheimer's disease, *CADASIL* cerebral autosomal dominant arteriopathy with subcortical infarcts and leukoencephalopathy, *CBD* corticobasal degeneration, *CMV* cytomegalovirus, *CNS* central nervous system, *EBV* Epstein-Barr virus, *ECG* electrocardiogram, *EEG* electroencephalogram, *ENMG* electroneuromyogram, *EBV* Epstein-Barr virus, *FTLD* frontotemporal lobar degeneration, *HIV* human immunodeficiency virus, *HSV* herpes simplex virus, *LP* lumbar puncture, *MND* motor neuron disease, *PSP* progressive supranuclear palsy, *PTH* parathyroid hormone

tremendously often. Some of the clinical indicators that may help differentiate confusional states, depression, and some of the more important dementias in the elderly are given in Table 21.3.

A number of clinical lighthouse syndromes may help orientate the aetiological diagnosis (Fig. 21.1).

It is, however, important to be aware that a given aetiology may present itself clinically in a quite heterogeneous way as a consequence, e.g. of different brain locations involved, a high interindividual variability, or the various comorbidities added on more often than not to the dementia syndrome.

So as to orientate the diagnosis according to the clinical features present, a thorough clinical investigation is warranted and ought to include a cognitive, psychopathological, physical, and functional assessment.

The differential diagnosis of dementia may take time and need a multidisciplinary approach and team. If available, it may therefore be advantageous to send the patient to a memory clinic or some other specialized setting such as an old-age psychiatric out-patient clinic. This may be particularly helpful in specific situations such as [21]:

- Results at screening unclear
- Persistent cognitive complaints requiring a more thorough neuropsychological assessment
- Cognitive impairment in a patient below 65 years of age
- Atypical or unclear symptomatology (e.g. early behavioural disturbance) or atypical evolution over
- Episode(s) of delirium (e.g. during a hospital stay)
- Multimorbidity reuniting a number of disorders with the potential to impact on cognition
- Divergence or contradiction of information during history taking
- Difficult family situation or relationships difficult to handle by any of the persons involved (patient, proxy, physician, other caregiver)

Table 21.3 Differential diagnosis including some relevant disorders

	Delirium	Dementia syndrome				Depression
		AD	DLBD	Vascular dementia	FTD	
Beginning	Quick (hours/days)	Insidious (months/years)	Insidious (months/years)	Variable (acute/months/years)	Insidious (months/years)	Variable (weeks/months)
Course	Fluctuating, lucid intervals (hours)	Progressive decline	Progressive decline	Variable	Progressive decline	Rather stable
Vigilance/orientation	Altered/altered	Normal/altered	Often fluctuating/altered	Variable	Normal	Normal/normal
Attention	Altered, fluctuating	No major deficit	Often fluctuating	No major deficit	No major deficit	Slightly altered
Memory	Short-term/working memory altered	Short-term memory altered	Short-term memory altered	Often altered, variable types	Little altered	Little altered
Behavioural changes	Frequent	Less frequent	Frequent	Less frequent	Frequent and early in course	Rare except for affective changes
Autonomy	Altered	Altered	Altered	Altered	Often altered	Sometimes altered

AD Alzheimer's disease, *DLBD* diffuse Lewy body disease, *FTD* frontotemporal dementia

Fig. 21.1 Some clinical lighthouse symptoms

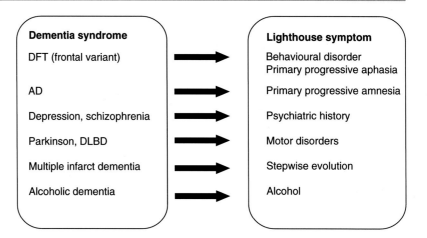

Dementia syndrome		Lighthouse symptom
DFT (frontal variant)	→	Behavioural disorder Primary progressive aphasia
AD	→	Primary progressive amnesia
Depression, schizophrenia	→	Psychiatric history
Parkinson, DLBD	→	Motor disorders
Multiple infarct dementia	→	Stepwise evolution
Alcoholic dementia	→	Alcohol

- Difficulty to evaluate or conclude regarding the impact of cognitive impairment on observed difficulties of basic and more particularly complex activities of daily living (e.g. driving, handling of complex financial issues, etc.).

21.2.2.3 Cognitive Investigations

The neuropsychological assessment quantifies the extent for each cognitive domain. Cognitive domains usually include executive functioning and attention, memory, language, and visuospatial capacities. Its usefulness lies in the profiling of the cognitive impairment that may add considerably to the differential diagnosis of disorders and helps distinguishing among the different neurodegenerative forms of dementia.

Attention deficit and of course lowered or changing vigilance may impact negatively on any cognitive domain. Thus, detailed cognitive assessment may not be useful in patients with delirium nor in the short-term aftermaths of delirium up to several weeks. However, attention deficit and fluctuations in the intensity of cognitive deficits is a constitutive and diagnostic criterion for LB dementias.

Executive dysfunction is usually secondary to a morphological or dynamic impairment of the frontal lobes and its subcortical connections. Executive functions are variously defined but often include a number of teleological capacities such as programming, anticipation, treatment of interferences, response inhibition, conceptualisa-

tion, and others. Therefore, executive deficits often impact negatively on other cognitive functions, in particular memory. Thus, subjects with executive dysfunction may have memory performance deficits (impaired use of memory capacities), while their basic memory competence is preserved (absence of a primary memory deficit). As once stated, these patients forget to remember.

Primary impairment or impairment secondary to executive dysfunction is most frequent though not always present and no more a requirement for the diagnosis of dementia. Clearly, investigating episodic memory is mandatory. A disorder of information encoding (e.g. AD, Korsakoff syndrome) or retrieval (e.g. Parkinson's disease, vascular subcortical encephalopathy) may hence be detected. Impaired retrieval usually corresponds to an executive deficit and thus of performance and is an indicator of a subcortical form of dementia, in particular when associated with motor basal ganglia deficits and marked retardation. However, a word of caution is necessary. The distinction between subcortical and cortical dementia is often more of a didactic interest rather than absolute as many overlaps exist.

Semantic memory encompasses the treasure of all the knowledge a person has been able to build. Its impairment is the consequence of a temporal lesion and constitutes the core element of semantic dementia, a temporal variant of FTD, a rare condition relative to AD. In this affection, autobiographical memory is eroded with recent memory being better preserved than remote memory as opposed to AD or Korsakoff syndrome that shows an inverse gradient.

Naming deficits are frequent in dementia. In AD, anomia will progressively be joined by difficulties of comprehension (transcortical sensory aphasia) to end in global aphasia characterized by the loss of both expression and comprehension. Different types of aphasia may represent the mode of beginning of various dementias including a sudden aphasia of multi-infarct dementia or the more progressive forms (primary progressive aphasia) of FDT and, more rarely, atypical AD.

Visuo-constructive deficits are more often a clinical expression of cortical dementias such as AD or LB or multi-infarct dementias, but they may also be the consequence of posterior cortical atrophy (Benson syndrome), this latter usually being associated with AD histopathology.

A specific training in neuropsychology is needed to perform a competent and thorough cognitive examination. This is hardly ever the competence of a primary care physician who would rather refer the patient to an experienced neuropsychologist or a dementia competence centre to obtain this assessment. Sadly enough, the possibility to refer to a competence centre depends on the level of development of the public health-care system which is weak or inexistent in many regions or countries.

As for a neuropsychological assessment, modifiers of test performance such as age and school level must be taken into account when using screening instruments of cognitive functioning such as the Mini-Mental Status Examination (MMSE) [22], MoCA [23], MiniCog [24], BrainCheck [25], and many others that have been published over the years. Indeed, unusual test results must be interpreted as they may not warrant a diagnosis of dementia. As an example, a maximum MMSE score of 30 precludes no beginning dementia syndrome in a young-old highly educated person, while a score of 23 may be entirely normal in the older-old with low-level schooling [26]. Thus, apparently normal results may still warrant further investigation in those with a history suspicious of possible cognitive decline despite a normal cognitive level at these screening tests.

21.2.2.4 Functional Investigation and Staging

Establishing the course over time of a person's cognitive and functional competency or decline is crucial. Indeed, any dementia is defined by both cognitive and functional decline starting at some previous higher level of performance either in a previously normal subject or a person with, e.g. a mental handicap. The practical relevance of dementia is related to the individual suffering emanating from functional impairment and, as discussed below, behavioural and psychological symptoms and signs of dementia.

Functional impairment as a consequence of cognitive impairment is the key feature to diagnose dementia and to distinguish it from mild cognitive impairment (MCI) in terms of disease staging [27]. In MCI, the decrease of cognitive functioning is not sufficient to result in an impairment of the activities of daily living. In a number of people, MCI will progress to dementia although in some others it may remain unaltered or reverse to normal.

Evaluating dependency or, positively speaking, autonomy is paramount. A number of tools or proxy questionnaires may be useful for the clinician and include, e.g. the Clinical Dementia Rating (CDR) [28], the Global Deterioration Scale (GDS) in the case of AD [29], or the ADL/IADL scales [30]. Taking the patient's history with a proxy who knows the patient well and who lives with is crucial. Obtaining information from professional caregivers is extremely useful. Surely, this approach requires as much as possible the patient's agreement, and this is usually easily obtained. A spontaneous narrative of the difficulties by the proxy is more often than not followed by a detailed assessment of the patient's activities of daily living, including both basic capacities (washing, dressing, eating, etc.) and more complex activities that require executive competence (taking medication, organizing the household, etc.). Specifically designed tool may be helpful and ease comparison of the evolution of these activities of daily living over time. These tools may include, e.g. the Informant Questionnaire on Cognitive Decline in the Elderly (IQ-CODE) [31], the Nurses' Observation Scale for Geriatric Patients (NOSGER) [32], as well as the (B)ADL [33] and the IADL [30], some of them being translated in a variety of languages. Difficulties using a phone and public transportation and difficulty to manage one's medication and one's payments may be particularly sensitive to the presence of a dementia syndrome.

Some simple and quickly administered questions may be helpful to screen for dementia-related functional difficulties and thus be useful both for screening cognitive impairment in the community and suggest the presence of significant functional impairment. Six questions appeared to be particularly useful as suggested by a study including 17,000 aged nurses with different levels of specificity and sensitivity for each question [34]: (1) recent modification of one's capacity to remember a new piece of information; (2) difficulty to remember a short list (e.g. shopping items); (3) difficulty to remember a recent event; (4) difficulty to understand or follow spoken instructions; (5) difficulty, due to memory, to follow a conversation in a group or a TV programme; and (6) difficulty to find one was in a known environment.

Sometimes, a simple but clinically useful distinction between mild, moderate, and severe dementia staging is suggested [21]. In mild dementia, the patient's cognitive deficits cause minor difficulties in complex activities of daily living such as organizing financial issues or unusual travels and preclude no independent living. In moderate dementia, the cognitive deficits result in significant difficulties in daily living such as dressing, eating, and taking their medication accurately and require at least occasional assistance although the patient may still be able to live at home. In severe cases, the changes of cognitive functioning are major and heavily impact on the activities of daily living such as nutrition, hygiene, and others, and constant or almost constant assistance is now required.

21.2.2.5　Psychopathological Investigations

The practical importance of dementia lies in the suffering it causes for both the patients and their proxies or caregivers. The psychopathological investigation is therefore paramount in every patient independently of the dementia stage. The identification of the more important caregivers and the assessment of their well-being are indispensable.

As to the patient, identifying what is referred to in the literature as behavioural and psychological symptoms of dementia (BPSD) [1] is crucial as these signs and symptoms are often amenable to efficient treatment and improve subjective and objective well-being of the patient and their caregivers.

ICD-10 acknowledges the importance of BPSD to some degree as it requires the presence of at least one noncognitive feature for the diagnosis of dementia, and this will be given, hopefully so, much more importance in the ICD-11 edition. Approximately 10–30% of all patients with AD will have depression at some point and 30% psychosis. Agitation may occur in half of the cases. Most patients will develop, earlier or later, some change in their personalities. Clearly, the evolution of BPSD is more difficult to predict than that of the cognitive and functional decline.

The semiology of BPSD is extremely rich and includes features of affective, psychotic, and behavioural disturbances [1].

Depression in dementia is often rather paucisymptomatic. The occurrence of depressive symptoms and signs seems associated with the existence of a family history of mood disorders. The intensity of depressive features does not seem to be correlated with the severity of cognitive impairment but rather with the degree of functional decline. Some clinical features are shared by depression and dementia (apathy, social retreat, loss of initiative, etc.), and primary depression may mimic dementia. Emotion regulation and its expression are frequently altered in dementia (catastrophic reactions in the case of overstimulation; pathological crying and laughing as a response to non-specific stimuli; emotional lability usually congruent with the patient's affect; the aprosodias as a language component that is not purely linguistic). The causes of depression during dementia are likely to be multiple. If awareness of cognitive impairment may lead to depression, in particular in the beginning of the disease, depression may also be the consequence of neurobiological modifications secondary to the neurodegenerative processes, e.g. in the case of changes of the production of neuromodulators (serotonin, noradrenalin, etc.).

Anxiety is tremendously prevalent in dementia and often independent of the severity of cognitive decline, but it is often associated with depressive and psychotic features. Anxiety may take a number of forms (panic attacks, apprehension of minor events, repetitive and stereotypical questioning (Godot syndrome), phobic manifestations, fear of being abandoned, etc.).

Psychotic features including delusions and hallucinations are among the more frequent BPSD (delusions of theft, infidelity, phantom boarder, mirror and TV sign, Capgras syndrome and other reduplicative paramnesias, and others). The presence of delusional ideas may be a risk factor for other BPSD, in particular aggressive behaviour. The presence of visual hallucinations suggests a LB disorder.

Agitation (repetitive attitudes and behaviours, shadowing, irritability, obstination, wandering and pacing, or, in the more extreme cases, verbal and physical aggressivity) may be the consequence of underlying depressive or psychotic features. This is, however, by no means always the case, but agitation is in all situations a source of major stress and burden both for the patient and their caregivers.

Sleep disorders are frequent in patients with dementia. Sometimes, a primary disorder such as sleep apnoea, restless legs syndrome, or REM sleep disorder is diagnosed. Inappropriate sleep habits must be looked for such in the case of patients who are forced into bed at an hour of the day unusual for them that provokes a shift of their sleep cycle. Often, patients with dementia present with difficulties falling asleep, or they have insomnias and sometimes sleep-wake inversions.

The identification and characterization of BPSD may be improved through the use of specific tools such as the Neuropsychiatric Inventory Questionnaire (NPI-Q) [35], the Behavioral Pathology in Alzheimer's Disease Rating Scale (BEHAVE-AD) [36], the Consortium to Establish a Registry for Alzheimer's Disease-Behavior Rating Scale for Dementia (CERAD-BRSD) [37], and, of course, others as well [38–40]. For affective symptoms, the Geriatric Depression Scale (GDS) [41] and the Cornell Scale for Depression in Dementia [42] may be helpful among others less specific for the demented [43–46].

A much under-researched area is the presence of multiple psychiatric pathologies in dementia, i.e. the cases of patients with a psychiatric disorder that later develop dementia. Similarly, there may well be a pathoplastic effect, e.g. of personality traits on the clinical expression of BPSD and an impact on cognitive decline [47].

It is of some importance to consider that behavioural and psycologial symptoms are often present in the pre-dementia stages, e.g. of AD, as they are estimated to occur in 35–75% of the persons having MCI [48].

21.2.2.6 Physical Examination

A complete routine physical examination including a neurological status is mandatory in every patient presenting with an active cognitive complaint or in whom cognitive impairment is suspected. This investigation will yield precious information in terms of the differential diagnosis or the detection of disorders related or not to the cognitive impairment. Furthermore, the causes of diminished activities of daily living due to sensory impairment, gait disorders, nutritional state, and others must be detected.

21.2.2.7 Paraclinical Investigations

Given the differential diagnosis of the various dementias and the frequent comorbidities, paraclinical investigations are usually mandatory even after a thorough history taking and clinical assessment including an interview with a proxy.

There may be some discussion and controversy as to what laboratory examinations may be useful. Usually, there is some reasonable degree of consent to proceed to a complete blood cell count, HbA1c, creatinine-based estimation of clearance, ASAT, ALAT, gamma-GT, electrolytes including calcium, vitamin B12, folate, and TSH.

In some clinically guided instances, complementary tests such as serology for syphilis (TPHA), HIV, and borreliosis may be indicated. With regard to infectious diseases that may at times lead to a picture of dementia, some further investigations partly depending on the locally prevalent epidemiology may be warranted (cf. chapter on prion and infectious diseases).

In high-income countries, the use of diagnostic neuroimaging has become a standard in the investigation of cognitive disorders. In the setting of memory clinics, the usual decision would be to do a MRI of the brain as it helps exclude primary disorders of dementia including, e.g. subdural haematomas, tumours, normal pressure hydrocephalus, and vascular load. Furthermore, it plays an increasingly important role in measuring local atrophy and thus determining brain atrophy patterns in a quantitative way. This assessment is useful to differentiate the various neurodegenerative disorders causing dementia. Even in high-income countries where this radiological device is now widely available, it is recommended to leave the decision to perform it to a specialized clinic such as a memory clinic.

Other sophisticated neuroimaging techniques of the functional type may be available in some places and be useful for specific cases. These techniques include PET and SPECT. Some authors have gone as far as to include these techniques as being part of the diagnostic criteria for some disorders [49] and even Alzheimer's disease [50, 51] notwithstanding the fact that in most places in the world this currently precludes a diagnosis of dementia according to these criteria for most patients as the necessary equipment or the funding to carry these investigations out are not available.

A careful history taking of sleep behaviour is part of any cognitive assessment. Specific sleep disorders may be associated with some dementias (REM sleep behaviour in the alpha-synucleinopathies) or contribute to cognitive deficits (depression) as may the use of drugs (BZP, anticholinergic drugs, antihistamines) that are frequently used to combat subjective sleep disorders. A frequent comorbidity of dementia is sleep apnoea that may cause cognitive impairment and perhaps dementia in some patients. On top of the clinical history and observation, it may be useful to proceed to a polysomnography. Some memory clinics now use small-scale somnographies before they send the patients to a more sophisticated investigation in a sleep centre.

In some rarer instances, further investigations may be useful or necessary. They usually require the assistance by a specialist. This may be the case, as mentioned above, of a specific polysomnography setting.

Doing a lumbar tap and analysing cerebrospinal liquid may be an indication to exclude inflammatory or infectious brain disorders (cf. chapter ad hoc on infectious dementias). More recently, the protein-based diagnosis of neurodegenerative disorders has been proposed and becomes more and more available [52].

An EEG may be helpful in the differential diagnosis of the dementias, particularly in the case of a suspicion of epilepsy, metabolic encephalopathy, or Creutzfeldt-Jakob disease.

Genetic investigations may be warranted in selected situations of a dementia that seems to run in a family. This is the case of Huntington's disease and some cases of FTD (many mutations described) or, more rarely, presenile forms of AD linked to mutations on chromosome 1, 14, or 21. In these cases, an appropriate genetic counselling by a knowledgeable professional is mandatory throughout the whole genetic diagnostic process.

Determining the ApoE status of a person with a diagnostic aim in mind is not appropriate, although ApoE is a risk factor for sporadic AD, given its lack of diagnostic selectivity or predictability.

In spite of all the diagnostic deployment described above, the aetiological classification remains probabilistic as it is usually not confirmed by neuropathological confrontation. However, the clinical and neuropathological match is as high as 80% in good memory clinics [53] though the error rate is often higher [54].

21.2.3 Treatment

It is often said that dementia cannot be treated. This is true if the statement refers to disease-modifying or curative treatments that, indeed, do not exist for any of the neurodegenerative disorders. However, they do exist for some cases of the rarer forms of dementia such as brain tumours, normal pressure hydrocephalus, or infectious disorders (cf. below).

However, it is entirely wrong to say that patients with dementia cannot be treated as there are many symptomatic treatment approaches that have been developed over the last decades. These treatments may target cognitive or functional signs and symptoms of dementia and they are often highly efficient in the treatment of the different forms of BPSD. Some of the treatment approaches available may be disease-specific treatments, while others are symptomatic treatments that target specific signs or symptoms of disease, but not a specific disease. BPSD, e.g. cut through the different diseases and the underlying disease, is often of little importance in the treatment decision tree. Other approaches may be specific to a disorder as in the case of antidementia drugs that have been approved for AD only.

21.2.3.1 Disease-Specific Treatments

Disease-specific treatments include disease-modifying treatments and those approved for some dementias only. There are disease-modifying and potentially curative treatments for the dementias secondary to infectious agents, and there are disease-specific treatments for AD and LB disorders. There are no disease-modifying nor disease-specific treatments for DFT.

However, we may consider the treatment of specific comorbidities as disease-specific treatments of the dementia syndromes. Surely, the diagnosis and subsequent treatment of diseases concomitant to the dementia syndrome are among the more important approaches when caring for a person suffering from dementia.

21.2.3.2 Treatment of Comorbidities

Numerous disorders may give rise to a dementia syndrome, and some of these disorders are extremely frequent in the elderly. This may be the case of hypothyroidism, anaemia, and many other diseases of internal medicine as well as of depression or substance use-related disorders. However, with the exception of depression and substance use-related cognitive disorders and despite their extraordinary high prevalence in the elderly population, they are rarely the cause of dementia in a given patient. In other words, they are usually not solely responsible for the dementia and turn out more often than not to be comorbidities grafted upon a neurodegenerative or vascular dementia syndrome.

Nevertheless, treating these conditions is usually mandatory as it improves a patient's quality of life and residual capacity although the dementia syndrome may remain irreversible. Comorbidities may at times worsen the cognitive or functional deficit, and they probably contribute quite often and to a substantial degree to the aetiology of the various BPSD that are often secondary to concomitant infections, urinary retention, faecal impaction, metabolic or electrolytic or endocrinological changes, flat earphone batteries that transform an auditory advice into an ear plug, and many others. Toxic effects of drugs both prescribed lege artis or not by physicians as well as over-the-counter prescriptions must always be suspected as a possible culprit of BPSD (cf. later chapters).

21.2.3.3 Symptomatic Psychosocial Care with an Emphasis on BPSD

Behavioural and psychological symptoms and signs (BPSD) are tremendously frequent in the dementias and are now the more focus of interest than in the past. This is fortunate as BPSD are paramount factors of suffering and burden both for patients and their caregivers.

Although a variety of interventions are used in different settings, there is insufficient evidence for most of these non-pharmacological treatments to be widely recommended individually as they have been mainly used in AD. However, the semiology of the BPSD is extremely rich and so are the possible aetiopathogenic processes underlying BPSD. Thus, overall there is a general agreement that psychosocial interventions are recommended and improve the patients' and caregivers' quality of life and may retard admission to a nursing home [55, 56].

Importantly, dementia is usually not a sufficient explanation of the occurrence of BPSD; it is often merely the conditio sine qua non. The histopathology of the underlying disease and its localization may be less important than for the cognitive dementia features, and this may allow for some generalization regarding treatment options across disease boundaries. Thus, if some new BPSD occurs in any type of dementia, it is mandatory to look for its cause that can be diverse and sometimes multiple and result from (a) physical incomfort, pain, or disease, (b) a drug side effect, (c) psychological ill-being, (d) environmental or caregiver inadequacy, or (e) any combination of the former.

Symptomatic psychosocial treatments require a person-centred approach [57–60] that is commonly considered central in the treatment of demented patients with or without concomitant pharmacological treatment of cognitive or non-cognitive features [59]. Indeed, the neuropathological process, whatever its nature, does not only impair a brain, but it impairs the brain of a person with their single history and individual characteristics. The better the personal story of a patient is known to the caregivers, the better they will be able to care for the patient. This helps tailoring each intervention individually according to disease stage, symptom pattern, needs [61–63], and available resources. Treatment is multidisciplinary and aims at improving daily functioning, managing symptoms, and preserving quality of life.

Thus, helping patients with BPSD requires a previous, often fine-grained analysis—if the degree of urgency allows for it—over 1–3 days of observation to install causative treatment. Looking for and treating some new or newly decompensate physical comorbidity are paramount. Disturbing features in the patient's physical environment need to be eliminated (obstacles, dark places, confinement, contention, visible locked doors) and the environment adapted and personalized which is most important in a nursing home (access to garden, personal features, photos, etc.) [59, 64]. Aromatherapy, snoezelen, music or musicotherapy, and basal stimulation therapy have shown some efficacy mostly in the more advanced stages of dementia [65, 66]. Physical activity may have a positive influence not only on BPSD but also on cognitive and functional capacities [67]. Physical activity adapted to the patient's residual capacities and their tastes is aimed at as opposed to performance.

Safety concerns are often associated with impaired cognitive functioning and impulsive behaviour. Environmental modifications may minimize risks and deleterious behaviour [68, 69]. They may include removal of dangerous items (e.g. firearms), rearrangement of furniture to prevent falls or access to stairs, covering door-knobs to discourage elopement, installing door alarms to alert elopement attempts, locking the kitchen door to prevent binge-eating, etc. Structuring the environment to facilitate participation may also prove useful (e.g. avoiding crowded or noisy places) [69]. Adapting to the patient's abilities and simplifying daily tasks (e.g. clearing area of all items except those related to the present task) may alleviate excessive stress and concomitant agitation [68, 70, 71]. Evaluation by an occupational therapist may contribute to securing the patient's physical surroundings.

Both hypo- and hyperstimulation—be they physical, environmental, or social—may increase BPSD. Favouring a stable day-night cycle, exposure to natural light, and the respect of personal rhythms and habits are of importance. Reality orientation therapy (ROT) is of limited value [72]. Limiting access to or eliminating TV and mirrors when a patient presents with a TV sign or mirror sign is far better than using neuroleptics. Favouring personalized social interactions is a well-being prerequisite for each and every member of the human species.

Delegate financial tasks may help eliminate persecutory or anxious symptoms in some patients who are not able any more to deal with the cognitive requirements of paying their bills. Financial problems may arise from neglected bills, impulsive or compulsive spending, or poor judgement (e.g. gifts to strangers), particularly in patients with frontal involvement [73].

General Attitude

A dignified approach of the patient is mandatory, and it helps caregivers to actively imagine how they would want to be treated if they were in the patient's situation. Most of us would insist very much on avoiding "elderspeak" such as "sweetie" or "good boy" [68]. Language must be simple with short sentences but dignified and empathic even if at times directive. However, it is important though often difficult to avoid projections of one's own personal belief systems onto those of the patient, a pitfall often encountered in caregivers of patients with dementia.

Behavioural Interventions

Much of the above-mentioned interventions and attitudes based on a meticulous behavioural analysis are of the behavioural type that target problematic behaviour identified by caregivers as most troublesome. Behavioural interventions are centre stage in dementia care. They aim at providing strategies to manage BPSD effectively but also to prevent them. Potential triggers and their temporal, spatial, or circumstantial characteristics are identified and eliminated or modified in order to improve well-being. Behavioural management training can be efficient [74].

Cognitive and Functional Interventions

From a theoretical stance, improving cognitive abilities will have positive effects on daily functioning and subsequently on emotional well-being, although no intervention can reverse the cognitive decline. Cognitive impairment may require external memory aids such as calendars, diary, photo albums, or electronic devices (e.g. tablets). A wide array of communication strategies and tools may prove useful for language deficits, for instance, written messages, drawing charts, photographs, etc. [68, 69, 75]. Cognitive interventions may also be helpful in the speech apraxia and linguistic variants of FTD [76, 77]. However, their efficacity on BPSD is at best limited [72]. These approaches aim at providing cognitive prostheses to the patient, but their successful implementation is often limited to a specific task, and their generalizability to untrained tasks and different settings is usually limited [78]. Cognitive training may be helpful as long as it respects the willingness of the patient to participate in these training activities, is implemented according to the personal reality and needs of a patient, and is accompanied by positive social interaction. These approaches are based on hypotheses or theories such as "use it or lose it", environmental enrichment, or the scaffolding theory of cognitive ageing based on neuroplasticity theories suggesting that the ailing brain may recruit intact neuronal areas to replace those damaged [79].

Cognitive therapy may be helpful in reducing dysfunctional thought processes in the demented with depression [80].

Implementing new adaptive strategies may compensate for lost or insufficient abilities and favour adequate functioning. The living environment should be simplified in order to promote self-reliance, and a stable daily routine made of structured activities should be implemented [68, 69]. Physical interventions include exercise, assessment of swallowing and advice on dietary modifications, and external aids for mobility and continence problems [68].

Life History Approach

Psychodynamic treatments sensu stricto may not be applicable any more in most demented patients but help them in the grieving process, e.g. after the diagnosis has been announced at an early dementia stage. It may also favour the establishment of directives for later dementia stages, which may at times be possible and give a sense of continuity of life into the last phase of the life cycle.

The influence of a patient's premorbid personality on the symptomatic expression of behaviours and psychopathology in dementia is still little investigated and our understanding therefore limited [47]. However, it seems likely that a patient's adaptational capacity to the announcement of a dementia diagnosis and further coping in everyday life are codetermined by their usual way of coping with adversities.

Diversion inspired by autobiographical and emotionally positive material to which the patient has still access in their memory may be useful in later stages of the dementias, e.g. those who show catastrophic reactions when confronted to specific situations of failure. However, reminiscence therapy may have some efficacy, and some benefit may be expected on affective BPSD [72, 81].

Safety and Risk Management

Within the realm of safety and risk management, environmental adaptations may be helpful as mentioned previously. Limiting access to bank accounts and credit cards may prove necessary as well as engaging in disability procedures. In the case of FTLD, as this disorder frequently begins before 65, it may bring about a loss of income along with growing health-care costs. Families should be advised by a lawyer or social worker about financial planning and to secure assets (e.g. life insurance).

Assessment of driving ability may prove necessary. Cessation of driving will restrict the patient's autonomy, can undermine the patient-doctor relationship, and cause conflicts between patient and family, and the decision should therefore never be made lightly [82]. Referral to the local jurisdiction for a formal driving assessment may be helpful to make the decision in some instances [73].

Caregiver Support

Caregiver burden is high in most dementia cases and higher in FTD as compared to AD [83, 84]. However, any dementia type affects, sometimes simultaneously, sometimes subsequently and progressively, a patient's cognitive, functional, or behavioural capacities as well as their identity. There is no exception to the observation that sooner or later a third party will have to help, and this third party is usually, certainly to start with, a family caregiver. The caregiving role is manifold and not limited to physical or functional help a caregiver provides. They also give moral, decisional, and identitory support to the patient and may end up substituting themselves for the patient in most aspects of their life. The progressive character of most dementias and the changing requirements emanating from it as well as BPSD are among the prime culprits of the toll the caregiver pays over time.

The caregiver's coping capacities are paramount and what may be reasonably easy to handle for one caregiver may be unbearable for another one. While patient-dependent variables contribute to carer burden, carer-dependent variables do so, too. Thus, young age, impaired anterograde memory and emotion recognition, diagnosis (FTD), low impulse control, and behavioural disturbances increase caregiver burden [84, 85], while this is less or not the case for the patient's gender, performance on general measure of cognition, disease duration, language skills, and the type of relationship (i.e. spouse versus other) between the patient and the carer do not influence carer burden [83]. Regarding carer variables in the case of FTD, young age, depression, social isolation, neglected personal needs, and inadequate coping style to problem behaviours are predictive of carer burden [83–85].

Helping a caregiver understand that the reality experienced by the demented is different from their own reality is crucial. Reassure rather than argue with the patient is usually the preferred way of communication. Improving caregiver communication skills reduces resistance to care among patients, e.g. informing patients about the upcoming task or avoiding "elderspeak" as mentioned above. Negative feedback loops between caregiver attitudes driven by misconceptions and misunderstandings and the patient's reactions leading to deleterious interactions must be disentangled. Feelings of guilt, lack of confidence in one's own capacities, emergence of previous conflicts, or invisible loyalties may be severe obstacles to harmonious relationships and can, and sometimes should, become targets of therapeutic interventions [86].

The learned dependency which occurs in the demented patients when the caregivers provide too much support is to be avoided. Whether by compassion or by irritation, caregivers may be tempted to do things for the patient instead of waiting for the person to do them by themselves. These overcompensatory interactions lead to reduced activities of daily living [68, 69]. Caregiver's information and education promotes activity and preserves skills.

Hence, support must be offered and support services developed to meet the needs of the caregiver population. Psychoeducation is a generally accepted approach and helpful to caregivers and patients [87, 88] better understand disease features, although group or individual information and education programmes may at times only be modestly successful in reducing stress and burden as in the case of FTD [84, 85]. Counselling regarding social and legal issues may be crucial for the caregivers. In some instances, e.g. in rare FTD or familial AD cases, genetic counselling done by experts may be useful [89]. Support groups for families, which may be internet-based, prove beneficial by providing mutual self-help and allowing verbalization of feelings [83, 84]. Mental healthcare professional counselling and case management also have positive effects on burden and satisfaction of caregivers [89]. In some instances, psychosocial support proves insufficient owing to high levels of carer distress. Referral to a mental health professional for psychotherapy should then be considered [73]. Practical issues, such as access to care facilities, disability procedures, financial advice, and evaluation of needs should be addressed systematically. Integration of the caregivers and family members into a team surrounding the patient ensures that everyone has a proper understanding of the situation.

At some point, formal help usually becomes necessary. Home-based interventions and visits are usually available in high-income countries. They consist of multidisciplinary teams with nurses, social workers and household maids, and others who provide support to patients and their families.

Specialized day hospitals and recreational centres benefit patients while giving families respite [81]. Respite facilities, for instance, short-duration nursing home placement, are another way to support families. Hospitalization may be required for cases which cannot be handled otherwise (e.g. violent behaviour). Residential care must be considered when care needs exceed the capacity of the carer. Families and patients often need time and active assistance to accept change and prepare emotionally for separation, so that early conversations about this topic are useful [73].

End-of-Life Issues

Inevitable decline and death and the goals of care are best discussed with patients and families when there is still time and ability to discuss these matters. The cognitive and physical decline should be addressed pre-emptively during the follow-up sessions. The expressed will of the patient helps diminish the stress and guilt that some caregivers may feel about not doing enough or making the right decisions, for instance, about measures of comfort or referral to palliative care.

Anticipatory grief in dementia is equivalent in intensity and breadth to death-related grief [90]. However, the grief process and the needs are different from one person to the other and differ according to some characteristics such as adult-child caregivers versus spouse caregivers or the dementia stage [90]. Support and guidance must therefore be adapted to fluctuating affective, intellectual, and existential needs. After the patient's death, contact with the family may address further issues, such as post-mortem brain examination, genetic implications of the disease, and bereavement [71]. Anticipatory grief appears to alleviate post-death grief initially, but not in the long run, emphasizing the need for psychological follow-up to be offered upon request [90, 91].

Overall, BPSD are of complex aetiopathogeny of multiple levels, and the interventions are usually combined to meet the needs of these patients and their caregivers. This is the case in particular of disruptive behaviours difficult to treat such as vocally and sexually disruptive ones [92, 93]. Behavioural management, caregiver support, cognitive stimulation and the offer of pleasant and structured activities are paramount [66, 94].

21.2.3.4 Symptomatic Biological Treatments with an Emphasis on BPSD

Symptomatic biological treatments may include psychoactive medication, light therapy, neuromodulation, and others.

Medication

The target of drug treatment may be impaired cognition and, possibly more importantly so, BPSD [21, 72, 95]. However, the first-line treatment of BPSD is psychosocial, but in numerous instances, the use of specific drugs will be indispensable. It is of paramount importance to realize that there still is a dearth of studies in the field of BPSD drug treatment leaving us with scarce knowledge especially as most studies carefully select patients that hardly correspond to the majority of polymorbid patients encountered in real-life settings. Although the theoretical prevalence of psychiatric comorbidities in demented patients must be tremendously high as this is the case in the general population, there is no literature on this topic and no treatment recommendations regarding patients with comorbid dementia and premorbid psychiatric illness. Pharmacokinetic and pharmacodynamic changes related to ageing or polymorbidity are serious difficulties for appropriate drug prescription in demented patients. Titration therefore starts at a lower dose and is slower than in young adults, but the maximum dose required for efficient treatment may at times be as high as in the young. It must be kept in mind that most studies have been done in patients with AD, and their findings may not be automatically extended to other forms of dementia. Furthermore, the use of many if not most recommended drugs may correspond to their off-label use in numerous countries. Indeed, many psychotropic drugs in use to counter BPSD are used off-label. This is often legally possible, depending on the national legislation, but is the sole responsibility of the physician [72].

It is recommended to individually plan drug prescription and favour psychotropic monotherapies and most importantly assure adherence, often possibly only if formal or informal caregivers are actively involved. Some web-based lists may be useful and guide drug prescription such as Beers Criteria (https://www.dcri.org/trial-participation/the-beers-list/), PRISCUS list (http://priscus.net/download/PRISCUS-Liste_PRISCUS-TP3_2011.pdf), or Mediq (http://www.mediq.ch/welcome_public).

Depression

Depression in dementia is often paucisymptomatic and subsyndromal and therefore underdiagnosed and undertreated. Thus, treatment should probably be initiated at a low depression threshold though this obviously holds some danger of overtreatment. At times, it is a comorbidity in patients with recurrent depression or bipolar disorder who develop dementia. It usually is a serious condition that needs treatment, and this holds also true for affective dysregulation syndromes such as emotionalism. The origin of depression in dementia is likely to be heterogeneous and needs some previous investigation to find the best balance between primary psychosocial and secondary drug treatment.

More often than not, one of the serotonin uptake inhibitors (citalopram, paroxetine, sertraline) will be the first-choice treatment given some level of efficiency [72] and their favourable adverse event profile in the elderly although initial gastrointestinal and further extrapyramidal side effects may be problematic. Given its tremendously long half-life, fluoxetine is best avoided. Other antidepressant agents may be used, but few studies exist, and some have not been tested, or results were negative [96, 97]. AChEI may have some preventive effect and also help alleviate affective symptoms related to dementia [98]. Tricyclic antidepressants are to be avoided due to their anticholinergic action. Ginkgo biloba may be efficient [72, 99].

After how long these drugs should be stopped is unclear but may depend on whether depression is related to the presence of a premorbid affective disorder or a first occurrence related to dementia.

Apathy

Apathy is a frequent syndrome in dementia and deserves treatment in the case of depression. Using psychostimulants is not generally recommended for the treatment of isolated apathy.

Anxiety

There are hardly any studies on anxious BPSD. Empiricism and scarce scientific evidence suggest that the use of serotonin reuptake inhibitors may be useful which may be advantageous as anxiety is often comorbid with depression. Other antidepressants may be tried, but there is little scientific evidence. Gabapentin may have some use in the treatment of anxiety [70]. Short-acting benzodiazepines and Z-drugs may occasionally be used in acute anxiety states.

Psychotic Symptoms

The nature and pathogenesis of psychotic BPSD may be very different from primary psychotic states such as those seen in younger adults with psychotic disease. Cognitive deficits and depressive symptoms may underlie these projections and treatment be chosen accordingly. However, the use of neuroleptics is often inevitable though caution must be taken given the potential of negative side effects including metabolic syndrome, extrapyramidal and anticholinergic features, or cerebrovascular events depending partially on the drug used. Typical neuroleptics are rather avoided although they can be efficient [100] as in the case of pipamperone [72]; haloperidol remains a drug of choice in the symptomatic treatment of acute delirium. Risperidone, olanzapine, and aripiprazole may be useful at low initial dose, e.g. a daily dose of 0.25–0.5 mg of risperidone. Quetiapine is often used in clinical practice with good empirical evidence, but scientific evidence is lacking and its use off-label, probably in most countries. In most situations, whatever the substance used, its usefulness must be checked every 6 weeks or so, and they should be tapered and possibly stopped after a few weeks or months.

Agitation and Aggressivity

As with most BPSD, agitation and aggressivity may be understand as the result of unmet needs and their treatment tailored individually based on a rigorous aetiopathogenic and behavioural analysis. The general attitude often encountered of prescribing neuroleptics in the case of agitation and aggressivity is wrong. Indeed, disruptive BPSD may be secondary to depression, anxiety, and other conditions and better respond to treatments using psychosocial treatments and, e.g. serotonin reuptake inhibitors such as citalopram or other drugs such as trazodone. The scientific evidence is low, however, possibly in part because drug trials are based on purely phenomenological disease classifications rather than on aetiopathogenic considerations. Neuroleptic drugs similar or identical to those chosen to treat psychotic features play an important part in the treatment of agitation and aggressivity [101, 102]. Gabapentin, lamotrigine, and carbamazepine may have some efficacy, though the side effect profile of the latter prohibits its use in most situations [70]. Memantine may reduce the incidence of BPSD as well as be helpful in the treatment of agitation and psychotic features [103, 104].

If pain is the underlying condition causing agitation or aggressivity, its adequate treatment may be efficient against agitation although scientific results are ambiguous [72]. Of course, a number of other psychotropic substances have been advocated as useful treatments, but their use is often secondary to the failure of the more common drugs mentioned above and left in the hands of specialists.

Sleep Disorders

Specific sleep disorder treatments include those for sleep apnoea or REM sleep disorder and sleep cycle adaptations, e.g. in those that are put to bed in nursing homes at inappropriate hours. However, sleep-favouring drugs may at times appear necessary. However, benzodiazepines and Z-drugs are not recommended except in acute situations and for short periods. Antidepressant or antipsychotic substances having a hypnotic action may sometimes be used and include, e.g. trazodone and doxepin. Antihistamine substances should not be used in the demented due among others to the concomitant anticholinergic action. There is currently no scientific recommendation to treat insomnia in the demented using melatonin or melatonin agonists (however, cf. treatment of DLB) or phytotherapeutics, chloral hydrate, or clomethiazole [72].

Other Biological Treatments

A number of other hypothetical treatments for BSPD can be mentioned. They include light therapy, sleep deprivation, or neuromodulatory treatments.

Thus, phototherapy may be helpful to treat insomnia and sundowning more so than depression [105]. Agrypnia has not been studied in dementia and is therefore not recommended. Electroconvulsive therapy may be useful [106] as well as, in the future, other neuromodulatory approaches such as transcranial magnetic stimulation for which research in dementia has only just begun.

21.3   Alzheimer's Disease (AD)

As for all dementias, estimation of AD is challenging. First, the diagnosis may at times be difficult, especially in the very old, as the interindividual variability increases with increasing age and the distinguishing normality from pathological cognitive decline becomes more difficult [107]. The schoolbook presentation of AD in the elderly is by no means the ordinary clinical picture encountered in the elderly as they often suffer from various diseases, some of which may cause dementia or have an impact on the clinical features exhibited by a patient. Often, features from AD and vascular dementia are found in neuropathological studies [108].

21.3.1 Epidemiology

Keeping these difficulties in mind, AD is the most common dementia, accounting for 50–75% of the total, with a greater proportion in the higher age ranges, an estimation based on neuropathologically defined cases [109]. The risk of developing AD reaches 50% for individuals beyond age 85, and the proportion of AD relative to vascular dementia in women is higher than in men [10].

21.3.2 Clinics

Alzheimer's disease (AD) is a brain disorder with identifiable clinical features at least if it presents as a typical monopathology. This is, however, not the most frequent case in the elderly, especially the very old as these patients often have mixed pathologies.

AD is a leading cause of morbidity in the elderly; yet, its origin is unknown. A great deal of knowledge has been accumulated, however, over the last three decades regarding the pathological cascades in the brain, but research makes it increasingly clear that the causes of AD will never be explained in a monocausal, mechanistic, and linear way. Numerous risk factors have been described, and, thus, a causal explanation of AD

is more likely to stem from a dynamic and epigenetic lifelong perspective in the context of increasing longevity pushed to its extreme in the human species with advanced age beginning the most important risk factor for sporadic AD. The rare genetically determined autosomal dominant young-onset cases related to APP, PS1, and PS2 mutations, usually starting long before 65 years of age, represent less than 1% of all cases [110] and cannot operate as a thorough model for the much more frequent sporadic late-onset cases although associations with other genes increase the risk for sporadic AD. In short, there is currently no thorough aetiological model of AD.

However, AD may be seen both as a neuropathologically defined brain disease and as a clinically defined syndrome suggestive of, but not confirming, the presence of specific neuropathological features. While the definite diagnosis of AD is based on neuropathological criteria, the clinical diagnosis of probable and possible AD in clinical settings is usually made according to the NINCDS-ADRDA criteria. Probable AD corresponds to a typical clinical syndrome, whereas possible AD is suggested when the observed clinical features are at odds with the typical syndrome [111]. As in most cases no histopathological confirmation of the presence of the typical neuropathological features is available, AD is mostly a clinical syndrome defined by a typical clinical constellation likely to be secondary to AD neuropathological features.

AD as a neuropathologically defined disease corresponds to the progressive invasion of the cerebral cortex by the two major pathological hallmarks of AD, neurofibrillary tangles and senile plaques, as well as neuronal and synaptic loss. Detailed analyses of AD lesion regional distribution have demonstrated that certain components of the neocortical and hippocampal circuits within the medial temporal lobe are particularly prone to degeneration. However, the first cited diagnostic criteria for AD elaborated by a National Institute on Aging (NIA) workshop [112] have since evolved in part because clinicopathological correlations were not as straightforward as initially thought, especially in the elderly, but also because precise quantification of neuropathological features may be technically difficult. The Consortium to Establish a Registry for Alzheimer's Disease (CERAD) [113] proposed another set of standardized neuropathological criteria adopting semiquantitative criteria as a function of the development of neuritic plaques in three age groups (less than 50, 50–75, and over 75). The diagnosis was based on a combination of clinical information and an "age-related plaque score" that reflected the maximal neocortical involvement, and a level of diagnostic certainty was assessed (i.e. definite, probable, or possible AD). A major weakness of CERAD criteria resides in that they have been inspired somewhat unilaterally by the amyloid cascade hypothesis and do not consider neurofibrillary tangles densities in the neocortex, even though these correlate strongly with the severity of dementia. The NIA-Reagan Consensus conference attempted to integrate the varying experience of neuropathologists in a comprehensive set of criteria for AD taking into account both the CERAD criteria and Braak staging system [114].

The typical clinical AD syndrome is a cognitive disorder characterized by an initially insidious and consequently progressive decline that affects first memory and later executive functions, language, and visuospatial skills. Several lines of evidence indicate that the primary progressive amnestic syndrome so characteristic of the initial stages of typical AD is the consequence of the neuropathological changes in the medial temporal structures, in particular the entorhinal cortex and the hippocampus. This sequence of cognitive deterioration is thought to reflect the progressive expansion of AD-type lesions in the brain starting in the mediotemporal brain regions and consequently invading the allocortex and isocortex [115].

Typical AD has been originally thought as an early and progressive amnestic syndrome mainly involving episodic memory which is accompanied by noncognitive features (i.e. depression, anxiety, psychotic signs and symptoms, as well as behavioural disturbances) in more advanced stages of the disease. Variations, however, occur mainly in late-onset forms and may be more pronounced than those suggested by early epidemiological studies [116]. Indeed, the diagnostic criteria for AD were heavily weighted towards memory impairment as the central deficit and may, therefore, prevent inclusion of cases with other patterns of cognitive decline. However, it is now well documented that certain cases of dementia do not meet the accepted clinical and neuropathologic criteria for the definition of AD, yet they show the same histopathologic features. They are referred to as atypical AD cases and may represent examples of clinicopathologic subtypes of AD [116]. The clinical heterogeneity of AD patients has long been recognized. Although AD is usually associated with early and prominent memory impairment, patients with neuropathologically confirmed AD may also display early deficits in language, musical skills and prosody, motor abilities, frontal and executive capacities, as well as visuospatial skills.

While AD is defined by a clinical syndrome suggestive of the presence of specific neuropathological lesions, dementia of the AD type is defined by the presence of both a dementia syndrome and a clinical syndrome suggestive of the presence of specific neuropathological lesions. Considering that AD is defined as a dementia syndrome, it is quite obvious that its investigation follows the general track laid out in the previous chapters.

In typical AD, the cognitive syndrome is usually characterized by beginning memory impairment. This impairment is usually of the amnestic type which means that a patient has difficulties in learning and retaining newly presented information that cannot be retrieved by hints or indicators as the memory trace has never been accurately encoded. However, executive problems may appear quite early in the course of AD, and prospective memory deficits may be among the first to become visible and clinically relevant. Thus, patients with prospective memory deficits are unable to anticipate future action and forget, e.g. to pay their bills at the end of the month. As the disease progresses, other cognitive deficits will become more apparent in the linguistic and visuospatial domains.

As a consequence of these cognitive deficits, a patient with AD will progressively have functional impairment that follows a typical pattern in pure cases which allows for functional staging of disease progression [29]. This staging approach has also some predictive power of what is to come once the patient has reached a given stage. It may also suggest the presence of some new or different condition if the disease progression fails to follow the predicted course.

BPSD have mainly been studied in AD which is tremendously frequently accompanied by BPSD (cf. previous chapters). As in any dementia, the aetiopathogeny of dementia should not be mixed up with the aetiopathogeny of BPSD. Indeed, as opposed to the predictable cognitive and functional decline in AD, there are no clear predictability patterns for the course of BPSD as AD progresses. This is a witness to the observation that dementia is, surely, the conditio sine qua non of BPSD, but not usually their immediate cause. As a corollary to this observation, a patient with new features of BPSD in the course of AD must be investigated.

As many patients with dementia do not show up in their doctors' offices with textbook features of AD, some aetiopathogenic investigation is warranted in many cases. Indeed, the polymorbidity with advancing age increases the likelihood of a patient to have two or more conditions, each of which may contribute to their cognitive decline. Detecting these comorbidities allows for their treatment (e.g. hypothyroidism) or secondary prevention (e.g. vascular subcortical encephalopathy) and may, in some cases, improve a patient's cognition and functioning. This stance has particular validity in cases of comorbid depression and substance abuse as treatment may lead to partial and sometimes complete reversal of the dementia syndrome.

The physical examination in the early stages of AD is usually within the normal boundaries except of course for any comorbidity the patient may present. As the disease progresses, extrapyramidal and pyramidal signs may appear, and at the late stages of the disorders, motor deficits progress according to a predictable pattern similar to that described in the GDS [29].

Standard laboratory assessment is usually bland, but vascular risk factors are often present as in the general population and given the observation that vascular risk factors are also risk factors for AD. However, more recently the search for AD biomarkers in the cerebrospinal liquid has somewhat changed the attitudes although dosing biomarkers is not available in most places. If available, dosing these biomarkers allows going some way in improving the accuracy of the diagnosis as there is a clear decrease of $A\beta_{1-42}$ and an increase of T-τ and P-τ_{181P} in typical AD although some overlap may exist between the results found during normal ageing, some other dementias, and the mixed forms [117].

The association between ApoE, coded on chromosome 19, and sporadic late-onset AD has been extensively studied and a higher risk found for ApoE4 carriers, in particular homozygotic carriers [118]. However, specificity and sensitivity of these polymorphisms are too low to be of any help in the usual clinical setting, and dosing ApoE is therefore not recommended.

21.3.3 Treatment

Despite more than two decades of intense biological research and regular newspaper announcements to the contrary, there is still no disease-modifying treatment of AD in sight. There are, however, some disease-specific treatments in the form of the different procognitive or antidementia drugs that have been approved for the treatment of AD although they are sometimes controversially discussed in the literature with national agency and expert recommendations that may come to different conclusions [21, 119–127]. However, more often than not, it is accepted or recommended that cognitive symptoms and signs of AD can or should be treated using the cholinergic and glutamatergic drugs available.

21.3.3.1 Cognitive Drug Treatment of AD

In many if not most countries, the acetylcholinesterase inhibitors (AChEIs) donepezil (Aricept®), galantamine (Reminyl®), and rivastigmine (Exelon®) are authorized for the treatment of cognitive signs of AD. The conditions under which and by whom they may be prescribed may differ between countries, and it is advisable to refer to the national legislation. Usually, the AChEI can be used in the beginning to moderate stages of AD which correspond to a MMSE score [22] between 10 and 30 [128] although some efficacy has also been shown for more severe dementia stages [27, 129, 130]. The AChEIs stimulate the cholinergic neurotransmitter system, and their beneficial clinical effects are usually not, if at all, immediately perceptible. It is impossible to predict which patients will respond. At that, telling a responder from a nonresponder may not be easy as slowing of the cognitive decline may already be a positive response. An individually obvious improvement is observed in rare instances only, and the main effect usually corresponds to a clinical stable state over 6 months relative to the pretreatment status.

Examining the usefulness of an AChEI prescription is even more important than usual when a patient is given anticholinergic or antimuscarinic drugs that counter the procholinergic effect of the AChEIs [131]. Many of the frequently prescribed drugs in the elderly have anticholinergic properties; they include neuroleptics, antidepressants, anti-incontinence drugs, and others.

Dropouts due to adverse events occur, and this further reduces the overall utility of these drugs. The pharmacokinetic and pharmacodynamic profile of the three available AChEIs being different, changing their form of application (capsules versus patch) or changing the molecules altogether in the case of intolerable side effects or inefficacity seems appropriate [132–135]. Titration is usually progressive over a few weeks, but this depends on the specific drug used (cf. Table 21.4).

There are no clear rules as to when to stop AChEI treatment. This usually occurs when side effects occur or the patient or caregivers observe no changes after several months of treatment in which case progressive tapering under careful clinical observation may be useful as some worsening may occur mostly in the domains of functional capacities or behavioural signs. Clearly, nursing home placement is not per se an indication to stop treatment.

Memantine (Axura®, Ebixa®) acts on the glutamatergic neurotransmitter system which has excitatory effects on the brain and may damage

Table 21.4 Comparison of commercialized antidementia drugs

	Donepezil	Galantamine	Rivastigmine	Memantine
Indications (Switzerland)	Mild to moderate AD		Mild to moderate AD and Parkinson's disease dementia	Moderate to advanced AD
Starting dose	5 mg	8 mg	1.5 mg	10 mg
Targeted dose	10 mg	24 mg	12 mg	20 mg
Efficacity starts at	5 mg	16 mg	6 mg	10 mg
Dosing pattern	oad	oad	tad for capsules 2× oad for patch	oad
Galenics	Tablets, orally dispersible	Capsules prolonged release	Capsules, solution, patch	Capsules, solution
Effects	Prevents synaptic acetylcholine decrease			Regulates glutamate
Main side effects	Nausea, vomiting, diarrhoea, bradycardia, syncope, weight loss (patch: skin irritation)			Vertigo, headache, constipation, somnolence
Limitations	MMSE ≥ 10 or equivalent; regular assessment (at outset, after 3 months, and then every 6 months; stop as soon as MMSE < 10), monotherapy only			MMSE 3–19; regular assessment (at outset, after 3 months, and then every 6 months; stop as soon as MMSE < 3), monotherapy only

This table describes the Federal Office rules in Switzerland as an example. These rules may be different in other countries neurones in the long run through calcium-mediated mechanisms. Memantine inhibits the postsynaptic NMDA (*N*-methyl-D-aspartate) receptor and is authorized for the treatment of AD in its moderate to more severe stages corresponding to an MMSE ranging between 3 and 19 (cf. Table 21.5) [126, 136, 137]. Here again, national regulation may differ between countries. Titration is progressive and the drug usually well tolerated.

Combined treatment using concomitantly AChEI and memantine has been advocated given the different neurotransmitters involved, but it is not unanimously used or authorized given both its costs and the results that are controversial [138–141].

Ginkgo biloba is a plant extract with studies based mostly on EGb761 use. However, no general recommendation of its use is made in AD as study results are considered not to be consistent enough [142], but there is some evidence that it may be useful in BPSD treatment (cf. later).

Table 21.5 General prescription guidelines for antidementia drugs

• Formal diagnosis of AD for donepezil, galantamine, rivastigmine, and memantine
• Formal diagnosis of PDD for rivastigmine
• Possibly donepezil, galantamine, and rivastigmine for DLBD; possibly donepezil and galantamine for vascular dementia
• No indication: *mild cognitive impairment*, subjective cognitive impairment
• Stop whenever possible any potentially amnesiant prescription (benzodiazepines, tricyclic antidepressants, neuroleptics, anticonvulsants— thymoregulators, β-blockers, quinidine, disopyramide, opiates, antihistamines, NSAI, antibiotics, interferons, and other drugs with a central anticholinergic action)
• Appropriate information given to both patient and caregivers
• Integrate drug prescription into a global care approach of both patient and caregivers
• Assure adherence to treatment (often dependent on formal or informal caregivers)
• Efficiency impossible to predict but at best modest in almost any case
• Make sure insurance issues depend on national policy

AD Alzheimer's disease, *DLBD* diffuse Lewy body disease, *PDD* Parkinson's disease dementia, *NSAI* nonsteroidal anti-inflammatory drug

Of course, there are numerous experimental drug trials using molecules based on a variety of pathophysiological hypotheses of AD, but none has so far proven useful in clinical practice [143].

21.3.3.2 Treatment of Mild Cognitive Impairment (MCI)

MCI is defined as a cognitive decline of one (amnestic MCI, single domain nonamnestic MCI) or several (multidomain MCI) cognitive domains not severe enough to interfere with daily activities of living. In patients in whom memory and/or several cognitive domains are impaired, the deficits may well evolve towards Alzheimer's dementia, in particular if apathy accompanies the clinical picture [144].

No pharmacological treatment described above and authorized for AD is recommended for MCI [145]. This holds also true for AChEIs which are of little benefit, if any, and for which side effects are significant [128]. Non-steroidal anti-inflammatory substances, hormone therapy, ginkgo biloba, vitamins, or omega fatty acids have not demonstrated, for the time being, their usefulness in the prevention or the treatment of MCI.

A healthy style of life including physical activity and the pursuit of intellectual activities, combined with the treatment of vascular risk factors, are likely to diminish the probability of developing cognitive disorders.

21.4 Frontotemporal Dementia (FTD)

21.4.1 Epidemiology

FTD is a neurodegenerative, either hereditary or sporadic, disorder with broad clinical and pathological variability. FTD is an important cause of dementia in adults and the young-old individuals where FTD is as frequent as AD. Although the age of onset is around 60, the range extends from those in their 30s to individuals in their 90s [146, 147]. Population-based studies investigating both FTD and AD come up with a point prevalence of FTD varying between 15 and 22 per 100,000 and incidence estimates ranging between 3.5 and 4.2 per 100.000/year [148]. The survival rate of FTD is shorter than that of AD, and cognitive and functional decline is more rapid [149, 150]. Some studies found a small preponderance in men [151].

Despite international collaborative effort to up-date diagnostic criteria, the prevalence and incidence of FTD in both community and clinical settings are more difficult to estimate than for AD because (1) diagnosis is challenging due to many clinical overlaps with psychiatric disorders and other dementias, (2) there is a lack professional training to identify cases, (3) clinical categorization is complex, and (4) population-based studies are seldom available as FTD is rare relatively to other dementias [152, 153].

21.4.2 Clinics

FTD is an aggregate of neurodegenerative disorders that results in progressive disturbances in behaviour, emotional regulation, and language. FTD is associated with focal degeneration in the frontal and temporal lobes. Three main syndromes have been characterized: behavioural variant (bvFTD), nonfluent primary progressive aphasia (nfPPA), and semantic dementia (SD). The wide variation of clinical presentations and complex symptomatology overlaps with many psychiatric and neurological disorders and makes diagnosis challenging.

Recent advances in neuroimaging and aetiological research (genetics, biomarkers) accompanied by a proliferation of terms and pathological classifications have so far resulted in little translational improvement for clinical practice. Thus, this review focuses on operative clinical characteristics with the aim to help primary care professionals to detect FTD with improved approaches to diagnosis and care.

FTD encompasses various syndromes that are qualified according to their main features and supportive criteria. The consensus criteria for behavioural and cognitive (language) syndromes related to frontotemporal lobar degeneration (FTLD) were updated in 2011 [154, 155].

21.4.3 bvFTD

The most frequent variant is bvFTD that is responsible for half of all cases. It is clinically different from most of dementias in that cognition is virtually unaffected in the initial phase. Its hallmark is a significant and persistent change in premorbid behaviour, emotion regulation, and personality characteristics [157, 158]. One of the most common symptoms of bvFTD is apathy with lower interest in common activities, which is sometimes difficult to differentiate from anhedonia due to depression. Apathy may also delay family perception and diagnosis, especially in cases where a "false quietness" is insidious. This is probably due to the compromised ability to perceive contextual social inadequacy as well as impaired insight. These characteristics of altered social cognition may be tentative indicators of bvFTD and help differential diagnosis with psychiatric disorders and AD [159, 160].

Loss of empathy is another important feature of bvFTD [161]. Disinhibition may lead to impulsive or invasive behaviours such as touching strangers and is associated with a demeanour of shamelessness. Periods of emotional lability or dysregulation may lead to a misdiagnosis of bipolar disorder. The differential diagnosis is important, but clinicians may also consider a comorbid diagnosis with an affective disorder episode, most often depression. Other examples of behaviours related to disinhibition include picking up other people's personal items or scribbling on inappropriate supports (utilization syndrome). Similarly, attempts to swallow objects or placing them in the mouth characterize hyperorality [162]. Compulsive behaviours (repetitive, simple, complex, or ritualistic) and disinhibition along with lack of insight are exhausting for families and increase the burden on caregivers [163]. Obsessive-compulsive personality traits may arise such as excessive organization, emotional rigidity, and excessive devotion to routines. However, obsessions such as preoccupations with contamination are rarer, and this may help differentiate it from primary obsessive-compulsive disorder where obsessions are preeminent and the compulsive behaviour component is commonly related to a mechanism of anxiety relief (e.g. excessive cleaning precipitated by a feeling of contamination). Including FTD in the differential diagnosis is crucial when mild symptoms appear (apathy, emotional lability, externalized inappropriate conduct) that may mimic late-onset affective disorders. The participation of family members and caregivers in consultations helps improve the information accuracy [164].

Patients with bvFTD may show Parkinsonism in more advanced stages of the disease although some patients may show secondary Parkinsonism due to antidepressant or antipsychotic use. Some motor syndromes are related to FTD and may emerge in the course of the disease. Motor neuron disease occurs in 15–20% of patients with bvFTD. Other FTD-related motor syndromes are corticobasal syndrome (CBS) and progressive supranuclear palsy (PSP). In these cases, specialized support may be necessary to characterize the aetiopathogeny of the motor features.

FTD is a dementia syndrome, and the clinical investigation is therefore similar to the multiaxial approach outlined above. Primary care professionals have a paramount role and can assert a clinical diagnosis of bvFTD with near 100% specificity and good sensitivity (80–85%) relying on the combination of inappropriate behaviour, stereotypies, eating disorders, and apathy without obvious memory or visual spatial deficits [162, 165–169]. Interviewing family members and caregivers is crucial given the patient's poor insight. Full diagnostic criteria for bvFTD updated in 2011 are summarized in Table 21.7, including clinical features, neuroimaging, neuropathology, and genetic testing [155].

Formally, the diagnosis of probable FTD requires the presence of a functional decline and structural or functional neuroimaging compatible with the diagnosis. A definite diagnosis is based on post-mortem pathology, confirmed genetic mutation, and tremendously rarely brain biopsy. None of this can be done outside specialized centres.

Caution is warranted as FTD semiology overlap with other psychiatric disorders. Confounding features include similar clinical presentations (e.g. depressive disorder, bipolar disorder, psychosis, anxiety disorder, obsessive-compulsive adjustment disorder), cognitive impairment (e.g. executive dysfunction), and imaging (e.g. frontal hypoperfusion). The prolonged latency of up to 20 years between the appearance of psychiatric symptoms and neurocognitive decline adds to the difficulty [156, 170, 171]. Cognitive impairment, lack of emotional distress, progressive treatment-resistant illness, unusual psychiatric presentation, new onset of a psychiatric disorder in middle-aged and older patients, positive family history of dementia, and neurological symptoms may point to the presence of FTD. Apathy associated with bvFTD is commonly confused with depression. Excluding medical illness, substance abuse, or other neurodegenerative disorders such as dementia with Lewy bodies and AD is crucial, and neuropsychological assessment may be helpful to tell them apart. Conversely, late-onset psychiatric disorders may be supported by a positive personal or family history of affective or psychotic disorder, a long-term clinical observation over one or more years (by health professionals, family, or caregivers), and the presence of specific symptoms rarely seen in FTLD. Examples of rare symptoms include feelings of worthlessness and poor self-esteem in depression, euphoria and insomnia in mania, obsessions in OCD, and complex delusions in schizophrenia [172]. A thorough assessment by a trained psychiatrist is highly advisable.

21.4.4 Primary Progressive Aphasia

Primary progressive aphasia (PPA) syndrome is characterized by a gradual and progressive impairment in language. This impairment is related to neurodegeneration in the language-dominant hemisphere and depends on the sites of atrophy. The syndrome encompasses nonfluent and semantic variants [173]. In PPA, language impairment is the earliest cognitive deficit to occur compared to other cognitive domains, including episodic memory which is relatively preserved. This feature differentiates PPA from AD. CBD and PSP may also be associated with PPA.

In the course of the disease, language impairment is the most prominent cognitive deficit, but other domains also decline. Language dysfunction may be perceived in common situations that require communication skills including difficulties in speaking, talking with a group, making phone calls, or problems in personal conversations. Language assessments are used to objectively identify the type of impairment [154].

The nonfluent variant of PPA (nfPPA) leads to deficits in articulating words and linguistic coordination resulting in hesitant speech, phonetic effort and errors, or the inability to use words properly. These language deficits can be observed in consultations or when testing articulatory skills. Such tests involve asking the patient to repeat specific words rapidly or brief sentences that are challenging to pronounce. Speech apraxia is more evident in group conversation than in individual conversation. Comprehension is typically spared, but difficulty with complex sentences can be seen [154].

Similar to other cognitive domains, memory is typically preserved in initial PPA [174]. The course of nfPPA is quite different from bvFTD though some patients develop behavioural changes, symptoms of motor neuron disease, or corticobasal degeneration [172, 173]. Deficits may be restricted to expressive language function for a few years to several years before a more global dementia supervenes [173, 175]. The clinical, imaging, and biological data to diagnose nfPPA were updated by consensus in 2011 [154].

Semantic variant PPA (svPPA) is characterized by the impairment of word comprehension. The earliest symptom is difficulty finding a word. A clear decline in comprehension is seen with a progressive loss of knowledge of intrinsic characteristics such as the function, similarity, and meaning of objects. However, the ability to understand sentences tends to be impaired later as the disease progresses [173]. A semantic rarefaction may be seen in dysgraphia or the loss of important details or parts in a drawing. Some patients experience early loss of facial recognition of famous people [176]. Other characteris-

tics related to disease progression are behavioural symptoms, impaired speech, loss of empathy, hypergraphia, and, later, memory decline [177].

21.4.4.1 Cognitive Features

Frontal lobe functions can be assessed by short bedside scales, such as the Frontal Assessment Battery, the Neuropsychiatric Inventory, or the Frontal Behavioral Inventory [178–180].

Early in the course of bvFTD, cognition is quite well preserved except for impairment of executive functions likely to be related to dorsolateral prefrontal cortex dysfunction. As mentioned, identification of social contexts, emotion recognition, and empathy are altered [89, 181]. Memory and visuospatial tasks decline at variable pace, and test results may be affected by impaired executive functions and attention. In prominent nfPPA, there is neither initial episodic or visual memory nor visuoperceptual or executive impairment. Except for the profound semantic loss, there is preserved phonology, syntax, elementary perceptual processing, spatial skills, and day-to-day memorizing for SD [154, 155]. Patients with nfPPA perform well on measures of social cognition such as recognition of sarcasm, empathy, and the ability to understand other peoples' perspectives. In svPPA, degeneration of the right anterior temporal lobe often emerges, leading to a decline in empathy and the emergence of coldness in personality profiles, increased rigidity, and interrupting others [161]. Examination of language helps differentiate among the nonfluent, semantic, and logopenic variants of PPA (cf. above).

21.4.4.2 Neuroimaging

Tremendously quickly increasing technical and scientific knowledge has not translated at the same pace to clinical practice. Among others, important barriers are restricted availability and prohibitive cost, especially for low- and middle-income countries. However, structural neuroimaging (especially magnetic resonance imaging (MRI)) plays an important role in excluding secondary causes and investigating vascular lesion load. The typical focal frontal or temporal atrophy is seen in slightly more than half of cases and is considered a supportive indicator of FTD, but brain imaging is often normal or unspecific [155, 162, 182].

The earliest regions of damage in bvFTD include the anterior insula in the right hemisphere, the pregenual anterior cingulate, and the orbito-frontal cortex. Some specific patterns of atrophy show clinical symptomatic correlations [161, 183]. A recent multicentre study using structural MRI neuroimaging associated with neuropsychological assessment examined participants carrying pathogenic genetic mutations (GRN, MAPT, or C9orf72) or having a first-degree relative with symptomatic disease identified promising imaging and cognitive techniques for presyndromic changes occurring 5–10 years before the expected disease onset in adults at genetic risk for FTD [184]. Functional neuroimaging including single-photon emission computed tomography (SPECT), perfusion MRI, or positron emission tomography (PET) has demonstrated frontal or frontotemporal hypoperfusion or hypometabolism as a sensitive early diagnosis tool before structural changes can be observed [155]. Functional neuroimaging is reserved for specific purposes for unspecific early-onset cases.

PPA structural imaging may demonstrate frontal and temporal lobe atrophy. Functional imaging may show hypometabolism (PET) or hypoperfusion (SPECT) in the same brain areas [154]. Specific cortical changes in different PPAs may correlate with typical symptoms. The clinical variants of PPA correspond to heterogeneous underlying neuropathologies. However, prediction of an individual patient's underlying pathological diagnosis remains challenging and has limited value outside of research and clinical trials. Clinical syndrome is thus determined not by the histopathology of the neurodegeneration but rather by its anatomic predilection for the language network of the brain [171].

21.4.4.3 Genetic, Biomarkers, and Neuropathology

Physicians should be aware that 10–15% of FTD cases are genetically determined (autosomal dominant inheritance) and have a strong family history (25–30%) [185, 186]. This may be important due to the need for referral for genetic investigation and counselling. Microtubule-associated protein tau (*MAPT*), progranulin (*GRN*), and chromosome 9 open reading frame 72 (*C9orf72*) are the most important genetic factors. Current recommendations suggest that genetic testing should be done in specialist centres with expertise in genetic counselling, with patient and caregiver consent [89]. No blood biomarker is currently recommended.

Neuropathological examination determining neuronal inclusions is required for a definite diagnosis and subtyping of FTLD as shown in Table 21.6 [187].

Table 21.6 Nomenclature for FTLD

Molecular class	Neuropathological diagnosis	Associated genes
FTLD-tau	Pick's disease Corticobasal degeneration Progressive supranuclear palsy Argyrophilic grain disease Multiple system tauopathy with dementia Neurofibrillary tangle predominant dementia White matter tauopathy with globular glial inclusions Unclassifiable	MAPT
FTLD-TDP	Types 1–4 Unclassifiable	GRN VCP C9orf72 TARDBP
FTLD-FUS	Atypical FTLD with ubiquitinated inclusions Neuronal intermediate filament inclusion disease Basophilic inclusion body disease	FUS
FTLD-UPS	Frontotemporal dementia linked to chromosome 3	CHMP2B
FTLD-no inclusions		

CHMP2B charged multivesicular body protein 2B, *C9orf72* chromosome 9 open reading frame 72, *FUS* fused in sarcoma, *MAPT* microtubule-associated protein tau, *TARDBP* transactive response DNA-binding protein, *TDP* transactive response DNA-binding protein 47, *UPS* ubiquitin-proteasome system, *VCP* valosin-containing protein
Table adapted from Mackenzie et al. 2010 [187]

If lumbar puncture and measurement of bio-markers in cerebrospinal fluid are available, low beta amyloid and high phosphorylated tau protein strongly suggest AD. Investigation with PET scan with amyloid ligands can identify amyloid pathology of AD. However, advanced neuroimaging and radiopharmaceutical agents need complex infrastructure and are very expensive, so they are usually only available in tertiary medical centres or research institutes. Delusions and hallucinations are more suggestive of dementia with Lewy bodies and atypical for FTD. However, psychosis may occur in 20–50% of bvFTD patients who carry the C9ORF72 hexanucleotide expansion, the most common genetic cause of sporadic and familial FTD and ALS.

21.4.5 Treatment

For the time being, there is no disease-modifying treatment of neurodegenerative dementias including FTD and non-AD dementias [87]. At that, no drug improves cognition, and neither acetylcholinesterase inhibitors nor memantine is indicated [183, 187–191].

As for BPSD some medications may be used in clinical practice despite insufficient scientific evidence [89]. Symptomatic therapy can enhance quality of life and provide relief to patients and caregivers. Decrease of serotoninergic receptors in frontotemporal regions and raphe nuclei suggests the use of selective serotonin reuptake inhibitors (sertraline, paroxetine, fluvoxamine, citalopram) that are considered safe and effective in treating mood and behavioural symptoms such as disinhibition, carbohydrate craving, compulsions, verbal and motor stereotypies, sexually inappropriate behaviours, apathy, and hyperorality [89, 188, 190–192]. Similarly, trazodone improves BPSD. Antipsychotic agents may be prescribed for aggression, psychosis, and agitation [89, 192]. Their efficacy must be carefully weighed against their side effects, especially extrapyramidal signs, higher mortality related to cardiac events, weight gain, stroke, and accelerated cognitive decline [89, 188, 191].

Recent studies on dopaminergic agonists showed decreased risk-taking and improvement in apathy and perseveration. Monoamine oxidase inhibitors might be useful given the serotoninergic and dopaminergic deficits, and selegiline has shown some efficacy [189, 192]. A number of other agents including mood stabilizers have been tested with little clinical usefulness although oxytocin may improve social behaviour [82].

21.5 Dementia with Lewy Bodies

Dementia with Lewy bodies (DLB) is a neurodegenerative disorder characterized histopathologically by the presence of cortical Lewy bodies (LB) beyond the substantia nigra as in Parkinson's disease (PD). Its main clinical features include visual hallucinations, cognitive fluctuations, dysautonomia, REM sleep disorder, Parkinsonism, and neuroleptic sensitivity.

21.5.1 Epidemiology

DLB is now considered the second most common neurodegenerative dementia in older adults after AD. It represents about 4% of all dementias in population-based studies [193, 194], but its prevalence may be as high as 15–35% in all forms of dementia [195, 196]. Thus, prevalence rates vary considerably and may be due to under- and misdiagnosis and different methodological problems in assessing and diagnosing DLB. Post-mortem studies tend to find higher prevalence rates than those reported in clinical series, which suggest misdiagnosis during life [197, 198]. DLB increases with age with a mean age at presentation of 75 years and, similarly with Parkinson's disease (PD), has a clear male preponderance of 4 to 1 [199, 200].

21.5.2 Clinics

The clinical features of DLB include as mentioned spontaneous Parkinsonism, visual hallucinations, cognitive fluctuations, dysautonomia, rapid eye movement (REM)-related sleep behaviour disorders, and neuroleptic hypersensitivity. International collaborative efforts have been made to regularly standardize and update diagnostic criteria for DLB that contribute to increase case identification and diagnostic precision to differentiate DLB from other dementias [193, 201–203].

Many patient complaints may lead to a consultation with the primary care physician. In this setting, it may be difficult to establish a precise diagnosis of DLB. However, a high degree of clinical suspicion arises when an elderly patient complains about sleeping problems associated with motor difficulties and dysautonomia in whom the physician finds evidence for parkinsonian features. In many cases, the differential diagnosis, initiation of treatment, as well as counselling and follow-up will have to be handled by primary care providers [204].

Cognitive impairment is found in the domains of attention, executive functioning, and visuospatial capacities that usually start early in the course of DLB. Thus, impaired spatial abilities are a common complaint observed in everyday or professional activities; these include missteps, bicycle falls, difficulty driving, or even car accidents.

DLB has three core clinical features, cognitive fluctuations, visual hallucinations, and Parkinsonism, of which two must be present for the diagnosis of probable DLB, and one must be present for the diagnosis of possible LBD (cf. Table 21.7).

Oscillations in alertness and attention are the most frequently observed symptoms and – together with fluctuations in other cognitive domains – they can be present in 60–80% of cases [205]. Cognition varies widely and may be marked and sudden or subtle and enduring. A lowered level of consciousness, intermittent somnolence and hypervigilance, confusion, uncommon motor reactions, or agitation may be one way how DLB presents. "False normal" or fleeting improvement along the line may also be seen. Thus, actively asking family members and caregivers as to changes in cognition and behaviour is mandatory.

Whenever possible, serial evaluations are useful to diminish the risk of confusing circadian

Table 21.7 Summary of bvFTD diagnostic criteria

Criteria	Rating
I. Progressive cognitive and/or behavioural deterioration	Compulsory
II. Possible bvFTD A. Early behavioural disinhibition B. Early apathy C. Early loss of empathy D. Early repetitive, stereotyped, or compulsive behaviour E. Hyperorality and dietary changes F. Specific neuropsychological profile	≥3 symptoms (A–F) compulsory
III. Probable bvFTD A. Meets criteria for II B. Functional decline C. Compatible imaging	All symptoms (A–C) compulsory
IV. bvFTD with definite FTLD pathology A. Meets criteria for II or III B. Histopathological evidence C. Known genetic mutation	≥2 symptoms compulsory (A + either B or C)
V. Exclusionary criteria A. Other non-degenerative nervous system or medical disorders B. Psychiatric disorders C. Incompatible biomarkers	A and/or B exclusionary C admissible for II, exclusionary for III

"Early" refers to symptom presentation within the first 3 years. Table adapted from Rascovsky et al. 2011 [155]

alterations found in many other dementias [206]. DLB can also mimic a delirium and, of course, be accompanied by delirium. Structured questionnaires objectively check for symptom fluctuation and may be useful when information is imprecise.

Visual hallucinations, often exuberant or complex hallucinatory visons, can be an early sign in DLB and are present in two-thirds of patients. They are absent in beginning AD and less frequent in other AD stages [207, 208]. Hallucinations most often generate an emotional response. Yet, they should be investigated since they tend to be underreported due to poor insight or shame. Importantly, dopaminergic medication used to treat extrapyramidal symptoms of DLB can exacerbate this symptom.

In DLB, Parkinsonism is present in 60–92% of cases and tends to be more bilateral and symmetrical with fewer signs and less often resting tremor than in typical PD [209, 210].

Suggestive features include REM sleep disorder, neuroleptic sensitivity, and low dopamine transporter uptake in the basal ganglia as seen on SPECT or PET. The presence of one suggestive feature with one core clinical feature supports a probable DLB diagnostic. If core clinical features are absent, more than one suggestive feature indicates the presence of possible DLB. REM sleep behaviour disorder is characterized by the presence of vivid dreams and movement in the REM phase that range in severity from benign to violent punching and kicking. In these cases, counselling to prevent injuries for patients and bed partners is necessary. Such signs may be relayed by bed partners for a decade before dementia onset occurs [211].

Neuroleptic sensitivity is not dose-related and may not emerge initially, but up to half of patients who use neuroleptics develop severe sensitivity and may include irreversible Parkinsonism, syncope, and features of neuroleptic malignant syndrome [212]. These medications are associated with increased mortality and may also precipitate confusion and dysautonomia. Conventional drugs such as typical antipsychotics tend to be more associated with neuroleptic sensitivity, but newer drugs also cause these reactions.

Supportive features are features that are not specific enough to reinforce a DLB diagnosis. However, they have clinical importance as they include repeated falls or even syncope due to postural imbalance, autonomic instability, or extreme cognitive fluctuations including loss of consciousness. Sometimes, mutism (i.e. a cataleptic-like syndrome) or even motor "freezing" as seen in idiopathic PD occurs. Autonomic dysfunctions encompass orthostatic hypotension, heart rate instability, urinary incontinence, sweating reactions, and constipation, among others. Autonomic symptoms are more prevalent and severe than in PD, but less than in multiple system atrophy [213]. Urinary incontinence occurs at later stages in AD, but is often an early sign of DLB [214]. Non-visual hallucinations, such as olfactory or tactile experiences, may occur, and most patients present delusions in the course of LBD [215]. As in PD, clinically significant depressive symptoms are seen in most patients throughout the course of the disease [215, 216].

The principal differential diagnosis of DLB is AD, PDD, vascular dementia (VD), and several psychiatric conditions. Differential diagnosis should take into account the fact that distinguishing between DLB and AD can be particularly difficult, since both neuropathological processes can occur simultaneously as observed in postmortem studies [217].

Distinguishing DLB and dementia associated with PD may be more a matter of taste than of different aetiopathogeny. However, diagnosing DLB is more difficult than PD dementia as dementia in PD begins after the movement disorder has been established, while in DLB, dementia occurs before Parkinsonism or no later than a year after the onset of movement disorder symptoms [203]. If Parkinsonism onset starts less than 1 year before the onset of dementia syndromes, then PDD is considered the diagnosis. Objectively investigating signs of both DLB and PDD improves detection of these Lewy body dementias [218]. Other dementias with psychosis and delirium are important on the differential diagnosis of DLB and include, e.g. Creutzfeldt-Jakob disease and normal pressure hydrocephalus. Health-care professionals who work in primary care settings are critical for early diagnosis or the identification of suspected cases that need referral for expert evaluation.

21.5.2.1 Cognitive Features

Impairment of attention as well as executive and visuospatial functions starts early in the course of DLB as opposed to AD where memory decline is the first and most prominent change [202, 208]. The onset of memory impairment varies in DLB but tends to emerge later than AD. Impairment in figure copying or clock drawing combined with the absence of memory impairment suggests DLB. The absence of visuospatial impairment in early dementia has a high negative predictive value of up to 90% for DLB [208]. Short cognitive tests do not discriminate between forms of dementia and have low validity with patients whose level of education is at the extreme ends of the spectrum [219]. Nonamnestic mild cognitive impairment (MCI) is more likely to progress to DLB than amnestic MCI [220].

21.5.2.2 Imaging

Structural neuroimaging (MRI is preferred) is recommended in order to rule out secondary causes of dementia. Structural neuroimaging may also help identify specific neurodegenerative disorders in the early stages but is of little value for patients with advanced dementia [221]. DLB presents with slower rates of brain atrophy and ventricular enlargement than AD and with atrophy of subcortical structures, including the basal ganglia, with relative preservation of medial temporal lobe [222].

Functional MRI (fMRI) may show focal occipital decrease similar to hypometabolism observed on PET and hypoperfusion on SPECT studies [223]. This finding correlates partly with clinical visuoperceptive impairment in DLB. PET and SPECT imaging using specific ligands shows low activity of dopamine transporters in the striatum and is considered suggestive of probable or possible DLB [224]. Noradrenalin analogue ([123]-I-metaiodobenzylguanidine) scintigraphy demonstrates reduced heart sympathetic innervation activity related to DLB and may occasionally be used where available to detect early DLB in amnestic MCI [225].

21.5.3 Treatment

As yet, no disease-modifying treatment for DLB exists. However, symptomatic drug treatments and non-pharmacological approaches as outlined earlier will usually be required to provide relief from distress for the patient, family members, and caregivers.

The initial treatment recommended for cognitive symptoms is acetylcholinesterase inhibitors (ACEIs) [226]. They can be effective for various disease manifestations including fluctuations, hallucinations, Parkinsonism, and mood disorders. Memantine was of little or no benefit [227].

REM sleep behaviour responds well to melatonin or clonazepam before sleep [228]. Melatonin is well tolerated and the first treatment choice as clonazepam may worse cognition.

The benefit of antipsychotics on DLB is limited to the treatment of psychotic symptoms, although these agents can attenuate mood swings. As mentioned, they are related to neuroleptic hypersensitivity, worsening dysautonomic repercussions, worsening cognition, increased risk of falls, and increased risk of death. Pronounced psychotic syndromes on DLB course may be also be related to use of antiparkinsonian drugs, and adjusting the dose should be tried first. Atypical neuroleptics are considered secondarily and should be used with caution for severe and/or persistent psychosis and agitation. They are used in the smallest possible doses, since hypersensitivity observation is mandatory even when using drugs usually considered safer such as quetiapine [226].

The evidence for the use of other psychotropic drugs in DLB is limited, but a number of them are sometimes indicated. They include selective serotonin reuptake inhibitors (SSRIs) and serotonin-norepinephrine reuptake inhibitors (SNRIs) to treat depression and anxiety [48]. In these cases, patient should be checked for mood response and worsening of Parkinsonism. In general, benzodiazepines, tricyclic antidepressants, and other drugs with anticholinergic effect should be avoided.

The treatment of Parkinsonism due to DLB is more difficult than in PD dementia due to the limited therapeutic range complicated by the conflict between motor improvement and worsening of BPSD. However, dopaminergic medications, especially carbidopa/levodopa, are often used and should be started at very low doses and with a slower titration [48, 226]. Patients with DLB show a lower response than those with PD, and it has been suggested that this is a distinguishing diagnostic feature between the two [48].

21.6 Prion Diseases

21.6.1 General Issues

Prion diseases are a group of transmissible neurodegenerative pathologies characterized by the presence and accumulation of a host-encoded misfolding cellular prion protein (PrP). The word *prion* derives from the combination of the words "protein" + "infection" since these protein particles have the capacity of transmitting the disease from one host to another. The pathological process is set off by a conformational alteration of the PrP, making it resistant to protease and leading to the accumulation of protein clusters in the brain tissue. The normal conformation of the *prion* protein (PrPC) and its pathogenic conformation (PrPSC) have the same sequence of amino acids, but they differ in their secondary and tertiary structures. In humans, this protein is coded by the PRPN gene. Histologically, the formation of vacuoles in the tissue is typical, giving the brain an appearance similar to a sponge, with this group of diseases also known as transmissible spongiform encephalopathies (TSE) [229–231].

The first prionic disease to be described was scrapie (mid-eighteenth century) seen with sheep and goats. The most recognized animal form of prionic disease is BSE (bovine spongiform encephalopathy), referred to as "mad cow disease", that spread throughout the United Kingdom at the end of the 1980s and which can be transmitted to humans. In humans, the best-known prionic disease is Creutzfeldt-Jakob disease (CJD), described in 1920. CJD can be sporadic (s-CJD), genetic (g-CJD), or acquired iatrogenically (i-CJD) or transmitted by food originating from cattle contaminated with BSE, referred to as the variant form of CJD (v-CJD). The other types of human prionic diseases are even rarer and include Gerstmann-Sträussler-Scheinker (GSS) disease which is genetically determined, fatal insomnia which is usually hereditary (FFI) and rarely sporadic (s-FI), as well as kuru, an acquired form that is no longer in existence [229, 230, 232].

The current classification of the prionic diseases that occur in humans is summarized in Table 21.8.

Below, the most common clinical form, i.e. sporadic CJD, will be described. Recently, a sporadic clinical form, often confused with CJD, presenting a prionic protein sensitive to protease, has been described as a distinct disease (PSPr) [234].

21.6.2 Sporadic Creutzfeldt-Jakob Disease (s-CJD)

21.6.2.1 Epidemiology

Based on the number of reported cases, it is estimated that the sporadic form of CJD afflicts one in every one million people throughout the world. However, it is possible that the incidence is underestimated, since many cases are likely to occur without diagnosis [235].

The most common type of human prionic disease is the sporadic form of CJD (s-CJD), being responsible for 85% of the cases of CJD reported in the United Kingdom in the past 10 years [233]. The mean age of onset of the disease is 70 years, without any difference between men and women [232].

21.6.2.2 Clinics

The clinical manifestation of CJD is quite heterogeneous, with countless clinical features having been described over time, such as Heidenhain's cortical blindness or thalamic, myoclonic, dyskinetic, ataxic, and amyotrophic forms [234]. The classification currently used associates the clinical features to two molecular parameters: (a) the electrophoretic mobility of the PrPSC fragment that is obtained after digestion by the K protein and which classifies the disease as type 1 or type 2 and (b) the polymorphism related to the codon 129 of the PRPN gene which can codify a valine or methionine amino acid, therefore presenting three types—MM, MV, and VV. Thus, there are six distinct clinical types, with the MM1 and MV1 types presenting the same clinical characteristics and therefore being grouped as only one type MM/MV1. MM2 can have two distinct clinical pictures, thalamic (MM2-T) or cortical (MM2-C) [232, 236].

The MM/MV1 type occurs most frequently, representing approximately 70% of s-CJD cases. Characteristic clinical features are a rapid progression over a few months towards dementia with early and prominent myoclonia, although this is not generally the first manifestation. Usually, walking and appendicular ataxia, as well as visual impairments, including hallucinations, are observed. Other psychiatric symp-

Table 21.8 Classification of human prionic diseases

Classification	Characteristics
Sporadic forms	
s-CJD (sporadic Creutzfeldt-Jakob disease)	Most frequent form with heterogeneous clinical presentation (cf. text)
s-FI (sporadic fatal insomnia)	Rare disease (24 cases reported until 2011) with presentation similar to FFI, no mutation identified
PSPr (protease-sensitive prionopathy)	Recently described protease-sensitive prionic disease with a clinical profile of atypical dementia with a more prolonged clinical course than CDJ. The presentation is dominated by BPSD, with progressive motor and cognitive decline, in most cases with ataxia and family history of dementia. No periodic complexes on EEG nor elevation of 14-3-3 protein in CSF
Acquired forms	
i-CJD (iatrogenic Creutzfeldt-Jakob disease)	CJD caused by iatrogenic transmission through contaminated materials or substances: intracerebral stereotaxic or EEG needles; neurosurgery instruments; graft of dura mater from a corpse; intramuscular injections of human growth hormones (hGH) and gonadotropin
v-CJD (variant Creutzfeldt-Jakob disease)	CJD variant with presence of kuru-type amyloid plaques surrounded by spongiform lesions ("florid plaques"). Disease associated with contaminants originating in cattle with BSE with four cases has been described of secondary transmission through blood transfusion. No cases in the past 2 years (the National Creutzfeldt-Jakob Disease Research & Surveillance Unit, 2016 [233]). It occurs in younger individuals and has a slightly longer duration than the sporadic form of CJD. Presence of psychiatric symptoms with the appearance of ataxia and involuntary movements. EEG without periodic sharp wave complexes; bilateral pulvinar MRI high signal
Kuru	First prionic disease described in humans. Occurrence restricted to Papua New Guinea and its surroundings, relating to cannibalistic rituals that no longer occur
Genetic forms	
g-CJD (genetic Creutzfeldt-Jakob disease)	Represents approximately 9% of CJD cases in United Kingdom. Autosomal dominant inheritance mutation in the PNRP; no identified family history in over 50% of cases. Heterogeneous clinical features, with slightly younger age of onset and longer disease duration
FFI (fatal familial insomnia)	Also known as thalamic dementia. Dominant autosomal disease with a mutation in the codon 178 of the PRNP gene. Severe insomnia or interrupted sleep and dysautonomia, generally associated with myoclonia, ataxia, dysarthria, dysphagia, and pyramidal signs. Age of onset between 20 and 70 (median of 49) with a median survival span of 18.4 months
GSS (Gerstmann-Sträussler-Scheinker) disease	Dominant autosomal disease; annual incidence 1/100 million. Onset between 30 and 60 years and slow evolution (3.5–9.5 years). Clinical features vary; occurs with cerebral ataxia, difficulty walking, dementia, dysarthria, ocular dysmetria, Parkinsonism, hyporeflexia, or distal areflexia. Usually no myoclonia. Possible alterations in sleep rhythms or body temperature. Apathy and depression are frequent

toms may occur, and generally pyramidal signs are found on neurological examination [229, 230, 236]. The EEG shows a characteristic pattern of periodic sharp wave complexes during the evolution of the disease [237]. MRI normally shows an increase in signal in the putamen and in the caudate nucleus and less frequently an increase in diffuse cortical signal [238]. An elevation of the 14-3-3 protein in the cerebral spinal fluid (CSF) can help define the

diagnosis [239]. The disease progresses towards death, with an average duration of 4 months [232, 236].

Type VV2 generally beings with ataxia, with features of dementia appearing later. It occurs in 15–16% of s-CJD cases, the median onset age being approximately 65, and it has a median duration of 6 months. It does not display the typical EEG findings, MRI normally shows alteration in the basal ganglia, and there is an increase of the 14-3-3 protein in the CSF. The MV2 type, which represents 8–9% of the cases, has clinical features similar to VV2, except for a longer duration of the disease. The other types also have longer durations, similar to MV2 (average of 15–16 months), are rarer, do not show typical alterations in EEG, and have various clinical features: MM2-T has an early presentation of insomnia, and MM2-C and VV1 have a presentation of progressive dementia [232, 236].

The diagnostic criteria for probable s-CJD requires a presentation of progressive dementia, with at least two of the four typical clinical characteristics (myoclonia, cerebellar or visual impairment, pyramidal or extrapyramidal signs, akinetic mutism) and one of the following additional findings (periodic discharges in EEG; elevated level of CSF 14-3-3 protein with the duration of the disease being shorter than 2 years; hyperintense lesions in the caudate and putamen or in two cortical regions, among temporal, parietal, and occipital; and absence of an alternative diagnosis during routine examination). If none of the additional findings are present but the duration of the disease is less than 2 years, there are criteria for possible s-CJD [229, 240].

21.6.2.3   Treatment

Currently there are no effective treatments that can alter the course of the disease. Symptomatic treatment is often necessary, with possible use of selective serotonin reuptake inhibitors for depression, clonazepam for severe myoclonia, and atypical antipsychotics such as quetiapine, being that all of them can be useful in controlling agitation [229].

21.7   Infectious Diseases

Numerous bacteria, viruses, or parasites can infect the CNS. In this chapter we only consider a few infectious diseases which we consider as examples of infectious diseases among many others and which seam of particular relevance to the issue on dementia in general or in relation to the elderly.

21.7.1   HIV-Associated Neurocognitive Disorders (HAND)

HAND is the term currently used to designate the cognitive impairment caused by the human immunodeficiency virus (HIV) which occurs in 20–50% of individuals infected by the virus depending on the stage of the disease and the response to treatment [241].

21.7.1.1   Epidemiology

According to the WHO, approximately 40 million people live with HIV worldwide [242]. The virus afflicts the CNS at the beginning of the infection and can affect the nervous system directly, leading to HANDs, or indirectly, through opportunistic infections or neoplasia. Before the advent of retroviral treatment, up to half of the patients developed a severe state of dementia before death [243].

Therapies have greatly improved the prognosis for the disease, but the concentration of drugs and the inhibition of viral replication are lower in the CNS [244]. Although a majority of cases do not show a loss of function that characterizes a state of dementia, well-conducted observational studies have shown a prevalence of up to 60% of neurocognitive decline in HIV-infected patients undergoing antiretroviral therapy [245]. Furthermore, approximately half of people infected throughout the world do not have access to treatment [242].

21.7.1.2   Clinics

HAND includes three levels of severity, according to the classification proposed by the National Institute of Mental Health and the National Institute of Neurological Diseases and Stroke of the United States [246]. Patients that show alterations in neuropsychological tests (more than 1 standard deviation below the median indicated for their age and education) in two cognitive domains (verbal/language, attention/working memory, abstraction/executive, memory learning/recall, speed of information processing, sensory-perceptual or motor skills) but do not have cognitive complaints nor loss of functionality are diagnosed as having HIV-associated asymptomatic neurocognitive impairment (ANI). Those with subjective cognitive complaints or whose caregiver observes cognitive changes interfering mildly in work, home, or social activities and who show an objective alteration in neuropsychological testing are diagnosed as having HIV-1-associated mild neurocognitive disorder (MND). HIV-1-associated dementia (HAD) is diagnosed when there is an important, objectively identified cognitive impairment, with significant interference on daily activities while excluding a diagnosis of delirium and other aetiology for dementia. Neuropsychological evaluation is not mandatory for the latter diagnosis [246].

Antiretroviral treatment has significantly changed the profile of the patient with HAND. The incidence of patients with dementia has been drastically reduced, and patients improve their cognitive state with treatment. On the other hand, therapy increases the lifespan of AIDS patients, therefore leading to an increase in the prevalence of less severe states (MND and mainly ANI) [244].

The clinical presentation of HAD is classically through an insidious subcortical dementia state with a progression over months. Normally, behavioural and motor alterations are observed in addition to cognitive decline. Initially, one can observe loss of short-term memory, slowing of psychomotor skills and cognitive processing, language alterations, and apathy. Motor alterations such as slow gait ataxia, tremor, and impairment of fine motor skill occur in the majority of cases. As the disease progresses, there is an intense global cognitive impairment, in addition to medullary and peripheral nervous system diseases. Three characteristic changes in the disease can be observed after the antiretroviral treatment era: a slower onset, a clinical manifestation of cortical and extrapyramidal impairment, and an approximation of the clinical state to the effects of ageing [241].

Imaging exams are necessary to exclude other aetiologies for the dementia state, such as opportunistic infections and neoplasia, among others not related to HIV. MRI is the most utilized exam and is also useful in identifying no specific alterations related to HAD: cortical and subcortical atrophy, with ventricular enlargement and confluent signal abnormalities compromising the deep white matter. These signal alterations of the white matter are related to interstitial oedema and can reduce or disappear with antiretroviral treatment [241, 244].

Differential diagnosis should be done with opportunistic infections such as toxoplasmosis, cryptococcal and tuberculous meningoencephalitis, progressive multifocal leukoencephalopathy, and primary CNS lymphoma, in addition to neurodegenerative diseases, particularly in the elderly.

21.7.1.3 Treatment

Currently, there are seven different classes of antiretroviral drugs with distinct action mechanisms, efficacy, and adverse effects. Adequate treatment requires a combination of drugs to which the virus is sensitive, avoiding the development of resistance. For patients with a compromised CNS, one factor to be taken into consideration is the drug's capacity to cross the haematoencephalic barrier. A treatment regime with drugs that have a higher CNS Penetration Effectiveness (CPE) is associated with a higher reduction in the viral load in the CSF. However, more robust studies are needed to prove that the use of drugs with higher CPE score is associated with a higher improvement in neuropsychological evaluations [245, 247]. In addition to the adequate antiviral treatment, non-pharmacological measures, as described above, can be useful in managing patients in a dementia state.

21.7.2 Neurosyphilis

Neurosyphilis is an infectious disease of the nervous system caused by *Treponema pallidum*. It is a sexually transmitted disease in which the systemic spread of the microorganism occurs, normally reaching the central nervous system, potentially causing various early and late forms of neurosyphilis.

The initial consequence, which appears on average between 3 and 18 months after infection, is a state of meningitis, which happens in approximately 20–25% of individuals who are infected with syphilis. The majority of cases are asymptomatic, but headache, vomiting, epileptic episodes, and lesions to cranial nerves may occur. This stage is followed by a latent period that can evolve, after an average period of 6–7 years, into a vascular impairment, becoming meningo-vascular syphilis, the most frequent clinical manifestation of neurosyphilis. The parenchymatic impairment of the CNS occurs after a period of 15–20 years, developing tertiary neurological forms of syphilis, the most frequent being tabetic neurosyphilis (tabes dorsalis) and paretic neurosyphilis (general paresis, dementia paralytica) [248, 249].

21.7.2.1 Epidemiology

There is no population-based epidemiological data that help define the epidemiological tendency of the disease. It is known that there was a dramatic reduction of its occurrence following the discovery of penicillin in the 1940s, turning the tertiary forms of the disease into rare occurrences. After the HIV pandemic, the occurrence of neurosyphilis increased again and early cases started to have a larger proportion [249].

21.7.2.2 Clinics of Syphilitic Dementia

The initial clinical stage can be similar to other more frequent causes of dementia, such as loss of memory, changes in personality, irritability, and sleep alterations [250]. In developing countries, serum VDRL is recommended in aetiological investigation for all patients with dementia [251]. Later a global cognitive decline occurs with progressive memory loss, disorientation, reasoning difficulty, and emotional instability, possibly presenting convulsions. Serious psychiatric disturbances are frequent, including psychosis, mania, and depression. Cerebellar signals may occur, such as ataxia, intention tremors and dysarthria, as well as pupillary abnormalities [250]. If not treated, the majority of cases lead to death within 5 years of the appearance of symptoms [249].

The diagnosis is clinical and based on the CSF exam. According to CDC recommendations [252], the diagnosis in individuals with signs and symptoms of neurological impairment can be made with a positive VDRL in the CSF or, when the VDRL is negative, an increase in the number of cells and proteins, as long as the FTA-ABS is positive in the CSF (VDRL is specific but not very sensitive, while FTA-ABS is sensitive but not as specific). In HIV+ patients, who can already have a slight cellular increase in CSF, a cellularity above 20 leukocytes per mm [3] for the diagnosis of neurosyphilis must be considered [249, 252].

An imaging examination is important to exclude other aetiologies as the signs that appear in the encephalic MRI are not specific to neurosyphilis. The exam can be normal in neurosyphilis patients, especially in the initial stages. The most frequent findings on MRI are cerebral atrophy, white matter lesions, cerebral infarction, and oedema [253].

21.7.2.3 Treatment

The treatment of neurosyphilis is with penicillin G IV 18–24 million IU/day (3–4 million every 4 h), for 10–14 days. Alternatives are procaine penicillin + probenecid or ceftriaxone. After initial treatment, a CSF exam should be done every 6 months. If the patient is without symptoms and the CSF exam shows normalization in the number of cells and a reduction in proteins and serological levels, patients are considered to be treated. The persistence of positive VDRL after normalization of cells and protein does not indicate a need for additional treatment. If the control CSF exam shows an increase in cells and proteins, a new treatment course is required [248, 252].

21.7.3 Other Dementia-Relevant Infectious Diseases

21.7.3.1 Neurocysticercosis

Neurocysticercosis is a parasitic disease still endemic to Latin America, Africa, and Asia, caused by the larva of the *Taenia solium* invading the CNS. Cognitive impairment is one of the manifestations of the disease, which is frequently asymptomatic or causes epileptic episodes and, sometimes, psychiatric symptoms. Dementia is less frequent but can occur during the acute phase of the disease, when there generally are multiple live cysts in the cerebral parenchyma and obstructive hydrocephalus can occur. The diagnosis is done through an imaging. Antiparasitic treatment can cause an extensive inflammatory process and untreatable epileptic crises, normally not being recommended when there are multiple active lesions [254].

21.7.3.2 Lyme Disease

Lyme disease is caused by a spirochete, *Borrelia burgdorferi*, normally transmitted through tick bites. It occurs predominantly in endemic regions of North America, Europe, and Asia. The typical initial manifestation of the infection is the erythema migrans. Encephalic impairment can occur months or years after the initial manifestation of the disease, potentially leading to dementia. Diagnosis is suggested by a compatible epidemiological history and corroborated by the identification of the intrathecal production of specific antibodies, the exclusion of other aetiologies, and response to treatment. Treatment is done with antibiotic IV for 28 days (ceftriaxone 2 g/day or cefotaxime 2 g TID or penicillin 24 million IU/day) [255, 256].

21.7.3.3 Other Infections

Rare cases of dementia have been described in association with cryptococcal meningitis [257, 258], Whipple disease [259], and tuberculosis [260, 261]. Recently, evidence has appeared suggesting an association of the herpes family with a higher risk in the development and progression of AD [262].

21.8 General Conclusion

Detecting cognitive impairment and diagnosing dementia are fundamentally important tasks for general practitioners all over the world given the worldwide dementia epidemics.

Dementia is a syndrome caused by a host of diseases of which mixed, neurodegenerative, and vascular aetiologies are the most common ones in the elderly. An aetiopathogenic assessment is crucial though complex and multidimensional including somatic, cognitive, psychopathological, functional, and paraclinical investigations

with the patient and their caregivers being the sources of information. Depression and substance-induced cognitive impairment are a central differential diagnosis as they may be treated causally and potentially be cured.

Behavioural and psychological features of dementia must be looked for actively as they are usually accessible to efficient treatment.

Taking care of a patient with dementia is complex and heavily depends on the patient's caregiver. Formal caregivers must collaborate one with the other. Antidementia drugs have a limited indication, and psychosocial treatment of behavioural and psychological features of dementia are paramount and often efficient. Medication, if required, complements psychosocial treatment and not the other way round. Treatment options have to be evaluated dynamically as the patient and caregiver needs are likely to change constantly.

References

1. International Psychogeriatric Association. Complete guide to behavioral and psychological symptoms of dementia (BPSD). IPA BPSD Educational Package. Milwaukee: International Psychogeriatric Association; 2010.
2. Alzheimer's Disease International. World Alzheimer Report 2010. The Global economic impact of dementia. London: Alzheimer's Disease International; 2010.
3. de Mendonça LC, Almeida C, Illife S, Rasmussen J. Dementia in primary care mental health. In: Ivbijaro G, editor. Companion to primary care mental health. London: Wonca and Ratcliff; 2012. p. 571–607.
4. Ballard C, Fossey J, Chithramohan R, Howeard R, Burns A, Thompson P, Tadros G, Fairbairn A. Quality of care in private sector and NHS facilities for people with dementia: cross sectional survey. BMJ. 2001;323(7310):426–7.
5. Pot AM. Improving nursing home care for dementia: is the environment the answer? Aging Ment Health. 2013;17(7):785–7.
6. World Health Organization. World report on ageing and health. Luxembourg: World Health Organization; 2015.
7. Rechel B. How can health systems respond to population aging? In: World Health Organization, on behalf of the European Observatory on Health Systems and Policies, editor. Health systems and policy analysis. Copenhagen: World Health Organization; 2009.

8. Ramaroson H, Helmer C, Barberger-Gateau P, Letenneur L, Dartigues JF, PAQUID. Prevalence of dementia and Alzheimer's disease among subjects aged 75 years or over: updated results of the PAQUID cohort. Rev Neurol (Paris). 2003;159:405–11.
9. Büla C, Joray S, Eyer S, Simeone I, Camus V. Vieillissement cérébral pathologique: les pathologies démentielles. In: Leuba G, Büla C, Schenk F, editors. Du vieillissement cérébral à la maladie d'Alzheimer: vulnérabilité et plasticité. 2nd éd ed. Bruxelles: De Boeck; 2013. p. 239–76.
10. Duthey B. Background paper 6.11. Alzheimer disease and other dementias. Geneva: World Health Organization; 2013.
11. Corrada MM, Brookmeyer R, Berlau D, Paganini-Hill A, Kawas C. Prevalence of dementia after age 90: results from the 90+ study. Neurology. 2008;71:337–43.
12. Lucca U, Tettamanti M, Lagroscino G, Tiraboschi P, Landi C, Sacco L, Garri M, Ammesso S, Bertinotti C, Biotti A, Gargantini E, Piedicorcia A, Nobili A, Pasina L, Franchi C, Djade CD, Riva E, Recchia A. Prevalence of dementia in the oldest old: the Monzino 80-plus population-based study. Alzheimers Dement. 2015;11:258–70.
13. Alzheimer's Disease International. World Alzheimer report 2009. London: Alzheimer's Disease International; 2009.
14. Alzheimer's Disease International. World Alzheimer report 2009. London: Alzheimer's Disease International; 2010.
15. Kraft E, Marti M, Werner S, Sommer H. Cost of dementia in Switzerland. Swiss Med Wkly. 2010;10:w13093.
16. American Psychiatric Association. Desk reference to the diagnostic criteria from DSM-5. Arlington: American Psychiatric Association; 2013.
17. World Health Organization. The ICD-10 classification of mental and behavioural disorders. Geneva: World Health Organization; 1992.
18. Blass DM, Rabins PV. In the clinic: dementia. Ann Intern Med. 2008;148(7):ITC4–16.
19. Gremaud F, Decrey H, Démonet JF, von Gunten A, Büla C. Cognitive impairment in elderly patients: what to do in primary care. Rev Med Suisse. 2013;9:2029–33.
20. Weytingh MD, Bossuyt PM, van Crevel H. Reversible dementia: more than 10% or less than 1%? A quantitative review. J Neurol. 1995;242:466–71.
21. Monsch AU, Büla C, Hermelink M, Kressig RW, Martensson B, Mosimann U, Müri R, Vögeli S, von Gunten A, et le groupe d'experts en Suisse. Konsensus 2012 zur Diagnostik und Therapie von Demenzkranken in der Schweiz. Praxis. 2012;101:1239–50.
22. Folstein MF, Folstein SE, McHugh PR. "Mini-mental state". A practical method for grading the cognitive state of patients for the clinician. J Psychiatr Res. 1975;12(3):189–98.
23. Nasreddine ZS, Phillips NA, Beédirian V, Charbonneau S, Whitehead V, Collin I, Cummings JL, Chertkow H. The Montreal cognitive assessment, MoCA: a brief screening tool for mild cognitive impairment. J Am Geriatr Soc. 2005;53(4):695–9.
24. Borson S, Scanlan J, Brush M, Vitaliano P, Dokmak A. The mini-cog: a cognitive 'vital signs' measure for dementia screening in multi-lingual elderly. Int J Geriatr Psychiatry. 2000;15(11):1021–7.
25. Ehrensberger M, Taylor K, Berres M, Foldi N, Dellenbach M, Bopp I, Gold G, von Gunten A, Inglin D, Müri R, Rüegger B, Kressig R, Monsch A. BrainCheck – a very brief tool to detect incipient cognitive decline: optimized case-finding combining patient- and informant-based data. Alzheimers Res Ther. 2014;6:69.
26. Crum RM, Anthony JC, Basset SS, Folstein MF. Population-based norms for the Mini-Mental State Examination by age and educational level. JAMA. 1993;269:2386–91.
27. Winblad B, Kilander L, Eriksson S, Minthon L, Båtsman S, Wetterholm AL, Jansson-Blixt C, Haglund A, Severe Alzheimer's Disease Study Group. Donepezil in patients with severe Alzheimer's disease: double-blind, parallel-group, placebo-controlled study. Lancet. 2006;367(9516):1057–65. Erratum in: Lancet 2006;368(9548):1650. Lancet 2006;367(9527):1980.
28. Morris J. The Clinical Dementia Rating (CDR): current version and scoring rules. Neurology. 1993;43:2412–4.
29. Reisberg B, Ferris SH, de Leon MJ, Crook T. The Global Deterioration Scale for assessment of primary degenerative dementia. Am J Psychiatry. 1982;139:1136–9.
30. Lawton MP, Brody EC. Assessment of old people: self maintaining and instrumental activities of daily living. Gerontologist. 1969;9:179–86.
31. Jorm AF, Jacomb PA. The Informant Questionnaire on Cognitive Decline in the Elderly (IQCODE): socio-demographic correlates, reliability, validity, and some norms. Psychol Med. 1989;19:1015–22.
32. Spiegel R, Brunner C, Ermini-Fünfschilling D, Monsch A, Notter M, Puxty J, Tremmel L. A new behavioral assessment scale for geriatric out- and in-patients: the NOSGER (Nurses' Observation Scale for Geriatric Patients). J Am Geriatr Soc. 1991;39(4):339–47.
33. Katz S, Ford AB, Moskowitz RW, Jackson BA, Jaffe MW. Studies of illness in the aged: the Index of ADL: a standardized measure of biological and psychosocial function. JAMA. 1963;185:914–9.
34. Amariglio RE, Townsend MK, Grodstein F, Sperling RA, Rentz DM. Specific memory complaints in older persons may indicate poor cognitive function. J Am Geriatr Soc. 2011;59:1612–7.
35. Kaufer D, Cummings J, Ketchel P, Smith V, MacMillan A, Shelley T, Lopez O, DeKosky S. Validation of the NPI-Q, a brief clinical form of the neuropsychiatric inventory. J Neuropsychiatr Clin Neurosci. 2000;12:233–9.

36. Reisberg B, Borenstein J, Salob S, Ferris S, Franssen E, Goergotas A. Behavioral symptoms in Alzheimer's disease: phenomenology and treatment. J Clin Psychiatry. 1987;48(suppl):9–15.

37. Tariot PN, Mack JL, Patterson MB, Edland SD, Weiner MF, Fillenbaum G, Blazina L, Teri L, Rubin E, Mortimer JA, Stern Y. Behavioral pathology committee of the consortium to establish a registry for Alzheimer's disease. Am J Psychiatry. 1995;152:1349–57.

38. Jeon Y, Sansoni J, Low L, et al. Recommended measures for the assessment of behavioral disturbances associated with dementia. Am J Geriatr Psychiatry. 2011;19:403–15.

39. Conn D, Thorpe L. Assessment of behavioural and psychological symptoms associated with dementia. Can J Neurol Sci. 2007;34(Suppl 1):S67–71.

40. Burns A, Lawlor B, Craig S. Rating scales in old age psychiatry. Br J Psychiatry. 2002;180:161–7.

41. Yesavage J, Brink T, Rose T, Lum O, Huang V, Adey M, Leirer O. Development and validation of a geriatric depression screening scale: a preliminary report. J Psychiatr Res. 1983;17:37–49.

42. Alexopoulos G, Abrams R, Young R, Shamoian C. Cornell scale for depression in dementia. Biol Psychiatry. 1988;23:271–84.

43. Beck A, Ward C, Mendelson M, Mock J, Erbaugh J. An inventory for measuring depression. Arch Gen Psychiatry. 1961;4:53–63.

44. Montgomery S, Asberg M. A new depression scale designed to be sensitive to change. Br J Psychiatry. 1979;134:384–9.

45. Radloff L, Teri L. Use of the center for epidemiological studies – depression scale with older adults. Clin Gerontol. 1986;5:119–37.

46. Hamilton M. A rating scale for depression. J Neurol Neurosurg Psychiatry. 1960;23:56–62.

47. von Gunten A, Pocnet C, Rossier J. The impact of personality characteristics on the clinical expression in neurodegenerative disorders - a review. Brain Res Bull. 2009;80:179–91.

48. Apostolova L, Cummings J. Neuropsychiatric manifestations in mild cognitive impairment: a systematic review of the literature. Dement Geriatr Cogn Disord. 2008;25:115–26.

49. McKeith IG, Dickson DW, Lowe J, Consortium on DLB, et al. Diagnosis and management of dementia with Lewy bodies: third report of the DLB Consortium. Neurology. 2005;65(12):1863–1872. Erratum in: Neurology 2005;65(12):1992.

50. Dubois B, Feldman HH, Jacova C, Dekosky ST, Barberger-Gateau P, Cummings J, Delacourte A, Galasko D, Gauthier S, Jicha G, Meguro K, O'Brien J, Pasquier F, Robert P, Rossor M, Salloway S, Stern Y, Visser PJ, Scheltens P. Research criteria for the diagnosis of Alzheimer's disease: revising the NINCDS-ADRDA criteria. Lancet Neurol. 2007;6(8):734–46.

51. McKhann GM, Knopman DS, Chertkow H, Hyman BT, Jack CR Jr, Kawas CH, Klunk WE, Koroshetz WJ, Manly JJ, Mayeux R, Mohs RC, Morris JC, Rossor MN, Scheltens P, Carrillo MC, Thies B, Weintraub S, Phelps CH. The diagnosis of dementia due to Alzheimer's disease: recommendations from the National Institute on Aging-Alzheimer's Association workgroups on diagnostic guidelines for Alzheimer's disease. Alzheimers Dement. 2011;7(3):263–9.

52. Mattsson N, Andreasson U, Persson S, Arai H, Batish SD, Bernardini S, Bocchio-Chiavetto L, Blankenstein MA, Carrillo MC, Chalbot S, Coart E, Chiasserini D, Cutler N, Dahlfors G, Duller S, Fagan AM, Forlenza O, Frisoni GB, Galasko D, Galimberti D, Hampel H, Handberg A, Heneka MT, Herskovits AZ, Herukka SK, Holtzman DM, Humpel C, Hyman BT, Iqbal K, Jucker M, Kaeser SA, Kaiser E, Kapaki E, Kidd D, Klivenyi P, Knudsen CS, Kummer MP, Lui J, Lladó A, Lewczuk P, Li QX, Martins R, Masters C, McAuliffe J, Mercken M, Moghekar A, Molinuevo JL, Montine TJ, Nowatzke W, O'Brien R, Otto M, Paraskevas GP, Parnetti L, Petersen RC, Prvulovic D, de Reus HP, Rissman RA, Scarpini E, Stefani A, Soininen H, Schröder J, Shaw LM, Skinningsrud A, Skrogstad B, Spreer A, Talib L, Teunissen C, Trojanowski JQ, Tumani H, Umek RM, Van Broeck B, Vanderstichele H, Vecsei L, Verbeek MM, Windisch M, Zhang J, Zetterberg H, Blennow K. The Alzheimer's Association external quality control program for cerebrospinal fluid biomarkers. Alzheimers Dement. 2011;7(4):386–95.

53. Au R, Seshadri S, Knox K, Beiser A, Himali JJ, Cabral HJ, Auerbach S, Green RC, Wolf PA, McKee AC. The Framingham Brain Donation Program: neuropathology along the cognitive continuum. Curr Alzheimer Res. 2012;9(6):673–86.

54. Beach TG, Monsell SE, Phillips LE, Kukull W. Accuracy of the clinical diagnosis of Alzheimer disease at National Institute on aging Alzheimer Disease Centers, 2005–2010. J Neuropathol Exp Neurol. 2012;71:266–73.

55. Prince M, Bryce R, Ferri C. The benefits of early diagnosis and intervention: World Alzheimer Report 2011. London: Alzheimer's Disease International; 2011 (www.alz.org).

56. Olazarán J, Reisberg B, Clare L, Cruz I, Peña-Casanova J, Del Ser T, Woods B, Beck C, Auer S, Lai C, Spector A, Fazio S, Bond J, Kivipelto M, Brodaty H, Rojo JM, Collins H, Teri L, Mittelman M, Orrell M, Feldman HH, Muñiz R. Nonpharmacological therapies in Alzheimer's disease: a systematic review of efficacy. Dement Geriatr Cogn Disord. 2010;30(2):161–78.

57. Alexopoulos GS, Silver IM, Kahn DA, Frances A, Carpenter D. Treatment of agitation in older persons with dementia. Expert Consensus Guideline Series. 2001;1–32. http://www.psychguides.com/gagl. html.

58. Lawlor BA. Behavioral complications in Alzheimer's disease. Washington, DC: American Psychiatric Press; 1995.

59. O'Connor D, Rabins P, Swanwick G. IPA complete guide to behavioral and psychological symptoms of dementia (BPSD): module 5, non-pharmacological treatments. Milwaukee: International Psychogeriatric Association; 2010.

60. Rybisar Van Dyke M, Kohler MC, Küng A, Camus V, von Gunten A. Prise en charge globale et thérapies actuelles de la démence de type Alzheimer. In: Schenk F, Leuba G, Büla C, editors. Du vieillissement cérébral à la maladie d'Alzheimer: vulnérabilité et plasticité. Bruxelles: De Boeck; 2013. p. 277–307.

61. Kolanowski A. An overview of the need-driven dementia-compromised behavior model. J Gerontol Nurs. 1999;25:7–9.

62. Kovach C. The serial trial intervention: an innovative approach to meeting needs of individuals with dementia. J Gerontol Nurs. 2006;32:18–25.

63. Kovach C, et al. Effects of the serial trial intervention on discomfort and behavior of nursing home residents with dementia. Am J Alzheimers Dis Other Demen. 2006;21:147–55.

64. Ayalon L, Gum AM, Feliciano L, et al. Effectiveness of nonpharmacological interventions for the management of neuropsychiatric symptoms in patients with dementia. Arch Intern Med. 2006;166:2182–8.

65. Thorgrimsen LM, Spector AE, Wiles A, et al. Aroma therapy for dementia. Cochrane Database Syst Rev. 2003;(3):CD003150. https://doi.org/10.1002/14651858.CD003150.

66. Livingston G, Johnston K, Katona C, et al. Systematic review of psychological approaches to the management of neuropsychiatric symptoms of dementia. Am J Psychiatry. 2005;162:1996–2021.

67. Heyn P, Abreu BC, Ottenbacher KJ. The effects of exercise training on elderly persons with cognitive impairment and dementia: a meta-analysis. Arch Phys Med Rehabil. 2004;85:1694–704.

68. Buchanan JA, Christenson A, Houlihan D, Ostrom C. The role of behaviour analysis in the rehabilitation of persons with dementia. Behav Ther. 2011;42(1):9–21.

69. Kortte KB, Rogalski EJ. Behavioural intervention for enhancing life participation in behavioural variant frontotemporal dementia and primary progressive aphasia. Int Rev Psychiatry. 2013;25(2):237–45.

70. Gitlin LN, Winter L, Dennis MP, Hodgson N, Hauck WW. A biobehavioral home-based intervention and the well-being of patients with dementia and their caregivers. JAMA. 2010a;304(9):983–91.

71. Gitlin LN, Winter L, Dennis MP, Hodgson N, Hauck WW. Targeting and managing behavioral symptoms in individuals with dementia: a randomized trial of a nonpharmacological intervention. J Am Geriatr Soc. 2010;58:1465–74.

72. Savaskan E, Bopp-Kistler I, Buerge M, Georgescu D, Giardini UM, Hatzinger M, Hemmeter U, Justiniano I, Kressig R, Monsch A, Mosimann U, Mueri R, Munk A, Schmid R, Wollmer M. Recommendations for diagnosis and therapy of behavioral and psychological symptoms in dementia (BPSD). Praxis. 2014;103:135–48.

73. Wylie MA, Shnall A, Onyike CU, Huey ED. Management of frontotemporal dementia in mental health and multidisciplinary settings. Int Rev Psychiatry. 2013;25(2):230–6.

74. Gormley N, Lyons D, Howard R. Behavioral management of aggression in dementia: a randomized controlled trial. Age Ageing. 2001;30:141–5.

75. Fried-Oken M, Beukelmann DR, Hux K. Current and future AAC research considerations for adults with acquired cognitive and communication impairments. Assist Technol. 2011;24(1):56–66.

76. Henry ML, Meese MV, Truong S, Babiak MC, Miller BL, Gorno-Tempini ML. Treatment for apraxia of speech in nonfluent variant primary progressive aphasia. Behav Neurol. 2013;26:77–88.

77. Jokel R, Anderson ND. Quest for the best: effects of errorless and active encoding on word re-learning in semantic dementia. Neuropsychol Rehabil. 2012;22(2):187–214.

78. Ballard C, Khan Z, Clack H, Corbett A. Nonpharmacological treatment of Alzheimer disease. Can J Psychiatr. 2011;56(10):589–95.

79. Goh JO, Park DC. Neuroplasticity and cognitive aging: the scaffolding theory of aging and cognition. Restor Neurol Neurosci. 2009;27(5):391–403.

80. Scholey KA, Woods BT. A series of brief cognitive therapy interventions with people experiencing both dementia and depression: a description of techniques and common themes. Clin Psychol Psychother. 2003;10:175–85.

81. Woods B, Spector A, Jones C, et al. Reminiscence therapy for dementia. Cochrane Database Syst Rev. 2005;18:CD001120.

82. Finger EC. New potential therapeutic approaches in frontotemporal dementia: oxytocin, vasopressin, and social cognition. J Mol Neurosci. 2011;45:696–701.

83. Shnall A, Agate A, Grinberg A, Huijbregts M, Nguyen MQ, Chow TW. Development of supportive services for frontotemporal dementias through community engagement. Int Rev Psychiatry. 2013;25(3):246–52.

84. Nunnemann S, Kurz A, Leucht S, Diehl-Schmid J. Caregivers of patients with frontotemporal lobar degeneration: a review of burden, problems, needs, and interventions. Int Psychogeriatr. 2012;24(9):1368–86.

85. Miller LA, Mioshi E, Savage S, Lah S, Hodges JR, Piguet O. Identifying cognitive and demographic variables that contribute to carer burden in dementia. Dement Geriatr Cogn Disord. 2013;36:43–9.

86. Pearce J. Systemic therapy. In: Heppel J, Pearce J, Wilkinson P, editors. Psychological therapies with older people. New York: Taylor and Francis; 2002. p. 76–102.

87. Bäuml J, Pischel-Wal G. Psychoedukation bei schizophrenen Erkrankungen. New York: Schattauer-Verlag; 2008.

88. Hepburn K, Lewis M, Tornatore J, et al. The Savvy Caregiver program: the demonstrated effectiveness of a transportable dementia caregiver psychoeducation program. J Gerontol Nurs. 2007;33:30–6.

89. Sorbi S, Hort J, Erkinjuntti T, Fladby T, Gainotti G, Gurvit H, et al. EFNS-ENS guidelines on the diagnosis and management of disorders associated with dementia. Eur J Neurol. 2012;19(9):1159–79.

90. Meuser TM, Marwit SJ. A comprehensive, stage-sensitive model of grief in dementia caregiving. Gerontologist. 2001;41(5):658–70.

91. Ettema EJ, Derksen LD, van Leeuwen E. Existential loneliness and end-of-life care: a systematic review. Theor Med Bioeth. 2010;31:141–69.

92. von Gunten A, Alnawaqil AM, Abderhalden C, Needham I, Schüpbach B. Vocally disruptive behavior in the elderly: a systematic review. Int Psychogeriatr. 2008;20:653–72.

93. Hajjar RR, Kamel HK. Sexuality in the nursing home, part 1: attitudes and barriers to sexual expression. J Am Med Dir Assoc. 2004;5:43–7.

94. Brodaty H. Meta-analysis of nonpharmacological interventions for neuropsychiatric symptoms of dementia. Am J Psychiatry. 2012;169:946–53.

95. Seitz D, Lawlor B. IPA complete guide to Behavioral and Psychological Symptoms of Dementia (BPSD): module 6, pharmacological treatment. Milwaukee: International Psychogeriatric Association; 2010.

96. Banerjee S, Hellier J, Dewey M, et al. Sertraline or mirtazapine for depression in dementia (HTA-SADD): a randomised, multicentre, double-blind, placebo-controlled trial. Lancet. 2011;378:403–11.

97. Lyketsos C, Carrillo M, Ryan J, et al. Neuropsychiatric symptoms in Alzheimer's disease. Alzheimers Dement. 2011;7:532–9.

98. Holmes C, Wilkinson D, Dean C, et al. The efficacy of donepezil in the treatment of neuropsychiatric symptoms in Alzheimer disease. Neurology. 2004;63:214–9.

99. von Gunten A, Schlaefke S, Überla K. Efficacy of *Ginkgo biloba* extract EGb 761® in dementia with behavioural and psychological symptoms: a systematic review. World J Biol Psychiatry. 2016;17:622–33.

100. Schneider LS, Pollock VE, Lyness SA. A metaanalysis of controlled trials of neuroleptic treatment in dementia. J Am Geriatr Soc. 1990;38:553–63.

101. Maher AR, Maglione M, Bagley S, et al. Efficacy and comparative effectiveness of atypical antipsychotic medications for off-label uses in adults: a systematic review and meta-analysis. JAMA. 2011;306:1359–69.

102. Ballard C, Waite J. The effectiveness of atypical antipsychotics for the treatment of aggression and psychosis in Alzheimer's disease. Cochrane Database Syst Rev. 2006;(1):CD003476.

103. Gauthier S, Loft H, Cummings J. Improvement in behavioural symptoms in patients with moderate to severe Alzheimer's disease by memantine: a pooled data analysis. Int J Geriatr Psychiatry. 2008;23:537–45.

104. Wilcock GK, Ballard CG, Cooper JA, Loft H. Memantine for agitation/aggression and psychosis in moderately severe to severe Alzheimer's disease: a pooled analysis of 3 studies. J Clin Psychiatry. 2008;69:341–8.

105. Zhou QP, Jung L, Richards KC. The management of sleep and circadian disturbance in patients with dementia. Curr Neurol Neurosci Rep. 2012;12(2):193–204.

106. Oudman E. Is electroconvulsive therapy (ECT) effective and safe for treatment of depression in dementia? A short review. J ECT. 2012;28(1):34–8.

107. Yates FE. Complexity of a human being: changes with age. Neurobiol Aging. 2002;23:17–9.

108. Gold G, Giannakopoulos P, Herrmann FR, Bouras C, Kövari E. Identification of Alzheimer and vascular lesion thresholds for mixed dementia. Brain. 2007;130:2830–6.

109. Braak H, Del Tredici K. Where, when, and in what form does sporadic Alzheimer disease begin? Curr Opin Neurol. 2012;25(6):708–14.

110. Cruchaga C, Kauwe J, Goate A. Alzheimer's disease. In: Nurnberger J, Berrettini W, editors. Priniciples of psychiatric genetics. Cambridge: Cambridge University Press; 2012. p. 371–81.

111. McKhann G, Drachman D, Folstein M, Katzman R, Price D, Stadlan E. Clinical diagnosis of Alzheimer's disease: report of the NINCDS-ADRDA Work Group under the auspices of Department of Health and Human Services Task Force on Alzheimer's Disease. Neurology. 1984;34:939–44.

112. Khachaturian Z. Diagnosis of Alzheimer's disease. Arch Neurol. 1985;42:1097–105.

113. Mirra S, Heyman A, McKeel D, Sumi S, Crain B, Brownlee L, Vogel F, Hughes J, van Belle G, Berg L. The Consortium to Establish a Registry for Alzheimer's Disease (CERAD). Part II. Standardization of the neuropathologic assessment of Alzheimer's disease. Neurology. 1991;41:479–86.

114. The National Institute on Aging, and Reagan Institute Working Group on Diagnostic Criteria for the Neuropathological Assessment of Alzheimer's Disease. Consensus recommendations for the post-mortem diagnosis of Alzheimer's disease. Neurobiol Aging. 1997;18:S1–2.

115. Braak H, Braak E. Neuropathological stageing of Alzheimer-related changes. Acta Neuropathol. 1991;82:239–59.

116. von Gunten A, Bouras C, Kövari E, Giannakopoulos P, Hof PR. Neural substrates of cognitive and behavioral deficits in atypical Alzheimer's disease. Brain Res Rev. 2006;51:176–211.

117. Blennow K, Hampel H, Weiner M, Zetterberg H. Cerebrospinal fluid and plasma biomarkers in Alzheimer disease. Nat Rev Neurol. 2010;6:131–44.

118. Smith M. Genetics of Alzheimer's disease. In: Ames D, Burns A, O'Brien J, editors. Dementia. London: Hodder Arnold; 2010. p. 451–8.

119. Deutsche Gesellschaft für Psychiatrie, Psychotherapie und Nervenheilkunde (DGPPN); Deutsche Gesellschaft für Neurologie (Hrsg.). Diagnose- und Behandlungsleitlinie Demenz. 1st ed. Berlin: Springer-Verlag; 2010. http://www.dgppn. de/publikationen/leitlinien/leitlinien10.html.

120. Hort J, O'Brien JT, Gainotti G, Pirttila T, Popescu BO, Rektorova I, Sorbi S, Scheltens P, EFNS Scientist Panel on Dementia. EFNS guidelines for the diagnosis and management of Alzheimer's disease. Eur J Neurol. 2010;17(10):1236–48.
121. NICE. NICE technology appraisal guidance 217: donepezil, galantamine, rivastigmine and memantine for the treatment of Alzheimer's disease - review of NICE technology appraisal guidance. London: National Institute for Health and Clinical Excellence; 2011.
122. NICE and SCIE. Dementia- Supporting people with dementia and their carers in health and social care. London: NICE and SCIE; 2006.
123. Birks J, Evans G. Ginkgo biloba for cognitive impairment and dementia. Cochrane Database Syst Rev. 2009;(1):CD003120.
124. Rolinski M, Fox C, Maidment I, McShane R. Cholinesterase inhibitors for dementia with Lewy bodies, Parkinson's disease dementia and cognitive impairment in Parkinson's disease. Cochrane Database Syst Rev. 2012;(3):CD006504.
125. O'Brien JT, Burns A, BAP Dementia Consensus Group. Clinical practice with anti-dementia drugs: a revised (second) consensus statement from the British Association for Psychopharmacology. J Psychopharmacol. 2011;25(8):997–1019.
126. Schneider LS, Dagerman KS, Higgins JP, McShane R. Lack of evidence for the efficacy of memantine in mild Alzheimer disease. Arch Neurol. 2011;68(8):991–8.
127. Hansen RA, Gartlehner G, Webb AP, Morgan LC, Moore CG, Jonas DE. Efficacy and safety of donepezil, galantamine, and rivastigmine for the treatment of Alzheimer's disease: a systematic review and meta-analysis. Clin Interv Aging. 2008;3(2):211–25.
128. Birks J, Flicker L. Donepezil for mild cognitive impairment. Cochrane Database Syst Rev. 2006;(3):CD006104. https://doi.org/10.1002/14651858.CD006104.
129. Black SE, Doody R, Li H, McRae T, Jambor KM, Xu Y, Sun Y, Perdomo CA, Richardson S. Donepezil preserves cognition and global function in patients with severe Alzheimer disease. Neurology. 2007;69(5):459–69.
130. Burns A, Bernabei R, Bullock R, Cruz Jentoft AJ, Frölich L, Hock C, Raivio M, Triau E, Vandewoude M, Wimo A, Came E, Van Baelen B, Hammond GL, van Oene JC, Schwalen S. Safety and efficacy of galantamine (Reminyl) in severe Alzheimer's disease (the SERAD study): a randomised, placebo-controlled, double-blind trial. Lancet Neurol. 2009;8(1):39–47.
131. Boudreau DM, Yu O, Gray SL, Raebel MA, Johnson J, Larson EB. Concomitant use of cholinesterase inhibitors and anticholinergics: prevalence and outcomes. J Am Geriatr Soc. 2011;59(11):2069–76.
132. Bullock R, Touchon J, Bergman H, Gambina G, He Y, Rapatz G, Nagel J, Lane R. Rivastigmine and donepezil treatment in moderate to moderately-severe Alzheimer's disease over a 2-year period. Curr Med Res Opin. 2005;21(8):1317–27.
133. Jones RW, Soininen H, Hager K, Aarsland D, Passmore P, Murthy A, Zhang R, Bahra R. A multinational, randomised, 12-week study comparing the effects of donepezil and galantamine in patients with mild to moderate Alzheimer's disease. Int J Geriatr Psychiatry. 2004;19(1):58–67.
134. Wilcock G, Howe I, Coles H, Lilienfeld S, Truyen L, Zhu Y, Bullock R, Kershaw P, GAL-GBR-2 Study Group. A long-term comparison of galantamine and donepezil in the treatment of Alzheimer's disease. Drugs Aging. 2003;20(10):777–89.
135. Wilkinson DG, Passmore AP, Bullock R, Hopker SW, Smith R, Potocnik FC, Maud CM, Engelbrecht I, Hock C, Ieni JR, Bahra RS. A multinational, randomised, 12-week, comparative study of donepezil and rivastigmine in patients with mild to moderate Alzheimer's disease. Int J Clin Pract. 2002;56(6):441–6.
136. Mecocci P, Bladström A, Stender K. Effects of memantine on cognition in patients with moderate to severe Alzheimer's disease: post-hoc analyses of ADAS-cog and SIB total and single-item scores from six randomized, double-blind, placebo-controlled studies. Int J Geriatr Psychiatry. 2009;24(5):532–8.
137. McShane R, Areosa Sastre A, Minakaran N. Memantine for dementia. Cochrane Database Syst Rev. 2006;(2):CD003154.
138. Tariot PN, Farlow MR, Grossberg GT, Graham SM, McDonald S, Gergel I. Memantine Study Group. Memantine treatment in patients with moderate to severe Alzheimer disease already receiving donepezil: a randomized controlled trial. JAMA. 2004;291(3):317–24.
139. Lopez OL, Becker JT, Wahed AS, Saxton J, Sweet RA, Wolk DA, Klunk W, Dekosky ST. Long-term effects of the concomitant use of memantine with cholinesterase inhibition in Alzheimer disease. J Neurol Neurosurg Psychiatry. 2009;80(6):600–7.
140. Howard R, McShane R, Lindesay J, Ritchie C, Baldwin A, Barber R, Burns A, Dening T, Findlay D, Holmes C, Hughes A, Jacoby R, Jones R, Jones R, McKeith I, Macharouthu A, O'Brien J, Passmore P, Sheehan B, Juszczak E, Katona C, Hills R, Knapp M, Ballard C, Brown R, Banerjee S, Onions C, Griffin M, Adams J, Gray R, Johnson T, Bentham P, Phillips P. Donepezil and memantine for moderate-to-severe Alzheimer's disease. N Engl J Med. 2012;366(10):893–903.
141. Porsteinsson AP, Grossberg GT, Mintzer J, Olin JT, Memantine MEM-MD-12 Study Group. Memantine treatment in patients with mild to moderate Alzheimer's disease already receiving a cholinesterase inhibitor: a randomized, double-blind, placebo-controlled trial. Curr Alzheimer Res. 2008;5(1):83–9.
142. Birks J. Cholinesterase inhibitors for Alzheimer's disease. Cochrane Database Syst Rev. 2006;(1):CD005593.
143. Salomone S, Caraci F, Leggio GM, Fedotova J, Drago F. New pharmacological strategies for treatment of Alzheimer's disease: focus on disease modifying drugs. Br J Clin Pharmacol. 2012;73(4):504–17.

144. Palmer K, Di Iulio F, Varsi AE, Gianni W, Sancesario G, Caltagirone C, Spalletta G. Neuropsychiatric predictors of progression from amnestic-mild cognitive impairment to Alzheimer's disease: the role of depression and apathy. J Alzheimers Dis. 2010;20(1):175–83.

145. Massoud F, Belleville S, Bergman H, Kirk J, Chertkow H, Nasreddine Z, Joanette Y, Freedman M. Mild cognitive impairment and cognitive impairment, no dementia: part B, therapy. Alzheimers Dement. 2007;3(4):283–91.

146. Rabinovici GD, Miller BL. Frontotemporal lobar degeneration: epidemiology, pathophysiology, diagnosis and management. CNS Drugs. 2010;24(5):375–98.

147. Johnson JK, Diehl J, Mendez MF, Neuhaus J, Shapira JS, Forman M, et al. Frontotemporal lobar degeneration: demographic characteristics of 353 patients. Arch Neurol. 2005;62:925–30.

148. Mercy L, Hodges JR, Dawson K, et al. Incidence of early-onset dementias in Cambridgeshire, United Kingdom. Neurology. 2008;71:1496.

149. Hodges JR, Davies R, Xuereb J, Kril J, Halliday G. Survival in frontotemporal dementia. Neurology. 2003;61:349–54.

150. Robertson ED, Hesse JH, Rose KD, Slama BA, Johnson JK, Yaffe K, et al. Frontotemporal dementia progresses to death faster than Alzheimer disease. Neurology. 2005;65:719–25.

151. Onyke CU, Diehl-Schimid J. The epidemiology of frontotemporal dementia. Int Rev Psychiatry. 2013;25(2):130–7.

152. Knopman DS, Robert RO. Estimating the number of persons with frontotemporal lobar degeneration in the US population. J Mol Neurosci. 2011;45(3):330–5.

153. Borroni B, Turrone R, Galimberti D, Nacmias B, Alberici A, Benussi A, Caffarra P, Caltagirone C, Cappa SF, Frisoni GB, Ghidoni R, Marra C, Padovani A, Rainero I, Scarpini E, Silani V, Sorbi S, Tagliavini F, Tremolizzo L, Bruni AC. Italian Frontotemporal Dementia Network (FTD Group-SINDEM): sharing clinical and diagnostic procedures in Frontotemporal Dementia in Italy. Neurol Sci. 2015;36:751–7.

154. Gorno-Tempini ML, Hillis AE, Weintraub S, et al. Classification of primary progressive aphasia and its variants. Neurology. 2011;76:1006.

155. Rascovsky K, Hodges JR, Knopman D, et al. Sensitivity of revised diagnostic criteria for the behavioural variant of frontotemporal dementia. Brain. 2011;134:2456–77.

156. Galimberti D, Fenoglio C, Serpente M, Villa C, Bonsi R, Arighi A, et al. Autosomal dominant frontotemporal lobar degeneration due to the C9ORF72 hexanucleotide repeat expansion: late-onset psychotic clinical presentation. Biol Psychiatry. 2013;74:384–91.

157. Rosso SM, Donker Kaat L, Baks T, Joosse M, de Koning I, Pijnenburg Y, et al. Frontotemporal dementia in the Netherlands: patients characteristics and prevalence estimates from a population-based study. Brain. 2003;126:2016–22.

158. Ducharme S, Price BH, Larvie M, Dougherty DD, Dickerson BC. Clinical approach to the differential diagnosis between behavioural variant frontotemporal dementia and primary psychiatric disorders. Am J Psychiatry. 2015;172(9):827–37.

159. Bertoux M, Delavest M, Souza LC, Fukiewiez A, Lépine JP, Fossati P, Dubois B. Sarazin social cognition and emotional assessment differentiates frontotemporal dementia from depression. J Neurol Neurosurg Psychiatry. 2012;83:411–6.

160. Bertoux M, Souza LC, O'Callaghan C, Greve A, Sarazin M, Dubois B, Hornberger M. Social cognition deficits: the key to discriminate behavioral variant frontotemporal dementia from Alzheimer's disease regardless of amnesia? J Alzheimers Dis. 2015;49(4):1065–74.

161. Rankin KP, Gorno-Tempini ML, Allison SC, et al. Structural anatomy of empathy in neurodegenerative disease. Brain. 2006;129:2945.

162. Piguet O, Petersén A, Yin Ka Lam B, et al. Eating and hypothalamus changes in behavioral-variant frontotemporal dementia. Ann Neurol. 2011;69:312.

163. Mioshi E, Foxe D, Leslie F, Savage S, Hsieh S, Miller L, Hodges JR, Piguet O. The impact of dementia severity on caregiver burden in frontotemporal dementia and Alzheimer disease. Alzheimer Dis Assoc Disord. 2013;27(1):68–73.

164. Warren JD, Rohrer JD, Rossor MN. Clinical review. Frontotemporal dementia. BMJ. 2013;347:f4827.

165. The Lund and Manchester Groups. Clinical and neuropathological criteria for frontotemporal dementia. J Neurol Neurosurg Psychiatry. 1994;57:416.

166. Perri R, Koch G, Carlesimo GA, et al. Alzheimer's disease and frontal variant of frontotemporal dementia – a very brief battery for cognitive and behavioural distinction. J Neurol. 2005;252:1238.

167. Kertesz A, Blair M, McMonagle P, Munoz DG. The diagnosis and course of frontotemporal dementia. Alzheimer Dis Assoc Disord. 2007;21:155.

168. Bathgate D, Snowden JS, Varma A, et al. Behaviour in frontotemporal dementia, Alzheimer's disease and vascular dementia. Acta Neurol Scand. 2001;103:367.

169. Piguet O, Hornberger M, Mioshi E, Hodges JR. Behavioural-variant frontotemporal dementia: diagnosis, clinical staging, and management. Lancet Neurol. 2011;10:162.

170. Floris G, Borghero G, Cannas A, Di Stefano F, Murru MR, Corongiu D, et al. Bipolar affective disorder preceding frontotemporal dementia in a patient with C9orf72 mutation: is there a genetic link between these two disorders? J Neurol. 2013;160:1155–7.

171. Woolley JD, Khan BK, Murthy NK, Miller BL, Rankin KP. The diagnostic challenge of psychiatric symptoms in neurodegenerative diseases: rates and risk factors for prior psychiatric diagnosis in patients with early neurodegenerative disease. J Clin Psychiatry. 2011;72(2):126–33.

172. Pose M, Cetkovich M, Gleichgerrcht E, Ibanez A, Torralva T, Manes F. The overlap of symptomatic dimensions between frontotemporal dementia and several psychiatric disorders that appear in late adulthood. Int Rev Psychiatry. 2013;25(2):159–67.

173. Mesulam MM, Grossman M, Hillis A, et al. The core and halo of primary progressive aphasia and semantic dementia. Ann Neurol. 2003;54(Suppl 5):S11.

174. Knibb JA, Xuereb JH, Patterson K, Hodges JR. Clinical and pathological characterization of progressive aphasia. Ann Neurol. 2006;59:156.

175. Le Rhun E, Richard F, Pasquier F. Natural history of primary progressive aphasia. Neurology. 2005;65:887.

176. Snowden JS, Thompson JC, Neary D. Knowledge of famous faces and names in semantic dementia. Brain. 2004;127:860.

177. Hodges JR, Patterson K, Ward R, et al. The differentiation of semantic dementia and frontal lobe dementia (temporal and frontal variants of frontotemporal dementia) from early Alzheimer's disease: a comparative neuropsychological study. Neuropsychology. 1999;13:31.

178. Dubois B, Slachevsky A, Litvan I, Pillon B. The FAB: a Frontal Assessment Battery at bedside. Neurology. 2000;55(11):1621–6.

179. Mathias JL, Morphett K. Neurobehavioral differences between Alzheimer's disease and frontotemporal dementia: a meta-analysis. J Clin Exp Neuropsychol. 2010;32(7):682–98.

180. Valverde AH, Jimenez-Escrig A, Gobernado J, Baron M. A short neuropsychologic and cognitive evaluation of frontotemporal dementia. Clin Neurol Neurosurg. 2009;111(3):251–5.

181. Shany-Ur T, Poorzand P, Grossman SN, et al. Comprehension of insincere communication in neurodegenerative disease: lies, sarcasm, and theory of mind. Cortex. 2012;48:1329.

182. Mendez MF, Shapira JS, McMurtray A, et al. Accuracy of the clinical evaluation for frontotemporal dementia. Arch Neurol. 2007;64:830.

183. Hodges JR. Hope abandoned: memantine therapy in frontotemporal dementia. Lancet Neurol. 2013;12:121–3.

184. Rohrer JD, Nicholas JM, Cash DM, et al. Presymptomatic cognitive and neuroanatomical changes in genetic frontotemporal dementia in the Genetic Frontotemporal dementia Initiative (GENFI) study: a cross-sectional analysis. Lancet Neurol. 2015;14(3):253–62.

185. Sieben A, van Langenhove T, Engelborghs S, Martin JJ, Boon P, Cras P, et al. The genetic and neuropathology of frontotemporal lobar degeneration. Acta Neuropathol. 2012;124:353–72.

186. Cerami C, Scarpini E, Cappa SF, Galimberti D. Frontotemporal lobar degeneration: current knowledge and future challenges. J Neurol. 2012;259:2278–86.

187. Mackenzie IR, Neumann M, Bigio EH, Cairns NJ, Alafuzoff I, Kril J, et al. Nomenclature and nosology for neuropathologic subtypes of frontotemporal lobar degeneration: an update. Acta Neuropathol. 2010;119:1–4.

188. Manoochehri M, Huey ED. Diagnosis and management of behavioural issues in frontotemporal dementia. Curr Neurol Neurosci Rep. 2012;12(5):528–36.

189. Kerchner GA, Tartaglia MC, Boxer AL. Abhorring the vacuum: use of Alzheimer's disease medications in frontotemporal dementia. Expert Rev Neurother. 2011;11(5):709–17.

190. Nardell M, Tampi RR. Pharmacological treatments for frontotemporal dementias: a systematic review of randomized controlled trials. Am J Alzheimers Dis Other Demen. 2014;29(2):123–32.

191. Weder ND, Aziz R, Wilkins K, Tampi RR. Frontotemporal dementia: a review. Ann General Psychiatry. 2007;6:15.

192. Portugal MG, Marinho V, Laks J. Pharmacological treatment of frontotemporal lobar degeneration: systematic review. Rev Bras Psiquiatr. 2011;33(1):81–90.

193. Vann Jones SA, O'Brien JT. The prevalence and incidence of dementia with Lewy bodies: a systematic review of population and clinical studies. Psychol Med. 2014;44:673.

194. Zaccai J, McCracken C, Brayne C. A systematic review of prevalence and incidence studies of dementia with Lewy bodies. Age Ageing. 2005;34:561.

195. Aarsland D, Rongve A, Nore SP, et al. Frequency and case identification of dementia with Lewy bodies using the revised consensus criteria. Dement Geriatr Cogn Disord. 2008;26(5):445–52.

196. Rahkonen T, Eloniemi-Sulkava U, Rissanen S, et al. Dementia with Lewy bodies according to the consensus criteria in a general population aged 75 years or older. J Neurol Neurosurg Psychiatry. 2003;74(6):720–4.

197. Fujimi K, Sasaki K, Noda K, et al. Clinicopathological outline of dementia with Lewy bodies applying the revised criteria: the Hisayama study. Brain Pathol. 2008;18:317.

198. Geser F, Wenning GK, Poewe W, McKeith I. How to diagnose dementia with Lewy bodies: state of the art. Mov Disord. 2005;20(Suppl 12):S11–20.

199. McKeith IG. Dementia with Lewy bodies. Br J Psychiatry. 2002;180:144.

200. Nelson PT, Schmitt FA, Jicha GA, Kryscio RJ, Abner EL, Smith CD, Van Eldik LJ, Markesbery WR. Association between male gender and cortical Lewy body pathology in large autopsy series. J Neurol. 2010;257:1875–81.

201. McKeith IG, Dickson DW, Lowe J, Emre M, O'Brien JT, Feldman H, Cummings J, Duda JE, Lippa C, Perry EK, Aarsland D, Arai H, Ballard CG, Boeve B, Burn DJ, Costa D, Del Ser T, Dubois B, Galasko D, Gauthier S, Goetz CG, Gomez-Tortosa E, Halliday G, Hansen LA, Hardy J, Iwatsubo T, Kalaria RN, Kaufer D, Kenny RA, Korczyn A, Kosaka K, Lee VM, Lees A, Litvan I, Londos E, Lopez OL, Minoshima S, Mizuno Y, Molina JA,

Mukaetova-Ladinska EB, Pasquier F, Perry RH, Schulz JB, Trojanowski JQ, Yamada M, Consortium on DLB. Diagnosis and management of dementia with Lewy bodies: third report of the DLB Consortium. Neurology. 2005;65(12):1863–72.

202. Metzler-Baddeley C. A review of cognitive impairments in dementia with Lewy bodies relative to Alzheimer's disease and Parkinson's disease with dementia. Cortex. 2007;43:583–600.

203. Emre M, Aarsland D, Brown R, Burn DJ, Duyckaerts C, Mizuno Y, et al. Clinical diagnostic criteria for dementia associated with Parkinson's disease. Mov Disord. 2007;22:1689–707.

204. Ihl R, Bunevicius R, Frölich L, Winblad B, Schneider LS, Dubois B, Burns A, Thibaut F, Kasper S, Möller HJ. World Federation of Societies of Biological Psychiatry guidelines for the pharmacological treatment of dementias in primary care. Int J Psychiatry Clin Pract. 2015;19(1):2–7.

205. McKeith IG, Galasko D, Kosaka K, et al. Consensus guidelines for the clinical and pathologic diagnosis of dementia with Lewy bodies (DLB): report of the consortium on DLB international workshop. Neurology. 1996;47:1113.

206. Bradshaw J, Saling M, Hopwood M, et al. Fluctuating cognition in dementia with Lewy bodies and Alzheimer's disease is qualitatively distinct. J Neurol Neurosurg Psychiatry. 2004;75:382.

207. Ala TA, Yang KH, Sung JH, Frey WH 2nd. Hallucinations and signs of parkinsonism help distinguish patients with dementia and cortical Lewy bodies from patients with Alzheimer's disease at presentation: a clinicopathological study. J Neurol Neurosurg Psychiatry. 1997;62:16.

208. Tiraboschi P, Salmon DP, Hansen LA, et al. What best differentiates Lewy body from Alzheimer's disease in early-stage dementia? Brain. 2006;129:729.

209. Burn DJ, Rowan EN, Allan LM, et al. Motor subtype and cognitive decline in Parkinson's disease, Parkinson's disease with dementia, and dementia with Lewy bodies. J Neurol Neurosurg Psychiatry. 2006;77:585.

210. Del Ser T, McKeith I, Anand R, et al. Dementia with Lewy bodies: findings from an international multicentre study. Int J Geriatr Psychiatry. 2000;15(11):1034–45.

211. Claassen DO, Josephs KA, Ahlskog JE, et al. REM sleep behavior disorder preceding other aspects of synucleinopathies by up to half a century. Neurology. 2010;75(6):494–9.

212. Ballard C, Grace J, McKeith I, Holmes C. Neuroleptic sensitivity in dementia with Lewy bodies and Alzheimer's disease. Lancet. 1998;351:1032.

213. Postuma RB, Gagnon JF, Pelletier A, Montplaisir J. Prodromal autonomic symptoms and signs in Parkinson's disease and dementia with Lewy bodies. Mov Disord. 2013;28:597.

214. Ransmayr GN, Holliger S, Schletterer K, et al. Lower urinary tract symptoms in dementia with Lewy bodies, Parkinson disease, and Alzheimer disease. Neurology. 2008;70:299.

215. Ballard CG, O'Brien JT, Swann AG, et al. The natural history of psychosis and depression in dementia with Lewy bodies and Alzheimer's disease: persistence and new cases over 1 year of follow-up. J Clin Psychiatry. 2001;62:46.

216. Ballard C, Aarsland D, Francis P, Corbett A. Neuropsychiatric symptoms in patients with dementias associated with cortical Lewy bodies: pathophysiology, clinical features, and pharmacological management. Drugs Aging. 2013;30(8):603–11.

217. Salmon DP, Galasko D, Hansen LA. Dementia with Lewy bodies. In: Hodes J, editor. Early-onset dementia: a multidisciplinary approach. Oxford: Oxford University Press; 2001. p. 305–18.

218. Galvin JE. Improving the clinical detection of Lewy body dementia with the Lewy body composite risk score. Alzheimers Dement. 2015;1(3):316–24.

219. Gnanalingham KK, Byrne EJ, Thornton A. Clock-face drawing to differentiate Lewy body and Alzheimer type dementia syndromes. Lancet. 1996;347:696.

220. Ferman TJ, Smith GE, Kantarci K, Boeve BF, Pankratz VS, Dickson DW, Graff-Radford NR, Wszolek Z, Van Gerpen J, Uitti R, Pedraza O, Murray ME, Aakre J, Parisi J, Knopman DS, Petersen RC. Nonamnestic mild cognitive impairment progresses to dementia with Lewy bodies. Neurology. 2013;81:2032–8.

221. von Gunten A, Meuli R. Delineating dementia with Lewy bodies: can MRI help? In: Giannakopoulos P, Hof PR. (editor). Dementia in clinical practice. Bogousslavsky J (series editor) Frontiers of neurology and neuroscience. Basel: Karger; 2009. p. 126–34.

222. Watson R, Blamire AM, O'Brien JT. Magnetic resonance imaging in Lewy body dementias. Dement Geriatr Cogn Disord. 2009;28(6):493–506.

223. Higuchi M, Tashiro M, Arai H, Okamura N, Hara S, Higuchi S, Itoh M, Shin RW, Trojanowsky JQ, Sasaki H. Glucose hypometabolism and neuropathological correlates in brains of dementia with Lewy bodies. Exp Neurol. 2000;162:247–56.

224. McCleery J, Morgan S, Bradley KM, et al. Dopamine transporter imaging for the diagnosis of dementia with Lewy bodies. Cochrane Database Syst Rev. 2015;(1):CD010633.

225. Fujishiro H, Nakamura S, Kitazawa M, Sato K, Iseki E. Early detection of dementia with Lewy bodies in patients with amnestic mild cognitive impairment using 123I-MIBG cardiac scintigraphy. J Neurol Sci. 2012;315:115–9.

226. Stinton C, McKeith I, Taylor JP, Lafortune L, Mioshi E, Mak E, Cambridge V, Mason J, Thomas A, O'Brien JT. Pharmacological management of Lewy body dementia: a systematic review and meta-analysis. Am J Psychiatry. 2015;172(8):731–42.

227. Emre M, Tsolaki M, Bonuccelli U, et al. Memantine for patients with Parkinson's disease dementia or dementia with Lewy bodies: a randomised, double-blind, placebo-controlled trial. Lancet Neurol. 2010;9:969.

228. Gagnon JF, Postuma RB, Montplaisir J. Update on the pharmacology of REM sleep behavior disorder. Neurology. 2006;67:742.

229. Takada LT, Geschwind MD. Prion diseases. Semin Neurol. 2013;33:348–56.

230. Imran M, Mahmood S. An overview of human prion diseases. Virol J. 2011;8:559.

231. Jackson WS, Krost C. Peculiarities of prion diseases. PLoS Pathog. 2014;10(11):e1004451.

232. Parchi P, Strammiello R, Giese A, Kretzschmar H. Phenotypic variability of sporadic human prion disease and its molecular basis: past, present, and future. Acta Neuropathol. 2011;121(1):91–112.

233. The National Creutzfeldt-Jakob Disease Research & Surveillance Unit (NCJDRSU). Creutzfeldt-Jakob Disease in the UK (by calendar year). 2016. http://www.cjd.ed.ac.uk/documents/figs.pdf.

234. Gambetti P, Dong Z, Yuan J, Xiao X, Zheng M, Alshekhlee A, Castellani R, Cohen M, Barria MA, Gonzalez-Romero D, Belay ED, Schonberger LB, Marder K, Harris C, Burke JR, Montine T, Wisniewski T, Dickson DW, Soto C, Hulette CM, Mastrianni JA, Kong Q, Zou W. A novel human disease with abnormal prion protein sensitive to protease. Ann Neurol. 2008;63(6):697–708.

235. Holman RC, Belay ED, Christensen KY, Maddox RA, Minino AM, Folkema AM, Haberling DL, Hammett TA, Kochanek KD, Sejvar JJ, Schonberger LB. Human prion diseases in the United States. PLoS One. 2010;5(1):e8521.

236. Parchi P, Giese A, Capellari S, Brown P, Schulz-Schaeffer W, Windl O, Zerr I, Budka H, Kopp N, Piccardo P, Poser S, Rojiani A, Streichemberger N, Julien J, Vital C, Ghetti B, Gambetti P, Kretzschmar H. Classification of sporadic Creutzfeldt-Jakob disease based on molecular and phenotypic analysis of 300 subjects. Ann Neurol. 1999;46(2):224–33.

237. Cyngiser TA. Creutzfeldt-Jakob Disease: a disease overview. Am J Electroneurodiagnostic Technol. 2008;48:199–208.

238. Collie DA, Sellar RJ, Zeidler M, Colchester AC, Knight R, Will RG. MRI of Creutzfeldt-Jakob disease: imaging features and recommended MRI protocol. Clin Radiol. 2001;56(9):726–39.

239. Gmitterova K, Heinemann U, Bodemer M, Krasnianski A, Meissner B, Kretzschmar HA, Zerr I. 14-3-3 CSF levels in sporadic Creutzfeldt–Jakob disease differ across molecular subtypes. Neurobiol Aging. 2009;30(11):1842–50.

240. Zerr I, Kallenberg K, Summers DM, Romero C, Taratuto A, Heinemann U, Breithaupt M, Varges D, Meissner B, Ladogana A, Schuur M, Haik S, Collins SJ, Jansen GH, Stoki GB, Pimentel J, Hewer E, Collie D, Smith P, Roberts H, Brandel JP, van Duijn C, Pocchiari M, Begue C, Cras P, Will RG, Sanchez-Juan P. Updated clinical diagnostic criteria for sporadic Creutzfeldt-Jakob disease. Brain. 2009;132(Pt 10):2659–68.

241. Brew BJ, Chan P. Update on HIV dementia and HIV-associated neurocognitive disorders. Curr Neurol Neurosci Rep. 2014;14(8):468.

242. UNAIDS. AIDS by the numbers 2015. 2015. http://www.unaids.org/sites/default/files/media_asset/AIDS_by_the_numbers_2015_en.pdf.

243. Grant I, Atkinson JH, Hesselink JR, Kennedy CJ, Richman DD, Spector SA, McCutchan JA. Evidence for early central nervous system involvement in the acquired immunodeficiency syndrome (AIDS) and other human immunodeficiency virus (HIV) infections. Studies with neuropsychologic testing and magnetic resonance imaging. Ann Intern Med. 1987;107(6):828–36.

244. McArthur JC, Steiner J, Sacktor N, Nath A. Human immunodeficiency virus-associated neurocognitive disorders: mind the gap. Ann Neurol. 2010;67(6):699–714.

245. Nightingale S, Winsto A, Letendre S, Michael BD, McArthur JC, Khoo S, Solomon T. Controversies in HIV-associated neurocognitive disorders. Lancet Neurol. 2014;13(11):1139–51.

246. Antinori A, Arendt G, Becker JT, Brew BJ, Byrd DA, Cherner M, Clifford DB, Cinque P, Epstein LG, Goodkin K, Gisslen M, Grant I, Heaton RK, Joseph J, Marder K, Marra CM, McArthur JC, Nunn M, Price RW, Pulliam L, Robertson KR, Sacktor N, Valcour V, Wojna VE. Updated research nosology for HIV-associated neurocognitive disorders. Neurology. 2007;69(18):1789–99.

247. The Mind Exchange Working Group. Assessment, diagnosis, and treatment of HIV-associated neurocognitive disorder: a consensus report of the mind exchange program. Clin Infect Dis. 2013;56(7):1004–17.

248. Hopper AH, Samuels MA, Klein JP. Infections of the nervous system (bacterial, fungal, spirochetal, parasitic) and sarcoidosis. In: Adams and victor's principles of neurology. 10th ed. New York: McGraw-Hill Education; 2014. p. 697–755.

249. Ghanem KG. Neurosyphilis: a historical perspective and review. CNS Neurosci Ther. 2010;16(5):157–68.

250. Rao A, Khan A, Singh K, Anderson DL, Malone ML. Neurosyphilis: an uncommon cause of dementia. J Am Geriatr Soc. 2015;63(8):1710–2.

251. Nitrini R, Caramelli P, Bottino CM, Damasceno BP, Brucki SM, Anghinah R. Diagnosis of Alzheimer's disease in Brazil: diagnostic criteria and auxiliary tests. Recommendations of the Scientific Department of Cognitive Neurology and Aging of the Brazilian Academy of Neurology. Arq Neuropsiquiatr. 2005;63(3a):713–9.

252. Workowski KA, Berman SM, Centers for Disease Control and Prevention. Sexually transmitted diseases treatment guidelines, 2015. MMWR Recomm Rep. 2015;64(RR-3):1–137.

253. Czarnowska-Cubała M, Wiglusz MS, Cubała WJ, Jakuszkowiak-Wojten K, Landowski J, Krysta K. MR findings in neurosyphilis – a literature review with a focus on a practical approach to neuroimaging. Psychiatr Danub. 2013;25(Suppl 2):153–7.

254. Rodrigues CL, de Andrade DC, Livramento JA, Machado LR, Abraham R, Massaroppe L, Lucato LT, Caramelli P. Spectrum of cognitive impairment in neurocysticercosis: differences according to disease phase. Neurology. 2012;78(12):861–6.

255. Blanc F, Philippi N, Cretin B, Kleitz C, Berly L, Jung B, Kremer S, Namer IJ, Sellal F, Jaulhac B, de Seze J. Lyme neuroborreliosis and dementia. J Alzheimers Dis. 2014;41(4):1087–93.

256. Nitrini R. Clinical and therapeutic aspects of dementia in syphilis and Lyme disease. Handb Clin Neurol. 2008;89:819–23.

257. Aharon-Peretz J, Kliot D, Finkelstein R, Ben Hayun R, Yarnitsky D, Goldsher D. Cryptococcal meningitis mimicking vascular dementia. Neurology. 2004;62(11):2135.

258. Hoffmann M, Muniz J, Carroll E, De Villasante J. Cryptococcal meningitis misdiagnosed as Alzheimer's disease: complete neurological and cognitive recovery with treatment. J Alzheimers Dis. 2009;16(3):517–20.

259. Sung VW, Lyerly MJ, Fallon KB, Bashir K. Isolated CNS Whipple disease with normal brain MRI and false-positive CSF 14-3-3 protein: a case report and review of the literature. Brain Behav. 2012;2(6):838–43.

260. Kesav P, Vishnu VY, Lal V, Prabhakar S. Disseminated tuberculosis presenting as rapidly progressive dementia. QJM. 2014;107(1):79–80.

261. Kobayashi K, Imagama S, Ito Z, Ando K, Yagi H, Shinjo R, Hida T, Ito K, Ishikawa Y, Matsuyama Y, Ishiguro N. Tuberculous meningitis with dementia as the presenting symptom after intramedullary spinal cord tumor resection. Nagoya J Med Sci. 2015;77(4):653–7.

262. Carbone I, Lazzarotto T, Ianni M, Porcellini E, Forti P, Masliah E, Gabrielli L, Licastro F. Herpes virus in Alzheimer's disease: relation to progression of the disease. Neurobiol Aging. 2014;35(1):122–9.

Neurocognitive Disorders in Older Adults (Vascular Dementia)

22

Olatunji Aina, Jenny Downes-Brydon, and Edmond Chiu

Abstract

Recent developments in the understanding of the relationship between vascular risk factors, vascular cognitive disorders and dementia have led to a renewed interest in these risk factors and their management. The role of the primary care physician in the prevention, control and management of all aspects of vascular diseases is highlighted. Diagnostic criteria in the DSM, ICD and VASCOG systems are examined, in particular their relevance and usefulness in primary care settings. Cognitive domains in a "bedside" testing schedule may be helpful for the primary care physician in their daily practice. Primary and secondary care for people with vascular cognitive disorders places the primary care physician in crucial roles.

Key Points

- Recent developments in the understanding of cerebral physiology, the advances of neuroimaging technology and the awareness of vascular risk factors as well as the clinical relationship between vascular and Alzheimer's dementia have led to a resurgence of interest in vascular cognitive impairment and vascular cognitive disorders (vascular dementia).
- The diagnostic criteria of vascular cognitive disorders in the ICD and DSM classification systems and that of the recent VASCOG update are described, as well as the subtypes seen in clinical practice.
- The relevance and usefulness in diagnostic application in primary care settings are discussed.
- The primary care management of vascular cognitive disorders and the related risk factors are explored.
- Secondary (out-of-home) care settings are sometimes necessary, and the optimal management in this setting is offered.
- Prevention of vascular risk factors and stroke, with the related social, cultural and political aspects, are highlighted.
- A suggested "bedside" testing schedule of cognitive domains is listed to assist the primary care physicians in their clinical practice.

O. Aina
College of Medicine of the University of Lagos, Lagos, Nigeria

J. Downes-Brydon
Peninsula Family General Practice, Frankston, VIC, Australia

E. Chiu (✉)
Department of Psychiatry, The University of Melbourne, Melbourne, VIC, Australia
e-mail: Edmond.Chiu@svha.org.au

© Springer Nature Switzerland AG 2019
C. A. de Mendonça Lima, G. Ivbijaro (eds.), *Primary Care Mental Health in Older People*,
https://doi.org/10.1007/978-3-030-10814-4_22

22.1 Introduction

Before Alois Alzheimer identified the pathology in a dementia which bears his name, cerebral arteriosclerosis and chronic cerebral ischaemia were considered to be the causes of brain degeneration which resulted in dementia. The ascendancy of Alzheimer's disease (AD) as a paradigm determined the criteria for the assessment and diagnosis of dementias. This relegated vascular pathology as a cause of dementia to a less considered status [1, 2]. Post-stroke dementia was first reported by Thomas Willis in the seventeenth century. In the late nineteenth century, arteriosclerosis and senile dementia were delineated as distinct syndromes with older patients being more likely to have vascular dementia [3].

The revival of interest in vascular aetiologies occurred in the 1960s when a strong association between vascular factors such as hypertension and arteriosclerosis with dementia were identified. Hachinski and colleagues proposed multi-infarct dementia [4]. The establishment of the NINDS-AIREN (National Institute of Neurological Disorders and Stroke and the Association Internationale pour la Recherche et l'Enseignement en Neurosciences) criteria furthered the interest into vascular dementia by bringing into focus the vascular contribution to cognitive impairment and dementia [5]. Recent developments in the understanding of the physiology of cerebral blood flow, the advances of neuroimaging technology and the heightened awareness of the clinical association between the two domains have led to a resurgence of interest in vascular cognitive impairment (VCI) and vascular dementia (VaD).

22.2 Diagnostic Criteria for Major Vascular Cognitive Disorder (Vascular Dementia)

A variety of scales have been used. Hachinski in 1975 developed the scale for multi-infarct dementias to distinguish between AD and vascular cognitive disorder [6].

DSM IV and ICD 10 defined VaD in their respective classificatory systems [2, 7]. The NINDS-AIREN criteria were probably the most used, although they had low sensitivity but high specificity [8, 9]. It can be used to establish a probable diagnosis (memory impairment + another cognitive domain + cerebrovascular disease, imaging evidence with clear association to decline) or possible diagnosis (memory impairment + another cognitive domain + CVD without imaging evidence or clear association to dementia). The reliance on imaging in the NINDS-AIREN criteria, however, limits its use in those clinical situations where there is not ready access to neuroimaging, such as in many primary care locations.

An advance in the development of diagnostic criteria of vascular cognitive disorder by the International Society for Vascular Behavioural and Cognitive Disorders (VASCOG) offers a more updated set of criteria which may be more useful in the primary care setting [10].

The following summarizes some of the salient features of diagnostic criteria appropriate for the primary care environment.

It requires both a *subjective* and an *objective* report of a cognitive disorder, plus the determination that vascular disorder is the dominant, if not the exclusive, pathology that accounts for the cognitive deficits.

The *subjective* report will typically be the presentation to the primary care physician (PCP) of an individual patient who has noted or been informed by family members of a change in the ability to plan, or to make decisions; has a decline in the ability to manage complex projects; needs frequent reminders for the task at hand; and has difficulty in navigating in familiar environments, difficulty with receptive and expressive language, and a clear disturbance of bodily schemata, calculation, reading or writing. The mild VCD is more subtle with the individual still able to function independently, although multi-tasking will be with greater effort.

Objective evidence of cognitive impairment would ideally be through a formal neuropsychological test battery administered by a trained practitioner. However, in the primary care setting, a short "bedside" test may be all that is available. Such a "bedside" test should include functions in a range of cognitive domains. Preponderance of disturbance is in the domains of slow information processing speed and frontal executive functions [11, 12].

1. Attention and processing speed (sustained attention, divided attention, selective attention, information processing speed)
2. Frontal executive function (planning, decision-making, working memory, responding to feedback/error correction, novel situations, over-riding habits, mental inflexibility, judgement)
3. Learning and memory (immediate memory, recent memory including free recall, cued recall and recognition memory)
4. Language (naming, expressive, grammar and syntax, receptive)
5. Visuoconstructional-perceptual ability (construction, visual perception and reasoning)
6. Praxis-gnosis-body schema (praxis, gnosis, right/left orientation, calculation ability, body schema, facial recognition)
7. Social recognition (recognition of emotions and social cues, appropriate social inhibitions, theory of mind, empathy)

To arrive at the diagnosis of major vascular cognitive disorder (VaD), *the cognitive deficits are sufficient to interfere with independence*, the individual requiring assistance with instrumental activities of daily living (IADL).

Where neuroimaging is available, the presence of large infarcts, multiple lacunar infarcts, strategically placed infarcts at the thalamus or basal ganglia, extensive and confluent white matter lesions, two or more cerebral haemorrhages or a strategically placed haemorrhage would confirm the presence of vascular lesions contributing to the disorder.

Should neuroimaging be unavailable, to establish the presence of cerebrovascular disease that is associated with cognitive disorder, the clinical history and a neurological examination may provide supporting information.

22.3 Subtypes

As the cerebrovascular lesions and their pathologies can be varied, the subsequent VCD will have differing clinical pathological subtypes.

1. Multi-infarct VCD with evidence of strokes and/or white matter infarcts.
2. Strategic infarcts where these are strategically located as to interfere maximally with memory and cognition (thalamic infarcts, anterior cerebral artery infarcts, parietal infarcts, cingulate gyrus infarcts).
3. Diffuse white matter lesions (leukoaraiosis).
4. Small vessel ischaemia with multiple lacunar infarcts. The clinical presentation will depend on the location of these lacunar lesions. Frontal dysexecutive symptoms and affective symptoms often accompany these lesions.
5. Haemorrhagic lesions. The location and size of these lesions will present a clinical picture consistent with such damage.
6. Hypo-perfusion from low cardiac output or decreased blood flow can affect the watershed area of the brain.
7. Mixed dementia where VCD can co-exist with AD. Overlap with AD and DLB are common [13–15]. This suggests a complex interaction between vascular and other pathology. It is known that lacunar infarcts in the basal ganglia, thalamus and deep white matter appear to greatly increase the risk of AD, and macrovessel strokes can double the rate of progression of dementia in AD [16, 17].

22.4 Making a Diagnosis in Primary Care Settings

Individuals and families managed in the primary care setting in Australia do not infrequently present with largely undifferentiated pathology or dysfunction, given that the primary care setting is the "first port of call" in the Australian healthcare system.

As such the diagnosis of vascular dementia in the primary care setting not infrequently emerges as part of a complex of presentations and diagnoses of older individuals, rather than as the primary presenting problem.

Typically the complex of presentations of a patient with vascular dementia may include:

- Other vascular comorbidities (ischaemic heart disease, renovascular disease, cerebrovascular disease/stroke)
- Risk factors for vascular comorbidities—diabetes, smoking, inactive lifestyle, lipid disorder, obesity, hypertension
- Mood disorder/anxiety in the older person
- Serious illness complicated by acute brain syndrome (such as surgery in the older person/metabolic disorder, hypoperfusion state, sepsis)

Individuals suffering vascular dementia may not be aware of their presenting symptoms and may not prioritize these symptoms. Amongst the complex of symptoms they themselves are concerned about, the primary care team may need to sift and sort out "vascular dementia" as part of the complex. Alternatively, within the primary care setting, families may raise the issue of altered cognition of their relative as either a primary concern or as part of a complex presentation.

In other instances, the primary care doctor may identify those individuals at risk of having or developing vascular dementia and proactively screen for emerging symptoms and signs of vascular dementia.

The primary care doctor, with the ability to observe and treat patients longitudinally and often over many years and in a variety of circumstances, may detect deterioration in an individual's cognition, function and capacity. The diagnosis of vascular dementia includes clinical evaluation and laboratory investigations. There is need to be exhaustive as studies have shown that using routine clinical history and examination alone by primary care physicians leads to wide range (29–76%) of missed diagnosis, hence advocating for the use of screening inventories to increase likelihood of diagnosis.

The primary care team in establishing a diagnosis of vascular dementia, in line with general principles of delivery of primary care, should be based on practical, scientifically sound and socially acceptable methods and technology made universally accessible to individuals and families in the community and at a cost that the community and country can afford to maintain.

22.4.1 Clinical Features

Symptoms of vascular dementia (VaD) often overlap with those of Alzheimer's disease, although impaired judgement is usually the initial symptom and memory may not be as seriously affected. The cognitive impairment in VaD is usually more acute than Alzheimer's disease, stepwise in progression and fluctuating in course. Cognitive disturbances include loss of memory, aphasia, apraxia, agnosia and disturbed executive functioning. A significant proportion of patients with VaD also develop focal neurological signs and symptoms such as exaggeration of deep tendon reflexes, extensor plantar response, pseudobulbar palsy, gait abnormalities and weak extremities, hemiparesis, ataxia, sensory change, dysphasia, dysarthria or visual disturbance. Furthermore, there may be a history of hypertension, diabetes, stroke and evidence of atherosclerosis.

Just as in other types of dementia, behavioural and psychological symptoms of dementia (BPSD) are part of the process of vascular dementia, most especially in moderate to severe cases. Such symptoms include affective symptoms most especially depressive type, disinhibition, agitation, apathy, disturbed nighttime behaviours, personality changes, regressive behaviours and frank psychotic symptoms such as hallucinations and delusion.

In clinical evaluation of VaD at the primary care level, high index of suspicion is important most especially in middle-aged to elderly subjects with cognitive impairment and underlying risk factors such as hypertension, diabetes and/or "repeated strokes". In addition to memory impairment are varying neurological signs such as paralysis, apraxia, dysphasia and visual field defects.

22.4.2 Clinical Examination

Full mental and physical state examinations are essential. Emphasis should be laid on cognitive assessment such as memory, judgement, executive functions, general knowledge and orientation. In physical examination, it is important to especially carry out thorough neurological evaluation.

22.4.3 Laboratory Investigations

- Routine laboratory tests such as full blood count, serum electrolytes and urea, lipid profiles, etc. are required.
- Neuroimaging studies: Neuroimaging techniques such as computerized tomography (CT) scan and magnetic resonance imaging (MRI) are the mainstay diagnostic investigations in VaD. However, this may not be available at the primary care level; hence referral to higher tier of healthcare may be necessary for this. It is not uncommon for healthcare practitioners in developing countries to neglect neuro-imaging investigation due to its prohibitive cost and non-availability in most facilities. However, it is strongly advised for patients with clinical diagnosis of dementia to have neuro-imaging investigations done.

In summary, the diagnosis of VaD is through:

- Clinical history
- Mental status examination
- Physical examination, in particular a full neurological examination
- Laboratory investigations, including neuroimaging studies, if available
- Use of screening inventories

Examples of Government Support for Primary Care

Dementia, particularly due to population ageing, is one of the most important global phenomena attracting attention in recent time.

Developed countries of the Western world have evolved different models for the management of dementia and elderly care. Examples include nursing home care and health insurance programmes in countries in Europe and America. A recent novel innovation is in the Australian Primary Care Government funding introduced over the last 10 years or so by way of "comprehensive medical assessments" which can be undertaken annually on patients over 75, which facilitates comprehensive medical, cognitive and mood assessments of patients by GPs and practice nurses using standardized Mini-Mental State Examination assessments to "triage" those who may have signs of vascular dementia. Uptake is variable amongst primary care teams and may be influenced by medical workforce, primary care workforce, demographics of the region of the primary care clinic (including patient age distribution and socio-economic status) as well as the desire of the primary care team to undertake complex health management and health prevention activities. Another example, this time from Asia, is the National Programme for the Health Care for the Elderly (NPHCE) developed in India, and whose objective amongst others is to identify health problems in the elderly and provide appropriate health interventions in the community based on primary healthcare approach with a strong referral backup support.

In sub-Saharan Africa (SSA), the situation is different. For now, with the exception of South Africa, there are only pockets of health services for dementia and geriatric care. Thus, in SSA, care for the elderly is largely the primary responsibility of the family and kinsmen. In recent times, this is supplemented in a number of cases by other informal services provided by non-governmental organizations (NGOs). A notable example from the West African subregion is the Geriatric Centre domiciled in the University College Hospital (UCH), Ibadan, Nigeria. The centre was donated by a Nigerian philanthropist with the mission to provide excellent clinical care of older persons through a patient- and family-centred care in a culturally sensitive environment.

In the pathway to the diagnosis of vascular dementia, serological tests undertaken in assessment of general vascular disorders are usually readily accessible. Vascular/cardiovascular imaging (such as echocardiography, carotid artery ultrasound/angiography) may be beneficial to establish any more reversible aspects of low cerebral perfusion, but the risk and cost benefit to the individual should be considered prior to this being undertaken. Definitively, MRI scanning of the brain is extremely valuable in differentiating vascular dementia from cognitive impairment of different etiologies and thereby assisting in discussions with patients and families regarding possible interventions, prognosis and management strategies. Interpretation of such MRI scanning ideally should be undertaken by a specialist with particular skills in the interpretation of such imaging.

Given the high incidence of coexistent vascular (and other) dementia with mood disorder/anxiety, psychiatric assessment of patients with vascular dementia is highly desirable, as treatment of underlying psychiatric diagnosis is likely to improve outcomes for patients and families of patients.

22.5 Management: General

The central management strategy is the energetic and thorough attention to vascular diseases and related risk factors, in particular the prevention of strokes which would also prevent the development of vascular dementia [18]. Both medication and lifestyle changes to control hypertension, hyperlipidaemia, diabetes and obesity are essential. Cessation of cigarette smoking, physical

activity and dietary intervention are strongly recommended [19]. Cholinesterase inhibitors have shown some modest benefits in control trials [20]. The NMDA receptor antagonist memantine also has small beneficial effects on cognition [21, 22]. In patients with co-existing Alzheimer's disease, cholinesterase inhibitors may have a stronger indication.

22.6 Management in Primary Care

The primary care team is ideally positioned to contribute to the management of risk factors for vascular dementia and potentially therefore the prevention of onset or progression of vascular dementia. The primary management of vascular dementia (VaD) is mainly preventive, that is, as much as possible to avoid development of the problem. Consequently, the management is subdivided into three groups: primary, secondary and tertiary.

22.6.1 Primary Management

This is a major area of emphasis in the management of VaD at the primary healthcare level.

– Much attention is paid to measures *to prevent VaD* through energetic vascular health maintenance. Primary care management of the symptoms of vascular dementia is integrally associated with management of all vascular parameters and will include optimization of blood pressure control, cardiac function, renal function and cerebrovascular perfusion. Whilst much of the primary care management will be pharmacological in nature, delivery of information and facilitation of lifestyle interventions by the primary care team to those at risk of and those suffering vascular dementia are an increasingly important role of primary care teams.
– *Health education*: Health enlightenment of the public over preventive measures such as routine medical check-up, with special emphasis on periodic measure of blood pressure, screening for diabetes mellitus, lipid profile

tests and abstinence from smoking, all go a long way to prevent VaD.

- Appropriate and prompt *treatment* of underlying disease risk factors such as hypertension, diabetes mellitus or hyperlipidaemia.

22.6.2 Secondary Management

Following the confirmation of the diagnosis of dementia, the following management steps are necessary:

- *Disclosure of diagnosis*: This requires tactful conversation on the part of the clinician. The disclosure of the diagnosis of VaD to the patient and relatives should be done personally and professionally because of the associated strong emotional reaction. The patient and the relatives must be educated on the necessary lifestyle modifications and prognostication of the disorder. In as much as the clinicians need not paint very gloomy picture of the disorder, it is also advised to avoid building false hope of "cure".

Medications in the management of VaD: This comprises of two modalities:

(a) Attempts to restore cognition or halts its deterioration
(b) Control of associated abnormal behaviours, that is, behavioural and psychological symptoms of dementia (BPSD)

Drug Treatment of the VaD Itself
- No known medication per se for the effective treatment of VaD, but certain groups of drugs are available in clinical practice as follows:
- Drugs to reduce rate of cognitive deterioration: Anticoagulants such as aspirin are recommended as they prevent further episodes of ischaemic stroke. Nicardipine, a dihydropyridine calcium channel blocker, is also used.
- Drugs that increase cerebral blood flow: Examples are ergoloid mesylate (Hydergine) and pentoxifylline.

Drug Treatment of Associated Behavioural and Psychological Symptoms of Dementia (BPSD)
- Antidepressants, most especially selective serotonin reuptake inhibitors (SSRIs) such as sertraline, fluoxetine and paroxetine, are useful in the treatment of any associated depression. In the elderly, caution should be applied if tricyclic antidepressants such as amitriptyline and imipramine are to be used because of untoward cholinergic and cardiac side effects.
- Antipsychotics, particularly second-generation antipsychotics (SGAs) such as olanzapine, risperidone or quetiapine, are recommended for most symptoms of BPSD such as psychotic symptoms and agitation.
- All these drugs should be used with caution, particularly using the minimum effective dose possible for as short duration as possible and be reviewed regularly.

22.6.3 Tertiary Management

As there is no cure for vascular dementia, emphasis is placed on rehabilitative and health maintenance measures, which include the following:

- Adequate nutrition and general health care.
- Regular physical exercise, sometimes with the aid of physiotherapy.
- Avoid wandering away from home.
- Forensic issues, such as management of asset by appointed attorney.
- Community/residential care.
- Non-governmental organizations (NGOs) with interest in rehabilitation of dementia.

22.7 Management in Secondary Care Settings

Many patients with vascular dementia are eventually placed in secondary care facilities as their disease and the associated management issues (including whilst not limited to wandering, incontinence, behavioural disturbances, difficulties managing hygiene, mobility issues) become too difficult or unsafe to be managed at home. Such facilities are staffed by registered nurses, enrolled nurses and untrained "carers" and may be visited regularly by allied health professionals and primary care doctors. A model of medical care in such facilities available in developed country such as Australia is for primary care doctors to undertake regular "visiting rounds" of the facilities. Government funding for such visits by doctors is considerably less than funding for doctors to see patients in clinics, and funding per patient reduces with each patient seen by the doctor, creating quite a disincentive for primary care doctors to visit low and high care facilities. Whilst the majority of staff in such facilities has education as carers, only a small percentage of staff on duty at any one time have nursing or paramedical education. Unfortunately, this has led to a high utilization of "episode-only" locum doctor attendance upon patients with vascular dementia in such facilities or of transfer of patients with vascular dementia that become unwell to emergency departments in hospitals. Such management of patients with vascular dementia is clearly not ideally patient-centric and is more likely to be suboptimal.

Interestingly, in a setting where non-pharmacological interventions including, whilst not limited to, gentle exercise and activity should be optimally utilized, there is very limited access for these patients to team care plans to access allied health support. Even more difficult is that, in such facilities where anxiety and depression are extremely prevalent as co-morbidities of vascular dementia, there is a need for residents to access psychological support or interventions and for staff to be supported and advised on management by psychologically trained and skilled professionals. Affordable access is extremely limited in most cases. Sadly behavioural disorders of residents suffering vascular dementia are all too often treated with sedative/antipsychotic and hypnotic pharmaceutical agents as currently there are no other available, accessible and socially acceptable options available. Clearly use of such drugs are unlikely to improve overall patient outcomes and/or wellbeing and may be distressing to families and carers.

Example of Government-Supported Strategies

Australian government funding which facilitates ongoing and comprehensive management of chronic disease by way of quarterly "care plan reviews" and annual "diabetes assessments", introduced over the last 10 years, has assisted the primary care team with funding to regularly and cyclically review patient risk factors including whilst not limited to blood pressure and cardiovascular indices, diabetes parameters and renal parameters. Annual/biannual government funding of pharmacist and primary care team collaboration in review of patient medications may also contribute to prevention of progression or inadequate management of risk factors for vascular dementia.

Since the introduction of government funding for "team care plans" as part of the management of patients with chronic disease over the last 10 years, primary care teams have become the "gatekeepers" for provision of funding for "start-up" lifestyle interventions to assist in the non-pharmacological management of chronic disease, including vascular dementia. Some primary care teams in Australia can and do now work collaboratively with exercise physiologists, dieticians and diabetes educators, podiatrists and physiotherapists to assist patients with vascular dementia to access funded education and supervision in establishing exercise, weight control, stop smoking, healthy eating and other lifestyle interventions as part of the management of their condition.

Uptake of the use of "care plans" and "team care plans" by primary care teams has been variable since the government funding was introduced. Factors which influence the uptake include whilst not limited to primary care doctors' motivation to manage patients with complex chronic disease, the availability of appropriate allied health services within the area of the primary care doctor and the "red tape" associated with primary care doctor accessing the funding for their patient (which is considerable). A diagnosis of vascular dementia attracts additional funds for the managing facility to deliver care, and it is possible that this has encouraged care providers to seek out such a diagnosis in their residents to maximize government subsidy. All of these factors therefore do and will have an impact on the effectiveness of prevention and management of vascular dementia in the primary care setting.

The primary care team has a role in managing not only the sufferer of the vascular dementia but in supporting the carer(s) of the patient. Primary care teams have the ability to refer patients with vascular dementia (and associated other chronic diseases) for assessment for eligibility for funded support for additional services (such as assistance with personal and home care), whilst the patient with vascular dementia continues to live within the community. Such assessment may also trigger eligibility for the patient to utilize periods of "respite care" within appropriate facilities should the need arise.

The ability of the patient with vascular dementia (and their supports) to optimally utilize and access available support services relies on the primary care team being aware of the services available and the pathways to access such services. The system is not always easy to navigate and relies on a level of interdisciplinary collaboration and co-operation.

Optimal management of the factors which influence the progress and fluctuation of the symptoms of the patient with vascular dementia ideally requires that the caregivers and treaters have a sound working knowledge of the basics of the physiological factors which influence vascular dementia, as well as longitudinal information on the response of the patient with vascular dementia to physiological variables. For example, a patient with vascular dementia who has a sudden reduction in cardiac output, causing reduced cerebrovascular perfusion, is likely to demonstrate deterioration in function. Ideally continuous care by a stable team for these "brittle" patients is ideal. Frequent medical and nursing care turnover, due to staff changing, low workforce issues, or patients and their families frequently changing providers, may have a significant negative impact on ongoing care of patients with vascular dementia.

22.8 Prevention

Patients with vascular cognitive impairment followed up over 5 years showed progression to a diagnosis of vascular dementia and a high rate of conversion from VCI to VaD [23, 24]. Thus the energetic and comprehensive management of vascular risk factors may prevent or delay the progression to VaD, and the primary care physician has a powerful role in such an intervention.

The high-risk group of older patients with vascular risk factors will benefit from prevention management [15, 19]. The prevention of CVD includes anti-platelet therapy for arteriosclerotic diseases, anticoagulation for cardio-embolic diseases and carotid endarterectomy for carotid stenosis.

22.9 Social, Cultural and Political Aspects of Dementia

Views about old age and associated health challenges vary from one culture to the other. In the Western world, the tendency to live a lonely life at old age is high; but in most developing nations particularly in Africa, community care for the elderly and cognitively impaired persons by the relations most especially in the extended family setting holds sway.

22.9.1 Sociocultural Constructs

Sociocultural constructs about dementia began to emerge in the 1970s/1980s. Across various cultures of the world, the term dementia evokes strong emotional feelings such as profound dread and horror. Dementia is seen as a very bewildering and frightening condition. The forgetfulness in persons with dementia, and most times their embarrassing behaviours, can cause a lot of distress on the part of the relatives. Thus, in most cultures, the regressive behaviour exhibited in dementia is seen as "second childishness and mere oblivion" [25].

22.9.2 Media and Political Descriptions of Dementia

For many decades now and with prominent political figures in the Western world developing dementia some years after their reign, political and media focus had been on dementia. Media metaphorical descriptions of dementia include derogatory terms as "Living dead", "A never ending funeral", "A private hell of devastation", "Plague", "Millennium demon", "Silent tsunami" and "Time bomb", amongst others [26, 27]. In movies, dementia has been animated as a monster [28].

22.9.3 Dementia and Stigma

Dementia is associated with stigma, most especially amongst subcategory of patients with prominent behavioural disturbances and gross personality changes. Furthermore, the media portrayal of dementia is believed to be partly responsible for the stigma [29, 30]. The primary care physician has a very strong role in educating the families and communities in de-stigmatization of vascular and other dementias.

22.10 Conclusion

This chapter discussed the relevance and usefulness of diagnostic application in primary care, exploring the risk factors and primary care management of vascular cognitive disorders. Secondary care settings are sometimes necessary, and the optimal management in this setting is

also discussed. It then highlights the prevention of vascular risk factors and stroke, with the related social cultural and political aspects. As primary care doctors see adults at risk of having or developing vascular dementia, they are encouraged to proactively screen those patients for emerging symptoms and signs of vascular dementia. The management strategy involves thorough attention to vascular diseases and related risk factors, in particular the prevention of strokes which would also prevent the development of vascular dementia.

Appendix

Suggested "bedside" testing of cognitive domains listed above.

For frontal dysexecutive testing, the Frontal Behavioural Inventory (FBI) provides a useful schedule of 24 items which can be used in primary care setting [31].

Screening Inventories

Numerous assessments exist, and many brief assessments have been developed which are easy to administer and score. An important aim of using these screening instruments is to pick up cases of dementia as early as possible, since studies have shown that more than 50% of cases of dementia, most especially the mild to moderate ones, are missed by clinicians during routine clinical evaluation. They are simple to administer and require little time to do so.

- Mini-Mental State Examination (MMSE) [31, 32]: Developed in 1975, with several modifications released since, the MMSE is the most widely known and researched screening tool. It is divided into two sections and takes 10–15 min to administer. Research indicates that it has satisfactory reliability and validity. It covers six areas of cognitive functioning: orientation, immediate recall, attention and calculation, language (including following verbal and written instructions and writing a spontaneous sentence) and copying interlocking pentagons. MMSE scores in the moderately impaired range can indicate either cognitive impairment associated with depression or an independent cognitive disorder [33].

- Clock-Drawing Test (CDT): CDT tests memory, adaptive functioning, information processing and visual-spatial and executive functioning. A person is asked to draw a clock face (with or without a pre-drawn circle) and indicate a specified time. The more distorted and inaccurate the drawings are, the more likely the person has dementia [34].

- Time and Change Test: This tests comprehension, working (or task completion) memory and planning and calculating skills. A person is given 60 s and two attempts to read the time on a clock and then is given 3 min and two attempts to make change for a dollar with three quarters, seven dimes and seven nickels [35]. Word recall: A person without memory problems should be able to remember at least three unrelated words and be able to recite them back after interruption with a distracting task. Someone who cannot remember at least two words out of three may have cognitive impairment. Another test is to ask a person to name as many items as possible in a given category, such as fruits or animals. Naming fewer than ten items in 1 min suggests slowed mental functioning [35].

- Mini-Cognitive Assessment Instrument (Mini-Cog): This test has been proven to assess a person's registration, recall and executive function and be effective culturally and educationally [36].

- General Practitioner Assessment of Cognition (GPCOG): This tool, developed in 2002, is used for screening cognitive impairment in the primary care setting. The GPCOG includes a 4-min patient assessment and a 2-min caregiver interview. A web-based tool is available. Research has shown it to perform at least as well as the MMSE [37].

Note: Most of these instruments are standardized screening tools for dementia in accordance with internationally recognized guidelines. It should however be noted that clinicians and researchers in multi-ethnic and diverse cultural societies in Asia and Africa have customized few of these screening tools to the culture, language and literacy level of their local populations, such as "Test of Senegal," developed for sub-Saharan African population. Other examples of such customized screening inventories are from the Indianapolis-Ibadan Dementia Project (IIDP) domiciled in Ibadan, Nigeria, that is, "Clinical Home-based Interview to assess Function" (CHIF), which measures activities of daily life drawing out statements from existing standard questionnaires, and "stick design", a questionnaire that measures visuo-constructional abilities. For indigenous Australians, the Kimberley Indigenous Cognitive Assessment (KICA) tool [38] has been well validated for this population.

References

1. American Psychiatric Association. Diagnostic and statistical manual of mental disorders. 3rd ed. Washington, DC: American Psychiatric Association; 1993.
2. World Health Organization. The ICD-10 classification of mental and behavioral disorders: diagnostic criteria for research. Geneva: World Health Organization; 1993.
3. Holstein M. Alzheimer's disease and senile dementia, 1885–1920: an interpretive history of disease negotiation. J Aging Stud. 1997;11:1–13.
4. Hachinski VC, Lassen NA, Marshall J. Multi-infarct dementia: a cause of mental deterioration in the elderly. Lancet. 1974;2:207–10.
5. Roman GC, Tatemichi TK, Erkinjuntti T, et al. Vascular dementia: diagnostic criteria for research studies. Report of the NINDS-AIREN International Workshop. Neurology. 1993;43:250–60.
6. Hachinski VC, Iliff LD, Zilhka A, et al. Cerebral blood flow in dementia. Arch Neurol. 1975;32:632–7.
7. American Psychiatric Association. Diagnostic and statistical manual of mental disorders. 4th ed, Text Revision ed. Washington, DC: American Psychiatric Association; 2000.
8. Chui HC, Mack W, Jackson JF, et al. Clinical criteria for the diagnosis of vascular dementia: a multicenter study of comparability and inter-rater reliability. Arch Neurol. 2000;57:191–6.
9. Chui HC, Zarrow C, Mack WJ, et al. Cognitive impact of subcortical vascular and Alzheimer's disease pathology. Ann Neurol. 2006;60:677–87.

10. Sachdev P, Kalaria R, O'Brien J, et al. Diagnostic criteria for vascular cognitive disorders: a VASCOG statement. Alzheimer Dis Assoc Disord. 2014;28(3):206–18.
11. Hachinski VC, Iadecola C, Peterson RC, et al. National Institute of Neurological disorders and Stroke - Canadian Stroke Network vascular cognitive impairment harmonization standards. Stroke. 2006;37:2220–41.
12. Looi JCL, Sachdev PS. Differentiation of vascular dementia from AD on neuropsychological tests. Neurology. 1999;53:670–8.
13. Barber R, Scheltens P, Gholkar A, et al. White matter lesions on magnetic resonance imaging in dementia with Lewy Bodies, Alzheimer's disease, vascular dementia, and normal aging. J Neurol Neurosurg Psychiatry. 1999;67:66–72.
14. Knopman DS, Parisi JE, Boeve BF, et al. Vascular dementia in a population based autopsy study. Arch Neurol. 2003;60:569–73.
15. Hankey GJ. Clinical update: Management of stroke. Lancet. 2007;369:1330–2.
16. Snowdon DA, Greiner LH, Mortimer JA, et al. Brain infarction and the clinical expression of Alzheimer's disease. The Nun Study. J Am Med Assoc. 1997;277:813–7.
17. Heyman A, Fillenbaum G, Welsh-Bohmer KA, et al. Cerebral infarcts in patients with autopsy- proven Alzheimer's disease: CERAD, part XVIII. Consortium to Establish a Registry for Alzheimer's disease. Neurology. 1998;51:159–62.
18. Goldstein L. Primary prevention of ischaemic stroke: a guideline. Stroke. 2006;37:1583–633.
19. Sacco RL, Adams R, Albers G, et al. Guidelines for prevention of stroke in patients with ischemic stroke or transient ischemic attack. Stroke. 2006;37:577–617.
20. Erkinjuntti T. Diagnosis and management of vascular cognitive impairment and dementia. J Neural Transm Suppl. 2002;63:91–109.
21. McShane R, Areosa Sastre A, Minakaran N. Memantine for dementia. Cochrane Database Syst Rev. 2006;(2):CD003154. https://doi.org/10.1002/14651858.
22. Orgogozo J, Riguad A, Stoffler A, et al. Efficacy and safety of memantine in patients with mild to moderate vascular dementia: a randomized, placebo-controlled trial (MMM300). Stroke. 2002;33:1834–9.
23. Wenzel C, Rockwood K, MacKnight C, et al. Progression of impairment in patients with vascular cognitive impairment without dementia. Neurology. 2001;57:714–6.
24. Meyer JS, Xu G, Thornby J, et al. Is mild cognitive impairment prodromal for vascular dementia like Alzheimer's disease? Stroke. 2002;33:1981–5.
25. Katzman R, Fox P. The world-wide impact of dementia. Projections of prevalence and costs. In: Mayeaux R, Christen Y, editors. Epidemiology of Alzheimer's Disease: from gene to prevention. Berlin: Springer; 1999. p. 1–17.
26. Kirkman AM. Dementia in the news: the media coverage of Alzheimer's disease. Australas J Ageing. 2006;25(2):74–9.
27. Peel E. The living death of Alzheimer's versus 'Take a walk to keep dementia at bay': representations of dementia in print media and career discourse. Sociol Health Illn. 2014;36:6. https://doi.org/10.1111/1.9566.12122.
28. Behuniak SM. The living dead? The construction of people with Alzheimer's disease as zombies. Ageing Soc. 2011;31(1):70–92.
29. Burgener SC, Buckwalter KC. Examining perceived stigma in persons with dementia. Iowa: US Department of Health and Human Services, National Institute of Health; 2008.
30. Riley RI, Burgener S, Buckwalter KC. Anxiety and stigma in dementia: a threat to aging in place. Nurs Clin North Am. 2014;49(2):213–31.
31. Kertez A, Davidson W, Fox H. Frontal behavioural inventory: diagnostic criteria for frontal lobe dementia. Can J Neurol Sci. 1997;24:29–36.
32. Folstein MF, Folstein SE, McHugh PH. Mini-mental state: a practical method for grading the cognitive state of patients for the clinician. J Psychiatr Res. 1975;12:189–98.
33. Osterweil D, Beck JC, Brummel-Smith K, editors. Comprehensive geriatric assessment. Castle Rock, Pittsford: McGraw-Hill Professional; 2000.
34. Agrell B, Review DO. The clock-drawing test. Age Ageing. 1998;27:399–403.
35. Inouye SK, Robinson JT, Froelich TE, Richardson ED. The time and change test: a simple screening test for dementia. J Gerontol. 1998;53:M281–6.
36. Borson S, Scanlan JM, Chen P, Ganguli M. The Mini-Cog as a screen for dementia: validation in a population-based sample. J Am Geriatr Soc. 2003;51:1451–4.
37. Brodaty H, Pond D, Draper B, et al. Assisting general practitioners to screen for cognitive impairment: The General Practitioner Assessment of Cognition website. Alzheimers Dement. 2009;5(5):e15–6.
38. LoGuidice D, Smith K, Thomas J, et al. Kimberly Indigenous Cognitive Assessment tool (KICA): development of a cognitive assessment tool for older indigenous Australians. Int Psychogeriatr. 2006;18(2):269–80.

Conceição Balsinha, Manuel Gonçalves-Pereira, Steve Iliffe, José Alexandre Freitas, and Joana Grave

Abstract

Dementia is a disabling, highly prevalent condition in older age. Complexities related to dementia care challenge the existing models of health and social services. Although for most people in Western Europe the first contact point for health-related concerns is a general practitioner, the role of primary care physicians and primary care teams regarding older people with dementia needs clarification. Primary care has much to offer to older people with dementia and their informal, family carers, but several challenges still need to be addressed. Given that the perspectives of people with dementia, their carers and staff regarding the role of primary care in dementia may share several points, it seems possible to define priority areas for intervention. Despite a growing number of studies on dementia care delivery in primary care, interventions addressing a wide range of important outcomes in dementia (e.g. falls, frailty) are overlooked in the research agenda; this probably hinders the quality of health care provided. At the end of the chapter, we finally discuss how current knowledge on dementia care fits into the Portuguese health and social care systems, as a case study example.

C. Balsinha (✉) · J. A. Freitas
CEDOC, Chronic Diseases Research Centre, NOVA Medical School/Faculdade de Ciências Médicas, Universidade Nova de Lisboa, Lisboa, Portugal

Unidade de Saúde Familiar Marginal, São João do Estoril, Portugal
e-mail: maria.balsinha@nms.unl.pt

M. Gonçalves-Pereira · J. Grave
CEDOC, Chronic Diseases Research Centre, NOVA Medical School/Faculdade de Ciências Médicas, Universidade Nova de Lisboa, Lisboa, Portugal
e-mail: gpereira@nms.unl.pt; joanagrave@ua.pt

S. Iliffe
Primary Care and Population Health, University College London, London, UK

Centre of Expertise in Longevity and Long-Term Care, Charles University, Prague, Czech Republic
e-mail: s.iliffe@ucl.ac.uk

Abbreviations

BPSD   Behavioural and psychological symptoms of dementia
PCP   Primary care physicians
PwD   People with dementia, or person with dementia

Key Points
- The role of primary care physicians and primary care teams regarding older people with dementia still needs clarification.

© Springer Nature Switzerland AG 2019
C. A. de Mendonça Lima, G. Ivbijaro (eds.), *Primary Care Mental Health in Older People*,
https://doi.org/10.1007/978-3-030-10814-4_23

- There are several challenges related to dementia care delivery for older people in primary care.
- The perspectives of people with dementia, their carers and staff regarding dementia care in primary care may have several common points.
- Interventions that could improve the quality of care for older people with dementia in primary care are overlooked in research.
- Primary care has much to offer to older people with dementia and their carers.
- How current knowledge on dementia care fits into the Portuguese health and social care systems.

23.1 Introduction

Our world faces continuous growth in ageing populations. In 2015, the population aged 65 years or older represented 7% or more of the total in many countries [1] and 18.9% of the population in the European Union [2]. These demographic changes are leading to a number of challenges for health and social care systems.

A great number of these challenges depend to a large extent on the health profile of the older population, but gaining knowledge of these health profiles has proved challenging, and evidence regarding future health trends is conflicting [3]. According to the OECD publication 'Health at a Glance 2017' [4], 51% of all over-65s on average across 26 European countries in 2015 reported that they were limited either to some extent or severely in their usual daily activities because of a health problem. Predicting the future prevalence of disability in the older population is the cornerstone of this debate. Population ageing and the greater longevity of individuals will lead to increasing numbers of people at older ages with disability and in need of long-term care [5]. On the other hand, a compression of morbidity (a shorter period of illness before death) in the future [6] will probably lead to a greater proportion of years lived without disability in older age.

One of the disabling conditions with a high prevalence in older age is dementia, broadly defined as loss of memory and problems in other cognitive functions causing impairment in everyday activities. Among chronic diseases, dementia is the fourth leading cause of burden of disease (DALYs) in high-income countries and is one of the major causes of disability and dependency among older people worldwide and therefore considered a public health priority [7]. It has extensive health consequences for the patients and their carers and a high financial impact on the patient, his family and society [8]. Although the incidence of dementia may be declining in some countries due to cardiovascular risk reduction and improved brain health [9, 10], dementia remains only partially preventable and is not a reversible condition in the great majority of cases. This puts pressure on health and social services to find solutions in order to deal with an increasing number of related challenges.

For most people in Western Europe, the first point of contact for health-related concerns is a primary care provider, most often a primary care physician (PCP). As a result, the quality of dementia health care that is delivered in primary care has been under scrutiny for decades. In 1996, Downs [11] wrote an editorial review in which she described the role that PCPs and primary care teams could play in dementia care and the difficulties they were facing and provided suggestions for supporting PCPs and primary care teams in dementia care delivery. Surprisingly, or not, those are the same issues that we are still debating today. It seems that primary care has been struggling to fulfil the expectations of health-care systems regarding dementia care in several countries for more than 25 years. It is not possible to discuss dementia care delivery in primary care without trying to frame it within a wider context that considers the interfaces between society and health care and health-care policies and health-care delivery (Fig. 23.1).

In this chapter, we will first review the role of primary care physicians and primary care teams in managing dementia. Secondly, we will explore the main challenges related to dementia care delivery for older people in primary care. Thirdly,

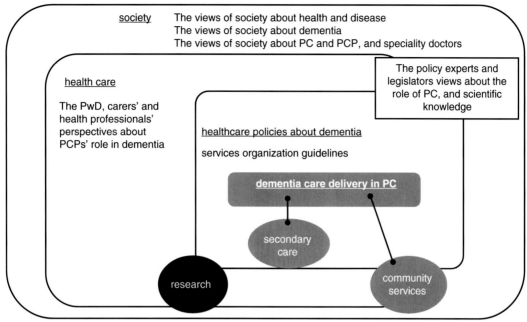

PC - primary care; PCP - primary care physicians; PwD - people with dementia

Fig. 23.1 Integrative model of interfaces that condition dementia care delivery in primary care. *PC* primary care, *PCP* primary care physicians, *PwD* people with dementia

we will explore the perspectives of people with dementia, their carers and health professionals on dementia care in primary care. Here we will try to define common ground and discrepancies, trying to pave the way for any possible interventions. Fourthly, we will review interventions that have been tested to improve the quality of care for older people with dementia in primary care. Fifthly, we will discuss what primary care has to offer to older people with dementia and their carers, considering the salience of specialist[1] services and prevailing ways of thinking about illness. Finally, we will discuss how current knowledge on dementia care fits into the Portuguese health and social care systems.

---

[1]In some countries (e.g. Germany, the UK), PCPs are not considered specialists. Therefore, in this chapter we will refer to 'specialists' meaning neurologists and psychiatrists (and geriatricians, in some countries) in charge of people with dementia, regardless of setting (public or private practice, hospital settings or not).

23.2 What Is the Role of Primary Care Physicians and the Primary Care Team in Managing Dementia?

The role of PCPs in health care, as defined by the World Organization of Family Doctors [12], is clear: to 'care for the individual within the context of the family, for the family within the context of the community, and for the community in the context of public health (…) for providing comprehensive and continuing, person-centred care (…), and in helping coordinate and integrate care' (p. 42). In addition, PCPs and other primary care professionals provide first contact to every person seeking health care and advice. Although this role applies to dementia care delivery, the roles and responsibilities of primary care providers with respect to dementia care have generally not been explicitly defined [13].

Despite the lack of definition of the PCP role in dementia care, it is expected that these care providers assume a wide range of responsibilities, such as ensuring early detection of dementia and diagnosis [14–18], initiating and managing pharmacological treatment [16, 19], providing ongoing support to the patients and their carers through the different stages of the disease [16–18], being able to assist in difficult decisions (e.g. medico-legal issues, driving) [16, 20–22] and having a central and coordinating role in collaborative care models [16, 17].

In each of the national dementia strategies of 14 European countries (UK, Norway, Finland, Netherlands, Denmark, Italy, Greece, Spain, Croatia, Bulgaria, Slovenia, Czech Republic, Switzerland, Belgium), the role of PCPs with respect to dementia is also mentioned [23]. The most well-established task is detecting new cases of dementia and maintaining the general health and safety of the patient, while the role in diagnosing dementia, initiating anti-dementia drugs and providing social support is more controversial. A recent EU-JPND study involving eight countries (Actifcare, i.e. ACcess to TImely Formal Care, www.actifcare.eu) focused on the access to and use of community care services for home-dwelling people with dementia (PwD) and their carers and issued best practice recommendations that also concerned the role of PCPs [24]. These professionals should have more knowledge and provide information about available community care services, have specific training to make timely diagnoses of dementia and to recognize the need of advanced diagnostic assessments (e.g. dementia subtypes) and have a comprehensive overview of the situation of the PwD. These recommendations also highlight the need for a well-defined pathway for PCPs' referrals regarding treatment of urgent cases and the need for PwD and their carers having a named contact person (e.g. PCP, case manager). These Actifcare best practice recommendations have been discussed taking into account each country's particular circumstances. The definition and roles of this 'contact person', along with implementation issues, are motivating an ongoing debate and generating further research questions within the consortium.

23.3 What Are the Main Challenges Related to Dementia Care Delivery for Older People in Primary Care?

The numerous challenges related to dementia care delivery for older people in primary care can be attributed to difficulties in drawing the line between the effects of ageing and those of the disease, as well as to the wide scope of action of primary care.

23.3.1 Primary Care Physicians Find It Difficult to Recognise Dementia

Underdiagnosis of dementia by PCPs has been identified as an important shortcoming in several countries [25–28]. A systematic review [29] of studies assessing the ability of PCPs to recognize dementia found that PCPs typically identify three out of four PwD but have more difficulties in the early stages (one out of two people with mild dementia) and record the correct diagnosis in medical notes infrequently.

A systematic review [30] of quantitative and qualitative studies on barriers to the recognition of dementia in primary care found factors related to physicians (diagnostic uncertainty or insufficient knowledge or experience disclosing the diagnosis, stigma attached to dementia and therapeutic nihilism), factors related to the patient or society (stigma and delayed presentation) and factors related to the health system (time constraints, lack of support and financial or remuneration issues). Dodd et al. [31] argued that PCPs' lack of confidence in making independent dementia diagnoses seems to be a major barrier to dementia diagnosis in primary care. In order to avoid inappropriate diagnoses, PCPs reported a modal average of four consultations with patients and their relatives before they make a conclusion.

It is important to acknowledge that there are different factors shaping PCPs' ability to diagnose dementia. The process of diagnosis and decision-making is not a linear one; instead it has been described in primary care as a three-step process [32]: (1) generating a list of diagnostic hypotheses, given the problem presented by the patient; (2) imposing a hierarchy on the list, based on the likelihood of each hypothesis; and (3) establishing a definite diagnostic conclusion, after excluding the hypotheses one by one. Dementia (as an overall condition) is not a disease but a syndrome (a group of symptoms that consistently occur together). However, subtypes of dementia such as Alzheimer's disease are associated with biomarkers that allow for a disease diagnosis [10]. Even if a diagnosis of subtype is not feasible in primary care, generally speaking, different factors pose specific challenges to PCPs regarding the dementia syndrome recognition. Cognitive performance at a defined moment of assessment is affected not only by normal ageing and education but also by, for example, depressive symptoms or stressful circumstances (like the death of a spouse). Moreover, the ability to live independently is also affected by physical conditions as well as by social expectations and not always easily ascertained as fulfilling the criterion for a diagnosis of dementia.

Another widely debated issue is the necessity of an early diagnosis [33–35]. The benefits of an early recognition of dementia include ending uncertainty regarding the cause of symptoms and behaviour change, giving access to appropriate support, promoting positive coping strategies, facilitating planning and developing the process of adaptation to the carer role [33, 36, 37]. On the other hand, negative consequences of unsupported diagnostic disclosure for PwD and their carers have also been identified: risk of causing emotional distress, inability of the person with dementia to understand and/or retain diagnosis, anxiety about increasing disability, negative effects on self-esteem and restricted activities [36]. In addition, attributing a range of behaviours or cognitive changes to dementia may lead to under-treatment of other conditions like depression [34]. It is important to consider that the drawbacks of an early diagnosis may outweigh the benefits if people are left with a diagnosis but are offered little support [33].

In fact, the focus on 'early diagnosis' is being overridden by a different emphasis on 'timely diagnosis', which means 'communicating a diagnosis at a time when the person with dementia and their carers will benefit from interventions and support' [38].

23.3.2   Multimorbidity and Frailty Are Highly Prevalent in Older People with Dementia

Throughout the discussions on the PCPs' role in managing PwD, there is surprisingly little focus on the integrated care of physical, mental and cognitive co-morbidities, given that most PwD have several co-morbidities [39, 40].

Effective provision of chronic health condition management may be compromised by prevailing views that the chronic disease burden is made up of individual diseases that are best managed independently (e.g. establishing a national diabetes or dementia strategy). Research [41] on co-occurrence of chronic diseases in older adults and geriatric syndromes highlighted the importance of providing comprehensive care to address multimorbidity. Given that the prevalence of chronic diseases increases in old age as does dementia [42], older PwD will also face the challenges of multimorbidity and most probably of geriatric syndromes (e.g. falls, urinary incontinence) [39, 40]. In addition, the co-existence of dementia and other conditions in older people increases the risk of disability and frailty and consequently of dependence; thus there will be a great diversity of care needs in an aged population with dementia [40]. Koroukian et al. [40] examined the prevalence of chronic conditions, functional limitations and geriatric syndromes across gradients of cognitive impairment in a representative sample of the US population aged 50 years or older. These authors have also defined a complex variable consisting of the co-occurrence of chronic conditions (minimum one), functional limitations and geriatric syndromes. Their findings showed an increased prevalence of multimorbidity in individuals with higher levels of cognitive impairment, but more interesting the same happened with the prevalence of the complex variable.

A recent systematic review [43] on the prevalence of frailty identified five studies including 543 patients with Alzheimer's disease and provided a pooled prevalence estimate of 31.9%.

The need to consider and optimize physical health in PwD (e.g. nutritional status, risks of falls) highlights the importance of a greater involvement of primary care in the delivery of dementia care [13]. On the other hand, the co-morbidities of dementia and their association with frailty increase the risk of dependence, which leads in turn to the wide variety and complexity of needs for care of PwD.

23.3.3 Older People with Dementia Often Have a Large Number of Highly Complex Needs

Previous research [44–48] on unmet needs (i.e. when a person is not receiving an appropriate support in a particular area of their life) have shown that they seem to predict important outcome measures, such as decreased quality of life, psychological and behavioural symptoms, institutionalization and mortality.

The comprehensive interview-based Camberwell Assessment of Needs for the Elderly [49, 50] has been used to map the needs and amount of help (received and needed) of PwD living in the community [46, 51]. Miranda-Castillo et al. [46] interviewed 125 PwD, with mild/moderate cognitive impairment, and their carers. The most frequent unmet needs identified by the carers (regarding PwD needs) were daytime activities (41.1%), company (29.8%), psychological distress (26.6%) and eyesight/hearing (20.2%). The most frequently met needs identified by the carers were memory (94.4%), looking after home (87.1%), food (86.2%) and money (81.5%). The European Actifcare cohort study [51] recruited 451 dyads of PwD and their carers. Most of these PwD (78%) had mild dementia and exclusion criteria included relying on significant amounts of formal care; thus the focus was on the intermediate stages of dementia. The most fre-

quently unmet needs identified by the carers were daytime activities and company, and the most frequently met needs were looking after home, food, memory and money.

A recent systematic mixed studies review [52] of studies that identified needs of patient-carer dyads found that the most frequently reported need was an earlier disclosure of dementia diagnosis, followed by needs related to education and counselling on the disease. Carers also pointed out the need for home support, and patients mentioned needs for meaningful activities where they could participate in and be assisted in daily activities.

Identifying unmet needs could help to identify who is at risk of an adverse outcome and to provide the care needed through tailored interventions. On the other hand, identifying the most frequently met needs, and the way they are met, could help policymakers to better design appropriate responses to support PwD and their carers. Evidence [46, 51] suggests that most needs are related to social support, highlighting the importance of the social model.

Sociology has much to tell us about health and illness and especially about chronic conditions, such as dementia. Sociology tends to be undervalued in medical training; therefore understanding about the experience and meaning of an illness eventually escapes physicians through the rush of consultations. Since medical sociology concerns the patient, their family and society as a whole, it has special relevance for PCPs providing dementia care.

Traditional views of illness put its investigation and treatment in the domain of medicine and the professions allied to medicine. The task of helping people to manage the personal and social consequences of illness is the domain of the social care professions [53]. Therefore, when we look at dementia mainly as a medical problem, we feel hopeless because it cannot be contained or cured; but if we see it as a disability, it can be accommodated into daily life [54]. However, in order to foster PwD's and their carers' wellbeing, we have to frame disability within the social model. The social model sees the problem experienced by people with disabilities as being the direct product of the physical, social and attitudinal environments. In the social perspective, the problem is a failure of the environment to adjust to the needs and desires of people with disabilities. In comparison, the medical model sees disability as a deviation from biomedical norms of structure and function, putting the solution in medical intervention to help the person adjust to their limitations.

The application of medical science cannot be ignored, but in the case of PwD, it is necessary to bring both the clinical and social perspectives together. By doing this, the lack of post-diagnostic support will be ameliorated, and many of the unmet needs currently identified by PwD and carers will be eventually met.

23.3.4 Informal Carers Are Not Only a Resource in Dementia Care

People with dementia most often need support from informal carers. Many older PwD are cared for at home, primarily by spouses and adult children [51, 55, 56]. These informal carers are frequently more actively involved in the caregiving process than their counterparts caring for patients with other illnesses, acting as care coordinators, information sources and front-line communicators for their relatives [57] and often being involved in medical encounters [58].

The negative consequences of informal caregiving in dementia have been widely studied, and the associated burden, in physical, emotional, social or financial terms, is uncontentious [55, 59, 60]. Cuijpers [61] reviewed the prevalence of depressive disorders in dementia caregivers and found a range of 15–32% prevalence rates and relative risks 2.8–38. A recent meta-analysis [62] found that carers of persons with Alzheimer's disease have a higher prevalence of mental health disorders, particularly depression and anxiety, as compared with the general population and with carers of patients with other health conditions. In sum, there is a consensus that about 40% of dementia caregivers may suffer from clinically significant anxiety or depression, while others present significant psychological symptoms [63]. It has also been acknowledged that taking care of an older relative with dementia places a heavy

burden on the general health of older carers [64]. Carers' somatic problems overall include cardiovascular issues and compromised immune function, with difficulties engaging in health behaviours and a higher mortality [55, 59, 60].

It is well established that neuropsychiatric, behavioural and psychological symptoms are particularly linked to carer burden in dementia [55, 65]. PCPs need better training in assessing and managing these behavioural and psychological symptoms of dementia (BPSD), but these professionals also should have better access to back up speciality services (e.g. geropsychiatry, occupational therapy) and be reimbursed for time spent on its prevention, assessment and management [66]. In conclusion, there is a rationale for the involvement of family members in clinical assessments of PwD. As informants, relatives are helpful, often decisive in the patient's evaluation. As informal carers, they may deserve to be assessed in their own right (concerning, e.g. psychological distress, ongoing ability to provide care). Finally, family dynamics must sometimes be evaluated or addressed; noteworthy, the family is seldom considered as a whole system in dementia caregiving research. Secondary carers may also be at risk and ought to be assessed in many situations [65]. The National Institute for Health and Care Excellence (NICE) clinical guidelines acknowledge that the diagnosis does not affect just one person but the whole family system [67].

In countries where PCPs are accountable for the whole family system, they are in a privileged position for a more comprehensive approach to PwD and their carer(s). This enables PCPs to 'think family' by empathically assessing and mobilizing family members, facilitating brief and simple family interventions [68].

23.3.5 Comprehensive and Coordinated Health-Care Systems Are Needed for Better Provision of Care in Dementia

The need for a continued management of such a complex condition as dementia in the community stresses the importance of a comprehensive and coordinated primary care system. It follows that primary care service organization must be adapted to the provision of dementia care and that primary care professionals must have a good enough knowledge about dementia.

In 1998, Starfield identified the four pillars of primary care practice, which are still used today as a measure of good primary care systems [69, 70]: first-contact care, continuity over time, comprehensiveness and coordination with other parts of the health system. First-contact care means that primary care is the point of entry into the health-care system. Continuity means that patients/families have a regular source of care over a significant period of time. However, this can be extended to incorporate a more comprehensive definition of continuity of care, as provided by the World Health Organization [70]: cross-sectional continuity (coherent interventions over the short term both within and among teams) and longitudinal continuity (uninterrupted series of contacts over the long term). Comprehensiveness is the extent to which different types of health services are provided (e.g. preventive, chronic, palliative). Finally, coordination involves the integration of all care, making it coherent for the individual patient.

More recently, other attributes (e.g. population-focused accountabilities for care, active patient engagement in care and team-based care) have been added to the aforementioned four pillars and together characterize high-performing primary care [69, 71].

These attributes sound promising in addressing the needs of PwD and their carers, although there are suggestions that primary care is struggling to keep up with these attributes of high-performing care. An integrative review [71] that included a broad range of published and grey literature between 2000 and 2013 identified three models of primary care for dementia:

- Carved-out models—they respond to the complexity of dementia care by referring patients and their carers to resources outside the practice (and focus exclusively on dementia care). It assumes that most of the needs of carers and patients are beyond the capacity of normal primary care and that the majority of needs need care plans built around dementia.

- Co-managed models—they respond to the complexity of dementia care by meshing external resources into primary care. This assumes that the patients require specialized attention but acknowledges the centrality of the primary care relationship. A robust electronic communication strategy is vital to ensure informational continuity in this model.

- Integrative-hub models—they respond to the complexity of dementia care by building capacity in primary care teams and incorporating resources to sustain the continuity of the primary care relationship.

The authors concluded that there has been a slow penetration of the high-performing primary care attributes into primary care delivery in the case of dementia. They note that the studies classified in the integrative-hub category were most consistent with providing comprehensive, relational and whole person-centred care. Nevertheless, most approaches described in the review still favour the dementia-specific care plans and interventions that focus on the coordination of disease-specific supports and services (with varying degrees of connection back to the primary care context), placing the disease in the foreground and fragmenting dementia care such that it fits within the constraints and time-compressed nature of primary care.

To our knowledge there has been little research on evaluating primary care comprehensiveness of dementia care, and the results have been limited by the small number of participants [20, 21, 72] and by audits to medical records [20, 22]. These studies showed an underuse of functional assessment tools and of community support [21], lack of home safety assessments [20], lack of attention to wandering, driving and medicolegal issues [20–22], unavailability of dementia-specific services [20, 72], lack of attention to carers' issues [21] and lack of registered information about signs and symptoms of dementia and treatment options [22]. The positive findings were general health assessments (vision, hearing, nutritional, continence and sleep) being done in 70% of cases

[20] and the presence or absence of BPSD and cognitive tests' results being documented in 30–40% of records [22].

A German national database analysis of pharmacological prescription showed that PCPs prescribe fewer anti-dementia drugs and more neuroleptics when compared with specialists [73].

23.4 Do People with Dementia, Their Informal Carers and Health Professionals Have Different Perspectives on Dementia Care Delivery in Primary Care?

To better understand the challenges of primary care regarding older PwD and their carers, it is important to know what their perspectives on dementia care delivered in primary care are.

Considering the early stages of the dementia diagnosis process, research [31, 74] suggests that carers were satisfied with primary care services. Nonetheless, some carers found the PCP reluctant to give a diagnosis, and many felt that their first concerns were not always addressed [31]. In addition, an association between perceived quality and the interpersonal skills of professionals was found (e.g. showing concern, being thorough) [74]. By contrast, when considering the care provided after the diagnosis, the carers and older PwD were found to be less satisfied with primary care services. The lack of support following the dementia diagnosis was identified by carers and older PwD alike [31, 75, 76]. The lack of information on available services provided by primary care professionals [31, 76] as well as on how to deal with carer burden and on how to manage dementia [75] has also been presented as negative aspects from the carer's perspective.

Regarding the perspective of PCPs, there is a growing body of evidence on constraints of dementia care delivery in primary care. The main barriers include:

- Structural and system-related factors: [77–79] insufficient consultation time, difficulty in accessing and communicating with special-

ists, low reimbursement, poor connections with community social service agencies and lack of interdisciplinary teams
- Family-related factors: [79] carers' fatigue/exhaustion/anger and planning for the patient's institution placement
- Medical-related factors: [30, 31, 77–79] inadequate clinician time, length of time needed to administer screening tools and limited treatment options
- Health-related factors: [30, 79] behavioural and psychological symptoms of dementia (e.g. aggressiveness, restlessness/agitation) and co-morbidities (e.g. falls, delirium, adverse reactions to medication, urinary incontinence)

The difficulties in coordinating with specialists seem to compromise the care for PwD and influence aspects of medical practice and may be due to three key factors [77]:

- Structural and system-related factors: managing care, carve outs (e.g. an approach to managing care that separates psychological and psychiatric services from medical care services, in order to reduce health costs), insurance/entitlements, poor geographical distribution, lack of trained providers and reimbursement policies.
- Patient/family and societal factors: ambivalence about treatment, frailty, neuropsychological symptoms, stigma, financial difficulties, cultural values and logistical problems.
- PCP/specialist factors: a lack of geriatric and psychiatric training for PCPs (increasing their need for referrals for complex diagnosis and treatment decisions), poor communication, lack of feedback from specialists and lack of coordinated care. PCPs preferred to use mental health specialists for consultations only and continue overall care management themselves in order to care for the co-morbid medical illness.

The attitudes and behaviours of primary care professionals towards informal carers have also been explored [80]. In general, the professionals perceive the informal carer as a resource and co-worker in dementia care; however, they fail to attend to carers' responses and attitudes to the caregiver role.

In our understanding, PwD and primary care professionals other than PCPs are underrepresented in research, particularly concerning the perceived role of primary care and primary care professionals regarding the provision of dementia care.

It is interesting to notice that PwD and carers identify some critical points that are related to the professionals' perspectives: lack of support following the diagnosis (PwD/carers) relates to lack of PCPs' geriatric/psychiatric training, lack of feedback from specialists and lack of coordinated care (PCPs); lack of information on available services (carers) relates to poor connections with community social service agencies and lack of interdisciplinary teams (PCPs); and lack of information on how to deal with carer burden (carers) relates to the professionals' perceptions of the informal carers as a resource and a co-worker in dementia care.

23.5 What Interventions Have Been Tested to Improve the Quality of Care for Older People with Dementia in Primary Care?

A systematic scoping review [13] to identify strategies for improving the quality and outcomes of primary healthcare regarding dementia may be found in the World Alzheimer Report 2016.

In this section, we would like to introduce our own review of intervention studies, identified by restricting the search scope of dementia in primary care with specific search terms related to ageing. Through this approach, we aimed to identify studies that considered other aspects of the health of PwD besides dementia itself (e.g. falls, co-morbidities assessment).

We identified eight studies that, aside from some overlapping strategies, share several common goals: to improve guideline adherence, to improve collaborative work, to manage symptoms more appropriately and to provide better carer support. These studies can be divided into three broad groups:

- Case management (also described as collaborative care) [52, 81–86]
- Implementing/improving clinical decision support systems [85–87]
- Educational interventions for PCPs [84]

Improving care delivery using a case manager appears to be a sensible option. Taking care of PwD is complex and requires experience that a PCP cannot easily achieve due to the low number of cases in their panels [88]. In addition, in a 15–20 min visit, physicians often do not have time to counsel patients and carers, and many do not know how to assess needs outside the scope of traditional medical management [83, 88, 89]. To overcome these barriers, it has been proposed that nurse practitioners specialized in dementia care could play a role in improving the quality of care for PwD and their carers in primary care. Through being dedicated to this role, they potentially have the time and knowledge to address medical and social aspects of care (e.g. counselling for safety concerns, managing dementia-related medication, referral to community resources, coordinate care). However, one systematic review [90] demonstrated that case management had limited positive effect on behavioural symptoms of dementia and length of hospital stay for patients and on burden and depression for carers. These heterogeneous results as well as the minimal benefits may imply that only highly intense case management is effective, which entails a small caseload, regular proactive patient-carer follow-up, regular contact between case managers and PCPs and effective communication between all healthcare professionals [90].

One study [82] that focused solely on collaborative care between primary care and community-based organizations found disappointing results. It assessed the effect of 'dementia care consultants' provided by local Alzheimer's Association chapters on nursing home placement and carer outcomes. Patients whose carers were in the intervention group were less likely than their control group counterparts to be admitted to a nursing home (AOR 0.40, 95% CI 0.14–1.18), but no effect on carer self-efficacy, carer depression, or strain was found. However, a sub-analysis showed that carer satisfaction with the intervention played a role in self-efficacy in symptom control and in using support services.

A combined approach between case management and collaborative care with community-based organizations was also found [81, 83]. In one study [81], an advanced practice nurse was integrated in a primary care team and worked with family carers in a case management model to assess its effect on neuropsychiatric symptoms. The intervention group showed lower BPSD and lower carer strain. The study found there was no effect on carer depression. The use of cholinesterase inhibitors and antidepressants was enhanced without increasing the use of antipsychotics or sedatives/hypnotics. The intervention was found to have no effect on PwD's cognition, depression, activities of daily living, hospitalization, nursing home placement, or death.

This combined approach was also tested at the University of California at Los Angeles in an Alzheimer's disease quality improvement programme (UCLA-ADC) [83]. A co-management model was developed with nurse practitioner dementia care managers working with PCPs and community-based organizations, to enhance adherence to guidelines. They verified an improvement in guideline adherence, regarding the assessment and screening for cognitive decline, co-morbidities, complications of dementia and counselling on various domains, but adherence to treatment guidelines did not improve. Carers' satisfaction with the programme was also assessed and showed high carer satisfaction with the care manager (help on decisions and listening to concerns) and with the support for their role.

A different way of optimizing delivery of care by the case manager is to use clinical decision support systems. This approach was shown to be effective in two large trials [85, 86]. One trial [86] tested the effect of a disease-based management programme implemented by case managers on quality of care and outcomes. The intervention group of this trial showed a twofold increase in guideline adherence, with higher care quality on 21 out of 23 guidelines and a higher proportion of assistance received from community agencies. An increase was found in PwD's quality of life, quality of caregiving and social support in the intervention group; conversely unmet caregiving assistance needs decreased. No effect on carer's quality of life was found. The second trial [85] tested the effectiveness and safety of dementia care management in the treatment and care of PwD as well as the carer burden. This used a computer-assisted assessment to create personalized intervention modules and subsequent success monitoring. The intervention resulted in significantly decreased behavioural and psychological symptoms of dementia and carer burden compared with usual care. In the intervention group, there was an increase in the use of anti-dementia drugs and a significant increase in quality of life for patients not living alone, but quality of life was not increased overall. Another study [87] analysed the results of the implementation of a computerized intervention-management-system that has been developed to facilitate dementia care management. The analysis showed that 72% of the unmet needs identified by the computer system were not recognized by the case manager, and, as a result, this improved the provision of recommendations for the PCP.

Finally, one study [84] assessed if a practice redesign intervention coupled with referral to local Alzheimer's Association chapters could improve the quality of dementia care. Adherence to guidelines by PCPs was used to measure the quality of care provided. One of the quality indicators of care for older people that has been used is the "Assessing Care of Vulnerable Elders" (ACOVE). In this study, a modified version of this instrument was used to redesign practice in primary care by improving PCPs' skills (ACOVE-AD); however, the results fell short of the required value to be clinically significant [84].

To sum up, we did not find evidence of measures concerning other aspects of the health of PwD besides dementia itself. The reviewed studies [52, 81, 83, 84, 86] do not refer to any co-morbidities other than depression.

Additionally, collaborative work with community-based organizations or using case managers as a single intervention seems to be ineffective. On the other hand, comprehensive approaches that combine different strategies (e.g. case managing with clinical decision support systems) may be of interest regarding guideline adherence and should be further explored.

Designing and testing innovative approaches with new services (e.g. carer schools) have been overlooked.

23.6 What Does Primary Care Offer to Older People with Dementia and Their Carers, Considering the Salience of Specialist Services and Ways of Thinking About Illness?

It is widely accepted that the initial identification of likely cases of dementia is an important function of primary care [7, 8, 13, 31, 91, 92]. In most countries, PCPs see their patients in their own environment, over a long period, with an understanding of the medical and non-medical life history of their patients [93]. The capacity that PCPs and other professionals in primary care have to assess co-morbidity in combination with dementia, to manage geriatric syndromes and to promote measures of primary and secondary prevention ensuring relational and management continuities has been seen as one of the major arguments for the greater involvement of primary care in the delivery of dementia care [13]. Furthermore, PCPs frequently see themselves as a provider of social care in some way, where symptoms must be interpreted in the context of the patient's life as a whole (as is required by the patient-centred care model) and attention should be given to the interplay between clinical and social factors. In addition, in countries such as Portugal, PCPs deliver care to several members of the same family, which gives them the opportunity to work with families more effectively, as previously discussed in Sect. 23.3 [68].

Despite the potential that primary care has for providing good quality care to older PwD and their carers, dementia specialists and dementia specialized services still have a major role in providing care. It is possible that this partially results from ways of thinking about illness. Medicine often has relatively few interventions that make a real difference to the patient with a chronic disabling condition (e.g. dementia). Nonetheless, physicians (and patients) dominate the management of the disease. This notion may be rooted in the stereotypical disease form, dominated by the methods and principles of the biological sciences, which it is the function of medicine to treat [94]. Furthermore, these concepts are subject to social, cultural and economic influences, and in recent years there has been a growing tendency to classify states of being as diseases and to medicalization [95, 96]. In this sense, it would matter to know how dementia is conveyed by the social media. A qualitative study [97] of UK national newspaper articles identified a 'panic-blame' framework where dementia was represented in catastrophic terms. Therefore, catastrophizing dementia in an era with so many technological and scientific developments can lead to increasing the demand for specialized medical care.

Given this situation, primary care professionals are in a privileged position to understand the experience and meaning of their patient's dementia, considering its social and emotional consequences for both patients and their family members. All of which enables them to deliver the most proper care to the patient (as a person) and the family.

23.7 Fitting the Current Knowledge on Dementia Care into Portuguese Primary Care

Portugal is a southern European country where the National Health Service (including primary care systems) has attained high standards in several areas of care, despite problems that are yet to be resolved. Dementia stands as an important public health problem where primary care services face major difficulties in tackling the needs of patients and families and remain to a large extent ineffective at this purpose. This picture contrasts with the potential of primary care in Portuguese settings, a case worth exploration in this last section.

In Portugal, the proportion of older people is expected to rise considerably in the forthcoming years, and the prevalence of dementia was esti-mated higher than the OECD-35 mean rate in 2017 [4]. A recent survey [98] reported a demen-tia prevalence rate of 9.2% (95% CI 7.8–10.9), using the 10/66 Dementia Research Group algo-rithm in community-dwelling older people. Despite lack of incidence data, awareness is increasing of the societal burden of dementia.

23.7.1 Brief Overview of Health and Social Care Systems

Everyone in Portugal has access to the mainly tax-funded National Health Service (NHS). In recent years, there have been a number of reform initiatives, and groups of primary health-care centres were created in 2008, aiming at a better use of resources and management structures [99].

However, and regardless of the promising findings of small-scale studies on the potential of brief evaluations, older people's needs assess-ment in primary care is not routine [100]. In dementia, particular challenges arise, concern-ing, e.g. diagnosis, home care and general support.

23.7.1.1 Diagnostic and Therapeutic Settings

The role of PCPs regarding dementia manage-ment is not formally defined, but these profes-sionals are considered to be the first point of contact for PwD and their families, and they usu-ally provide an important gatekeeping function. PCPs are allowed to prescribe anti-dementia medication, although they do it infrequently and this is not reimbursed as with neurologists or psy-chiatrists' prescriptions. The prevalence of PwD in primary care has doubled in the last 5 years, from 0.4% to 0.8% of all users [101]. Access to specialized physicians (in the NHS) is limited by waiting time for consultations, mandatory refer-ral, out-of-pocket payment and, in some cases, traveling long distances. There are disparities in GPs' dementia knowledge and skills, along with insufficient support from specialized care and non-medical staff. GPs' gatekeeping functions may actually contribute to diagnosis delay: when

referred to neurology or psychiatry, most patients are already at moderate or severe stages [102].

Outpatient clinics specifically for cognitive impairment/dementia are available in public hos-pitals (mainly connected to neurology services and of the 'memory clinic' type), but access is conditioned by long waiting times and some-times long traveling distances [103].

23.7.1.2 Home Care and Support for People with Dementia

There is no formal contact person for PwD and their families although the PCP is generally con-sidered the main reference person for NHS users. Team-based community mental health care for older people is rarely available and is not dementia-specific. Most day centres deliver social care for older people in general, and the few dementia-specific day centres are only regionally available. The provision of care at home to meet PwD's basic needs or assist in basic activities of daily living is available nation-wide, and in the area of home care, standards have increased significantly during the last decade, from a low level in 2005 [4]. Nursing homes for older people in general are available nationwide, while for PwD they are scarce and only available at regional level. Respite care is available nationwide through the National Network for Integrated Long-Term Care (RNCCI), but not in NHS hospitals [103].

23.7.1.3 Information and Counselling

Information structures aiming to provide informa-tion for PwD and their carers regarding dementia and support services are regionally available, mainly through Alzheimer Portugal [103].

On the whole, relationships between health and social care systems are complex, and bound-aries overlap [103]. This represents a major prob-lem, more so as case management does not exist in community dementia care, and there is no current official definition of professionals' roles or of standard pathways to health and social care. As a consequence, there are difficulties in timely access to community health/social formal services and insufficient support for carers and families [103].

There have been strong claims that primary care should be much more involved in early diagnosis of dementia and its appropriate disclosure, among other areas (e.g. treatment monitoring in collaboration with specialized care, counselling and support, monitoring carers' health) [102]. This could help meeting the complex biopsychosocial needs in dementia [104].

Nevertheless, opinions may differ on whether primary care services should be more proactive in dementia management or if current focus should be solely on optimizing referral systems and improving follow-up according to indications from highly specialized hospital centres.

23.7.2 A Portuguese Dementia Policy Is Urgently Needed

There is still no official dementia policy in Portugal (either as a strategy or a plan), although an initial proposal [105] was drafted in 2017 by a workgroup of experts in different health and social areas, nominated by the Health Ministry. These experts put forward examples of what should be done in primary care:

- To early identify cognitive impairment and consider referral for specialized assessment or follow-up when appropriate
- To foster collaborations between primary and secondary care, enabling integrated diagnoses (dementia subtype and functional assessment)
- To implement an Individual Care Plan (it is still to be defined if the care manager should be a PCP, nurse, or social assistant)
- To deliver more person-centred and tailored therapeutic interventions to PwD and their families, in coordination with health and social care community services

It must be recognized that this endeavour implies firm, two-way and continuing collaborations between primary, secondary and tertiary care, as well as between primary care and the social sector.

23.7.3 The Complexity of Practice Can Hinder the Implementation of Dementia Policy

The utilization of knowledge, be it a policy or research evidence, necessarily requires the active involvement and skills of health-care professionals, which means it must be adapted locally. In Table 23.1 we frame the current knowledge available and the generic goals advanced for the role of primary care in dementia, taking into account the complexity of primary care practice in Portugal.

In Portugal as elsewhere, as pointed out in major international reports [8, 13], primary care must take a more important role in the delivery and optimization of dementia care. Overall it has been internationally recognized that dementia (often occurring along with frailty and multiple somatic morbidities) calls for integrated, comprehensive, evidence-based and friendly person-centred approaches to prevent nutritional problems, falls, infection, or *delirium*. This calls for a major involvement of primary care, where staff are best acquainted with PwD and their families, while also implying better resourced services, and a serious discussion of task-shifting versus task-sharing approaches [13, 60].

The wide scope of action of primary care is, perhaps, the main challenge for primary care professionals to ensure quality of care for PwD and their carers. The literature concerning dementia care delivery in primary care has evolved so far around the core notion of enhancing primary care professionals' (namely, PCPs') education and of better service coordination regarding dementia (including case management programmes). Unfortunately, approaches focusing on comprehensive, whole-person primary care have been overlooked. In fact, attributing specific roles to PCPs without better understanding PwD's, carers' and professionals' expectations of the roles and responsibilities of PCPs can lead to policy failure.

In order to understand the limited success of primary care in struggling to fulfil the expectations of health-care systems in the last decades,

Table 23.1 Policy aspirations and theoretical expectations and the complexity of practice in Portuguese primary care

	Policy aspirations/theoretical expectations	Complexity of practice in primary care
Under-recognition of dementia in primary care	PCPs should early identify cognitive impairment	Diagnosis processes in primary care do not fit the complexities of ageing
		Lack of education in geriatrics and cognitive impairment in particular
		Lack of non-medical staff in primary care teams (e.g. neuropsychologists)
Coordination/collaboration between primary and secondary care	To accomplish an integrated diagnosis and follow-up	Feedback information from specialists is not mandatory
		Access to patients' health hospital records depends on faulty informatics
		Conflicting relationships between primary and secondary care
		Patients' and professionals' views may compromise policy's aspirations
Case management	To implement an Individual Care Plan Coordination/collaboration with social care (and with secondary/tertiary care)	Large increase in complexity and intensity of clinical and bureaucratical work in the recent years
		Non-clinical activity is undervalued by administration
		Possible funding limitations
		Lack of community resources specific for dementia
Therapeutic interventions	To deliver more person-centred and tailored care (PwD and families) Reframing dementia according to the social model of disability or the biopsychosocial model	Available 'skill mix' is insufficient in primary care
		Lack of community resources specific for dementia

PCP primary care physicians, *PwD* people with dementia

we seriously need to address these concerns through high-quality mixed method health services research.

References

1. Wan H, Goodkind D, Kowal P. An ageing world: 2015. Washington, DC: U.S. Census Bureau; 2016.
2. Eurostat. Proportion of population aged 65 and over. 2016. http://ec.europa.eu/eurostat/web/population-demography-migration-projections/population-data/main-tables. Accessed 12 Jan 2018.
3. Parker MG, Thorslund M. Health trends in the elderly population: getting better and getting worse. Gerontologist. 2007;47(2):150–8.
4. OECD. Health at a glance 2017: OECD indicators. Paris: OECD; 2017.
5. Lafortune G, Balestat G. Trends in severe disability among elderly people: assessing the evidence in 12 OECD countries and the future implications. Report No. 1815-2015. Paris: OECD; 2007.
6. Fries JF. The compression of morbidity. Milbank Q. 2005;83(4):801–23.
7. WHO. Dementia: a public health priority. http://apps.who.int/iris/bitstream/10665/75263/1/9789241564458_eng. pdf?ua=12012 Date Accessed. Available from:http://apps.who.int/iris/bitstream/10665/75263/1/9789241564458_eng. pdf?ua=1.
8. WHO. Global action plan on the public health response to dementia 2017–2025. Geneva: World Health Organization; 2017. Available from: http://www.who.int/mental_health/neurology/dementia/action_plan_2017_2025/en/.
9. Prince M, Ali G-C, Guerchet M, Prina AM, Albanese E, Wu Y-T. Recent global trends in the prevalence and incidence of dementia, and survival with dementia. Alzheimers Res Ther. 2016;8:23.
10. Scheltens P, Blennow K, Breteler MMB, de Strooper B, Frisoni GB, Salloway S, et al. Alzheimer's disease. Lancet. 2016;388(10043):505–17.
11. Downs MG. The role of general practice and the primary care team in dementia diagnosis and management. Int J Geriatr Psychiatry. 1996;11(11):937–42.
12. WONCA. In: Kidd M, editor. The contribution of family medicine to improving health systems. London: Radcliff; 2013.
13. Prince M, Comas-Herrera MA, Knapp M, Guerchet M, Karagiannidou MM. World Alzheimer Report 2016: improving healthcare for people living with dementia - coverage, quality and costs now and in the future. London: Alzheimer's Disease International; 2016.

14. Fossan G. Dementia in the elderly: the role of the general practitioner. Scand J Prim Health Care. 2009;7(1):3–4.

15. Koch T, Iliffe S. Editorial: the role of primary care in the recognition of and response to dementia. J Nutr Health Aging. 2010;14(2):107–9.

16. Massoud F, Lysy P, Bergman H. Editorial: care of dementia in Canada: a collaborative care approach with a central role for the primary care physician. J Nutr Health Aging. 2010;14(2):105–6.

17. Villars H, Oustric S, Andrieu S, Baeyens JP, Bernabei R, Brodaty H, et al. The primary care physician and Alzheimer's disease: an international position paper. J Nutr Health Aging. 2010;14(2):110–20.

18. Warshaw GA, Bragg EJ. Preparing the health care workforce to care for adults with Alzheimer's disease and related dementias. Health Aff. 2014;33(4):633–41.

19. Petrazzuoli F, Vinker S, Koskela TH, Frese T, Buono N, Soler JK, et al. Exploring dementia management attitudes in primary care: a key informant survey to primary care physicians in 25 European countries. Int Psychogeriatr. 2017;29(9):1413–23.

20. Bridges-Webb C, Giles B, Speechly C, Zurynski Y, Hiramanek N. Patients with dementia and their carers. Ann N Y Acad Sci. 2007;1114:130–6.

21. Parmar J, Dobbs B, McKay R, Kirwan C, Cooper T, Marin A, et al. Diagnosis and management of dementia in primary care: exploratory study. Can. Fam. Physician. 2014;60(5):457–65.

22. Wilcock J, Iliffe S, Turner S, Bryans M, O'Carroll R, Keady J, et al. Concordance with clinical practice guidelines for dementia in general practice. Aging Ment Health. 2009;13(2):155–61.

23. Alzheimer-Europe. National dementia strategies. Alzheimer Europe; 2017. http://www.alzheimer-europe.org/Policy-in-Practice2/National-Dementia-Strategies. Accessed 23 Feb 2018.

24. Actifcare-Consortium. Best practice recommendations from the Actifcare Study. http://actifcare.eu/wp-content/uploads/2017/09/Short-version-Best-Practice-Recommendation-without-supporting-findings-1.pdf. 2016.

25. Aminzadeh F, Molnar FJ, Dalziel WB, Ayotte D. A review of barriers and enablers to diagnosis and management of persons with dementia in primary care. Can Geriatr J. 2012;15(3):85–94.

26. Iliffe S, De Lepeleire J, van Hout H, Kenny G, Lewis A, Vernooij-Dassen M, et al. Understanding obstacles to the recognition of and response to dementia in different European countries: a modified focus group approach using multinational, multi-disciplinary expert groups. Aging Ment Health. 2005;9(1):1–6.

27. Maeck L, Haak S, Knoblauch A, Stoppe G. Early diagnosis of dementia in primary care: a representative eight-year follow-up study in Lower Saxony, Germany. Int J Geriatr Psychiatry. 2007;22(1):23–31.

28. Vernooij-Dassen MJFJ, Moniz-Cook ED, Woods RT, De Lepeleire J, Leuschner A, Zanetti O, et al. Factors affecting timely recognition and diagnosis of dementia across Europe: from awareness to stigma. Int J Geriatr Psychiatry. 2005;20(4):377–86.

29. Mitchell AJ, Meader N, Pentzek M. Clinical recognition of dementia and cognitive impairment in primary care: a meta-analysis of physician accuracy. Acta Psychiatr Scand. 2011;124(3):165–83.

30. Koch T, Iliffe S. Rapid appraisal of barriers to the diagnosis and management of patients with dementia in primary care: a systematic review. BMC Fam Pract. 2010;11(1):52.

31. Dodd E, Cheston R, Fear T, Brown E, Fox C, Morley C, et al. An evaluation of primary care led dementia diagnostic services in Bristol. BMC Health Serv Res. 2014;14(1):592.

32. Dinant G-J, van Leeuwen YD. Clinical diagnosis: hypothetico-deductive reasoning and other theoretical frameworks. In: Jones R, Britten N, Culpepper L, Gass D, Grol R, Mant D, et al., editors. Oxford textbook of primary care, vol. I. New York, NY: Oxford University Press; 2005.

33. de Vugt ME, Verhey FR. The impact of early dementia diagnosis and intervention on informal caregivers. Prog Neurobiol. 2013;110:54–62.

34. Iliffe S, Manthorpe J. Sooner or later? Issues in the early diagnosis of dementia in general practice: a qualitative study. Fam Pract. 2003;20(4):376–81.

35. Iliffe S, Jain P, Wong G, Lefford F, Warner A, Gupta S, et al. Dementia diagnosis in primary care: thinking outside the educational box. Aging Health. 2009;5(1):51–9.

36. Bamford C, Lamont S, Eccles M, Robinson L, May C, Bond J. Disclosing a diagnosis of dementia: a systematic review. Int J Geriatr Psychiatry. 2004;19(2):151–69.

37. Pratt R, Wilkinson H. A psychosocial model of understanding the experience of receiving a diagnosis of dementia. Dementia. 2003;2(2):181–99.

38. Livingston G, Sommerlad A, Orgeta V, Costafreda SG, Huntley J, Ames D, et al. Dementia prevention, intervention, and care. Lancet. 2017;390(10113):2673–734.

39. Browne J, Edwards DA, Rhodes KM, Brimicombe DJ, Payne RA. Association of comorbidity and health service usage among patients with dementia in the UK: a population-based study. BMJ Open. 2017;7:e012546. https://doi.org/10.1136/bmjopen-2016-012546.

40. Koroukian SM, Schiltz NK, Warner DF, Stange KC, Smyth KA. Increasing burden of complex multimorbidity across gradients of cognitive impairment. Am J Alzheimers Dis Other Demen. 2017;32(7):408–17.

41. Lee PG, Cigolle C, Blaum C. The co-occurrence of chronic diseases and geriatric syndromes: the health and retirement study. J Am Geriatr Soc. 2009;57(3):511–6.

42. Sinnige J, Korevaar JC, Westert GP, Spreeuwenberg P, Schellevis FG, Braspenning JC. Multimorbidity patterns in a primary care population aged 55 years and over. Fam Pract. 2015;32(5):505–13.

43. Kojima G, Liljas A, Iliffe S, Walters K. Prevalence of frailty in mild to moderate Alzheimer's Disease: a systematic review and meta-analysis. Curr Alzheimer Res. 2017;14(12):1256–63.

44. Ferreira AR, Dias CC, Fernandes L. Needs in nursing homes and their relation with cognitive and functional decline, behavioral and psychological symptoms. Front Aging Neurosci. 2016;8:72.

45. Gaugler JE, Kane RL, Kane RA, Newcomer R. Unmet care needs and key outcomes in dementia. J Am Geriatr Soc. 2005;53(12):2098–105.

46. Miranda-Castillo C, Woods B, Galboda K, Oomman S, Olojugba C, Orrell M. Unmet needs, quality of life and support networks of people with dementia living at home. Health Qual Life Outcomes. 2010;8:132.

47. Miranda-Castillo C, Woods B, Orrell M. The needs of people with dementia living at home from user, caregiver and professional perspectives: a cross-sectional survey. BMC Health Serv Res. 2013;13(1):43.

48. Slade M, Leese M, Cahill S, Thornicroft G, Kuipers E. Patient-rated mental health needs and quality of life improvement. Br J Psychiatry. 2005;187(3):256.

49. Orrell M, Hancock GA. CANE: Camberwell assessment of need for the elderly. London: Gaskell; 2004.

50. Reynolds T, Thornicroft G, Abas M, Woods B, Hoe J, Leese M, et al. Camberwell Assessment of Need for the Elderly (CANE). Development, validity and reliability. Br J Psychiatry. 2000;176:444–52.

51. Kerpershoek L, de Vugt M, Wolfs C, Woods B, Jelley H, Orrell M, et al. Needs and quality of life of people with middle-stage dementia and their family carers from the European Actifcare study. When informal care alone may not suffice. Aging Ment Health. 2018;22(7):897–902.

52. Khanassov V, Vedel I. Family physician-case manager collaboration and needs of patients with dementia and their caregivers: a systematic mixed studies review. Ann Fam Med. 2016;14(2):166–77.

53. Baldwin S. Social care and its place in primary care. In: Jones R, Britten N, Culpepper L, Gass D, Grol R, Mant D, et al., editors. Oxford textbook of primary care, vol. I. Italy: Oxford University Press; 2005.

54. Manthorpe J, Iliffe S. The dialectics of dementia. London: King's College; 2016. https://www.kcl.ac.uk/sspp/policy-institute/publications/The-dialectics-of-dementia.pdf.

55. Ferri C, Sousa R, Albanese E, Ribeiro W, Honyashiki M. World Alzheimer report 2009. London: Alzheimer's Disease International; 2009.

56. Liu S, Li C, Shi Z, Wang X, Zhou Y, Liu S, et al. Caregiver burden and prevalence of depression, anxiety and sleep disturbances in Alzheimer's disease caregivers in China. J Clin Nurs. 2017;26(9-10):1291–300.

57. Schoenmakers B, Buntinx F, Delepeleire J. What is the role of the general practitioner towards the family caregiver of a community-dwelling demented relative? A systematic literature review. Scand J Prim Health Care. 2009;27(1):31–40.

58. Fortinsky RH. Health care triads and dementia care: integrative framework and future directions. Aging Ment Health. 2001;5(Suppl 1):S35–48.

59. Brodaty H, Burns K. Role of family caregivers. In: Draper B, Brodaty H, Finkel S, editors. The IPA complete guides to behavioral and psychological symptoms of dementia. Milwaukee: IPA; 2015. p. 4.1–4.30.

60. Prince M, Wimo A, Guerchet M, Gemma-Claire Ali M, Wu Y-T, Prina M. World Alzheimer Report 2015: the global impact of dementia - an analysis of prevalence, incidence, cost and trends. London: Alzheimer's Disease International; 2015.

61. Cuijpers P. Depressive disorders in caregivers of dementia patients: a systematic review. Aging Ment Health. 2005;9(4):325–30.

62. Sallim AB, Sayampanathan AA, Cuttilan A, Chun-Man HR. Prevalence of mental health disorders among caregivers of patients with Alzheimer Disease. JAMDA. 2015;16:1034–41. https://doi.org/10.1016/j.jamda.2015.09.007.

63. Livingston G, Barber J, Rapaport P, Knapp M, Griffin M, King D, et al. Clinical effectiveness of a manual based coping strategy programme (START, STrAtegies for RelaTives) in promoting the mental health of carers of family members with dementia: pragmatic randomised controlled trial. BMJ. 2013;347:f6276.

64. Schulz R, Martire LM. Family caregiving of persons with dementia: prevalence, health effects, and support strategies. Am J Geriatr Psychiatry. 2004;12:240–9.

65. Gonçalves-Pereira M, Marques M, Grácio J. Family issues in behavioral and psychological symptoms of dementia: unraveling circular pathways? In: Verdelho A, Gonçalves-Pereira M, editors. Neuropsychiatric symptoms in cognitive impairment and dementia. Berlin: Springer; 2017. p. 331–48.

66. Kales HC, Gitlin LN, Lyketsos CG. Assessment and management of behavioral and psychological symptoms of dementia. BMJ. 2015;350:h369.

67. NICE. Dementia: supporting people with dementia and their carers in health and social care | guidance and guidelines. London: NICE; 2006. https://www.nice.org.uk/guidance/cg42/.

68. Gonçalves-Pereira M. Toward a family-sensitive practice in dementia. In: Verdelho A, Gonçalves-Pereira M, editors. Neuropsychiatric symptoms of cognitive impairment and dementia. Berlin: Springer; 2017. p. 349–68.

69. Bodenheimer T, Ghorob A, Willard-Grace R, Grumbach K. The 10 building blocks of high-performing primary care. Ann Fam Med. 2014;12(2):166–71.

70. WHO. Primary care evaluation tool. Europe: WHO; 2010. http://www.euro.who.int/__data/assets/pdf_file/0004/107851/PrimaryCareEvalTool.pdf.

71. Spenceley SM, Sedgwick N, Keenan J. Dementia care in the context of primary care reform: an integrative review. Aging Ment Health. 2015;19(2):107–20.

72. Morgan DG, Kosteniuk JG, Stewart NJ, O'Connell ME, Kirk A, Crossley M, et al. Availability and primary health care orientation of dementia-related services in rural Saskatchewan, Canada. Home Health Care Serv Q. 2015;34(3-4):137–58.

73. Bohlken J, Schulz M, Rapp MA, Bätzing-Feigenbaum J. Pharmacotherapy of dementia in Germany: results from a nationwide claims database. Eur Neuropsychopharmacol. 2015;25(12):2333–8.

74. Downs M, Ariss SMB, Grant E, Keady J, Turner S, Bryans M, et al. Family carers' accounts of general practice contacts for their relatives with early signs of dementia. Dementia. 2016;5(3):353–73.

75. De Cola MC, Lo Buono V, Mento A, Foti M, Marino S, Bramanti P, et al. Unmet needs for family caregivers of elderly people with dementia living in Italy: what do we know so far and what should we do next? Inquiry. 2017;54:46958017713708. https://doi.org/10.1177/0046958017713708.

76. Dello Buono M, Busato R, Mazzetto M, Paccagnella B, Aleotti F, Zanetti O, et al. Community care for patients with Alzheimer's disease and non-demented elderly people: use and satisfaction with services and unmet needs in family caregivers. Int J Geriat Psychiatry. 1999;14(11):915–24.

77. Franz CE, Barker JC, Kim K, Flores Y, Jenkins C, Kravitz RL, et al. When help becomes a hindrance: mental health referral systems as barriers to care for primary care physicians treating patients with Alzheimer's disease. Am J Geriatr Psychiatry. 2010;18(7):576–85.

78. Hinton L, Franz CE, Reddy G, Flores Y, Kravitz RL, Barker JC. Practice constraints, behavioral problems, and dementia care: primary care physicians' perspectives. J Gen Intern Med. 2007;22(11):1487–92.

79. Stewart TV, Loskutova N, Galliher JM, Warshaw GA, Coombs LJ, Staton EW, et al. Practice patterns, beliefs, and perceived barriers to care regarding dementia: a report from the American Academy of Family Physicians (AAFP) national research network. J Am Board Fam Med. 2014;27(2):275–83.

80. Manthorpe J, Iliffe S, Eden A. Testing Twigg and Atkin's typology of caring: a study of primary care professionals' perceptions of dementia care using a modified focus group method. Health Soc Care Community. 2003;11(6):477–85.

81. Callahan CM, Boustani MA, Unverzagt FW, Austrom MG, Damush TM, Perkins AJ, et al. Effectiveness of collaborative care for older adults with Alzheimer disease in primary care: a randomized controlled trial. JAMA. 2006;295(18):2148–57.

82. Fortinsky RH, Kulldorff M, Kleppinger A, Kenyon-Pesce L. Dementia care consultation for family caregivers: collaborative model linking an Alzheimer's association chapter with primary care physicians. Aging Ment Health. 2009;13(2):162–70.

83. Jennings LA, Tan Z, Wenger NS, Cook EA, Han W, McCreath HE, et al. Quality of care provided by a comprehensive dementia care comanagement program. J Am Geriatr Soc. 2016;64(8):1724–30.

84. Reuben DB, Roth CP, Frank JC, Hirsch SH, Katz D, McCreath H, et al. Assessing care of vulnerable elders – Alzheimer's disease: a pilot study of a practice redesign intervention to improve the quality of dementia care. J Am Geriatr Soc. 2010;58(2):324–9.

85. Thyrian JR, Hertel J, Wucherer D, Eichler T, Michalowsky B, Dreier-Wolfgramm A, et al. Effectiveness and safety of dementia care management in primary care: a randomized clinical trial. JAMA Psychiat. 2017;74(10):996–1004.

86. Vickrey BG, Mittman BS, Connor KI, Pearson ML, Della Penna RD, Ganiats TG, et al. The effect of a disease management intervention on quality and outcomes of dementia care: a randomized, controlled trial. Ann Intern Med. 2006;145(10):713–26.

87. Eichler T, Thyrian JR, Fredrich D, Köhler L, Wucherer D, Michalowsky B, et al. The benefits of implementing a computerized Intervention-Management-System (IMS) on delivering integrated dementia care in the primary care setting. Int Psychogeriatr. 2014;26(8):1377–85.

88. Iliffe S, Robinson L, Brayne C, Goodman C, Rait G, Manthorpe J, et al. Primary care and dementia: 1. diagnosis, screening and disclosure. Int J Geriatr Psychiatry. 2009;24(9):895–901.

89. Pimlott NJG, Persaud M, Drummond N, Cohen CA, Silvius JL, Seigel K, et al. Family physicians and dementia in Canada: part 2. Understanding the challenges of dementia care. Can Fam Physician. 2009;55(5):508–9.e7.

90. Khanassov V, Vedel I, Pluye P. Barriers to implementation of case management for patients with dementia: a systematic mixed studies review. Ann Fam Med. 2014;12(5):456–65.

91. Iliffe S. Commissioning services for people with dement how to get it right. Psychiatrist. 2013;37(4):121–3.

92. Köhler L, Meinke-Franze C, Hein J, Fendrich K, Heymann R, Thyrian JR, et al. Does an interdisciplinary network improve dementia care? Results from the IDemUck-Study. Curr Alzheimer Res. 2014;11(6):538–48.

93. Boeckxstaens P, De Graaf P. Primary care and care for older persons: position paper of the European Forum for Primary Care. Qual Prim Care. 2011;19:369–89.

94. Blaxter M. How is health embodied and experienced? Health. 2nd ed. Cambridge: Polity Press; 2010. p. 54–5.

95. Moynihan R. Medicalization. A new deal on disease definition. BMJ. 2011;342:d2548.

96. Scully JL. What is a disease? EMBO Rep. 2004;5(7):650–3. https://doi.org/10.1038/sj.embor.7400195.

97. Peel E. 'The living death of Alzheimer's' versus 'Take a walk to keep dementia at bay': representations of dementia in print media and carer discourse. Sociol Health Illn. 2014;36(6):558–901. https://doi.org/10.1111/1467-9566.12122.

98. Gonçalves-Pereira M, Cardoso A, Verdelho A, Alves da Silva J, Caldas de Almeida M, Fernandes A, et al.

The prevalence of dementia in a Portuguese community sample: a 10/66 Dementia Research Group study. BMC Geriatr. 2017;17:261.

99. Barros PP, Machado SR, Simões JA. Portugal - health system review. Health Syst Transit. 2011;13(4):1–156.

100. Balsinha C, Marques MJ, Goncalves-Pereira M. A brief assessment unravels unmet needs of older people in primary care: a mixed-methods evaluation of the SPICE tool in Portugal. Prim Health Care Res Dev. 2018;19(6):637–43.

101. Directorate-General-of-Health. Programa Nacional para a Saúde Mental. Lisboa, Portugal: Directorate General of Health; 2017.

102. Gonçalves-Pereira M, Leuschner A. Portugal. In: Burns A, Robert PE, editors. Dementia care: inter-national perspectives. Oxford: Oxford University Press; 2018.

103. Meyer G, Bieber A, Broda A, Stephan A, Verbeek H, Actifcare-Consortium. Structural aspects of access to formal dementia care services across the European countries. [Deliverable D2.1 - The EU-JPND Actifcare Project]. 2014.

104. Spector A, Orrell M. Using a biopsychosocial model of dementia as a tool to guide clinical practice. Int Psychogeriatr. 2010;22(6):957–65.

105. Bases para a Definição de Politícas Públicas na Área das Demências [Internet]. Serviço Nacional de Saúde. 2017. Available from: https://www.sns.gov.pt/2017/08/10/bases-para-a-definicao-de-politicas-publicas-na-area-das-demencias/. Accessed 05 Mar 2018.

Agitation

24

Anne P. F. Wand and Brian Draper

Abstract

Agitation, a term that includes behaviour such as excessive motor activity, verbal and physical aggression, is common in people with dementia. The assessment and management of agitation in older people can be challenging in primary care. Agitation may be the initial presentation of an early dementia, with a differential diagnosis that includes delirium, agitated depression, late life psychoses and anxiety disorders. In persons with established dementia, factors that contribute to agitation include acute medical problems, physical discomfort, communication difficulties, misinterpretations, carer and environmental problems and psychiatric comorbidity. Prevention of agitation by appropriate training of carers to provide person-centred care and by adapting the physical environment to meet the needs of people with dementia is paramount. Interventions to manage agitation should focus on non-pharmacological strategies first including addressing physical needs (e.g. pain relief), providing individualized psychosocial activities (e.g. physical exercise, music therapy, aromatherapy) in a regular structured program, educating and supporting the carers and optimizing the environment. In general, pharmacotherapy with psychotropic medication should be reserved for the more severe forms of agitation not responding to non-pharmacological interventions or when safety is seriously compromised and initially be used in trials of up to three months duration.

Key Points

- Agitation in older adults is not normal ageing.
- Agitation can occur in a range of mental disorders including dementia, delirium, depression, anxiety and psychoses.
- Agitation in dementia is often multifactorial in aetiology including neurobiological substrates, premorbid personality, psychological reactions and social interactions with carers and the environment.
- Assessment of agitation needs to focus on establishing the likely causal factor(s) in each individual case.
- Acute agitation is usually due to a medical condition.
- Interventions for agitation should initially be non-pharmacological, based on identified causal factors and include strategies to minimise carer stress.
- Apart from emergencies, psychopharmacotherapy of agitation should usually

A. P. F. Wand · B. Draper (✉)
School of Psychiatry, University of New South Wales, Sydney, Australia
e-mail: b.draper@unsw.edu.au

© Springer Nature Switzerland AG 2019
C. A. de Mendonça Lima, G. Ivbijaro (eds.), *Primary Care Mental Health in Older People*,
https://doi.org/10.1007/978-3-030-10814-4_24

only be considered after an adequate trial of psychosocial interventions.

- Adoption of person-centred care practices, staff and carer training and appropriate environmental design in facilities might prevent agitation.

Case Vignette

A couple in their late 70s visited their family doctor, and the wife reported that her husband had recently become increasingly agitated: 'doctor: please do something'.

As a primary care physician, how would I handle this?

24.1 Introduction

The term 'agitation' is used in this chapter to describe behaviour associated with dementia and other cognitive disorders. In this context, agitation has been provisionally defined by an 'Agitation Definition Working Group' of the International Psychogeriatric Association as behaviour that is consistent with emotional distress and is a change from the person's normal behaviour. It includes excessive motor activity, verbal or physical aggression and causes excess disability and is not solely attributable to another primary mental disorder such as depression, psychosis or stress disorder or due to a medical disorder causing delirium [1]. Indeed, these exclusions form important differential diagnoses that are addressed later in the chapter.

There are many other terms used in the literature instead of agitation, and these include 'behavioural and psychological symptoms of dementia (BPSD)', 'neuropsychiatric symptoms', 'challenging behaviour', 'behavioural problems' and 'behavioural disturbances'. There are concerns that some of these terms are pejorative and stigmatizing; hence they are now less frequently used.

Agitation featured in historical descriptions of the dementia syndrome. When Alois Alzheimer described his patient Auguste Deter in 1907,

symptoms of psychosis and vocal disruption were present in addition to cognitive impairment. Despite this, for many years the focus of clinical dementia research was on the cognitive features, and it was only in the 1980s that an increase in research into the non-cognitive symptoms occurred [2].

Agitation in people with dementia and other cognitive disorders is often very challenging for family carers, as well as for nurses and other care providers in hospital and long-term institutional settings. Family carers can become very distressed in their efforts to cope with agitation, and for many it can be a major factor that contributes to placement decisions. Primary care physicians have the opportunity to intervene in managing the behaviour as well as to provide support for distressed carers.

This chapter will provide an overview of agitation from a primary care perspective including the epidemiology, relationship to the ageing process, aetiological factors, behavioural types, assessment and management issues. It will provide guidance on working with specialist and multidisciplinary teams involved with dementia care.

24.2 Epidemiology

Agitation is common in people with dementia. The types of behaviour covered by this term are listed in Table 24.1. In the community-based Cache County Study, there was 97% five-year prevalence of any type of behaviour as measured by the Neuropsychiatric Inventory (NPI) in people with dementia [3]. In population-based studies the prevalence of the NPI domain behaviours that are captured within the agitation definition includes agitation/aggression 20–35%, disinhibition 8–17%, irritability 20–31% and aberrant motor behaviour (commonly described as 'wandering') 10–32% [4]. Of course, in clinic populations the prevalence is higher with agitation/aggression 29–60%, disinhibition 10–36%, irritability 25–66% and aberrant motor behaviour 22–47% [4]. Many types of behaviour persist, for example, aberrant motor behaviour persisted for

Table 24.1 Types of agitated behaviour

These behaviours should be associated with emotional distress, e.g. irritability, emotional lability, mood changes, outbursts
Excessive motor activity
Pacing
Rocking
Restlessness
Gesturing
Pointing fingers
Repetitious mannerisms
Verbal aggression
Yelling
Speaking in very loud voice
Using profanity
Screaming
Shouting
Physical aggression
Grabbing
Shoving
Pushing
Resisting
Hitting others
Kicking objects or people
Scratching
Biting
Throwing objects
Hitting, cutting or otherwise physically injuring self
Slamming doors
Tearing things
Destroying property

Adapted from Ref. [1]

18 months in 56% of participants in the Cache County Study [5].

In individuals with mild cognitive disorders, the prevalence of agitation is higher than in the normal population but much lower than in people with dementia [6]. The presence of agitation in mild cognitive disorders is associated with an increased risk of subsequent cognitive decline and conversion to dementia [7, 8]. In general, the prevalence of agitation increases with severity of cognitive impairment and dementia [2]. This is one of the factors that contribute to agitation being common in long-term residential care, with the point prevalence ranging from 69 to 92% in studies from Australia, Norway, the Netherlands and the United States [2]. Other prominent factors in long-term care include the physical envi-ronment, with too few facilities designed appropriately for the care of people with demen-tia, and care practices, where too few organiza-tions ensure their staff follow the principles of person-centred care [9]. There are likely to be cultural factors that impact upon the prevalence of agitation in dementia. For example, there is a large difference in the prevalence of agitation/aggression in studies from the United Kingdom (9%), Brazil (20%), Spain (28%), the United States (30%), Japan (35%) and Korea (41%) [10]. Gender issues are prominent in specific types of behaviour, with aggression being more prevalent in males and verbal agitation more prevalent in females [2].

There has been a paucity of research that has explored the relative prevalence of agitation in different types of dementia [11]. However, early behavioural disinhibition is a diagnostic criterion for frontotemporal dementia, which is distin-guished from other types of dementia in most studies by the presence of disinhibition, apathy and aberrant motor behaviour. Comparisons of vascular dementia and Alzheimer's disease have had inconsistent findings [11].

24.3 Nature of Agitation Using a Life Course Approach

24.3.1 How It Differs from the Normal Ageing Process

Agitation is not part of the normal ageing pro-cess. However, across the life cycle, some people are more prone to become agitated when under life stress, often related to their personality, past life experiences, post-traumatic stress disorder (PTSD) or chronic anxiety disorders. This will tend to persist into late life, and the primary care physician will be aware that certain patients will be prone to become agitated when stressed.

The observation that an older adult is becom-ing agitated in situations that would not have resulted in such behaviour previously should alert the primary care physician to review the patient. Agitation that appears in late life for the first time is usually associated with a psychiatric disorder (such as major depression, late life psychosis) or a cognitive disorder (such as delirium or dementia). Acute change over a few days, even in a person with dementia, suggests the possibility of delirium, particularly if accompanied by fluctuating level of attention, increased confusion and symptoms of an acute medical condition. In the early stages of mild cognitive disorders and dementia, neuroticism increases, and this may have accompanying agitated behaviour [12]. The assessment of the differential diagnosis of agitation is covered in more detail later.

Agitation in people with dementia tends to occur later in the course of the disorder when cognitive and functional decline has already become quite noticeable. However, agitated behaviour will accentuate the impairment through its effects on concentration, attention and memory. Sometimes the older adult can barely keep still long enough to focus on the task at hand. Psychosocial function tends to decline with the older adult feeling restless, less adept in social and interpersonal situations and less able to self-care. With mild agitation the effects are less pronounced, and it may be unclear whether impairment is due to the behaviour change itself or just from the underlying dementia.

There is potential to improve cognition and function by reducing agitation; hence it is imperative to identify the underlying cause(s) promptly so that effective interventions can be introduced. The aetiology of agitation is multifactorial and often involving an interaction of neurobiological substrates (such as genetic polymorphisms, neurotransmitter changes, neuropathology, medical comorbidity), premorbid personality, psychological reactions and social aspects including carer and environmental issues [13].

24.3.2 Aetiological Factors

Aetiological factors can vary with the different types of agitation. For example, physical aggression, which is more common in males, is often associated with other frontal symptoms such as disinhibition and may be a reflection of executive dysfunction. Other factors commonly associated with aggression include medical comorbidities, history of head injury, premorbid personality, alcohol/substance misuse and discomforts related to pain. Carer intrusion into physical space might provoke an aggressive response if the person with dementia perceives it as a threat or if they feel embarrassed. Neurobiological substrates of aggression in Alzheimer's disease are multiple and complex. Genetic factors include polymorphic variations in serotonergic and dopaminergic genes. Dopaminergic, cholinergic, serotonergic and noradrenergic neurotransmitter changes have been reported in the brain [13].

A second example, vocally disruptive agitated behaviour, is more common in females and may be secondary to pain, physical discomfort (e.g., constipation, thirst, overheating), depression, boredom, loneliness and other health issues. Neurotic features in the premorbid personality are not uncommon. These behaviours are often best interpreted as a form of communication of distress [13].

Three explanatory models of how carer interactions and the environment might contribute to agitation in dementia provide some insights into potential management strategies. People with dementia have a lower threshold to coping with stress. The 'stress threshold' model hypothesizes that agitation occurs when this threshold is exceeded. Hence strategies that optimize exposure to potential stressors (such as noise, large groups, physical discomforts, etc.), which are likely to vary with the individual, may reduce agitation [13].

In learning theory, the likelihood of a behaviour occurring is increased if it is reinforced by the provision of rewards. For a bored and lonely person with severe dementia, the realization that a staff member will provide attention to them (the 'reward') if they call out can reinforce the behaviour. The 'learning theory model' emphasizes the importance of inadvertent reinforcement of inappropriate behaviours. By providing quality time with the person when they are quiet, it is hypothesized that over time, they will learn that they will have the pleasurable experience of being with the carer at those times rather than when they call out [13].

The 'unmet needs model' recognizes that people with more severe dementia cannot always communicate their needs through comprehensible language [13]. Behaviour is a form of communication, and in much the way that mothers learn the meanings of their baby's different cries and behaviours, the challenge is for carers to learn what unmet needs are represented by different behaviours in the person with severe dementia. For some individuals, restlessness might be a sign of tiredness; in others it might indicate a toileting need or be an indication of boredom. Similarly, verbal abuse and irritability might suggest that the person is hungry, but physical aggression might only occur if they are in pain.

The models are not mutually exclusive. Each model offers insights into behaviour that might operate simultaneously, for example, behaviour might be a communication of unmet need that has been inappropriately reinforced by the way in which a carer responds. The individual circumstances of the person with dementia perhaps indicate which factors might be more relevant in their situation.

An approach to assess the possible cause(s) of agitation in the primary care setting is provided in Table 24.2.

24.3.3 Implication for the Individual's Autonomy, Independence and Human Rights

Moderate to severe agitated behaviour in a person with dementia can be difficult for family carers to manage at home. Acute agitation may require short-term hospitalization to control the behaviour and treat the underlying cause(s), while persistent chronic agitation often results in the need for placement into a residential care facility as carers become burnt-out with stress. In either circumstance, the behaviour can be so severe and the capacity of the person with dementia so impaired that it requires involuntary detention under a mental health or guardianship framework depending on the circumstances and jurisdiction.

Unfortunately many hospital and long-term residential care settings are less than ideal in their design and staff capacity to manage agitated behaviour. Worldwide there is overprescription of antipsychotic drugs to control behaviour, and these are associated with increased risk of morbidity and mortality [9]. Frequently they have been prescribed without appropriate consent [14]. Physical restraints are still used, usually

Table 24.2 Six steps for determining the aetiology of agitation in dementia

Step 1	Is the behaviour new?	Any new behaviour that develops over a few days is due to an acute medical problem until proven otherwise
Step 2	Is the person in pain or discomfort, e.g. constipation, cramps?	Most people get irritable if in pain or discomfort from a chronic disability
Step 3	Is the behaviour due to misidentification, misinterpretation or disorientation?	Behaviour often reflects the underlying cognitive changes from the dementia
Step 4	Does the behaviour represents a particular distress or is the person unable to otherwise verbally express their needs?	Behaviour is a form of communication in the person with dementia and may be a way of drawing attention to unmet need
Step 5	Would *you* be happy to live in this physical and care environment?	If you have reservations about the quality of the environment, then it is likely that the person with dementia does too, and the behaviour may represent a reaction to it
Step 6	Does the person with dementia have a comorbid mood disorder or primary psychiatric disorder such as schizophrenia?	Agitation may be due to a comorbid psychiatric disorder such as severe depression, psychosis or anxiety

inappropriately, to control behaviour in some facilities despite the lack of evidence of efficacy and the undoubted ill effects on the individual. Most agitated behaviour can be adequately managed by non-pharmacological strategies provided adequately trained staff adopt a person-centred approach to care, use a range of pleasurable diversional activities and are supported by management [15].

Our anecdotal observation of good quality special care dementia units, which specialize in the management of people with the most severe forms of agitation, indicates that the residents usually appear to be, superficially at least, happy older adults behaving normally. Their human rights are being respected by the way in which the trained staff and the environment strive to meet their needs. In contrast, facilities in which residents are frequently agitated and distressed are likely to have a systemic problem hindering the provision of the type of care required to address their long-term needs.

24.4 Management of Agitation Using a Stepped Care Framework

24.4.1 Diagnostic Criteria Including Assessment Tools

The term agitation is a phenomenological description and not a diagnosis in itself. It may be present in a wide range of medical and psychiatric conditions, necessitating consideration of a broad differential diagnosis. The main diagnostic clusters are cognitive disorders, psychiatric illness, organic illness and substance misuse. With each diagnostic possibility, a detailed history, including corroborative history, focused physical examination, screening tool and/or indicated investigations, is important (see Table 24.3).

Delirium must be excluded first when there is an acute change in cognition, behaviour or mental state in someone with dementia or indeed any older adult. It is characterized by fluctuation in level of consciousness and cognition and inattention. Motor subtypes of delirium have been

Table 24.3 Key investigations for agitation

Physical examination	Sensory impairment, pain, temperature, hypotension, hypoxia, dentition
Delirium	Urinalysis, electrolytes (including glucose, calcium, magnesium, phosphate), liver function tests, full blood count, B12, folate, thyroid function tests, C-reactive protein
Dementia	Cognitive testing (mini-mental status examination, General Practitioner Assessment of Cognition, clock-draw test)
Psychiatric illness	Rating scales: Geriatric Depression Scale, Cornell Scale for Depression in Dementia, Beck Depression Inventory, Depression Anxiety Stress Scale Exclude organic illness: as per delirium investigations, electroencephalogram, syphilis and viral serology and cerebral imaging
Substance misuse	Physical examination for signs of intoxication or withdrawal, urine drug screen

described, namely, hyperactive (which may present with an excess of movement and speech and lack of sleep), hypoactive (where the person appears sleepy, withdrawn and there is a paucity of movement and speech) and the 'mixed' subtype [16]. Screening tools may assist in detecting delirium. Two brief screening tools suitable for primary care are the Confusion Assessment Method (CAM) and the 4A's test [17, 18]. The former requires some training and essentially operationalises the DSM III-R criteria for delirium. The 4A's test does not require any operator training, or require physical responses from the patient and may be used for someone with severe agitation or drowsiness. Any medical condition, surgery and numerous medications may precipitate a delirium, so thorough history (including medication review particularly focused on anticholinergic drugs, opiates and benzodiazepines) and physical examination are required. Screening investigations (such as urinalysis, blood tests of electrolytes, liver function and blood count) and specific tests (such as an electrocardiograph, chest X-ray or cerebral imaging) as indicated by the patient's comorbidities may further elucidate the underlying cause(s).

Various psychiatric illnesses may present with agitation, mood or behavioural changes. Grief may also be associated with confusion, guilt and anxiety [19]. Mood disorders to consider include agitated or psychotic depression, mania and anxiety disorders. Agitated depression is a form of melancholic major depression with features including pervasive low mood (often with diurnal variation), anhedonia, anxiety or irritability, changes in sleep, energy, concentration, appetite and weight, psychomotor signs and depressive cognitions such as helplessness, hopelessness, worthlessness and suicidal ideation. Psychotic depression may include (usually) mood-congruent delusions (of poverty, guilt and nihilism), hallucinations and thought disorder and may be associated with behavioural and functional change. Screening tools for depression include the Geriatric Depression Scale for people with only mild cognitive impairment and the Cornell Scale for Depression in Dementia, rated separately by a clinician and a carer [20, 21]. The Beck Depression Inventory is useful in people with major medical conditions such as post-stroke, as it relies less on somatic or memory symptoms [22]. Agitated depression might also be due to organic illnesses (e.g. cerebral tumours, anaemia, hypothyroidism) or medications. Mania may occur in a person with bipolar disorder or de novo secondary to certain medications (e.g. high-dose steroids) or physical illness. Common features are elevated, angry or irritable mood, lack of need for sleep, excessive energy and activity, grandiosity, pressured speech and thought disorder and behaviour which is disinhibited, impulsive or risky.

Anxiety disorders are common and may be associated with agitation, both physical and psychological. Anxiety is a common presentation of depression in older adults but may also be due to an underlying anxiety disorder (such as panic disorder, agoraphobia and generalized anxiety disorder), medical conditions (such as chronic obstructive pulmonary disease or thyroid disorders) and substance abuse (see later). Fear of falling is also common in older adults, who may become agitated and fearful when needing to mobilize. In making a diagnosis, it is important to determine the duration of symptoms and temporal relationship with other illnesses, the focus of anxiety (to classify the type of anxiety disorder), associated functional impairment (such as avoidance or constraints on activities of daily living) and contributory physical factors (e.g. hypoxia) and to review their medication. The Depression, Anxiety and Stress Scale (DASS-21) is a simple self-rated tool which may be used to screen for depression, anxiety and stress and is valid in people with comorbid physical illness [23].

Psychotic disorders such as schizophrenia or delusional disorder may also cause agitation and may be longstanding or have an onset in late life. Key features include delusions, hallucinations, disordered thoughts and disturbed behaviours, which have developed over several months.

Organic illnesses may also cause agitation, for example, secondary to physical symptoms such as pain, hypoxia and dyspnoea, or due to the underlying cause, for example, epilepsy (associated with psychosis), neurosyphilis, neuroendocrine and other carcinomas. Poor dental and general hygiene, sensory impairment (vision, hearing) and malnutrition may also cause agitation. Psychiatric illness secondary to medications for general medical conditions should also be considered, for example, steroid-induced mania, hormonal treatment of cancers (e.g. depression secondary to goserelin) or interferon-induced depression and anxiety. As the onset of psychiatric illness is most common in youth or early adulthood, patients who present with new onset of psychiatric symptoms in later life should be carefully investigated for an underlying organic illness. A systems review when taking the history and a physical examination should be conducted. Screening investigations should include a urinalysis, blood biochemistry (including electrolytes, glucose, calcium, magnesium and phosphate), liver function tests, full blood count, B12, folate, thyroid function and cerebral imaging. Additional tests may be guided by the history, for example, screening blood tests for autoimmune and vasculitic conditions (erythrocyte sedimentation rate, C-reactive protein, antinuclear antibody, antineutrophil cytoplasmic antibody), infectious diseases (e.g. syphilis and HIV serology, lumbar puncture) and malignancy (endoscopy, faecal occult blood, computerized tomography). An electroencephalogram may be reserved for complex cases, e.g. when a seizure disorder or atypical delirium is considered.

Substance intoxication or withdrawal can also present with agitation. People intoxicated with substances such as amphetamines, cocaine, caffeine and cannabis may be agitated. Agitation may also be a feature of withdrawal from benzodiazepines, nicotine, opiates and alcohol. A thorough substance use history should be particularly evaluated whether the person is dependent and the route of administration, amount and last time of use. Physical examination for specific signs of intoxication or withdrawal, a corroborative history from family or carers and a urine drug screen may assist with diagnosis. Prescribed medicine should also be reviewed, for example, sudden cessation of antidepressant medication may cause discontinuation symptoms such as irritability, agitation, restlessness, anxiety and sleep disturbance [24], which may be mistaken for anxiety or relapse of depression [25].

24.4.2 Specific Issues for Primary Care Assessment

Longer consultations or a series of appointments may be required to enable adequate time for assessment of agitation and other BPSD. Although evaluation for the common differential diagnoses of agitation is important, the component causes of the behaviour may be complex and multiple. Therefore, understanding the person, interactional factors and environment are important—why this person, why this behaviour and why now? Individual factors include the person's cultural background, previous employment, personality traits, medical comorbidities and current physical concerns (e.g. thirst, hunger, constipation). Interactional factors may include whether communication is impaired secondary to dysarthria or difficulties using language with progression of dementia, changes to routines, activities not well matched to the person's interest or intellect, insufficient or excessive stimulation, and

encroachment upon personal space. Environmental considerations include poor lighting, insufficient visual prompts, lack of personal belongings, lack of privacy, visual distraction (e.g. patterns on flooring) and clutter [19].

Following assessment of agitation, the primary care clinician should inform the patient and their family/carer of the diagnosis made, options for management and prognosis. Informed consent should be obtained before treatment is commenced. Referral for specialist assessment may be indicated if, after comprehensive assessment, the diagnosis or cause of agitation is still uncertain; the presentation is unusual; the patient is young or atypical; there are multiple complex comorbidities, there is severe behavioural disturbance or psychosis; the person has learning difficulties or intellectual disability; or medication is being considered [26].

24.4.3 Health Promotion

According to the World Alzheimer Report, the prevalence of dementia internationally is expected to rise dramatically with the ageing of the population [27]. Accordingly, rates of BPSD, including agitation, which are almost universal in dementia and may occur throughout the disease process, are also expected to rise [2]. The association between agitation and adverse outcomes such as increased financial costs, carer stress (family and residential care staff), excess disability, premature institutionalisation and reduced quality of life for the person with dementia and their carers [2] makes this a priority for healthcare services in general and especially dementia care.

Health promotion in dementia applies across the spectrum from primary to tertiary prevention [28], with public health opportunities for agitation falling predominantly in the secondary and tertiary levels. Dementia is under-recognized and under-disclosed in the community [29]. A variety of reasons have been proposed to explain this fact including patient and carer factors (lack of knowledge about dementia, stigma, fear, denial, attribution to normal ageing), disease factors (slow progression), primary health care providers lack of knowledge or time to diagnose dementia and limited access to specialist confirmation of diagnosis, and systemic factors (e.g. no definitive diagnostic test or accurate biomarkers) [29]. Each of these factors represents an opportunity to intervene, particularly through educational interventions and public health campaigns.

People with dementia report significant delays in the diagnosis being made, with significant implications for exercising their autonomy and decision-making capacity and receiving timely support [30]. For example, most people identify memory loss as a symptom of dementia, but may not recognize BPSD symptoms such as agitation or apathy [31]. Conversely, memory loss may be viewed by families as a normal part of ageing, and so medical advice is not sought [31]. The impact on carers of undiagnosed dementia and agitation, in particular, is multifactorial and may include carer stress or mental illness and isolation, potential for abuse, misattribution of causes of agitation and premature placement of the person with dementia in care facilities [2]. To improve understanding about the early diagnosis of dementia, the Alzheimer's Association in the United States developed the "Know the 10 signs" campaign [32].

A recent report from the Alzheimer's Society, the United Kingdom, identified key areas of health promotion for people with dementia [30]. The areas included improving community awareness and understanding, the provision of information and support to people with dementia, ensuring that people with dementia are seen as active individuals who may have a good quality of life in the community and improving health and social care services and related research [30]. Stigma about dementia is a key public health issue. A World Health Organization dementia survey revealed that people with dementia may be hidden or isolated due to shame or the potential for agitation and other BPSD to be observed by others [31]. Improved health literacy regarding dementia and agitation may help reduce stigma through greater public awareness [31]. For people with dementia, this might result in more opportunities to socialize and engage in community activities, greater tolerance and patience from others and improved community spirit [30].

In general hospital settings, dementia and agitation are also under-recognized [33]. Hospital inpatients with dementia have longer lengths of stay and greater care costs [33]. The environment can be overstimulating, unfamiliar and distressing to the person with dementia, resulting in or exacerbating challenging behaviours [33]. Difficulties communicating and engaging in care may contribute to the adverse outcomes [34]. People with dementia are at greater risk of delirium, which in itself is often not detected, may be untreated and is associated with high morbidity and mortality [35]. Initiatives to improve the care of people with dementia in hospital include strategies to reduce admissions (e.g. hospital in the home, healthcare services delivered in residential aged care settings), rapid specialist assessments in the emergency department and general hospital liaison services, appropriate 'dementia-friendly' environments and better discharge planning and integration of care [33].

24.4.4 Self-Care

A number of strategies have been suggested to promote self-care in people with dementia. Research evidence indicates that cardiovascular disease predisposes to both Alzheimer's and vascular dementia [31]. Longitudinal population-based studies suggest the potential for risk reduction through regular exercise, more education and addressing cardiovascular risk factors (e.g. through healthy diet, smoking cessation, tight control of diabetes and hypertension and reducing obesity) [36]. Some of these general lifestyle interventions may be important in slowing progression of dementia, particularly exercise and preventing vascular events [36]. The primary care clinician is also well placed to conduct general health screening and preventative medicine (e.g. blood pressure, skin checks, weight).

Meaningful activities in line with the person's ability and interests provide an outlet for expression and stimulation and optimizing quality of life in people with dementia [31]. Having a daily routine for the person with dementia can also provide structure and reduce anxiety. The benefits of participating in creative arts, although modest, include improving self-esteem and social interaction [37]. Access to social networks and peer support are also important [30].

The functional decline which occurs in people with dementia may be addressed through carers and services providing support with activities of daily living and home modifications for people living in the community. This may enable the person to stay in their own residence longer and improve their quality of life [30]. Information should also be provided about respite (in home or a residential aged care facility), local services and facilities [30].

It is important for the person with dementia to plan ahead for the time when decision-making capacity may be impaired. Primary care clinicians may assist this process and enhance patient autonomy by discussing issues such as driving, options for care (medical, services and accommodation) as dementia progresses, decision-making (e.g. appointment of an Enduring Guardian and Enduring Power of Attorney) and financial issues (creation of a will) early and in an ongoing way [38]. Conversations about advanced care planning may also be initiated by the primary carer clinician and should detail the person's values, wishes and preferences for end of life or emergency care in the event that they cannot make a choice [26].

24.4.5 Biopsychosocial Interventions

The causes of agitation and other BPSD are varied and often multiple, necessitating multimodal interventions which take into account biological, social, psychological, environmental, cultural and interpersonal factors. The key psychosocial interventions for agitation are outlined in Table 24.4. As it may be difficult for the person with dementia to communicate their needs, a holistic and broad approach is needed. General principles of assessment include clearly describing the behaviour or symptom and deciding whether intervention is

Table 24.4 Psychosocial interventions for agitation

Physical	– Correct sensory impairment – Address physical needs, e.g. thirst, hunger, temperature, physical inactivity, bowel movements – Treat underlying physical illnesses and delirium
Environmental	– Appropriate lighting and visual contrast – Use interpreters when required
Behavioural	– Structured routine – Aromatherapy – Individualized music – Daily physical exercise – One-to-one clinical contact – Pet therapy – Snoezelen rooms – Sleep hygiene strategies
Psychological	– Psychoeducation for carers – Train carers in behavioural management – Cognitive stimulation therapy – Cognitive behavioural therapy
Social	– Day-care programmes – Domiciliary care packages – In-home respite – Residential aged care facilities – Carer health and support

required. A person-centred approach is important to best understand the individual, their symptoms, behaviour and situation and in order to select the most appropriate interventions.

24.4.6 Pharmacological

Although non-pharmacological approaches are recommended as first line for managing agitation, medications may be used in certain circumstances [2]. For example, they may be used as an adjunct to non-pharmacological measures or when the latter has been unsuccessful and when the agitation poses risks to safety, is severe or adversely affects quality of life and function of the patient or carer [13]. However, there is only modest evidence for the use of medications to treat various forms of agitation but significant risk of serious side effects [39].

After careful assessment of need and indication, prescribing medications for people with agitation includes a number of important considerations. The adverse effects of the drug must be weighed against potential benefits and individual circumstances (medical comorbidity, medications, supervision, cost) and informed consent obtained from the patient or substitute decision-maker. The duration of the medication trial and a plan for review should be determined. Doses should be titrated slowly and polypharmacy avoided. Prescriptions of antipsychotics to people with dementia with Lewy bodies or Parkinson's disease require particular caution due to neuroleptic sensitivity [13].

Various medications have been trialled for different types of agitation and are summarized in Table 24.5. For aggression, there is modest evidence for the antipsychotics haloperidol, risperidone or aripiprazole and the antidepressant citalopram [40]. Quetiapine may cause greater cognitive decline in Alzheimer dementia as well as being ineffective for agitation with Alzheimer or Lewy body dementia [39]. Risks of antipsychotics in people with dementia include extrapyramidal effects, falls, metabolic problems, stroke and neurological symptoms and greater mortality [13]. Some antipsychotics also have anticholinergic (which may precipitate delirium or worsen cognition) or cardiac effects. Although benzodiazepines are often used for agitation, there is no good evidence to support this, and adverse effects such as falls, sedation, delirium and ataxia are common. Effective use of analgesics for pain may reduce agitation in moderate to severely demented nursing home residents. There is modest evidence for carbamazepine for agitation in dementia.

Cholinesterase inhibitors may be useful when targeting specific symptoms such as motor behaviours, apathy, anxiety and depression, and hallucinations and delusions [41]. There is good evidence for rivastigmine for agitation and visual hallucinations in particular, in dementia with Lewy bodies. Side effects of cholinesterase inhibitors include anorexia, gastrointestinal upset, diarrhoea, bradycardia, dizziness and agitation. Additionally, agitation may worsen within six weeks of withdrawal of cholinesterase inhibitors. The glutamate receptor antagonist memantine may be useful for aggression and agitation, irritability and delusions and hallucinations. Adverse effects include drowsiness, constipation, dizziness, anorexia, headache, hypertension and

Table 24.5 Pharmacological interventions for agitation

General principles	• Weigh up risks and benefits and seek informed consent • Low doses with gradual titration • Avoid polypharmacy • Determine the duration of the trial and schedule interim reviews
Aggression	Citalopram, memantine, risperidone, aripiprazole, haloperidol
Agitation	Analgesia, carbamazepine, melatonin, rivastigmine (dementia with Lewy bodies), memantine, citalopram
Motor behaviours, apathy, anxiety and depression, psychosis	Cholinesterase inhibitors, memantine
Insomnia	Cholinesterase inhibitors, ginkgo biloba, melatonin

anxiety. There is meta-analytic evidence for melatonin improving some types of agitation, but effect on mood requires more study, and it does not appear to improve impaired cognition [42].

24.4.7 Physical

The optimization of physical and sensory functioning is an important aspect of addressing agitation. Basic unmet physical needs such as thirst, hunger, comfortable temperature, physical activity and constipation may cause agitation and distress. Additionally, visual and hearing impairment may predispose to misinterpreting the environment and hallucinations and should be screened for and addressed. Attention to appropriate lighting and visual contrast is also helpful [13]. If the person with dementia does not speak the local language, inability to communicate may exacerbate agitation. Regular use of interpreters or placement in culturally appropriate facilities may be useful.

There are several non-pharmacological approaches to managing behavioural changes, especially agitation, in people with dementia. Those with some evidence include developing a structured routine, aromatherapy, music matched to individual preference, daily physical activity (minimum 30 minutes), one-to-one engagement with a clinician, animal-assisted therapy (pets), Snoezelen rooms and therapeutic activities [13].

24.4.8 Physiological

Delirium is very common in people with dementia and may lead to agitation, aggression, mood changes and psychotic symptoms. Therefore, any acute change in behaviour or psychological symptoms in someone with dementia should be considered a delirium until proven otherwise. Delirium is characterized by sudden onset, fluctuations in cognition and level of consciousness and inattention. Surgical procedures, any medical condition and many medications may contribute to development of a delirium. Management requires a broad approach incorporating identification and treatment of acute medical illness, optimization of sensory function and physical health (e.g. hydration, nutrition, constipation) and mobility, medication review, environmental measures and staff interventions [43]. People with dementia may take longer to recover from a delirium, even once the contributory factors have been addressed.

24.4.9 Psychological

A few psychotherapeutic strategies have been evaluated for the management of agitated behaviour. Effective strategies for carers include psychoeducation and behavioural management approaches targeting challenging behaviours or carer responses [44]. The effect is greater for individual sessions than groups.

The evidence for psychotherapy in people with agitation in dementia is poor, and studies are generally of poor methodological quality [44]. One promising approach is cognitive stimulation therapy [45]. The purpose of this structured therapy is to improve cognition and social function through a variety of enjoyable activities, usually in a small group social setting, which stimulate memory, thinking and concentration [45]. Beneficial outcomes include better quality of life and less symptoms of depression.

Cognitive behavioural therapeutic approaches may be useful for people with dementia and anxiety. For example, the small Peaceful Mind pilot study demonstrated less anxiety and improved quality of life in people with dementia and anxiety and reduced related carer distress [46]. However, positive effects were not maintained at six months. Other psychotherapeutic approaches for agitation have included reminiscence therapy, validation therapy and reality orientation therapy; however, evidence of effectiveness is limited [13].

24.4.10 Social (Housing Support)

Accommodation options depend upon the person's level of function, availability of carer support and supervision, preferences and particular needs. People with dementia may be able to live in their own home with formal community services or carers providing assistance with activities of daily living tailored to their cognitive or functional impairment. Occupational therapists may assess the home environment and suggest modifications to improve safety and meet the person's needs.

Residential aged care facilities are an option for people with dementia whose care needs cannot be met at home. Facilities may be chosen depending on need for low or high care, and there may be dementia-specific units available, with highly trained staff and lower staff-to-resident ratios. There is evidence for placement in a home-like environment reducing aggression [47], but as these units are usually small with highly skilled staff, familiar environments and particular models of care, it is difficult to know which specific elements confer benefit [47].

Looking after someone with dementia can be stressful and burdensome. Carers may neglect their own health and have poor mental and physical health. They face numerous challenges such as lack of time for themselves, guilt, grief for aspects of the person they have known, social isolation and may have difficulty coping with challenging behaviours and the demands of care [48]. A primary care physician is well placed to enquire about how the carer is managing and to evaluate their health, the need for additional help or respite and supports available [48]. Their health and needs can be monitored along with the patient.

24.4.11 Day Care

Adult day centres offer a safe environment where the person with dementia can take part in activities and social contact. They vary in hours, services provided, support with personal care, cost and staffing skills and availability. Day centres may cater for specific cultural, language and religious groups. For the carer, a day centre provides an opportunity for respite. In-home or residential respite is another option, which provides care for the person with dementia in their own environment from a qualified person or relative/friend, thus giving the usual carer a break.

24.4.12 Night Support

Disturbances in circadian rhythm and sleep are common in dementia, especially dementia with Lewy bodies, and are associated with depressive symptoms, greater carer burden, poor quality of life and premature placement in residential aged care facilities [49]. While there are a variety of causes, it is important to exclude and address environmental (e.g. temperature, changes to routine, noise) and medical factors (e.g. pain, illness, delirium, depression or anxiety or medication effects). Carers may be taught sleep hygiene strategies such as limiting caffeine, adequate exercise, appropriate lighting, adequate hydration and keeping a regular night time routine [49]. Attention to safety is also important for wandering at night, for example, removing trip hazards and leaving a night light on. Studies of light stimulation have inconsistent results.

There is little evidence for pharmacological approaches and risks must be considered. Atypical antipsychotics have some evidence but are not recommended unless psychosis underlies the nocturnal disruption [49]. Cholinesterase inhibitors have some evidence in Alzheimer's disease. Ginkgo biloba and melatonin have limited evidence for improving sleep [49], and melatonin may worsen early morning waking [42].

24.4.13 Management of Frailty

Dementia, particularly vascular type, is strongly associated with frailty in people aged over 75 [50]. Dementia and frailty are both associated with greater risk of mortality, falls and fractures [50]. Population based initiatives in midlife to prevent disability, dementia and frailty target public policy, educational campaigns and legal regulatory frameworks. The key areas of intervention include smoking cessation, increasing physical activity/reducing sedentary behaviour, achieving a healthy weight and diet and reducing alcohol consumption [51]. The individual management of frailty includes exercise (resistance, aerobic, balance and dual tasking), high-protein diet, vitamin D and leucine-enriched essential amino acids supplements [52]. One example of an intervention which prevents frailty in older adults is resistance and balance training programmes combined with nutritional counselling [53]. However, specific programmes for people with dementia, agitation and frailty are lacking.

24.4.14 Spirituality

Spirituality may involve the search for meaning and purpose, connectivity with others, sense of an Other or organized religion. The ability to practice religion or faith is an important element of quality of life in people with dementia, even those with advanced disease in care facilities [54]. Religion may help the individual find purpose and meaning or assist with coping [55]. Given the potential value and diversity of ways in which spirituality may be experienced, people should be asked directly how they would like to stay connected with their faith [55].

24.4.15 Management of Emergencies

Primary care physicians will often be requested to urgently attend a residential aged care facility because one of the residents has become severely agitated. A behavioural emergency is any situation in which the safety of the person with dementia, their carers or other persons is potentially seriously compromised. The types of agitation include severe physical aggression and self-injurious behaviour. Usually by the time the primary care physician has been called the opportunity for an early intervention to de-escalate, the situation has either passed or has been attempted with varying degrees of success. An early intervention involves the carers (family or professional) being able to recognize the early warning signs that agitation is escalating. This should result in the prompt use of a de-escalation strategy involving protecting the person and others from coming to harm by using a calm, attentive approach, removing objects, such as knives, which could cause harm, manoeuvring the person into a safe quiet location with supervision, removing other persons who might be harmed and summoning assistance from others. Frequently this approach might suffice to settle the emergency.

The most important task for the primary care physician is to determine the possible cause(s) of the emergency, even before pharmacotherapy is used to control unresolved severe agitation, as the likely aetiology could influence the medication to be administered. In this regard, the possibility of the behaviour being symptomatic of delirium (as described in 4.1) is a priority consideration partic-ularly when the behaviour has only emerged in the previous few days. The identification and treatment of the medical cause need to occur promptly and include a physical examination. Other possible causes, as previously described, include unmet need, the person being a 'victim' who has reacted to the behaviour of someone else and a chronic recurring pattern of behaviour that has not been adequately addressed before (as described in 3.2).

There is very little empirical evidence to guide choice of pharmacotherapy for treatment of behavioural emergencies. If possible, oral medication is preferred as first-line treatment. If the person has Lewy body dementia, antipsychotic drugs should be avoided. Caution is required if the patient is delirious, hypotensive or frail. Suggested pharmacotherapy options are in Table 24.6.

Consideration needs to be given regarding consent for medication. In most jurisdictions, emergency administration can occur without prior consent, but it is expected that the substitute decision-maker is informed, usually within 24 hours, and consent for subsequent pharmacotherapy obtained. This implies that a treatment plan is required that includes prevention of further episodes, treatment of new episodes and perhaps a short-term regular course for up to three months depending on the cause.

Safe administration of emergency sedation requires close monitoring afterwards as there is a high risk of adverse effects due to the likelihood that a higher than usual dose will be required to settle the behaviour, the presence of medical comorbidity and the possibility that the person is medication naïve. The main concerns are oversedation, hypotension, extrapyramidal side effects and falls.

Table 24.6 Emergency pharmacotherapy for severe agitation

Oral pharmacotherapy		
First line	Short-acting benzodiazepine	E.g. lorazepam 0.5–1.25 mg (maximum 7.5 mg in 24 h)
Second line	Atypical antipsychotic	E.g. risperidone 0.5–1 mg (maximum 4 mg per event) *or* Olanzapine 2.5–5 mg (maximum 10 mg in 24 h)
Third line	Traditional antipsychotic	E.g. haloperidol 0.5–1 mg (maximum 4 mg in 24 h)
Parenteral pharmacotherapy		
First line	Short-acting benzodiazepine	Lorazepam 1 mg IMI 2 hourly (maximum 3 mg in 24 h)
Second line	Atypical antipsychotic	Olanzapine 2.5 mg IMI 2 hourly (maximum 7.5 mg in 24 h)
Third line	Traditional antipsychotic	Haloperidol 1 mg IMI 2 hourly (maximum 3 mg in 24 h)

IMI intramuscular injection, *mg* milligrams
Table based on Refs. [39, 41]

24.4.16 Evaluation of Interventions Made

It is important to provide ongoing review and set a timeline for evaluating whether an intervention has been successful. This is especially true for any pharmacological interventions, where risks may outweigh benefits [39]. Any ineffective treatment should be withdrawn. Staff at residential care facilities may be asked to complete a behaviour diary, which records the nature, frequency and type of agitation, as well the intervention used and outcome. The Antecedent, Behaviour and Consequences (ABC) approach is commonly used to describe challenging behaviours and evaluate the effectiveness of management interventions. This approach involves the carer or staff documenting the antecedent, behaviour and consequences of the behaviour.

Formal assessment tools improve the differentiation of agitated behaviour which facilitates targeted treatment [56]. Rating scales are also useful in objectively quantifying change in symptoms and behaviours from pre-intervention levels. They are particularly helpful in residential aged care facilities. A variety of rating scales have been devised to evaluate specific (e.g. depressive symptoms, agitation, apathy) and general agitation and other BPSD [56]. For example, the Cohen-Mansfield Agitation Inventory [57], Behavioural Pathology in Alzheimer's Disease [58] and the NPI [59]. Tools may be scored by carers (family or professional), self-report by the person with dementia, or physicians' direct observations. However, to achieve consistency and reliability in ratings, staff must be trained in the use of the rating scale.

24.4.17 Specific Recommendations for Management in Primary Care

It is important to consider and screen for cognitive impairment in older adults. This should include taking a history from the person and their carer including regarding the onset, nature and progression of cognitive symptoms, functional impairment (i.e. activities of daily living),

whether they are driving and other safety considerations (such as access to weapons, becoming lost, accidental injury or self-neglect) and mood [48]. Agitation can also be a potent cause of carer stress, which should be evaluated. Formal tools to assess and monitor cognition such as the mini-mental status examination [60], clock-draw test and the General Practitioner Assessment of Cognition (GP-Cog) should be conducted [61]. The GP-Cog is a valid, quick screening tool for dementia developed for primary care and consists of objective cognitive tests combined with historical reports from an informant [61].

The key issues in managing agitation and other BPSD in primary care are to elucidate the underlying causes and address them. Assessment may take time and is necessarily broad, including corroborative information from families, carers and residential care staff. Once an intervention has commenced, there should be a plan for regular review. It may be necessary to sequentially try different approaches to management before an effective intervention is found for the individual. While behavioural, environmental or psychological interventions may continue indefinitely, pharmacological strategies should have a time frame determined for use, relevant monitoring and be withdrawn if ineffective. Families and carers may benefit from additional information and support, for example, through the local Alzheimer's Association branch, carers organizations and Dementia Services.

24.5 Conclusion

Agitation is a common complication of dementia that will be frequently encountered by primary care physicians. It is often a manifestation of distress in the person with dementia, can be very stressful for their carers and results in premature institutionalization. Early assessment and appropriate interventions by primary care physicians can ameliorate the distress, assist carers in coping with the situation and delay placement into institutional care. For those persons already in residential care, well-trained staff using person-centred care practices in a well-designed facility can reduce the likelihood of agitation development.

References

1. Cummings J, et al. Agitation in cognitive disorders: International Psychogeriatric Association provisional consensus clinical and research definition. Int Psychogeriatr. 2015;27(1):7–17.
2. Draper B, Finkel SI, Tune L. Module 1-an introduction to BPSD. In: Draper B, Brodaty H, Finkel SI, editors. The IPA complete guides to BPSD-specialists guide. 4th ed. Northfield: International Psychogeriatric Association; 2015. p. 1.1–1.16.
3. Steinberg M, et al. Point and 5-year prevalence of neuropsychiatric symptoms in dementia: the Cache County study. Int J Geriatr Psychiatry. 2008;23:170–7.
4. Bergh S, Selbaek G. The prevalence and the course of neuropsychiatric symptoms in patients with dementia. Norsk Epidemiol. 2012;22(2):225–32.
5. Steinberg M, et al. The persistence of neuropsychiatric symptoms in dementia: the Cache County Study. Int J Geriatr Psychiatry. 2004;19:19–26.
6. Peters ME, et al. Prevalence of neuropsychiatric symptoms in CIND and its subtypes: The Cache County Study. Am J Geriatr Psychiatr. 2012;20(5):416–24.
7. Stella F, et al. Neuropsychiatric symptoms in the prodromal stages of dementia. Curr Opin Psychiatry. 2014;27:230–5.
8. Brodaty H, et al. Neuropsychiatric symptoms in older people with and without cognitive impairment. J Alzheimers Dis. 2012;31:411–20.
9. Conn D. Module 8 - long-term care. In: Draper B, Brodaty H, Finkel SI, editors. The IPA complete guides to BPSD-specialists guide. 4th ed. Northfield: International Psychogeriatric Association; 2015. p. 8.1–8.33.
10. Wang H, et al. Module 7 - cross cultural and transnational considerations. In: Draper B, Brodaty H, Finkel SI, editors. The IPA Complete Guides to BPSD-Specialists Guide. 4th ed. Northfield: International Psychogeriatric Association; 2015. p. 7.1–7.51.
11. Ford AH. Neuropsychiatric aspects of dementia. Maturitas. 2014;79:209–15.
12. Waggel SE, et al. Neuroticism scores increase with late life cognitive decline. Int J Geriatr Psychiatry. 2015;30(9):985–93. https://doi.org/10.1002/gps.4251.
13. Draper B, Wand APF. Behavioural and psychological symptoms of dementia. In: Pachana N, editor. Encyclopedia of geropsychology. in press.
14. Rendina N, et al. Substitute consent for nursing home residents prescribed psychotropic medication. Int J Geriatr Psychiatry. 2009;24:226–31.
15. O'Connor D, Rabins P, Swanwick G. Module 5 - non-pharmacological treatments. In: Draper B, Brodaty H, Finkel SI, editors. The IPA complete guides to BPSD-specialists guide. 4th ed. Northfield: International Psychogeriatric Association; 2015. p. 5.1–5.13.
16. Meagher DJ, et al. Phenomenology of delirium. Assessment of 100 adult cases using standardized measures. Br J Psychiatry. 2007;190:135–41.
17. Inouye SK, et al. Clarifying confusion: the confusion assessment method. A new method for detection of delirium. Ann Intern Med. 1990;113:941–8.
18. Bellilli G, et al. Validation of the 4AT, a new instrument for rapid delirium screening: a study in 234 hospitalised older people. Age Ageing. 2014;43:496–502.
19. The Royal Australian College of General Practitioners. Medical care of older persons in residential aged care facilities. In: Silver book. 4th ed. East Melbourne: National Taskforce, The Royal Australian College of General Practitioners Victoria; 2006.
20. Yesavage JA, et al. Development and validation of a geriatric depression screening scale: a preliminary report. J Psychiatr Res. 1982–1983;17:37–49.
21. Alexopoulos GS, et al. Cornell scale for depression in dementia. Biol Psychiatry. 1988;23:271–84.
22. Beck AT, Ward C, Mendelson M. Beck Depression Inventory (BDI). Arch Gen Psychiatry. 1961;4:561–71.
23. Lovibond SH, Lovibond PF. Manual for the depression anxiety stress scales. 2nd ed. Sydney: Psychology Foundation; 1995.
24. National Collaborating Centre for Mental Health. Depression. The NICE guideline on the treatment and management of depression in adults (updated edition) (National Clinical Practice Guideline 90). London: British Psychological Society and Royal College of Psychiatrists; 2010.
25. Jenkins C, McKay A. A collaborative approach to health promotion in early stage dementia. Nurs Stand. 2013;27:49–57.
26. Brodaty H, et al. Dementia: 14 essentials of assessment and care planning. Med. Today. 2013;14:18–27.
27. World Alzheimer's Report 2009. London: Alzheimer's Disease International; 2009.
28. Mrazek PJ, Haggerty RJ, editors. Reducing risks for mental disorders: frontiers for preventive intervention research. Washington, DC: National Academy Press; 1994.
29. Australian Institute of Health and Welfare. Dementia in Australia. Cat. no. AGE 70. Canberra: AIHW; 2012.
30. Lakey L, et al. Dementia 2012: a national challenge. London: Alzheimer's Society; 2012.
31. World Health Organization and Alzheimer's Disease International. Dementia: a public health priority. Chapter 6 Public understanding of dementia: from awareness to acceptance. http://www.who.int/mental_health/publications/dementia_report_2012. Accessed 4 Oct 2015.
32. Know the 10 signs. Chicago: Alzheimer's Association. http://www.alz.org/alzheimers_disease_know_the_10_signs.asp. Accessed 4 Oct 2015.
33. Australian Institute of Health and Welfare. Dementia care in hospitals: costs and strategies. Cat. no. AGE 72. Canberra: AIHW; 2013.
34. Draper B, et al. The Hospital Dementia Services Project: Age differences in hospital stays for older people with and without dementia. Int Psychogeriatr. 2011;23:1649–58.

35. Siddiqi N, House A, Holmes J. Occurrence and outcome of delirium in medical in-patients: a systematic literature review. Age Ageing. 2006;35:350–64.

36. Farrow M. Dementia risk reduction. A practical guide for health and lifestyle professionals. Alzheimer's Australia; 2010.

37. Douglas S, James I, Ballard C. Non-pharmacological interventions in dementia. Adv Psychiatr Treat. 2004;10:171–9.

38. Decision-making capacity and dementia. A guide for health care professionals in NSW. Mini-legal kit Series 1.7 ACCEPD (Capacity Australia). 2013.

39. Royal Australian and New Zealand College of Psychiatrists. Assessment and management of people with behavioural and psychological symptoms of dementia (BPSD): a handbook for NSW health clinicians. North Ryde: NSW Ministry of Health; 2013.

40. Schneider LS, Dagerman K, Insel PS. Efficacy and adverse effects of atypical antipsychotics for dementia: meta-analysis of randomized, placebo-controlled trials. Am J Geriatr Psychiatr. 2006;14:191–210.

41. Seitz D, Lawlor B. Module 6 - pharmacological management. In: Draper B, Brodaty H, Finkel SI, editors. The IPA complete guides to BPSD-specialists guide. Northfield: International Psychogeriatric Association; 2015. p. 6.1–6.35.

42. Jansen SL, et al. Melatonin for the treatment of dementia (review). Cochrane Database Syst Rev. 2011;3:CD003802.

43. Wand APF, et al. A multifaceted educational intervention to prevent delirium in older inpatients: a before and after study. Int J Nurs Stud. 2014;51:974–82.

44. Livingston G, et al. Systematic review of psychological approaches to the management of neuropsychiatric symptoms of dementia. Am J Psychiatr. 2005;162:1996–2021.

45. Woods B, et al. Cognitive stimulation to improve cognitive functioning in people with dementia. Cochrane Database Syst Rev. 2012;2:CD005562.

46. Stanley MA, et al. The Peaceful Mind Program: a pilot test of a CBT-based intervention for anxious patients with dementia. J Geriatr Psychiatry. 2013;21:696–708.

47. Fleming R, Crookes P, Sum S. A review of the empirical literature on the design of physical environments for people with dementia. Kensington: University of NSW; 2009. http://www.dementiaresearch.org.au/images/dcrc/output-files/147-summary_of_a_review_of_the_empirical_literature_on_the_design_on_physical_environments_for_people_with_dementia.pdf. Accessed 21 Jan 2015.

48. Brodaty H, et al. Dementia: 14 essentials of management. Med Today. 2013;14:29–41.

49. Burns K, Jayasinha R, Brodaty H. Managing behavioural and psychological symptoms of dementia (BPSD). A Clinician's Field Guide to Good Practice. Sydney: Dementia Collaborative Research Centre, UNSW; 2014.

50. Kulmala J, et al. Association between frailty and dementia: a population-based study. Gerontology. 2014;60:16–21.

51. National Institute for Health and Care Excellence. Dementia, disability and frailty in later life – mid-life approaches to prevention. NICE guidelines [NG16]. London: National Institute for Health and Care Excellence; 2015.

52. Morley JE. Frailty: diagnosis and management. J Nutr Health Aging. 2011;15:667–70.

53. Chan DC, et al. A pilot randomised controlled trial to improve geriatric frailty. BMC Geriatr. 2012;12:58.

54. Alzheimer's Society. My name is not dementia. London: Alzheimer's Society; 2010.

55. Higgins P. The spiritual and religious needs of people with dementia. Cathol Med Q. 2011;61:24–9.

56. Grossberg G, Luxemberg J, Tune L. Module 2 - clinical issues. In: Draper B, Brodaty H, Finkel SI, editors. The IPA complete guides to BPSD-specialists guide. 4th ed. Northfield: International Psychogeriatric Association; 2015. p. 2.1–2.29.

57. Cohen-Mansfield J, Marx MS, Rosenthal AS. A description of agitation in a nursing home. J Gerontol. 1989;44:M77–84.

58. Reisberg B, et al. Behavioral symptoms in Alzheimer's disease: phenomenology and treatment. J Clin Psychiatry. 1987;48(Suppl):9–15.

59. Cummings J, et al. The neuropsychiatric inventory: comprehensive assessment of psychopathology in dementia. Neurology. 1994;44:2308–14.

60. Folstein MF, Folstein SE, McHugh PR. Mini-mental state: a practical method for grading the cognitive state of patients for the clinician. J Psychiatr Res. 1975;12:189–98.

61. Brodaty H, et al. The GPCOG: a new screening test for dementia designed for general practice. J Am Geriatr Soc. 2002;50:530–4.

Part VII

Strategies in Rehabilitation

Carlos Augusto de Mendonça Lima and Nicolas Kuhne

Abstract

Psychosocial rehabilitation (PR) in old age psychiatry is the set of direct and indirect processes, mobilizing individuals and their environment, in order to allow adults at retirement age presenting a disability, a capacity limitation, or a difficulty of performance related to a mental health problem to recover an optimal functioning. PR for older adults doesn't differ from that of younger adults. But their specific needs require special skills of professionals and specific resources too. In older adults, the social reintegration and rehabilitation aspects are more valued than vocational ones. Solutions are required for the participation of retirees in all kind of activities within the community. Two complementary dimensions must be taken into account: the psychological well-being and individual resilience. The reduction of stigma and discrimination is central. By acting on social determinants of health, it is possible to improve a better subjective mental health and well-being, to build the capacity of communities to manage adversity, and to reduce the burden and consequences of mental health problems. Primary care teams should be included in all PR program as a cost-effective valuable resource able to deliver and manage important steps of such programs in the respect of local cultural rules.

Key Points

- In order to cope with older adults with mental disorders number increase and with the problems related to them, innovative approaches are needed for their treatment and care: the application of the psychosocial rehabilitation (PR) principles in the care of the older adults with mental disorders may be a response to that.
- PR in old age psychiatry is the set of direct and indirect processes, mobilizing individuals and their environment, in order to allow adults at retirement age presenting a disability, a capacity limitation, or a difficulty of performance related to a mental health problem to recover an optimal functioning.
- PR in old age psychiatry does not differ essentially from that of younger adults. But the complexity and the specific needs of older adults require the development of special skills of mental health professionals and the implementation of specific resources.

C. A. de Mendonça Lima (✉)
Unity of Old Age Psychiatry, Centre Les Toises, Lausanne, Switzerland

N. Kuhne
University of Applied Sciences Western Switzerland, Lausanne, Switzerland

© Springer Nature Switzerland AG 2019
C. A. de Mendonça Lima, G. Ivbijaro (eds.), *Primary Care Mental Health in Older People*,
https://doi.org/10.1007/978-3-030-10814-4_25

- In older adults, it is only the social reintegration and rehabilitation aspects that will be more valued. Solutions for the participation of retirees in paid or voluntary activities within the community should be found.
- To achieve the highest possible level of quality of life for older adults, two complementary dimensions must be taken into account: the psychological well-being and individual resilience.
- The reduction of stigma and discrimination against older adults with mental disorders occupies an important place in a PR project.
- By acting on social determinants of health, it is possible to contribute to a better subjective mental health and well-being of older people, to build the capacity of communities to manage adversity, and to reduce the burden and consequences of mental health problems.
- Primary care teams should be included in all PR program as a cost-effective valuable resource able to deliver and manage important steps of such programs in the respect of local cultural rules and habits.

25.1   Introduction

The number of older adults in the world is increasing at varying speeds, depending on the country income level where they live: the life expectancy of the world's population has increased by 30 years throughout the twentieth century [1, 2]. This success of humanity is also transforming itself into an enormous challenge: to become able to cope with this population of older adults, with its specific needs and problems. Indeed, the living conditions of people at retirement age (in general, after age 65) are undergoing profound changes. The place and the role of these older adults in the community require a redefinition, and a transformation is essential in all sectors of society [2–4].

Many older adults are left on their own without the health care and social support they need. On the other hand, many others are kept in expensive housing structures and in often inadequate conditions: they could be treated at home with minor adaptations of the care system or in institutions better prepared to meet their needs, in respect of their dignity [3, 4]. Everyone, especially the older adults, has the right to enjoy a good quality of life and to have a recognized role as a member of society.

The number of older adults with mental disorders is also increasing not only because of demographic pressure but also because of the life expectancy increase of younger people with chronic mental disorders, particularly with psychotic disorders [2]. Indeed, for the first time in history, the effective care they have received since the beginning of their illness allows these people to reach very advanced ages [5].

Mental disorders in older adults are a source of great suffering for the individual and for his/her family. They also are an important burden for the community. The patient thus fears becoming a burden for others. Affected families are usually required to provide material and emotional support while experiencing the discrimination associated with the mental disorder. Many family members have to adapt, to make compromises, and to spend a good deal of their time caring for the sick person. This charge hampers their full personal development. They are socially embarrassed—often also financially—and live in fear of relapses that would disrupt their daily lives [6]. Finally, older adults with mental disorders often suffer from a double prejudice: one related to their age and the other related to mental disorder [7].

Thus, in order to cope with older adults with mental disorders number increase and with the problems related to them, innovative approaches are needed for their treatment and care. One of these innovations could still be the application of the psychosocial rehabilitation principles in the care of the older adults with mental disorders [8, 9].

25.2 Toward a Psychosocial Rehabilitation (PR) in Old Age Psychiatry of the Elderly

25.2.1 Concept Development

Old age psychiatry is a branch of psychiatry. It is part of the multidisciplinary mental health-care system for older adults. Its field of competence is the psychiatric care for older adults at retirement age (usually people over 65), and it is characterized by community orientation and a multidisciplinary approach of assessment, diagnosis, and treatment [10].

The complexity of older adults' needs, assessment, and individual care and long-term follow-up require all the collaboration of health and social services with volunteer organizations and families. The specialty deals with the full range of mental disorders and their consequences and is particularly concerned with older adults who have developed chronic mental disorders at a younger age [10].

In its basic concept, PR in old age psychiatry does not differ essentially from that of younger adults, especially since PR has been extended beyond the scope of reintegration to work [11, 12]. But the complexity and the specific needs of older adults require the development of special skills of mental health professionals and the implementation of specific resources (policies, programs, and services). These special needs are related to aspects of prevention, early detection of disorders, and reduction of impairments (capacity limitations or performance problems associated with mental and behavioral disorders). The organization of PR services in old age psychiatry aims to facilitate the access to care and to introduce effective interventions while reducing stress for the ill person and his/her entourage [13].

It is difficult to develop a project of integration into society for people who are often in loss of life project. This difficulty is even greater for a family group in which there are three or four different generations living together, each presenting specific needs and problems, for which à la carte rehabilitation project must be developed.

In general psychiatry, PR involves vocational/social reintegration and rehabilitation [14–16]. In the case of older adults, it is only the social aspects that will be more valued. However, the increase in the number of pensions to be financed, and the increase in life expectancy, means that projects have to be studied to find new solutions for the participation of retirees in paid or voluntary activities within the community. We claim a place within these projects for older adults with mental disorders: any exclusion should not be accepted.

The PR in old age psychiatry is highly sensitive to the role and place that older adults hold in a given society. This role and place are currently being transformed in the present moving societies wherever families are breaking up, the number of places for dependent older adults in nursing homes is being reduced, the economic power of older adults is being loss as well as their role as potential consumers, while the weight of their role in political life in modern democracies should be increasing. All these points can question the place of older adults in society and therefore their role as citizens [17–19].

25.2.1.1 Quality of Life, Well-Being, and Resilience

Improving patients and informal caregivers' quality of life, while taking into account the needs of the support network, is central to a PR project [20, 21]. In addition, interventions must take into account the wishes of the patient in the respect of his/her autonomy and dignity [22]. To achieve the highest possible level of quality of life, two complementary dimensions must be taken into account: the psychological well-being and individual resilience.

Psychological well-being is an integral part of an individual's capacity to lead a fulfilling life, including the ability to form and maintain relationships, to study, to remain active inside the community or pursue leisure interests, and to make day-to-day decisions about the management of the social determinants of his/her own life [23]. To achieve this state of well-being, some values inherent to the human condition have to be promoted and protected [23]:

- The *independent thought and action*, which is the capacity of each one to manage their interactions with others.
- *Pleasure, happiness, and life satisfaction*: happiness represents the ultimate goal in life and is the truest measure of well-being [24, 25].
- *Family relations, friendship, and social interaction*: own self-identity and capacity to be happy are deeply related to the social surroundings, including the opportunity to form relationships and engage with those around them (family members, friends, colleagues).

Resilience, on other side, refers to a pattern of sufficient functioning indicative of positive adaptation in the context of significant risk of adversity [26, 27]. It is a process of effectively negotiating, adapting to, or managing significant sources of stress or trauma. Assets and resources within the individual, the close environment, and the community as a whole may facilitate this capacity for coping. This capacity may change along the life course and depend also on the past experiences facing to adversity.

Well-being is related to resilience, but it is possible to have individuals—and communities—with high level of well-being and low resilience [26]. Higher emotional well-being, optimism, self-related successful aging, social engagement, and fewer cognitive complaints are strongest predictors of good resilience [26].

In the case of very older adults, an important capacity of resilience is used to cope with physical and health changes—as well as perceived well-being fluctuation—in order to focus in what is really essential in life contributing to own happiness. In this case, perfect physical health is not indispensable nor enough for the perception of a successful aging. The self-satisfaction involves much more emphasis on psychological factors, such the capacity to cope (resilience), optimism, and well-being, in absence of important mental health symptoms of anxiety and depression [26].

25.2.1.2 Stigma and Discrimination

The reduction of stigma and discrimination against older adults with mental disorders occupies an important place in a PR project. Stigma is the result of a process, whereby some individuals are unwarranted to feel ashamed, excluded, and discriminated. Discrimination includes all forms of distinction, exclusion, or preference that result in the abolition or reduction of equitable rights [7]. Discrimination can manifest itself in terms of poor quality of care, marginalization within health systems, poor housing conditions for the people concerned, but also devaluation of professionals and services providing care, difficulties with financing, unfairness in the reimbursement of health costs, negative impact on families, abuse, preventable institutionalization, social exclusion, poor quality of life, discriminatory legislation, negligence on the part of authorities, etc. [7].

The reduction of stigma involves complex educational actions to change beliefs and attitudes, while the reduction of discrimination mainly involves a legislative and judicial approach [7]. The main goals of a strategy to reduce stigma and discrimination in the context of mental disorders in older adults are to:

- Ensure the existence and the effectiveness of social and health services for these people and their caregivers.
- Ensure that the mental health of older adults receives the same attention that of other age groups.
- Promote a better understanding and acceptance of these people.
- Create more supportive environments for them.
- Encourage the search for effective and non-stigmatizing treatments, care, and access to sufficient occupational activities.

While government authorities have primary responsibility for reducing stigma and discrimination, other sectors also have an important role to play. They must act in a coordinated way; carry out realistic actions, limited in time; and if possible regularly evaluate their actions [28].

25.2.1.3 Social Determinants of Health [29–32]

Mental well-being is an asset of individuals, communities, and populations whose value can change throughout the life course. Someone's mental health is affected by a range of determinants throughout life, such as the genetic heritage, personal experiences, and the environment in which the person lives [29, 30]. Social determinants of health are the conditions in which people are born, grow, live, work, and age and which are shaped by the distribution of money, power, and resources at global, national, and local levels [29, 30]. These social determinants are associated with mental disorders by contributing to its onset or its course. Social determinants may play a role as risk factors for mental health (poverty, inequalities, stigma and discrimination, poor housing, poor early years experience, violence, abuse, neglect, drug and alcohol abuse, poor general health, caring duties), while others may be protective factors (social protection, resilience, social networks, positive community engagement, positive spiritual life, hope, optimism, good general health, good quality parenting, positive relationships in old age) [29, 30].

Social determinants of health are the conditions in which people are born, grow, live, work, and age and which are shaped by the distribution of money, power, and resources at global, national, and local levels [29, 30]. These social determinants are associated with mental disorders by contributing to its onset or course. A list of these social determinants should include at least [29, 32]:

– Cultural and spiritual references
– Education and literacy
– Physical environment
– Social status and security
– Financial resources including income security
– Food and housing security and quality
– Health system
– Justice system, including respect of human rights
– Employment and working conditions
– Access to occupational activities
– Leisure and personal development
– Spiritual development
– Discrimination and stigma
– Inequalities

– Social, political, and physical exclusion and marginalization
– Violence, abuse, neglect, and abandon

Social determinants of health are primarily responsible for disparities in health. They are influenced by policy choices which influence the development of public service systems. These systems, in their turn, shape the social determinants of health through the development of programs, resource allocations, and organization of services. The influence of negative social determinants of health often is caused by bad political choices and the consequent unequal distribution of resources [29, 30].

Older adults' mental health relates both to earlier life experiences and also to experiences, conditions, and contexts specific to aging and the postretirement period. Older adults' mental health is related to socioeconomic status, educational status, gender, ethnicity, age, and levels of physical health. The aging process varies by country, related to their social, political, and economic arrangements and particular levels of social protection. Some of the life events that can trigger mental disorders are likely to be experienced in older age—bereavement, perceived loss of status and identity, poor physical health, loss of contact with family and friends, lack of exercise, and living alone. In fact, social isolation among older people is particularly significant (especially for women) in raising the risk of mental disorders [32].

By acting on social determinants of health, it is possible to contribute to a better subjective mental health and well-being of older people, to build the capacity of communities to manage adversity, and to reduce the burden and consequences of mental health problems [33]. Disadvantages because of mental health problems damage the social cohesion of communities and societies by decreasing interpersonal trust, social participation, and civic engagement [33].

The interventions which contribute to prolong and/or improve older people's social activities, well-being, life satisfaction, resilience, and quality of life can significantly reduce mental disorders symptoms and protect against risk factors, such as social isolation. Effective interventions exist, including psychosocial interventions, interventions to reduce social isolation and to improve exercise and physical activity programs, and programs promoting lifelong learning, in addition to actions aimed at reducing poverty and improving physical health. Furthermore, interventions that improve heating at home, help older people make new friends, and provide opportunities for older people to volunteer are effective in improving and protecting mental health [17, 18, 33].

To achieve the objectives to offer to older adults with mental disorders the best quality of life and the best possible well-being perception, to develop their resilience skills, and to ensure their place as citizens in the community, in the respect of their autonomy and their protection against stigma and discrimination, it must be recognized that the PR is therefore waiting for a definition to better set benchmarks for rehabilitation in old age. This definition must be made within each cultural context, at a local level, by all those involved.

25.2.1.4   Proposal of a Definition

The literature on psychosocial rehabilitation in old age psychiatry is insufficient [11], while the care of chronic diseases and disabilities remains the great challenge of modern medicine. Jones proposed that the rehabilitation of older persons with mental disorders should "restore and maintain the highest possible level of psychological, physical and social functioning despite the presence of incapacitating effects of disease" [11]. This definition implies the prevention of preventable disadvantages associated with diseases and maladaptive responses to diseases. It is also concerned with the fight against the harmful effects of negative prejudices toward older adults, present in patients, in families, and in society in general.

Taking into account the various works published for psychiatry in general [12, 14–16, 34] and more recent concepts on the functioning of the sick person and on the handicap [35], we propose here a definition:

Psychosocial rehabilitation in old age psychiatry is the set of direct and indirect processes, mobilizing individuals and their environment, in order to allow adults at retirement age (generally, with over 65 years) presenting a disability, a capacity limitation, or a difficulty of performance related to a mental health problem to recover an optimal functioning. The use of their own preserved skills and resources, in terms of autonomy and independence, is the base of all actions in psychosocial rehabilitation. Individuals are encouraged to learn how to cope with capacity limitations, or performance issues, by developing their individual functional skills—particularly those related to:

- Personal care (hygiene, eating habits, etc.)
- Social exchanges
- Their meaningful commitment to all different kinds of activities

The general objective of psychosocial rehabilitation is achievement of the highest level of satisfaction with life, at the living place of the person's choice and, as far as possible, within the community. Compensation for their disadvantages is obtained, on the one hand, by internal psychological work aimed on reinforcing resilience skills and adapting personal aspirations to its preserved capacities and resources but also by providing a supportive and adaptive environment and, in particular, through the development of real-life opportunities within the community. The reduction of stigma toward them is done by promoting actions in various sectors of society and by providing accessible means to defend against discrimination. Finally, improving their status as citizens and achieving the highest possible level of well-being are the ultimate goals of psychosocial rehabilitation.

25.3 Strategies

Good quality of care for older adults with mental health problems should consider the person as a whole and take into account the needs and wishes of the patient at the psychological, physical, and social level. Care services must be accessible from geographical, financial, political, cultural, and linguistic points of view. The answers provided must correspond to the problems addressed and provided as quickly and adequately as possible. The care delivered must be centered on the person. They must take into account the problem of mental health in the context of the individual's life and must aim, as far as possible, to maintain the person in his or her usual environment. The approach to care is transdisciplinary. The exchanges among professionals as well as the exchanges between professionals and the other members of the community participating in the patient's care and treatment must to be facilitated. The services must ensure the quality of the services delivered and be sensitive to the ethical and cultural aspects of the interventions. The systemic approach flexibly integrates all available services in order to ensure the best possible continuity of care [10].

If diagnostic procedures are quite similar to that used in other age groups, it should be realized as often as possible in the living area where the person lives. It is suitable that it includes the collection of a collateral anamnesis. The diagnostic formulation must emphasize the abilities preserved, the limitations of capacity, and the difficulties of participation. It must also highlight the impact of the disease in the life of the patient and his family. The wide range of available services must consider the patient, the family, and other caregivers in the community providing the ongoing care and treatment. This care and support must be flexible, complementary, and integrated, in order to provide the best possible quality of life. Structural barriers have to be minimized to allow the patient to cope when transferring from one service to another, as soon as this transfer is necessary [10].

The PR efficiency is higher when deployed as part of a community-based activity [13]. If the PR for the older adults is to be deployed in their usual place of residence, it will have to be deployed also in long-stay institutions (nursing homes). One of the roles of PR for the elderly is to prevent unnecessary institutionalizations. But another one is to define the criteria to propose this institutionalization at the right time, in the best interest of the person. At this particular time, PR must help the dependent person who cannot anymore live independently at home to participate in the process of choosing the institution that will host him/her. It should also help to give to the hosting institution the means to adapt to this person's needs. These long-stay institutions must fully assume their role as a place to live and avoid the isolation of residents: the long-stay institutions must participate in the life of the community, and the community should participate in the life of the institution as well.

The diverse components of intervention strategies in PR can be described according to several levels of intervention, the most important of which are the individual level and the level of services and the environment.

25.3.1 Strategies at Individual Level

Pharmacological Treatments Their proper use is often essential to reduce symptoms and prevent relapse. In the elderly, these treatments involve special knowledge of age-related pharmacokinetic and pharmacodynamic changes and the management of drug interactions in the presence of other common diseases and treatments in this group of older adults.

Social Skills Training (methods that use specific principles of the learning theory to promote the acquisition, generalization, and long-term preservation of the necessary skills for social and interpersonal situations) Available interventions depend on the living environment, but they must be proposed both for people living in the community and for people living in institutions. They can range from simple participation in speaking groups to participation in media-related activities around a specific topic.

Training in Activities of Daily Living to Live Independently (Food, Hygiene, Dressing, Cleaning, Transport, Communication) This training allows the development of skills to achieve a level of quality of life and independence favorable for a life in the community but also, for the residents of the institutions, in order to avoid too much regression. For patients living alone with limitations in their skills to perform activities of daily living, appropriate help must be provided. Particular attention must be paid to improving home security and setting up an effective warning system for crisis or accident.

Psychological Support for Patients and Families Regardless of the technique used, intensive and ongoing psychological support to patients and families is a key component of PR programs. Self-help groups for caregivers of patients with chronic conditions are also an effective strategy. Adequate information should be provided on diagnosis, alternative care, the individual implications of each one of them, the rights of users and families, and the available psychological resources. In particular, the need of caregivers for respite has to be recognized. An adapted response can be given in terms of taking care of certain tasks by prepared staff (hygiene care, preparation and consumption of meals, home visit for a few hours of the week to allow family members to rest), attendance at day-care facilities, or short-term stays in adapted institutions.

Accommodation For older adults who can no longer stay at home, alternative accommodation must be offered in order to ensure their safety and the best possible quality of life. A significant effort must be made to prevent psychiatric hospital from becoming a permanent place of accommodation. In situations where an alternative does not exist, the psychiatric hospital must be adapted to ensure this exceptional accommodation. Different hosting strategies can be adopted, depending on local cultural resources and rules. Ideally, individual accommodation with support from trained personal should be made available to the patient. If the necessary resources are not available to meet individual needs, alternatives for collective housing must be found. But in this case, the risks of keeping people together in institutions should not be overlooked.

Financial Resources Every older adult with a mental disorder must have a pension that ensures at least the minimum subsistence level, taking into account the own difficulties. Access to basic care should not be limited by personal financial hardship. Legal protection must be available to protect human rights and prevent exploitation by others. In particular, measures must be taken to ensure the protection of the personal interests in case of incapacity to manage the own affairs.

Meaningful Occupations and Spiritual Needs The ability to participate in and enjoy the leisure activities chosen by the individual, regardless of his or her environment, is also an element of PR. Access to appropriate, freely chosen activities is a prerequisite for activities with a positive impact on health. Physical activities should be promoted. Opportunities to express their spiritual needs must be offered to the sick older adults. They must be able to freely practice the rites related to their convictions in this field.

25.3.2 Strategies for Mental Health and Human Resources Services

Mental Health Services and Resource Allocation Policies PR has been considered an essential component of any mental health service policy. In formulating these policies, it is important to avoid the separation between services oriented toward specific (pharmacological) treatments and those oriented toward PR. The integration of the two components is essential, and adequate resources must be provided for PR programs. A community-based mental health service must become a care center that can not only provide treatment but also be ready to facilitate access to community resources for users and their families. Integrating health system resources with those of the community increases the exchange of knowledge and the chances of success for rehabilitation.

The Improvement of Institutional and Residential Services The promotion of the human resources and the improvement of material conditions at the institutions where PR users live are essential prerequisites for any program in PR. Both must progress together regardless of the user's place of life. There is an urgent need for guidance on minimum and/or optimal care standards for patients and users.

Staff Education and Training The usual training programs for health professionals are insufficiently geared toward PR. Thus, specific components of PR must be introduced in all courses of graduate training, postgraduate training, and continuing education. These aspects are important in the field of rehabilitation because they involve not only the training of professionals but also the dissemination of appropriate information to patients, their caregivers, and family members as well as to the general public [36].

Quality Assurance Health professionals always feel that they are delivering the best quality of care, from their own point of view. However, users insist not only on having care of quality but also on having easy access to a diverse range of care options. As the definition of quality of care is still under discussion, a negotiated agreement must be reached in each case. A key to the success of quality assessment is the provision of standards and quality indicators that cover the full range of essential RP services. These indicators and standards must be formulated in such a way to let them adapted to local needs and contexts [37, 38].

25.3.3 Strategies at Societal Level

Improving the Relevant Legislation In most cases, improvements at the existing legislation for the organization and access to the mental health-care system, or the formulation of a new legislation, create a formal structure in which PR programs can achieve maximum efficiency. Persons with disabilities must enjoy the same rights and benefits as those without disabilities, regardless of the cause of the disability. Legislation should cover aspects such as involuntary treatment and hospitalization, patients' rights, access to the labor market, accommodation, education, and other social benefits.

Advocacy Advocacy is a component and a purpose of PR. Users must actively participate in the planning, delivery, and evaluation of programs in PR. This empowerment of users is not simply a realization of the formal rights of patients: they also allow greater access to community resources for users and their families. This strengthening of advocacy power is one of the main strategies to enable psychiatric patients, independently of their age, to increase their citizenship status [39].

Improving Public Opinion and Attitudes Toward Mental Disorders Stigma associated with mental disorders affects not only people with mental disorders but also those who care for them, their families, and professionals. Stigma and discrimination are based on negative attitudes toward people with mental disorders and mistaken beliefs about mental disorders. These attitudes and beliefs are sometimes even present among health professionals. Changing attitudes toward mental disorders can take a long time, but legislative interventions can produce results much more quickly. The dissemination of appropriate information to patients, to their caregivers, to family members, and to the general public provides a better understanding of mental illness, of their treatment and care. It increases the capacity of individuals to participate in the organization of care and services.

25.4 Role of Primary Care

The primary care team has the initial responsibility for identifying, assessing, and managing mental health problems in older adults. The decision to refer to a specialist team is usually made in primary care. But in many countries, the current configuration of services for older adults with mental health problems will not cope with the consequences of the demographic shift that is now underway. Primary care, which has traditionally referred to specialist provision for diagnosis and management of older people with mental health problems, will need to adopt a more active role. This will entail the acquisition of new skills, particularly around psychosocial interventions, and the development of systematic care packages and pathways.

Improving the ability of primary care practitioners to identify mental health problems in older adults depends, therefore, first on recognition of the necessary preconditions for acquiring new skills. Whole health system changes would need to include policy changes at the macro-level of funding bodies, efforts at systematization of care at the meso-level of specialist service providers, and educational interventions aimed at individual professionals and workgroups at the micro-level. These changes would be different in different jurisdictions, depending on funding streams, the presence or absence of a gatekeeper function in primary care, and the availability in the community of other disciplines, like clinical psychology.

Second, practitioners' pattern recognition abilities need to be enhanced and their illness scripts made richer and deeper. The diagnostic task is rarely an easy one in the early stages of mental health problems, but it is one that primary care practitioners can master once they know what it is they are facing and what resources they can call upon.

Third, it should be given resources and skills to develop effective, and at affordable cost, management of the older adult's mental health problems in the community. Primary care professionals know much better than specialists which resources are available in the community that can be useful in a PR perspective. Primary care professionals often have also in charge the management of other health issues that may be related with the mental health problems. Too much often, the mental disorders in older adults are caused by somatic disorders and/or their treatments. Primary care professionals are in good position to detect these issues and manage the drug interactions.

For all these reasons, Primary care teams should be included in all PR program as a cost-effective valuable resource able to deliver and manage important steps of such programs in the respect of local cultural rules and habits.

25.5 The Research

Given the various aspects involved in PR, it is necessary to develop research projects that cover all the topics mentioned above. Universities, research institutes, and professionals are invited to consider the possibility of developing research activities in this area, while governments and funding agencies are strongly encouraged to consider the creation of funds specifically for activities related to PR [8].

25.6 Conclusion

Only 48% of countries in the world have developed specific mental health programs for older adults [30]. This probably explains why many people are not yet benefiting from the progress made by the PR. The most basic rights of patients are still insufficiently insured—whatever the age group—and patients are still too often victims of stigma and discrimination. That is why, in 1991, the United Nations General Assembly adopted the Principles for the Protection of People with Mental Illnesses and for the Improvement of Mental Health Care [40].

Access to care and continuity of care, especially outside the institutional circuit, are not yet sufficiently assured. Many professionals working in older adult mental health are still underqualified. On the other hand, health services remain underutilized, mainly because of the fear of stigma and discrimination related to the condition of the mentally ill [5]. The role of primary care is essential here to offer early detection of mental health problems, to start their management and support the natural caregivers in the community.

The complex interaction among physical disorders, mental disorders, and social difficulties in old age can change very quickly. That's why the rehabilitation of older adults is never completely finished. Careful planning of continuity of care, follow-up, and permanent availability of care in case of need are unavoidable necessities to ensure dignified living conditions for these people.

Indeed, it is our own dignity that is at stake: that of ensuring for older adults with mental difficulties the promotion of a life of quality and the best well-being perception.

References

1. World Health Organization. Atlas: mental health resources in the world. Geneva: WHO; 2014.
2. Organisation Mondiale De La Santé. Rapport Mondial sur le Vieillissement et la Santé. Genève: WHO; 2015.
3. de Mendonca Lima CA, Camus V. Aging and mental health: epidemiological considerations. Psiquiatr Biológica. 1996;4(4):193–8.
4. de Mendonca Lima CA, Camus V. Envelhecimento das populações e saúde mental. Informação Psiquiátr. 1995;14(3):97–9.
5. Brundtland GH. Director-General, World Health Organization. Second World Assembly on Ageing-Main Assembly Statement. Madrid, 9 avril 2002.
6. World Health Organization. World health report 2001. Geneva: WHO; 2001.
7. World Health Organization/World Psychiatric Association. Reducing stigma and discrimination against old persons with mental disorders. Geneva: WHO; 2002 (WHO/MSD/MBD/02.3).
8. de Mendonca Lima CA, Kühne N, Bertolote JM, Camus V. Psychose, réadaptation psychosociale, psychiatrie de la personne âgée: concepts et principes généraux. L'Année Gérontol. 2003;1:347–68.
9. Camus V, de Mendonca Lima CA. Psychosocial rehabilitation of the elderly with early- or late-onset schizophrenia: general principles. In: Hasset A, Ames D, Chiu E, editors. Psychosis in the elderly. London: Taylor and Francis; 2005. p. 85–96.
10. World Health Organization/World Psychiatric Association. Psychiatry of the elderly: a consensus statement. Geneva: WHO; 1996 (WHO/MNH/MND/96.7).
11. Jones R. Rehabilitation. In: Copeland JRM, Abu-Saleh MT, Blazer DG, editors. Principles and practice of geriatric psychiatry. Chichester: Wiley; 1994. p. 889–994.
12. Morin L, Franck N. Historique et fondamentaux. In: Franck N, editor. Outils de la réhabilitation psychosociale. Issy-les-Moulineaux: Elsevier Masson; 2016. p. 1–18.
13. World Health Organization/World Psychiatric Association. Organisation of care in psychiatry of the elderly: a technical consensus statement. Geneva: WHO; 1997 (WHO/MSA/MNH/MND/97.3).
14. Vidon G. La réhabilitation psychosociale en psychiatrie. Paris: Éditions Frison-Roche; 1995.
15. Pratt CW, Gill KJ, Barrett NM, Roberts MM. Psychiatric rehabilitation. San Diego: Academic Press; 1999.
16. Tessier L, Clément M. La réadaptation psychosociale en psychiatrie. Québec: Gaëtan Morin Éditeur; 1992.
17. de Mendonça Lima CA, Ivbijaro G. Editorial: mental health and wellbeing of older people: opportunities and challenges. Ment Health Fam Med. 2013;10(3):125–7.
18. de Mendonça Lima CA, Mintzer J. World Mental Health Day 2013: a day to reflect on the mental health and well-being of older people around the world. WPA News, September 2013.
19. Saraceno B. Préface. In: Vidon G, editor. La réhabilitation psychosociale en psychiatrie. Paris: Édition Frison-Roche; 1995. p. 13–5.
20. Orley J, Kuyken WQ. Quality of life assessment: international perspectives. Berlin: Springer-Verlag; 1994.
21. Guerlan B, Katz S. Quality of life and mental disorders of elders. In: Katschnig K, Freeman H, Sartorius S, editors. Quality of life in mental disorders. Chichester: Wiley; 1997.
22. World Federation for Mental Health. Dignity in mental health. WMHD Report 2015. In: Leplège A, editor. Les mesures de qualité de vie. Paris: PUF; 1999.
23. Nakagawa T. Psychological well-being in older adults. Angew Gerontol Appl. 2017;2(17):9–10.
24. Perrin T, May H. Assessing occupational capacity and wellbeing. In: Perrin T, May H, editors. Wellbeing in dementia. An occupational approach for therapists and carers. Edinburgh: Churchill Livingstone; 2000. p. 123–44.
25. Fava G. Well-being therapy. Treatment manual and clinical applications. Basel: Karger; 2016.
26. Richardson JC, Chew-Graham CA. Resilience and well-being. In: Chew-Graham CA, Tay M, editors. Mental health and older people: a guide for primary care practitioners. Switzerland: Springer; 2016. p. 9–17.
27. Hurst S. Vulnérabilité et résilience dans le grand âge. Angew Gerontol Appl. 2017;2(17):39–40.
28. Gaebel W, Rössler W, Sartorius N. The stigma of mental illness – end of the story? Switzerland: Springer; 2017.
29. World Health Organization, Commission on Social Determinants of Health. Closing the gap in a generation: health equity through action on the social determinants of health. Final Report of the Commission on Social Determinants of Health. Geneva: WHO; 2008.
30. World Health Organization and Fundacao Calouste Gulbenkian. Social determinants of mental health. Geneva: WHO; 2014.
31. O'Sullivan C. Social determinants of mental health. In: European Communities. Background document for the thematic conference: "Promoting Social

Inclusion and Combating Stigma for better Mental Health and Well-being". Luxembourg: European Communities; 2010. p. 9–14.

32. de Mendonça Lima CA. Lifespan perspective: social determinants of health and promotion of mental health in old age. In: Bährer-Kholer S, editor. Social determinants and mental health. New York: NOVA; 2012. p. 203–13.

33. World Health Organization. Investing in mental health: evidence for action. Geneva: WHO; 2013.

34. World Health Organization. Psychosocial rehabilitation: a consensus statement. Geneva: WHO; 1996 (WHO/MNH/MND/96.2).

35. Organisation Mondiale De La Santé. Classification internationale du fonctionnement, du handicap et de la santé. Genève: OMS; 2001 (WHO/EIP/GPE/CAS/ICIDH-2 F1/01.1).

36. World Health Organization/World Psychiatric Association. Education in psychiatry of the elderly: a technical consensus statement. Geneva: WHO; 1998 (WHO/MNH/MND/98.4).

37. World Health Organization. Quality assurance in mental health care. In: Check-lists and glossaries, vol. 1. Geneva: WHO; 1994 (WHO/MNH/MND/94.17).

38. World Health Organization. Quality assurance in mental health care. In: Check-lists and glossaries, vol. 1. Geneva: WHO; 1997.

39. Stengard E. Key principles for mental health promotion and mental disorder prevention in older people: ProMenPol and DataPrev projects. In: European Communities, editor. Mental health and well-being in older people–making it happen. Conclusions from the thematic conference. WHO/MSA/MNH/MND/97.2. Luxembourg: European Communities; 2010. p. 5–6.

40. United Nations. Principles for the protection of persons with mental illness and for the improvement of mental health care. Résolution 46/119 de décembre 1991 adoptée par l'Assemblée Générale des Nations Unies.

Cognitive Intervention for Patients with Neurocognitive Impairments

26

Genevieve Gagnon and Marjolaine Masson

Abstract

The prevalence of neurocognitive disorders is rising. In the last 20 years, there has been increased interest for the development of cognitive interventions to prevent the onset and/or delay the progression to dementia in at-risk older adults. Cognitive interventions are not a unitary concept. It comprises several varieties of interventions such as cognitive stimulation, cognitive training, and cognitive rehabilitation. Research suggests these treatment approaches may have a chance at improving or stabilizing cognition in patients with mild cognitive impairment. Moreover, it seems cognitive intervention would be most efficient with patients who are aware, motivated and able to remember and apply the learned skills. Indeed, data from recent literature suggests cognitive intervention should begin before the onset of manifest memory impairment and should be implemented as a form of *cognitive prevention* where patients are educated about the *modifiable risk factors* for Alzheimer's while performing cognitive training and learning new strategies.

Key Points
- Neurocognitive disorders are increasing in prevalence and in incidence due to the expanding senior demographic. Hence, there is a growing interest to develop cognitive interventions to prevent the onset and/or delay the progression to dementia in at-risk older adults.
- Cognitive intervention is not a unique concept and includes several kinds of interventions such as cognitive stimulation, cognitive training and cognitive rehabilitation.
- Cognitive training and cognitive rehabilitation should involve a skilled therapist to have a better chance of improving cognition or functioning of patients.
- Cognitive intervention would be most efficient with patients who are aware, motivated and able to remember and

G. Gagnon, Ph.D. C.Psych. (✉)
Department of Psychiatry, McGill University, Montreal, QC, Canada

Department of Psychology, McGill University, Montreal, QC, Canada

Douglas Mental Health University Institute, McGill University, Montreal, QC, Canada
e-mail: ggagnon@neuro-consults.com

M. Masson, Ph.D.
Douglas Mental Health University Institute, McGill University, Montreal, QC, Canada

© Springer Nature Switzerland AG 2019
C. A. de Mendonça Lima, G. Ivbijaro (eds.), *Primary Care Mental Health in Older People*,
https://doi.org/10.1007/978-3-030-10814-4_26

apply the learned skills. Therefore, cognitive intervention should begin before the appearance of large memory impairment and could be implement as *cognitive prevention*.

- Including information about *modifiable risk factors* (e.g., healthy life habits) in cognitive interventions could help reduce the risk of cognitive decline and dementia.

26.1 Introduction

The last few decades have been one of exponentially growing interest for neuroscience and human cognition, which led to precise characterizations of cognitive profiles in various psychiatric and neurological disorders. This allowed clinicians with an interest in intervention to use this new knowledge to develop cognitive interventions to help their patients with cognitive difficulties and complaints. Interventions can range, for example, from working with a computer, practicing a task every week, to learning how to use an agenda.

In fact, just like psychotherapy, cognitive intervention includes several types of approaches and strategies. All cognitive interventions would target cognition, but the various programs available would use different methods and have different goals. A recent literature review suggests a nomenclature: cognitive stimulation, cognitive training, and cognitive rehabilitation [1]. This nomenclature has been used in a few literature reviews [2, 3] and provides a precise shared language to refer to the various interventions in the field of cognition.

- Cognitive stimulation attempts to improve cognitive and social functioning using general mental activation (e.g., conversation, games, quizzes) [4]. This category implies using cognition without necessarily seeking metacognition (thinking about one's own mental processes). It can be used without the need of a therapist [1].
- Cognitive training aims to maintain or improve specific cognitive functions (e.g., attention or

memory), with the help of guided execution and repetition of standardized tasks [5].

- Cognitive rehabilitation aims at maintaining or improving everyday skills [5] with the use of compensatory strategies, ranging from an adaption of the environment to the use of external aids (e.g., automatic reminders). Cognitive rehabilitation is generally an individualized approach, but it also offered in group [6–9].

26.2 Epidemiology

With the growing population of older adults (aged 65 years or older) in the USA and in Canada, as well as the increased incidence of Alzheimer's disease (AD) and other progressive neurocognitive disorders, researchers and healthcare practitioners have worked collaboratively to develop and implement novel clinical care practices aimed at preventing the onset and/or delaying the progression to dementia in at-risk older adults.

Traditionally, cognitive interventions for adults with cognitive difficulties were used in rehabilitation centers, mostly with patients who were recovering from acquired brain injuries. The goal was to help these patients improve their cognition and get back to their life with compensating strategies to help, if necessary. Various approaches were used and are still used in rehabilitation centers: cognitive stimulation, cognitive training, and cognitive rehabilitation. Selecting one approach over another usually depends on (1) the level of cognitive functioning of the patient and (2) the patient treatment goals in light of (3) the expected progression of the cognitive difficulties.

Over the last two decades, with the proliferation of memory clinics and aging consortium across North America, efforts are continuously being deployed to understand and treat neurocognitive diseases. Many memory clinics and clinicians also share interests to develop and implement evidence-based cognitive intervention techniques, to help remediate the emerging cognitive deficits. The hope is such that interventions would help prevent and/or delay the progression of symptoms to dementia. Even if this field seemed promising 10 years ago [1, 10–12], few interventions have consistently proved their efficacy in AD or in MCI. Details are shown below.

26.3 Nature of the Problem Using a Life Course Approach

26.3.1 How It Differs from the Normal Aging Process Including Its Likely Effects on Cognitive, Psychological, Social, and Physical Functioning

With the growth of the aging population, neurocognitive disorders prevalence has increased. Hence, older patients tend to progressively decline cognitively and need more support. Loss of declarative memory is among the first symptoms reported by patients suffering from AD (patients struggle to form new declarative memories) [13]. Difficulties with forming new memories and learning are the hallmark of AD [14, 15]. Depending on the patient, this difficulty might interfere significantly with their ability to learn from the interventions. Moreover, those who experience difficulties with executive functioning [16–18] might struggle to transfer these learning's to daily life [19]. This is indeed a major critic to this field of intervention—patients sometimes improve on some cognitive tasks but fail to show improvement in activity of daily living [20].

In the first stages, two factors might predispose patients to experience feelings of anxiety and symptoms depression. First, at these stages, patients are generally aware that they are declining, which causes great stress, also predisposing them to depression. Secondly, as the efficiency of their problem-solving skills decline, they may be less able to address some of their daily challenges, which may further challenge their mental health [16, 19, 21]. Hence, the presence of a mood disorder is seen by many as a telling-tell signs that cognition may have to be assessed as this could be the sign of a very early cognitive decline [15, 22].

As the neurocognitive disease progresses, the patient's ability to learn new information progressively worsens, this new reality may interfere with the attempted work of the clinician. Patients also progressively lose their ability to look at themselves with perspective [18]. As the cognitive difficulties progress, patients lose insight into their difficulties, lose interest in treatment and therefore may withdraw from the intervention program. For some, there may be mild frustration of not being able to learn new material which could indeed also be discouraging for the patient, the family, and the clinicians. Interventions have to be tailored to the progressive stage of the disease, so patients could experience those little successes that are crucial to motivation. All these aspects have to be taken into consideration by the clinician who whishes to help aging patients with progressive neurocognitive diseases.

26.4 Description of the Implication for the Individual's Autonomy, Independence, and Human Rights

Autonomy One of the greater goals of such intervention is to help patients become more autonomous and independent in daily life. Therefore, some interventions target functional activities and revolve around learning how to use an electronic agenda or reminders [23, 24] which could provide reminders for appointments or cues for taking medication, for instance. Other interventions teach patients strategies to learn new information or remember the content of texts [10], while some others teach navigation strategies [25] to help patient with orientation in familiar and unfamiliar spaces. For many, the goal of the intervention is to improve cognitive functioning in activities of daily living or improve use of strategies in daily living [6, 20, 26]. Details are in the next section.

Independence Including a family member or a caregiver in the intervention, to teach this person the same strategies could help transfer the skills in daily life. Some interventions will formally include participation of a member of the family. Most interventions will at least suggest it because the help of the spouse, for example, increases the likelihood of transfer into daily life. In Canada, for instance, the program "Learning the Ropes for Living with MCI™" is offered to Toronto patients in the hope to optimize cognitive health through lifestyle choices, memory training, and psychosocial support. It is aimed at older adults with MCI and their family. Including a family member could help patients eventually become independent from the intervention.

Human Rights Eventually, for patients who experience more serious cognitive decline and lost insight into their difficulties, it becomes important to respect that their perception of the situation becomes increasingly different from those of clinicians. It is the clinician's role to accept that their own desire to help the patient may, at some point, make them become more anxious.

26.5 Management of the Problem Using a Stepped Care Framework to Include

When implementing a cognitive intervention program, one of the first steps is to identify personally relevant goals and then select strategies to achieve these goals, with respect to the existing and projected cognitive impairments [12].

Patient should be assessed soon after they start to complain about cognitive difficulties [15, 27–29]. This will not only help with diagnosis, but it will also help define the nature and the importance of their cognitive difficulties, so that the relevant interventions will be set up.

Different goals could be pursued. For instance:

- Improve cognition [10, 30].
- Improve awareness and understanding of cognition (metacognition and psychoeducation) [31].
- Improve cognitive *functioning* in activities of daily living or improve use of strategies in daily living [30].
- Improve empowerment/perceptions of cognitive abilities [30] or well-being [10].

Once realistic goals have been established, then, an array of therapeutic interventions and strategies can be put in place or taught to the patient and his family. These strategies will vary depending on the nature and severity of the deficits.

We also advise that memory clinics interested in such intervention should use the help of an expert in cognition for leading the intervention program. Neuropsychologists are trained in human psychology and cognition which enables them to adjust and understand the subtle differences between a problem with anxiety, attention, or memory, so they can understand the patients' complaints and suggest relevant interventions.

26.5.1 Diagnostic Criteria Including Assessment Tools

Before the beginning of the intervention, it is crucial to have a recent cognitive evaluation, which could be used as baseline to assess the effects of the intervention. In some cases, the screening diagnostic evaluation could be used, if recent. However, there could be variable time between the diagnostic evaluation and the beginning of the intervention, in which cases dated evaluations have to be updated. The use of alternate versions of the same test could be useful.

As mentioned before, patient should be assessed soon after they start to complain about cognitive difficulties. This will not only help with diagnosis [32, 33] but also with tailoring the intervention.

Moreover, all patients will not respond to the intervention in the same way because of inter-individual characteristics, just like in psychotherapy. Hence, baseline measures could be added, to better understand the variety of patients taking part in the intervention. Levels of (1) insight, (2) motivation, (3) openness to change, (4) number of session attended, and (5) participation during sessions could be assessed. This will help better understand the variable effect of the intervention and will help the definition of inclusion criteria in order to target the responders.

26.5.2 Specific Issues for Primary Care Assessment

Cognitive intervention would be most efficient with patients who have *subjective* cognitive complaints [3]. To insure the intervention is useful, patients have to be aware, motivated, able to remember, and apply the learned skills [34]. Therefore, it is crucial to offer the intervention as *cognitive prevention*. In cases where the cognitive symptoms become apparent and the diagnosis is clear, it means that the AD pathology has been present for many years already [32, 33, 35] and that it may be late for taking part in a cognitive intervention.

A formal diagnosis is not always needed to take part in the intervention. Depending on the type of intervention, some will be designed for patients with memory impairment [6, 10], while others could be more appropriate for patients with *subjective* memory impairments or only concerns about aging and human memory [6].

Current data shows mixed results for interventions in individual with MCI and AD. One possible explanation is that the intervention has taken place when memory and insight had already declined, limiting the possible benefits from the interventions. Future research should focus on *cognitive prevention*. Such intervention may target promotion of good life habits (e.g., the modifiable risk factors for Alzheimer's disease [36]) and teach strategies to optimize human memory [6, 37]. To hope for an impact, cognitive prevention should take place well before the onset of the first symptoms [35, 38].

In *cognitive prevention*, the intervention will not promote the idea that participants have a cognitive disorder. Rather, it should explain the basis of cognitive functioning and suggests ways to optimize its functioning (e.g., limiting distraction, using internal or external strategies, etc.). Thus, *cognitive prevention* program should be offered by a professional who has an expertise in cognitive intervention, such as a neuropsychologist [39]. Consequently, almost any concerned individual could participate in such program.

On the other hand, interventions for patients with objective memory impairment (most often MCI), the intervention could include psychoeducation [6] and could even tailor a set of interventions around acceptance of this diagnosis, for instance.

In summary, patients presenting in primary care might not always necessarily need to wait for a formal MCI diagnosis before they can receive cognitive interventions. Early *cognitive prevention* program may have greater impact if offered at the prodromal stage of the disease [35, 38].

26.5.3 Health Promotion

Current body of literature strongly suggests a link between several modifiable risk factors and a risk for cognitive decline [36, 40–43]. Some will also argue that there is sufficient evidence to suggest that some modifiable risk factors may be associated with reduced risk of dementia [40].

For instance, the Alzheimer's Association believes there is sufficiently strong evidence, from a population-based perspective, to conclude that regular physical activity and management of cardiovascular risk factors (diabetes, obesity, smoking, and hypertension) reduce the risk of cognitive decline and may reduce the risk of dementia [40]. The Association also believes there is sufficiently strong evidence to conclude that a healthy diet and lifelong learning/cognitive training may also reduce the risk of cognitive decline [40]. Hence, including information about these *modifiable risk factors* [41, 43, 44] in cognitive interventions has become central to help patients make positive changes in their life habits [45–47]. Possibly, these changes could be longer lasting when adopting a collaborative attitude with the patient while avoiding shaming and guilt. Psychoeducation followed by motivational interviewing could be useful in this context [48–50].

26.5.4 Evaluating the Cognitive Interventions

As interventions for cognitive deficits are a relatively new field, it is important to assess the impact of the intervention [6]. Several *dimensions* should be assessed: cognitive performance, daily functioning, and neuropsychiatric symptom severity. The tools used for assessing the effectiveness of cognitive rehabilitation are cognitive tests and questionnaires on activities of daily living, quality of life, and subjective perceptions.

The outcome measures should reflect the rehabilitation *goals* and expectations. If the goal of the intervention was to increase knowledge about cognition, improvement should be expected on knowledge, sense of control, perhaps mood, but little improvement should be expected in daily functioning and use of compensatory strategies in daily living.

Moreover, as patient's insight can vary with the presence of some cognitive deficits, clinical trials should include a combination of objective measures, collateral report measures, and self-report measures. Especially in psychiatry, literature on patient's *perspective* reminds the importance of assessing with both views [51]. Thus, studies should also explore aspects other than the symptoms, like the representations of illness or improvements in older adults [51]. For instance, the perceived improvement questionnaire (PIQ) is a good indicator to assess symptomatic change by patients and clinicians [51, 52].

Repeated measures could also be included within the intervention, to (1) help the patient and the clinician see potential changes, (2) identify domains of struggle, and (3) keep the troops motivated. For instance, one could use a questionnaire about self-efficacy or subjective symptoms, to help patients see the changes.

Finally, selecting tools that have good psychometric properties will help better capture and understand the effect of the intervention. Tools that are sensitive and specific will help in that sense. For example, if an improvement or maintenance of functioning within everyday context is realistically expected, then scales such as the

IADL and the ADL [53] make sense to use. However, it might not offer the most sensitive measure of reality as very large effects will be picked up by its short range.

26.5.5 Specific Recommendations for Management in Primary Care

Many studies using cognitive stimulation or cognitive training have failed to find a transfer of benefice to real-life situation [20]. This was hypothesized to be related to the lack of similarities between the practiced tasks and the reality of the patients. Moreover, patients with executive difficulties might have a hard time transferring these learnings to real-life, personal situations. Indeed, to recognize which situation is appropriate for which strategy takes good reasoning/executive functioning. Similarly, taking the initiative of applying the learned strategies to new situations that arise also requires preserved executive skills. Cognitive rehabilitation, a slightly more recent approach, addresses this problem more directly by teaching patients strategies that would be closer to their reality. An additional assumption about the difficulty of transfer is that tasks were not tailored enough to the patient's level in many cognitive programs [54]. Just like therapy, cognitive intervention approaches have to be suited to the experienced cognitive difficulties. Finally, others have argued that the failure to produce transferable benefits was also related to the assessment tools. Indeed, it is really important to select assessment methods that are coherent with the goal: if the goal is to improve cognition but the content of the intervention focuses on improving knowledge about cognition, effects of the intervention might be disappointing.

According to recent literature reviews, the *cognitive rehabilitation* approach would be better suited for training MCI participants on how to use external aids to compensate for memory difficulties because the strongest effect is in relation to compensatory strategies (i.e., cognitive rehabilitation) [55]. Another review of the literature on the efficacy of cognitive rehabilitation in MCI patients showed that compensatory methods (i.e., cognitive rehabilitation) seem to be associated with higher long-term effects on memory performance compared to restorative approaches (i.e., cognitive training) [6]. Finally, an important review about cognitive interventions for mild to moderate Alzheimer's disease did not provide evidence to support the efficacy of cognitive training, whereas cognitive rehabilitation found promising results in relation to a number of participants and caregiver outcomes and was generally of high quality [20]. According to recent literature review, *cognitive stimulation* has failed to show improvements in cognition of MCI patients, while effects of *cognitive training* are parsimonious in MCI patients [5, 20], perhaps because cognitive stimulation does not tap on metacognition, while both cognitive training and cognitive rehabilitation does. Whether the approach is cognitive training or cognitive rehabilitation, interventions that target functions such as reasoning may support top-down cognitive processes and have better chance on improving cognition in patients with MCI [56].

Also, the *expected progression* has to be taken into account. A few years ago, cognitive interventions was seen as a hopeful approach to delay, reduce, or prevent cognitive decline [57, 58] as early literature reviews on the topic were encouraging [1, 59]. Previous studies have targeted MCI in the hope to slow progression to AD, perhaps preventing or delaying further cognitive decline [60]. Currently, the research supports the application of cognitive rehabilitation for people with MCI [18, 55, 61, 62], but more and more, the field of cognitive interventions is moving toward earlier stages of the disease, pushed by literature suggesting that they have better changes of improvements [5, 20]. Recent reviews of literature [5, 20] suggest that *pre-MCI* (patients with subjective cognitive complaints) could also be a good target for prevention as they are often quite motivated and have relatively preserved cognitive abilities. Large studies with community-dwelling adults aged 65 and older showed improvements on task of memory and attention [30], speed of processing, reasoning, and memory [63]. Moreover, these training gains remained statisti-

cally and practically significant at the 5 year follow-up [64].

Technically, most patients with subjective and/or mild objective cognitive complaints could benefit from some form of cognitive intervention, if the intervention is realistically *tailored* to the patient's needs/complaints and if the patient is motivated. Working with older adults, the nature and severity of the cognitive difficulties, the learning potential, in relation to the goals of the intervention have to be kept in mind [5], to avoid missing targets! For instance, if patients show mild impairment of declarative memory and executive functioning, the learning potential of a group-base, academic style, and intervention is impeded. Also, it is recommended that patients have sufficient remaining cognitive skills to learn from the selected cognitive intervention program [5], especially if the offered intervention is a group setting, teaching approach where patient has to be attentive to a speaker and memorizing the verbally transmitted information. At the term of their literature review [5], some authors suggest patients should be enrolled at earlier stages of cognitive decline (such as pre-MCI and MCI), in order to benefit from intervention. In other words, cognitive intervention may benefit persons with milder (or preclinical) cognitive difficulties because they have the attentional, memory, and executive skills to listen, learn, and apply sets of new strategies in everyday life. These strategies could be useful immediately and/or in the future (e.g., implement the use of an electronic agenda). An eloquent example is the fact that positive observed effects of a specific cognitive intervention are not always transferable to another group of patients especially if they are cognitively more impaired that the other group.

Cognitive rehabilitation is certainly appropriate for primary care. Current literature suggests that multidisciplinary work and good communication during the referral process are key points. Because cognitive rehabilitation is a neuropsychological intervention, consultation with a neuropsychologist about the patient's cognitive profile is very often warranted. The cognitive intervention could be offered in multidisciplinarity (with occupational therapist or recreational therapist), with the involvement of the neuropsychologist, to insure that intervention is relevant and appropriate to clientele. If neuropsychological data are not available, careful description of the patients functional or subjective complaints have to be included in the referral. In a group setting, tailoring the intervention to the needs of different patients will help patient gain from this intervention. In a primary care setting, cognitive rehabilitation seems to be the most recommended intervention. If MCI or AD is suspected, referral to memory clinic should be made.

Unfortunately, clinics rarely offer cognitive rehabilitation—if only memory clinics. In these cases, arrangements should be made for primary care patients go to local memory clinics only to attend to cognitive rehabilitation programs. If the cognitive rehabilitation program is indeed offered by a neuropsychologist, this professional shall be in relevant position to detect, through the cognitive rehabilitation intervention, patients at further risk cognitive decline or patients that already have significant cognitive difficulties. Similarly, a neuropsychologist should be included in cognitive rehabilitation research projects and recruitment. The neuropsychologist could also be in charge of including the patient in a research project about cognitive rehabilitation or in a clinical group in memory clinic.

It is recommended to use a standardized "manualized" cognitive remediation program which already has shown its effectiveness. Ideally, if the program is meant to be used by many types of professionals, some background and cognitive information should be provided to guide the clinicians [39].

Suggested inclusion criteria to target good respondents (for clinical setting):

- Someone who is very motivated and wants to learn memory strategy
- Someone who has the sufficient cognitive skills to learn
- Someone who is able to concentrate for enough time

Limitations:

- We do not know how long the benefits last over time. Few studies that followed participants did show encouraging data [12, 64]. Yet, longitudinal studies are rare in this field. Moreover, in patients with neurodegenerative disease, sometimes, the benefit can be only expressed with stability in cognitive deficits but no improvement. Without proper follow-up, this hypothesis cannot be validated.
- There are a number of methodological issues including small samples, absence of longitudinal studies, lack of functional impact measures, and generalization effects [61].
- Many studies do not follow the same nomenclature (cognitive stimulation, cognitive training, cognitive rehabilitation), limiting the literature review and meta-analysis that would help the field evolve [3].

Ultimately, more *longitudinal* studies will be warranted to evaluate whether interventions are associated with a reduced conversion rate to dementia in the future. Working with MCI patients, cognitive rehabilitation therapies seem to have the potential to maintain cognitive status (i.e., prevention of dementia) rather than to reverse cognitive decline (i.e., treatment of MCI) [6]. Encouragingly, some cognitive rehabilitation studies have shown improved hippocampal thickness. Interestingly, some cognitive training studies also suggest that practicing a mental representation of space can improve hippocampal thickness [65].

26.6 Conclusions

Cognitive interventions emerged and rapidly gained popularity over the last few decades. Like psychotherapy, cognitive intervention techniques are varied and need to be constituously tailored to the patient's specific and evolving needs. Research has provided initial insight into the effectiveness of cognitive interventions. New programs are continually emerging as ongoing research is sheading new light on these treatment approaches.

References

1. Clare L, Woods RT. Cognitive training and cognitive rehabilitation for people with early-stage Alzheimer's disease: a review. Neuropsychol Rehabil. 2004;14(4):385–401.
2. Bahar-Fuchs A, Clare L, Woods B. Cognitive training and cognitive rehabilitation for persons with mild to moderate dementia of the Alzheimer's or vascular type: a review. Alzheimers Res Ther. 2013;5(4):35.
3. Jean L, Bergeron M-È, Thivierge S, Simard M. Cognitive intervention programs for individuals with mild cognitive impairment: systematic review of the literature. Am J Geriatr Psychiatry. 2010;18(4):281–96.
4. Aguirre E, Woods RT, Spector A, Orrell M. Cognitive stimulation for dementia: a systematic review of the evidence of effectiveness from randomised controlled trials. Ageing Res Rev. 2013;12(1):253–62.
5. Kasper E, Ochmann S, Hoffmann W, Schneider W, Cavedo E, Hampel H, Teipel S. Cognitive rehabilitation in Alzheimer's Disease – a conceptual and methodological review. J Prev Alzheimers Dis. 2015;2(2):142–52.
6. Huckans M, Hutson L, Twamley E, Jak A, Kaye J, Storzbach D. Efficacy of cognitive rehabilitation therapies for mild cognitive impairment (MCI) in older adults: working toward a theoretical model and evidence-based interventions. Neuropsychol Rev. 2013;23(1):63–80.
7. Storzbach D, Twamley EW, Roost MS, Golshan S, Williams RM, O'Neil M, et al. Compensatory cognitive training for operation enduring freedom/operation iraqi freedom/operation new dawn veterans with mild traumatic brain injury. J Head Trauma Rehabil. 2017;32(1):16–24. https://doi.org/10.1097/htr.0000000000000228.
8. Twamley EW, Jak AJ, Delis DC, Bondi MW, Lohr JB. Cognitive Symptom Management and Rehabilitation Therapy (CogSMART) for veterans with traumatic brain injury: pilot randomized controlled trial. J Rehabil Res Dev. 2014;51(1):59–70. https://doi.org/10.1682/jrrd.2013.01.0020.
9. Twamley EW, Thomas KR, Gregory AM, Jak AJ, Bondi MW, Delis DC, Lohr JB. CogSMART compensatory cognitive training for traumatic brain injury: effects over 1 year. J Head Trauma Rehabil. 2015;30(6):391–401. https://doi.org/10.1097/htr.0000000000000076.
10. Belleville S, Gilbert B, Fontaine F, Gagnon L, Menard E, Gauthier S. Improvement of episodic memory in persons with mild cognitive impairment and healthy older adults: evidence from a cognitive intervention program. Dement Geriatr Cogn Disord. 2006;22(5-6):486–99. https://doi.org/10.1159/000096316.
11. Londos E, Boschian K, Lindén A, Persson C, Minthon L, Lexell J. Effects of a goal-oriented rehabilitation program in mild cognitive impairment: a pilot study. Am J Alzheimers Dis Other Demen. 2008;23(2):177–83.
12. Troyer AK, Murphy KJ, Anderson ND, Moscovitch M, Craik FI. Changing everyday memory behaviour in amnestic mild cognitive impairment: a randomised controlled trial. Neuropsychol Rehabil. 2008;18(1):65–88.
13. Nestor PJ, Fryer TD, Hodges JR. Declarative memory impairments in Alzheimer's disease and semantic dementia. NeuroImage. 2006;30(3):1010–20. https://doi.org/10.1016/j.neuroimage.2005.10.008.
14. McKhann G, Drachman D, Folstein M, Katzman R, Price D, Stadlan EM. Clinical diagnosis of Alzheimer's disease: report of the NINCDS-ADRDA Work Group under the auspices of Department of Health and Human Services Task Force on Alzheimer's Disease. Neurology. 1984;34(7):939–44.
15. Storey E, Slavin MJ, Kinsella GJ. Patterns of cognitive impairment in Alzheimer's disease: assessment and differential diagnosis. Front Biosci. 2002;7:e155–84.
16. Alves MR, Yamamoto T, Arias-Carrion O, Rocha NB, Nardi AE, Machado S, Silva AC. Executive function impairments in patients with depression. CNS Neurol Disord Drug Targets. 2014;13(6):1026–40.
17. Harrington MG, Chiang J, Pogoda JM, Gomez M, Thomas K, Marion SD, Fonteh AN. Executive function changes before memory in preclinical Alzheimer's pathology: a prospective, cross-sectional, case control study. PLoS One. 2013;8(11):e79378. https://doi.org/10.1371/journal.pone.0079378.
18. Vannini P, Amariglio R, Hanseeuw B, Johnson KA, McLaren DG, Chhatwal J, Sperling RA. Memory self-awareness in the preclinical and prodromal stages of Alzheimer's disease. Neuropsychologia. 2017;99:343–9. https://doi.org/10.1016/j.neuropsychologia.2017.04.002.
19. Arean PA, Perri MG, Nezu AM, Schein RL, Christopher F, Joseph TX. Comparative effectiveness of social problem-solving therapy and reminiscence therapy as treatments for depression in older adults. J Consult Clin Psychol. 1993;61(6):1003–10.
20. Bahar-Fuchs A, Clare L, Woods B. Cognitive training and cognitive rehabilitation for mild to moderate Alzheimer's disease and vascular dementia. Cochrane Database Syst Rev. 2013;6:CD003260.
21. Cotrena C, Branco LD, Shansis FM, Fonseca RP. Executive function impairments in depression and

bipolar disorder: association with functional impairment and quality of life. J Affect Disord. 2016;190:744–53. https://doi.org/10.1016/j.jad.2015.11.007.

22. Ganguli M. Depression, cognitive impairment and dementia: why should clinicians care about the web of causation? Indian J Psychiatry. 2009;51(Suppl 1):S29–34.

23. Gillette Y, DePompei R. The potential of electronic organizers as a tool in the cognitive rehabilitation of young people. NeuroRehabilitation. 2004;19(3):233–43.

24. Hart T, Hawkey K, Whyte J. Use of a portable voice organizer to remember therapy goals in traumatic brain injury rehabilitation: a within-subjects trial. J Head Trauma Rehabil. 2002;17(6):556–70.

25. Konishi K, Bohbot VD. Spatial navigational strategies correlate with gray matter in the hippocampus of healthy older adults tested in a virtual maze. Front Aging Neurosci. 2013;5:1. https://doi.org/10.3389/fnagi.2013.00001.

26. Kinsella GJ, Mullaly E, Rand E, Ong B, Burton C, Price S, et al. Early intervention for mild cognitive impairment: a randomised controlled trial. J Neurol Neurosurg Psychiatry. 2009;80(7):730–6. https://doi.org/10.1136/jnnp.2008.148346.

27. Traykov L, Rigaud AS, Cesaro P, Boller F. Neuropsychological impairment in the early Alzheimer's disease. Encéphale. 2007;33(3 Pt 1):310–6.

28. Wolfsgruber S, Wagner M, Schmidtke K, Frolich L, Kurz A, Schulz S, et al. Memory concerns, memory performance and risk of dementia in patients with mild cognitive impairment. PLoS One. 2014;9(7):e100812. https://doi.org/10.1371/journal.pone.0100812.

29. Snitz BE, Wang T, Cloonan YK, Jacobsen E, Chang CH, Hughes TF, Ganguli M. Risk of progression from subjective cognitive decline to mild cognitive impairment: the role of study setting. Alzheimers Dement. 2018;14(6):734–42. https://doi.org/10.1016/j.jalz.2017.12.003.

30. Smith GE, Housen P, Yaffe K, Ruff R, Kennison RF, Mahncke HW, Zelinski EM. A cognitive training program based on principles of brain plasticity: results from the Improvement in Memory with Plasticity-based Adaptive Cognitive Training (IMPACT) study. J Am Geriatr Soc. 2009;57(4):594–603. https://doi.org/10.1111/j.1532-5415.2008.02167.x.

31. Carretti B, Borella E, Zavagnin M, De Beni R. Impact of metacognition and motivation on the efficacy of strategic memory training in older adults: analysis of specific, transfer and maintenance effects. Arch Gerontol Geriatr. 2011;52(3):e192–7. https://doi.org/10.1016/j.archger.2010.11.004.

32. Morris JC. Early-stage and preclinical Alzheimer disease. Alzheimer Dis Assoc Disord. 2005;19(3):163–5.

33. Sperling RA, Aisen PS, Beckett LA, Bennett DA, Craft S, Fagan AM, Phelps CH. Toward defining the preclinical stages of Alzheimer's disease: recommendations from the National Institute on Aging-Alzheimer's Association workgroups on diag-

nostic guidelines for Alzheimer's disease. Alzheimers Dement. 2011;7(3):280–92. https://doi.org/10.1016/j.jalz.2011.03.003.

34. Kallio EL, Ohman H, Hietanen M, Soini H, Strandberg TE, Kautiainen H, Pitkala KH. Effects of cognitive training on cognition and quality of life of older persons with dementia. J Am Geriatr Soc. 2018;66(4):664–70. https://doi.org/10.1111/jgs.15196.

35. Caselli RJ, Reiman EM. Characterizing the preclinical stages of Alzheimer's disease and the prospect of presymptomatic intervention. J Alzheimers Dis. 2013;33(Suppl 1):S405–16. https://doi.org/10.3233/jad-2012-129026.

36. Flicker L. Modifiable lifestyle risk factors for Alzheimer's disease. J Alzheimers Dis. 2010;20(3):803–11. https://doi.org/10.3233/jad-2010-091624.

37. McGough E, Kirk-Sanchez N, Liu-Ambrose T. Integrating health promotion into physical therapy practice to improve brain health and prevent Alzheimer Disease. J Neurol Phys Ther. 2017;41(Suppl 3, Supplement, IV STEP Special Issue):S55–s62. https://doi.org/10.1097/npt.0000000000000181.

38. Barnett JH, Hachinski V, Blackwell AD. Cognitive health begins at conception: addressing dementia as a lifelong and preventable condition. BMC Med. 2013;11:246. https://doi.org/10.1186/1741-7015-11-246.

39. Masson M, Franck N, Cellard C. Objectifs et enjeux de la remédiation cognitive en psychologie. J Neuropsychol Clin Appl. 2017;1:22–35.

40. Baumgart M, Snyder HM, Carrillo MC, Fazio S, Kim H, Johns H. Summary of the evidence on modifiable risk factors for cognitive decline and dementia: a population-based perspective. Alzheimers Dement. 2015;11(6):718–26. https://doi.org/10.1016/j.jalz.2015.05.016.

41. Chen ST, Siddarth P, Ercoli LM, Merrill DA, Torres-Gil F, Small GW. Modifiable risk factors for Alzheimer Disease and subjective memory impairment across age groups. PLoS One. 2014;9(6):e98630. https://doi.org/10.1371/journal.pone.0098630.

42. Kamer AR, Janal MN, de Leon M. Letter to the editor regarding: summary of the evidence on modifiable risk factors for cognitive decline and dementia: a population-based perspective. Alzheimers Dement. 2015;1(4):385–6. https://doi.org/10.1016/j.dadm.2015.08.003.

43. Xu W, Tan L, Wang HF, Jiang T, Tan MS, Tan L, Yu JT. Meta-analysis of modifiable risk factors for Alzheimer's disease. J Neurol Neurosurg Psychiatry. 2015;86(12):1299–306. https://doi.org/10.1136/jnnp-2015-310548.

44. Galvin JE. Prevention of Alzheimer's Disease: lessons learned and applied. J Am Geriatr Soc. 2017;65(10):2128–33. https://doi.org/10.1111/jgs.14997.

45. Farhud DD. Impact of lifestyle on health. Iran J Public Health. 2015;44(11):1442–4.

46. Gardner B, Lally P, Wardle J. Making health habitual: the psychology of 'habit-formation' and general prac-

tice. Br J Gen Pract. 2012;62(605):664–6. https://doi.org/10.3399/bjgp12X659466.

47. Young S. Healthy behavior change in practical settings. Perm J. 2014;18(4):89–92. https://doi.org/10.7812/tpp/14-018.

48. Ng JY, Ntoumanis N, Thogersen-Ntoumani C, Deci EL, Ryan RM, Duda JL, Williams GC. Self-determination theory applied to health contexts: a meta-analysis. Perspect Psychol Sci. 2012;7(4):325–40. https://doi.org/10.1177/1745691612447309.

49. Soderlund LL, Madson MB, Rubak S, Nilsen P. A systematic review of motivational interviewing training for general health care practitioners. Patient Educ Couns. 2011;84(1):16–26. https://doi.org/10.1016/j.pec.2010.06.025.

50. Britt E, Hudson SM, Blampied NM. Motivational interviewing in health settings: a review. Patient Educ Couns. 2004;53(2):147–55. https://doi.org/10.1016/s0738-3991(03)00141-1.

51. Potes A, Gagnon G, Toure EH, Perreault M. Patient and clinician assessments of symptomatology changes on older adults following a psycho-educational program for depression and anxiety. Psychiatr Q. 2016;87(4):649–62. https://doi.org/10.1007/s11126-016-9416-4.

52. Perreault M, Pawliuk N, Veilleux R, Rousseau M. Qualitative assessment of mental health service satisfaction: strengths and limitations of a self-administered procedure. Community Ment Health J. 2006;42(3):233–42.

53. Lawton MP, Brody EM. Assessment of older people: self-maintaining and instrumental activities of daily living. The Gerontologist. 1969;9(3):179–86.

54. Jaeggi SM, Buschkuehl M, Jonides J, Shah P. Short- and long-term benefits of cognitive training. Proc Natl Acad Sci. 2011;108(25):10081–6.

55. O'Sullivan M, Coen R, O'Hora D, Shiel A. Cognitive rehabilitation for mild cognitive impairment: developing and piloting an intervention. Aging Neuropsychol Cognit. 2015;22(3):280–300.

56. Mudar RA, Chapman SB, Rackley A, Eroh J, Chiang HS, Perez A, et al. Enhancing latent cognitive capacity in mild cognitive impairment with gist reason-

ing training: a pilot study. Int J Geriatr Psychiatry. 2017;32(5):548–55. https://doi.org/10.1002/gps.4492.

57. Mowszowski L, Batchelor J, Naismith SL. Early intervention for cognitive decline: can cognitive training be used as a selective prevention technique? Int Psychogeriatr. 2010;22(4):537–48. https://doi.org/10.1017/s1041610209991748.

58. Naismith SL, Glozier N, Burke D, Carter PE, Scott E, Hickie IB. Early intervention for cognitive decline: is there a role for multiple medical or behavioural interventions? Early Interv Psychiatry. 2009;3(1):19–27. https://doi.org/10.1111/j.1751-7893.2008.00102.x.

59. Gates NJ, Sachdev PS, Fiatarone Singh MA, Valenzuela M. Cognitive and memory training in adults at risk of dementia: a systematic review. BMC Geriatr. 2011;11:55. https://doi.org/10.1186/1471-2318-11-55.

60. Albert MS, DeKosky ST, Dickson D, Dubois B, Feldman HH, Fox NC, Petersen RC. The diagnosis of mild cognitive impairment due to Alzheimer's disease: recommendations from the National Institute on Aging-Alzheimer's Association workgroups on diagnostic guidelines for Alzheimer's disease. Alzheimers Dement. 2011;7(3):270–9.

61. Belleville S. Cognitive training for persons with mild cognitive impairment. Int Psychogeriatr. 2008;20(01):57–66.

62. Clare L, van Paasschen J, Evans SJ, Parkinson C, Woods RT, Linden DE. Goal-oriented cognitive rehabilitation for an individual with Mild Cognitive Impairment: behavioural and neuroimaging outcomes. Neurocase. 2009;15(4):318–31.

63. Tennstedt SL, Unverzagt FW. The ACTIVE Study: study overview and major findings. J Aging Health. 2013;25(8):3S–20S. https://doi.org/10.1177/0898264313518133.

64. Willis SL, Tennstedt SL, Marsiske M, Ball K, Elias J, Koepke KM, Wright E. Long-term effects of cognitive training on everyday functional outcomes in older adults. JAMA. 2006;296(23):2805–14. https://doi.org/10.1001/jama.296.23.2805.

65. Konishi K, Bohbot VD. Spatial navigational strategies correlate with gray matter in the hippocampus of healthy older adults tested in a virtual maze. Front Aging Neurosci. 2013;20(5):1.

Part VIII

From Theory to Practice

Gabriel Ivbijaro, Carlos Augusto de Mendonça Lima,
Lucja Kolkiewicz, and Yaccub Enum

Abstract

Families play a significant role in the care of older adults. Some of these family carers are older adults themselves and have their own healthcare needs. This 'informal care' is usually provided 24 h a day and often goes unnoticed and can have detrimental effects on the mental and physical health of family carers. Health and social care services need to be mindful of this and put systems in place to support family carers. The cases presented here highlight the need for primary care services to work with other stakeholders providing health and social care services, including families in order to provide holistic care for older adults.

G. Ivbijaro (✉)
NOVA University, Lisbon, Portugal

Waltham Forest Community and Family Health
Services, London, UK

C. A. de Mendonça Lima
Unit of Old Age Psychiatry, Centre Les Toises
Lausanne, Lausanne, Switzerland

L. Kolkiewicz
NOVA University, Lisbon, Portugal

East London NHS Foundation Trust, London, UK

Y. Enum
East London NHS Foundation Trust, London, UK

Public Health Department, London Borough
of Waltham Forest, London, UK

27.1 Introduction to Case Vignettes

The following six case examples come from those who plan and pay for services and clinicians who work with older adults with mental health difficulties.

They have been brought together to highlight some of the challenges in the delivery of mental health care to older adults in different parts of the world and demonstrate some of the possibilities.

Some of the case examples may resonate with your practice and provide you with an opportunity to reflect upon your own daily practice. All the case vignettes irrespective of country and economic development remind us that families continue to carry the greatest burden for the care of older adults when they are ill. Efforts and initiatives need to be developed to support families and carers in order to avoid mental ill health in carers and carer burnout.

Case Vignette One from London in the UK has been chosen to demonstrate the value of joint working in order to provide a rapid response when older adults suffer deterioration in their health. It also highlights the need to support carers. It provides a framework that others can adopt if they wish to develop a similar service.

Case Vignette Two from Argentina has been chosen because it reminds us that older adults who present with mental distress can also be carers for others. It also highlights that chronic benzodiazepine usage in the older population should

C. A. de Mendonça Lima, G. Ivbijaro (eds.), *Primary Care Mental Health in Older People*,
https://doi.org/10.1007/978-3-030-10814-4_27

be managed to decrease the morbidity and mortality associated with this medication.

Case Vignette Three from Brazil has been chosen to highlight the need to recognize that loneliness occurs in older adults even though they may be living with members of their family. It also reminds us that staff in emergency departments need to be trained to diagnose and manage delirium which was missed at this ladies first presentation to the emergency department.

Case Vignette Four from Romândia has been chosen to highlight the need for end-of-life care when dealing with dementia.

Case Vignette Five from Turkey has been chosen because it highlights the need for hope when we manage older adults with dementia, particularly those with vascular type dementia.

Case Vignette Six from Poland was chosen because it shows the need to respect the patient's dignity and autonomy, and shows that older adults are never too old to study.

The key messages are a quick guide to each case vignette which highlight the need for primary, community and secondary care collaboration including the role of families as partners. Collaborative care works and is cost-effective because each partner in the collaboration brings their own unique skills to support the individual.

27.2   Case Vignette One

27.2.1 Reducing Emergency Hospital Admissions for People with Dementia: A Case Study from the London Borough of Waltham Forest in London

Janice Richards, Gabriel Ivbijaro, Yaccub Enum, Lucja Kolkiewicz and Christopher Soltysiak

Key Messages
- Older adults are prone to multi-morbidity leading to recurrent hospitalization. Many admissions are preventable with appropriate care packages and support.

- Collaborative care is a useful model for managing people with dementia and preventing inappropriate emergency hospital admissions.
- Unpaid family carers play an important role in the care of people with dementia. Care plans for the person with dementia should include support for the carer.
- A logic model provided a useful framework by looking at the care pathway and considering inputs, interventions and outputs.
- It is important to have a rapid escalation process to deal with UTIs (urinary tract infections) to prevent unnecessary emergency hospital admission.

Case Vignette Mrs. A suffers from dementia, lives at home with her son and receives five visits a day from a care worker as part of her care package. Her son is an unpaid, informal carer and keeps his mother company throughout the day, and cares for her throughout the night.

During a visit from the care worker Mrs. A's son described feeling isolated and was finding it increasingly difficult to cope with his mother's condition and said that at times he had felt like walking away from the situation he found himself in.

The care worker noticed that Mrs. A was aggressive towards her son who told the care worker that his mother was shouting during the night and appeared to be experiencing visual hallucinations. The care worker suspected that a urinary tract infection was causing this behaviour.

The care worker reviewed the plan and asked for the rapid response team to be contacted to carry out a home visit and manage Mrs. A's physical health.

The rapid response team is a nurse led team who are able to deliver oral and parenteral treatment in the community and whose role is to work in collaboration with the general practitioner and local authority services with patient who is too complex for the general practitioner alone to manage in order to avoid hospital admission.

The rapid response team diagnosed and treated the urinary tract infection and liaised with the memory service mental health team who were also providing Mrs. A with care.

The rapid response team provided Mrs. A's son with information and education about his mother's condition and because he said that he was finding it difficult to cope he was referred to the local carer support service.

This type of presentation is not unusual when working with older adults and services need to be designed to support older adults to remain in the community. Because older adults often have multiple conditions they need a team of people around them who are able to work collaboratively to ensure that all the needs an older adult and their carers can be met.

Introduction There has been emphasis on the need for collaborative care in many chapters of this book because many older adults have multiple medical and social problems. Getting the best outcomes requires systems that can support the multiple needs of older adults.

A Cochrane review provides evidence to support collaborative care in health systems but notes that it is more difficult to demonstrate that this is the case for health and social care working together [1].

The Waltham Forest model from the UK is being presented to demonstrate that it is possible for health and social care to work collaboratively for the benefit of the older adult population. The Waltham Forest model is based on collaborative care between general practitioners and their team who are responsible for providing primary care, community mental health nurses for older people, the Memory Clinic comprising psychologists and psychiatrists that care for older adults, Adult Social Care provided by local government and the voluntary sector (non-government organizations) including Carers First and Alzheimer's Society who provide education and support for older adults with dementia to their families and carers.

The emphasis of this service re-design has been to ensure that older adults with dementia receive holistic care that takes into account all their needs by using community assets to ensure that appropriate social and clinical resources are available to the older adult using a collaborative care model.

The intervention has been developed using the Institute for Health Improvement's Plan-Do-Study-Act (PDSA) [2] approach to transformation. This approach focuses on testing a change by planning it, trying it and observing the results, then acting on what is learned.

This case study demonstrates that with the patients' needs at the centre, collaboration is achievable across health, social care and the voluntary sector by addressing clinical needs in parallel with social needs and by task shifting. In the Waltham Forest new model of care older adults at risk of dehydration are identified early using a joint health and social care assessment. Appropriate plans are put in place to support adequate hydration. Such tasks can be performed by any appropriately trained member of the team who is tasked to ensure that this happens.

Older adults are at increased risk of falls and many falls are preventable. In the Waltham Forest example falls risk assessments that have been traditionally carried out by health staff have been shifted to the Alzheimer's Society (a voluntary sector non-government organization) so that health staff can be deployed to deal with more complex medical tasks.

This UK example demonstrates how a local Clinical Commissioning Group (those who commission and pay for health services) has worked with its key health and social care partners to address high levels of emergency care and treatment in hospital for older adults with the diagnosis of dementia.

National Context There were an estimated 850,000 people living with dementia in the UK in 2015, with numbers projected to rise to over one million by 2025 and to two million by 2051 [3].

Box 27.1: UK Dementia Facts
- An estimated 1 in 6 people over the age of 80 has dementia.
- Two-thirds of the cost of dementia is paid for by people with dementia and their families.

- Unpaid carers supporting someone with dementia save the economy £11 billion a year.
- Dementia is one of the main causes of disability later in life, ahead of cancer, cardiovascular disease and stroke.

Alzheimer's Society [4].

The impact on hospitals of rising emergency admissions poses a serious challenge to both dementia services and the financial position of the NHS. Older adults accounted for more than half of the growth in emergency admissions between 2013 and 2014 and 2016 and 2017. Some of this is down to demographic change. Between 2013 and 2014 and 2016 and 2017, the number of people aged 65 and over grew by 6.2%. However, over the same period, emergency admissions for people aged 65 and over grew by 12%, almost twice the rate of population growth. The demographic pressure will only increase as the number of people aged 65 and over is projected to increase by a further 20% between 2017 and 2027 [5–9].

27.2.1.1 Local Context

Background: Overview of London
London is the capital of England and is divided into 32 boroughs. London's population of over 8.6 million makes up 13% of the UK's population. The city's population is growing faster than the rate of the UK as a whole. There are health inequalities and high levels of Black and Minority Ethnic Groups within London boroughs compared to the rest of England, which are manifested in variation in life expectancy at birth—from 82.4 years to 86.2 years in females and 77.5 years to 82.6 years in males. The top five risk factors contributing to disability and premature death in London are smoking, obesity, alcohol, high blood pressure and prediabetes [10].

Waltham Forest
The London Borough of Waltham Forest is in the North East of London, with an estimated 2018 population of 283,500. The older adult (age 65+) population estimate is 29,500 (10.4% of the population). Waltham Forest is an ethnically diverse borough with a relatively young population. The 2011 Census data show that Waltham Forest's Black, Asian and Minority Ethnic (BAME) population represents 47.8% of the total population. This is the eighth highest BAME percentage in London [11].

The overall population of Waltham Forest is expected to continue growing; however, the rate of increase is projected to be highest in children of school age (5–19 years) and oldest (80+) sections of the population. The population aged 65+ is estimated to increase by 61% over the next 20 years. This increase in the population of older adults has implications for health and social care, in particular dementia services, as the prevalence of dementia increases with age.

The gender split in the borough is about 50/50 with an equal number of women and men living here. However, there is a gender imbalance with roughly 3000 more women than men in the older cohort aged 65 and older. Women also live longer than men by 5 years on average in the borough.

The 2015 Index of Multiple Deprivation (IMD) scores show that Waltham Forest is the seventh most deprived borough in London, and 35th in England. Even though this is a slight improvement compared to the previous ranking in 2011, many areas in the borough still face very high levels of deprivation, and the associated problems for health and well-being.

Life expectancy varies significantly within the borough. For example, the difference in life expectancy between the most affluent and poorest parts of the borough is 5.3 years for men and 5.5 years for women.

Summary of Health Needs Waltham Forest in the Older Adults
Cardiovascular disease (CVD) is the biggest killer of those aged 75 and under. This is not significantly different to the London averages but the mortality rate is not evenly distributed across the borough. There are significantly higher rates in the poorer wards compared to more affluent areas. In addition, cardiovascular disease mortality is

significantly above both the London and national average [11]. High prevalence of CVD has implications for dementia, as CVD increases the risk for dementia. For example, reduced cerebral blood flow due to heart disease of any kind worsens the vascular homeostasis of the brain and has been seen as a precursor to vascular dementia and Alzheimer's disease.

Health related quality of life for older adults is equal to the London average but below the national average, and excess winter deaths are above average. There are poor outcomes for falls patients. Hospital admissions for falls and associated injuries, and mortality from fracture of femur for the 65 to 84 years age group in Waltham Forest are significantly higher than similar areas.

The Waltham Forest Health and Wellbeing Strategy 2016–2020 notes that on average 4956 years of life are lost annually in Waltham Forest due to causes that are amenable to healthcare [12]. These are deaths that should not occur in an environment of timely and effective healthcare.

Dementia Admissions

Recorded prevalence of dementia in Waltham Forest GP practices ranges from 1.5% to 10.2%. Older adults make up a significant proportion hospital admissions. The most common reasons for admission to hospital for people with Dementia are urinary tract infection, pneumonia and falls. People with Dementia should not be admitted to hospital with urinary tract infections if their care planning is robust. This is a quality and outcomes framework (QOF) requirement for GPs but Alzheimer's Society staff is also involved in care planning.

We also know that dementia diagnosis and related depression is under recorded. Depression is often diagnosed in the early stages of dementia, but it may come and go, and may be present at any stage. Depression is also common among family carers supporting a person with dementia. Nationally there has been a big push to improve psychiatric liaison services in order to provide integrated services between acute and mental health services.

Waltham Forest CCG published its Mental Health Strategy "Better Mental Health" in 2014 and this included investment for improved psychiatric liaison services at Whipps Cross Hospital, in Leytonstone, London.

Despite this, Waltham Forest has a higher spend on emergency department attendance compared to similar areas. Secondary uses services (SUS) data show that there has been an increase in emergency hospital admissions for people with dementia. The total cost of emergency admissions for people with dementia was £5.4 m in 2017/18. That was a 10% increase from the previous year. In addition, cost per episode of inpatient stay for people with dementia is higher in Waltham Forest than other boroughs. A comparison of inpatient cost per episode in seven CCGs found that Waltham Forest had the second highest cost—11% more than the lowest.

As these emergency admissions are preventable, stakeholders came together to find ways of addressing the problem. The Waltham Forest example illustrates how multi-agency collaboration involving commissioners, primary care, social care and NGOs working in partnership with carers can help reduce emergency admissions for UTI in people with dementia which in turn will reduce admissions for UTI, sepsis, pneumonia, and falls.

Interventions and Model of Care

The logic model in Fig. 27.1 derived from IHI Qi methodology shows (from right to left) the inputs, activities/interventions and outputs. A multipronged approach was used, starting from the award of care package contracts through brokerage. Dehydration was found to be a key feature in many of these patients. To address this, care packages for people with dementia, whether cared for in their own homes or in institutions, were designed to include a requirement for fluid monitoring. Providers of these services are being urged to ensure they monitor hydration, which is a good practice and support dignity in the care of older adults (Fig. 27.2).

To embed this change and scale it up across the whole local health economy the CCG and local authority are working together to introduce incentives in future to scale up the intervention across the whole of our local older adult population.

Fig. 27.1 Map of London showing the boroughs

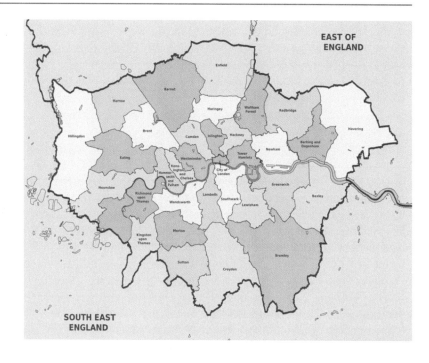

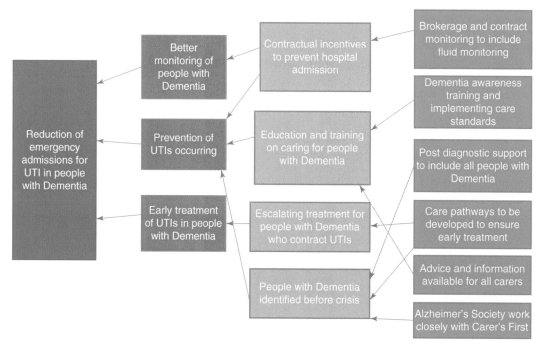

Fig. 27.2 Public Health England (2019) Introduction to Logic Models

This will be made possible by the savings released due to a decrease in hospital admissions. Many payments and incentives in health care are for treatment interventions but the emphasis in this model is on incentives for prevention.

The period following a diagnosis of dementia is often very challenging and could be traumatic for families, leading to increased use of emergency services. Therefore post-diagnostic support, which is available to anyone diagnosed with dementia and their families, now includes risk assessment as well as the service being first point of contact if there are problems.

Minimum care standards have been agreed and in the near future care providers will be required to provide dementia awareness training for all their staff. Alzheimer's Society, a leading NGO in dementia, are working with people who have a diagnosis of dementia living at home and their carers to ensure that advice and relevant information are made available to the carers, who are mostly family members. These initiatives have resulted in more people with dementia being identified before crisis.

Care pathways were developed to ensure seamless transitions between different levels of care, for example, primary and secondary care. This included developing a simplified tool to ensure that carers and people with dementia understand the risk factors of UTIs and prevent them. However if UTIs still occur, families are supported in rapid escalation to the rapid response team, a nurse led cost-effective service that is easy to set up, or to their general practitioners.

Outcomes
The collaborative approach benefits the whole health and care economy with three main outcomes:

- Better monitoring of people with dementia.
- Reduction in admission and readmission to hospital for UTIs, pneumonia, falls and sepsis in people with dementia, not just UTIs. Quick access to the rapid response team leading to avoidance of hospital admission where appropriate.

The first 3 months of this service re-design resulted in a reduction in emergency admissions for UTI in people with dementia and over 50% of the target reduction set for the first 6 months of this project was achieved in 3 months.

Conclusion This example demonstrates that multi-agency collaboration at a local level helps prevent inappropriate hospital admission for dementia patients whilst providing improved access to practical and emotional patient and carer support.

The case summary set the wider context of dementia in the UK and locally in London and Waltham Forest. It then set out how a logic model was used in a multi-pronged approach to improve outcomes for people living with dementia and their families. The project is only a few months old but already showing encouraging results. The target 6-month reduction in hospital admissions that was set at the beginning is on course to being achieved, as over 50% had been achieved in the first 3 months,

This case example from the UK shows that it is possible for health and social care to work collaboratively for the benefit of the older adult population.

27.3 Case Vignette Two

27.3.1 Generalized Anxiety Disorder in an Older Adult

Alicia Beatriz Kabanchik

27.3.1.1 Reason for Choosing This Case Example

This case from Argentina has been chosen because it helps to remind us that older adults who present with mental distress can also be carers for others and chronic benzodiazepine usage in the older population should be managed to decrease the morbidity and mortality associated with this.

National Context Argentina
According to the 2010 National Census (INDEC in Argentina) of the 40,117,096 inhabitants, 20,593,330 are women, and 19,523,766 are men. 9.8% are 60 to 74 years old and 4.5% are 75 and over.

A characteristic of the older adult population in Argentina is that women are in the majority and life expectancy in Argentina is 77 years for men and 81 years for women.

There have been no specific epidemiological studies of older adults in Argentina until the 2015 Argentine Study of

Epidemiology in Mental Health carried out by APSA (The Association of Argentine Psychiatrists, the University of Buenos Aires). This confirmed a treatment gap in the mental health care of older adults.

This highlights the need to improve collaboration between the community, primary care and secondary care to ensure that more people who require treatment receive it.

Key Messages

Late onset anxiety disorders are common in older adults.

Late onset anxiety disorder has high comorbidity with depression, medical illness, alcoholism and dementia.

Use of benzodiazepines (BZ) can worsen symptoms of anxiety disorder and their use should be avoided when possible.

Case History and Mental State Examination

A 79-year-old retired female. She married when she was 24 years old and lives with her 82-year-old husband who has cognitive impairment. She has a good relationship with her three grown up daughters and 5 years ago was treated with psychotherapy for 1 year following the onset of her husband's illness.

She was the victim of a robbery 3 years ago and lost her cardiologist who she had known for many years when he recently died.

She is a non-smoker.

She presented for psychiatric assessment accompanied by her daughter in June 2018 and reported a 7 month history of anxiety, insomnia, pains, fears, excessive worries about her hypertension and her economic future because she had become aware of her age.

She had a past medical history of hysterectomy aged 38 years and renal stones aged 50 years. She was suffering from hypertension, hypertrophic cardiomyopathy, irritable bowel syndrome and hypothyroidism.

On presentation the patient it was prescribed:

- Levothyroxine (50 mcg) for hypothyroidism
- Verapamil (160 mg) and Atenolol (50 mg) for her cardiac pathology
- Myopospan (400 mg) for irritable bowel syndrome
- Alprazolam (1 mg) for anxiety

Mental state examination revealed a well presented lady with decreased attention and concentration. Speech was coherent and spontaneous. Subjective mood was sad and anxious. Objectively she appeared depressed with decreased motivation, altered sleep and diminished appetite. She denied suicidal ideation. There was no evidence of hallucination, delusions or passivity experiences at the time of examination. She was well orientated with no evidence of cognitive impairment and had insight into her condition.

Differential Diagnosis

- Generalized anxiety disorder DSM V (300.02) and ICD 10 (F 41.1)
- Persistent depressive disorder (dysthymia) DSM V (300.4) and ICD 10 (F 34.1)
- Caregiver burnout syndrome

Investigations

Psychological testing:

- Hamilton anxiety rating scale, (HARS): score 16 (moderate to severe anxiety)
- Geriatric depression scale (GDS) 15 items: score 7 (moderate depression)
- MMSE: 29/30
- Clock drawing test (CDT): score 8/10
- Zarit Care Burden Interview (ZCBI): score 50/88 (moderate to severe burden)

Laboratory testing:

- Urea and electrolytes
- Liver function tests
- Blood sugar
- Uric acid
- Cholesterol and triglycerides
- VDRL
- Thyroid function tests including thyroid antibodies
- Calcium and phosphate
- Full blood count
- Erythrocyte sedimentation (ESR)
- B12
- Folic acid
- 25 hydroxy vitamin D
- Homocysteine
- Creatinine phosphokinase (CPK)
- Urinalysis

   All laboratory testing normal

Other investigations:

- Brain CAT without contrast: No pathology
- ECG: Findings were in keeping with the patients cardiac pathology

Management Plan

- The patient had been taking 1 mg of Alprazolam for several years and the use of benzodiazepines is not advisable in the elderly because it is addictive and increases the risk of delirium and falls and their complications.

- A plan to withdraw benzodiazepines was developed in consultation with the patient and her daughters who are her carers.
- Alprazolam has a half-life of 6–12 h in adults and up to 20 h in older adults and was discontinued following washout.
- It was initially substituted with clonazepam which was gradually discontinued in order to avoid benzodiazepine withdrawal syndrome taking into account the half-life of this medication.
- Following ECG and consultation with the cardiologist the patient was commenced on a serotonin reuptake inhibitor (SSRI) sertraline at a starting dose of 25 mg daily gradually increased to 50 mg daily.
- Weekly psychodynamic psychotherapy re-commenced including movement therapy, relaxation music and a symbiotic food diet.
- With the support of her daughters the patient re-established her social networks and activities.
- Her hypertension, hypertrophic cardiomyopathy, irritable bowel syndrome and hypothyroidism were managed in collaboration with the specialists already known to her and managing these conditions.

Outcome

The patient made a good recovery with decreased anxiety because her daughters brought her to see the psychiatrist early in the presentation and participated in her treatment plan. They recognized that their mother was also experiencing caregiver burnout and were able to provide additional support by assisting with the care of their father. This care package helped to reduce symptoms and prevent the patient's condition becoming chronic.

Wider Lessons

- Older adults who present to specialists can also be carers and this must be taken into account in the formulation and management plan.
- Engaging families and carers in the management plan is essential to achieve the best outcomes.
- Collaborative care between mental health specialists, primary care and other secondary care specialists who manage older adults is essential to manage multi-morbidity because it is cost-effective and enables better decision making.
- It is very important to raise awareness of the need for interdisciplinary work with the primary care physician so that this becomes the detector and referral to the psychiatrist for diagnosis and appropriate therapeutic approach avoiding the pathology becoming chronic.

27.4 Case Vignette Three

27.4.1 Delirium in an Older Patient Who First Presented with Major Depressive Disorder

Lilian Scheinkman

27.4.1.1 Reason for Choosing This Case Example

This case vignette from Brazil has been chosen to highlight the need to recognize that loneliness occurs in older adults even though they may be living with members of their family. The diagnosis of delirium was missed at this ladies first presentation to the emergency department which highlights the need for staff in emergency departments to be trained to diagnose and manage this condition.

National Context Brazil

Whilst the aging of the population is a worldwide phenomenon, in Brazil the number of individuals aged 60 or above rose from three million in 1960 to seven million in 1975 and 14 million in 2002 representing an increase in 500% in 40 years. It is expected to reach 32 million in 2020. One of the consequences of this process is an increasing demand of this rapidly growing population for health services [13].

The Health Ministry created the "Política Nacional de Saúde do Idoso—PNSI (Health Policy for the elderly)" in 1999 to promote healthy aging, prevent diseases and preserve, improve and rehabilitate functional capacity in order to ensure that the elderly can function independently in the society [14].

The "Estatuto do idoso", a federal law regulating the rights and needs of the elderly, in effect since January 2004, was another important step. In 2006, the Health Ministry created the National Policy for the Health of the Elderly Person—PNSPI, emphasizing the implementation of actions and the institutional responsibilities required to achieve preservation of functional capacity, autonomy and quality of life of the elderly person, in accordance with the principles of the SUS (Sistema Único de Saúde), Brazilian Unified Health Care system.

Despite these advances, the SUS (Sistema Único de Saúde) is not yet able to meet the needs of this population [15]. Health care delivery is fragmented, health information is not shared among health care providers and there is a lack of coordinated care [16].

Case History

Mrs. R is a 90-year-old widowed lady from Rio de Janeiro, Brazil who, in 2017, was brought to the Geriatric Outpatient Clinic by her son in a wheelchair, drowsy and not interacting having fallen and hit her head 2 days before.

Her son reported that 2 days before this fall Mrs. R had started seeing little animals and said "they were so real that she tried killing them with her slippers". She had to be fed by family members and was no longer capable of taking care of activities of daily living (ADLs). She was taken to the emergency care unit of a local hospital, diagnosed with hyponatremia and dehydration, received treatment and was discharged home. Two days after being discharged, her family brought her to a geriatric clinic and she was immediately transferred to the emergency room at Pedro Ernesto University Hospital (HUPE) and a psychiatric consultation was requested.

Mrs. R's level of consciousness was decreased, attention was impaired, she had very little interaction, was lethargic and unable to engage in the interview. Speech was slow and she was disoriented to time. Her son's report was consistent with recent visual hallucinations but there was no evidence of hallucinations or delusional beliefs during the psychiatric evaluation. Hypoactive delirium was diagnosed.

Mrs. R had a past history of depression treated by a private psychiatrist from 2013 to 2016 and had previously presented to the geriatric outpatient clinic of the Pedro Ernesto University Hospital in September 2016 accompanied by her daughter complaining of "dizziness, difficulty hearing, urinary incontinence and a lack of interest and pleasure in her daily activities". She presented with low body weight and a history of four falls during that same year.

Her husband had died in May 2014, following a 6-month illness during which Mrs. R was his main carer. She described having no friends and feeling lonely. She spent her days at home watching television, listening to the radio and doing crossword puzzles. She lived with her two unemployed sons, one with COPD and the other with bipolar affective disorder.

Her past medical history included bilateral cataract surgery approximately 10 years before, hypertension, irritable bowel syndrome and osteoporosis and physical examination showed a systolic murmur and she met criteria for age-related frailty.

Mini-mental state examination (MMSE) was 28/30, and registration and recall were 3/3. Clock drawing test was normal. In order to evaluate Mrs. R's functional status and help with planning her care, the KATZ (index of independence in activities of daily living) was used and she scored 5/6, indicating slight impairment, and the Lawton scale of instrumental activities of daily living was administered, in which she scored 7/8.

Mrs. R was diagnosed with major depressive disorder (MDD) and managed with escitalopram, psychotherapy and psychosocial interventions. She experienced an episode of agitation and disorientation which responded to a change in antidepressant medication from sertraline to mirtazapine with resolution of these symptoms. Five months later Mrs. R was asymptomatic. She was also attending psychotherapy and was followed by the Social Work Services to help with her situation at home.

Investigations
Laboratory testing:
- Full blood count
- Electrolytes and blood sugar
- Renal tests
- Liver function tests
- Thyroid function tests
- Urinalysis

The only abnormalities found were:

- Sodium 128 mEq/L
- Blood glucose 188 mg/dL

Other investigations:
- Brain CT scan: No acute changes

Differential Diagnosis
Hypoactive delirium

Management Plan
- There was no evidence of urinary tract infection.
- Her sodium and glucose levels were managed.
- Her cardiovascular medication was also reviewed.

Outcome
- She was successfully discharged from hospital and was seen for follow-up 1 month later.
- She walked in unaided, was alert, her level of consciousness was normal.
- She described her mood as "a bit sad".

Wider Lessons
- Since the elderly are more prone to developing delirium and this diagnosis can carry serious or even fatal consequences, it should always be kept in mind when evaluating older adults.
- A previous diagnosis of any mental illness does not preclude a future diagnosis of delirium. Mood symptoms can and many times are present in a delirious patient as part of the neurocognitive disorder, regardless of whether the patient had presented with these symptoms before or has/had a psychiatric disorder.
- Early detection of cognitive changes is crucial for prompt identification and treatment of delirium. Studies have revealed that most patients referred for psychiatric consultation services with purported depression are ultimately found to have delirium [17].
- The use of screening protocols by clinicians and referring these patients for psychiatric consultation are important tools for improving care.
- A multi-professional, interdisciplinary team of geriatricians, nurses, social workers, nutritionists, physical therapists, speech therapists, psychologists and pharmacists who work with older adults with the goal of health promotion, prevention and rehabilitation improves quality of care.
- Brazil has made definite advances in health care delivery to the elderly, but there is still room to improve and a need to integrate and coordinate care throughout each patient's trajectory in the health system because interdisciplinary, coordinated care is key to a good outcome and should be our ultimate goal in delivering optimal health care.

27.5 Case Vignette Four

27.5.1 Dementia in Alzheimer's Disease

Nicoleta Tătaru

27.5.1.1 Reason for Choosing This Case Example

This case from România has been chosen because it considers the need for planning for end-of-life care when managing cases of dementia.

National Context România

România is a developing former communist country in Eastern Europe with a population of 21.794.793 (2002) and covers 237.500 square km with 42 districts. National statistics for 2002 showed infant death rate 17, 3/1000 and life expectancy at birth 67.6 years for males and 71.1 year for female. In România around 12–14% of the general population are over 65, compared with the rest of Europe, where 14–16% is over 65 (WHO). It is estimated that the number of person with dementia in România will be approximately 600,000 in 2025 (WHO).

România remains currently in a period of transition from communism to democracy. România like other Eastern Europe countries is at the geographical border between the West, the Middle East and Asia. Like other former communist countries, România remained behind the Iron Curtain until December 1989. In January 2007, România became member of EU. In the last few years, in most countries the psychiatric services have been more and more orientated towards the community [18–20].

Historically, the special needs of the mentally ill were not always respected and recognized by generic services. In line with this trend, stigma continues to be an obstacle in ensuring that mentally ill patients have access to good care.

The Mental Health Law appeared in România only in August 2002. This was the first step towards reform of Romanian mental health services and its care system of mentally ill patients alongside the country's care standards for people with mental disorders [21]. România has recently begun to transform its mental health system to add community mental health care services to the traditional system of psychiatric hospital care with the involvement of social services. The scientific organizations such as the Romanian Alzheimer Society (1996) and Romanian Association of Geriatric Psychiatry (1999) provide postgraduate training courses for doctors to enable them to provide better care of the older adults.

Key Messages

- Normal aging is accompanied by multiple somatic diseases; mental illnesses are common and their diagnosis is quite difficult.
- Older adults with dementia often receive suboptimal care and are often neglected.
- The use of an educational prevention programs can improve the quality of life for older adults throughout the course of dementia in primary care in collaboration with specialist services and should include a plan for end-of-life care.

Case History

A 79-year-old retired priest who is married with three children came to the local outpatient hospital clinic accompanied by his wife and one of his daughters with multiple complaints including:

- Not recognizing his friends or neighbours
- Feeling depressed and anxious
- Feeling agitated and wanting to go home

He was noted to have good hygiene, and he was able to complete simple chores and could dress himself. His wife reported deterioration in judgement and thinking, planning and organizing and described that he had symptoms of irritability, psychomotor agitation and wandering.

The patient had completed a theology and history degree and worked as a teacher before becoming a priest and his family had noticed that the current problems began when he was about 74 years old and had progressed slowly. This was managed by his family doctor and psychiatrist.

The family reported that they were concerned about his safety because he once drank a toxic substance because he didn't recognize what it was and the family was afraid to leave him on his own. He disliked being alone and is always accompanied by his wife.

Early in his presentation he was managed on:

- An antidepressant sertraline 50 mg/daily
- An anticholinesterase donepezil 5 mg–10 mg/daily

This combination of medication was helpful but there was a break in treatment when donepezil was unavailable because of an economic crisis. The patient developed side effects when eventually re-started donepezil and this was changed to rivastigmine 6 mg/daily.

The patient had a past history of surgery for renal stones, an inguinal hernia and appendectomy. He had ischemic heart disease and a cardiac pacemaker. The family reported that the patient's father also had cognitive impairment.

Mental state examination revealed a polite, clean gentlemen who appeared irritable, anxious and depressed. There was no evidence of hallucinations or delusions. He had moderate cognitive impairment and according to his family was no longer able to shop or handle money. He was disorientated in time and place and did not recognize his family or that he was seeing a doctor. He lacked insight and did not recognize his cognitive problems or that he had an illness.

Investigations

Psychological testing:

- MMSE
- Clock test
- GDS-geriatric deterioration scale

Laboratory testing:

- Full blood count (FBC)
- Erythrocyte sedimentation (ESR)
- Blood sugar
- Urea and electrolytes
- Creatine
- Liver function tests
- Transaminases (GOT, GPT)
- Uric acid
- Creatinine phosphokinase (CPK)
- Cholesterol
- Lipids and triglycerides
- Urinalysis

All laboratory testing were normal

Other investigations:
- CT and MRI: Global cortical atrophy

There is no evidence from history, physical examination, psychiatric and neurological examination or special investigations as laboratory testing, EEG, CT and MRI for any other form of dementia, a systemic disorder, or alcohol or drug abuse.

Differential Diagnosis
- Alzheimer's dementia BPSD (behavioural and psychological symptoms of dementia) moderate with late onset.

Management Plan
- Patient was continued on sertraline antidepressant and rivastigmine.
- Patient's care team ensured that the patient's basic psychosocial and spiritual needs were met through continued collaboration between the family doctor, psychiatrist, family psychotherapist and family carers.

Outcome
- This patient was able to be managed at home despite the increasing severity of his cognitive impairment in collaboration with the family, family doctor, psychiatrist and family therapist.

Wider Lessons
- Patients should be managed at home supported by the family doctor for as long as possible. The role of NGOs and spiritual providers in the provision of community care for the older adult is increasing in many developing countries such as Romania but remains limited [22, 23].
- Stigma remains an obstacle in ensuring access to good care for the mentally ill patients. Stigma against the mentally ill leads to the development of negative attitudes, including to professionals and services in term of poor quality treatment and care, and inadequate funding at national and local level [24].
- Standards of basic mental health care must be raised, and adapted in relation to the patients' needs and his/her quality of life. Action against stigma and discrimination of older people with mental disorders should be a major component of all levels of a health and social care program.
- Assessing and improving end-of-life care for people with dementia presents particular challenges. Respect for the individual's expressed wishes and interest should guide all end-of-life care decisions.
- It is necessary to recognize the role of spirituality in the well-being of the older adults and those with dementia at the end of their life. This means the physicians must attend not only on patients' physical complaints or their somatic problems, but sensitively to include an awareness of their cultural, moral and spiritual convictions.
- Old age psychiatry has been a recognized subspecialty of psychiatry in Romania since 2001 but the number of professionals working in the field is still too low to satisfy the needs of care of the older adults with mental disorders.

27.6 Case Vignette Five

27.6.1 Vascular Dementia

Şahinde Özlem Erden Aki

27.6.1.1 Reason for Choosing This Case Example

This case from Turkey was chosen because it highlights the need for hope when we manage older adults with dementia, particularly those with vascular type dementia.

National Context Turkey

The older population is rapidly increasing in Turkey as in the other countries. Older adults people are much respected in our culture, but due to modern life and its necessities, extended families of the past which the older adults are the main part are disappearing, nuclear family increasing in both rural and urban regions; as the result of social changes the social care and health care needs of older people are increasing.

Many geriatrics fellowship programs have been founded under the roof of the internal medicine departments of state universities, but no official geriatric psychiatry training has been started yet in the psychiatry residency.

Turkish Ministry of Health is working with universities and related parties to plan a national health care program for older adults, but this program is fragmented yet.

Family physicians are actively participating in the care of their elder population (home visits, immunization, and routine care).

Municipalities are very active in providing home healthcare programs for the populations in need including older adult people. But there is still a long way to fully cover the needs of older population in our country.

Key Messages

- Vascular dementia is a common form of dementia in older adults particularly those with cardiovascular and cerebrovascular disease.
- Late life depression could be a harbinger of emerging vascular dementia.
- Patients with vascular dementia are more aware about their condition than people Alzheimer's type dementia.
- Vascular dementia commonly co-occurs with Alzheimer's type dementia and patients with vascular dementia require close follow-up for emerging signs of Alzheimer's type dementia.

Case History

A female, 79-year-old, retired school teacher, married and living with her husband.

Her first consultation was in September 2016, accompanied by her husband. Both the patient and her husband are complaining about her depressed mood, inability to plan activities and recent memory difficulties. The patient reveals that she has not been feeling well lately and lost interest in her usual activities such as being with friends, going to a hand-crafting course, shopping and gardening. She blames her occasional urinary incontinence for stepping down from these activities, and also admits that sometimes she overreacts in certain situations, such as bursting into tears even with a little stimulation. She is aware about her memory difficulties and admits that she cannot remember many things.

Her husband confirms and adds that she has lost interest almost in everything and become insensitive. She generally forgets important information such as doctors' appointments, family meetings, payment of bills, etc. She cannot remember a list of shopping items and she seems hard to understand explanations. Once a very skilled organizer, now she cannot plan even a basic meal for her children and gets anxious. He also tells that her movements become very slow for the last year; and due to a fear of falling, she keeps indoors most of the time. No sleep or appetite problems.

During the psychiatric examination the patient's speech was slow, she appeared apathetic, inattentive to surroundings, but still with a reactive affect and mildly depressed mood; no thought disorder and no perceptual disturbance.

On physical examination no rigidity or ataxic gait was detected, but bradykinesia was noted.

Past medical history: Hypertension for 40 years poorly controlled for the last few years, diabetes mellitus controlled with oral antidiabetics for 20 years, hypothyroidism, gall-bladder surgery a year ago, and cardiac angiography 10 and 2 years ago. Heavy smoker until 10 years ago, and no alcohol use.

Medications:

- Telmisartan and hydrochlorothiazide (for hypertension),
- Metoprolol (for tachycardia),
- Furosemide (for edema due to cardiac insufficiency),
- Aspirin (for prophylaxis against cardiovascular events),
- Metformin, and Repaglinide (for type II diabetes mellitus), and
- Atorvastatin (for hypercholesterolemia).

Family history: Father with forgetfulness in late 70s, diagnosed with senile forgetfulness.

Investigations
Neuropsychiatric Evaluation:
- MMSE 26/30 (lost 2 points from attention, lost 2 points from recall)
- Clock drawing test: ¾
- California verbal learning test: free recall 3/15, cued recall 12/15, total recall 15/15, no false recognition
- Trail making test A: 57 s, trail making test B: 289 s, 4 errors
- Controlled Oral Word Association Test: 12 for phonemic fluency, 18 for categorical fluency (animal naming)
- Geriatric depression scale: 12/30

Laboratory Evaluation:
- Full blood count,
- Aspartate aminotransferase (AST),
- Alanine aminotransferase (ALT),
- Blood urea nitrogen (BUN),
- Creatinine,
- Plasma sodium and potassium,
- Magnesium,
- Erythrocyte sedimentation rate,
- Thyroid stimulating hormone (TSH), free T4, and free T3, and
- Vitamin B12, vitamin D levels, and folic acid.

All within normal limits

- Fasting blood glucose slightly above normal limit.
- Cholesterol values (LDL, VLDL, and total cholesterol) above limits.

Neuroimaging:
- Brain MRI without contrast (September 2016): Widespread bilateral white matter hyperintensities, a few lacunar infarcts in the left temporal lobe, and hippocampal atrophy on coronal sections.
- Fluorodeoxyglucose-positron emission tomography (FDG-PET) (September 2016): Bilateral frontal hypometabolism and slight temporo-parietal hypometabolism reported.

Differential Diagnosis

- Vascular cognitive impairment/vascular dementia vs mixed vascular and Alzheimer's type dementia (VaD and AD).

Management Plan

- The patient had multi-morbidity and required collaboration with other specialists in managing her condition.
- Cardiology consultation requested for blood pressure control.
- Endocrinology consultation requested for blood sugar control.
- Neurology consultation for bradykinesia—no Parkinson disease diagnosed.
- Sertraline 50 mg/day started (for apathy and pseudobulbar symptoms).
- Donepezil (an acetylcholinesterase inhibitor) offered but the family rejected the activity program created by the help of occupational therapy department, regular physical exercise recommended, and husband instructed to become supportive and initiative in daily activities.

Outcome

3-month follow-up:

Affect stabile and reactive, less depressed mood, began to enjoy daily life, less forgetful

6-month follow-up:

Less forgetful, almost as old-self

1-year follow-up:

Stable as in 6-month follow-up

2-year follow-up:

Became forgetful for the last few months, began to ask the same questions, difficulty in remembering shopping list items and doctors' appointments, mood-wise fine

A follow-up brain MRI planned and neuropsychological tests will be repeated due to suggestive symptoms of Alzheimer's type cognitive impairment

Wider Lessons

- Vascular dementia is the second most common type of dementia among older adults.
- Mood disturbances, attention and executive function disorder and the difficulty in recall but not the recognition of the information (subcortical involvement) are the prominent features of vascular cognitive impairment.
- Not uncommonly vascular cognitive impairment and dementia of Alzheimer's type are diagnosed together.
- Extensive cerebrovascular impairment may play the catalyst role for the conversion of low-grade Alzheimer's disease to an overt dementia syndrome.
- The vascular risk factors and vascular diseases should be recognized early and treated aggressively in inclined individuals, and these patients should be followed-up closely for an emerging AD type dementia.

27.7 Case Vignette Six

27.7.1 Suicide Attempt

Dorota Szcześniak and Joanna Rymaszewska

27.7.1.1 Reason for Choosing This Case Example

This case example from Poland was chosen because it shows the need to respect the patient's dignity and autonomy, and shows that older adults are never too old to study.

National Context Poland

According to Polish Central Statistical Office Poland has a population of 38.4 million individuals, of whom 48% were men and 52% were women at the end of 2014 (Polish Central Statistical Office, 2014) [25]. Although the number of people aged 65 and older in Poland is lower than the European average (17%), this percentage in Poland is expected to increase slowly but steadily so that by 2030, 27% of the population is projected to be 65 or older [26].

According to WHO, globally, suicide rates are highest in people aged 70 years and over (WHO 2014) [27]. In 2016 in Poland, more people died by suicide than by road accidents. People between 50 and 69 years old undertook 2827 suicide attempts, of which 2027 ended in death. This represents 38% of fatal suicide, whilst 12.1% of suicides are committed by people over 70 years of age (Polish Central Statistical Office, 2016) [28].

Poland provides free healthcare to all citizens through the National Health Fund (NFZ). However, due to limited financing, the NFZ limits the number of procedures health care professionals can perform. Consequently, it results in common complains about long wait time to access spe-

---

cialized services. Therefore, individuals who want to quickly gain access to specialist outpatient services such as psychiatrists use private healthcare [29].

Key Messages

- Depressive episode in the elderly may manifest unusual symptoms that are not classically associated with depression. Older patients often show irritability, strong anxiety and lack of complaints about sadness. Somatic complaints dominate, sometimes leading are sleep disturbances, decreasing interest and limiting social contacts as well as increase in medical consultations and visits to the family doctor or GP and other specialists.
- Never underestimate symptoms of mood disorders, including atypical ones, and always ask the patient and, if possible, his or her closest relatives about thoughts of resignations, reluctance to live or thoughts and suicidal tendencies.
- Termination of employment, change of social roles and position in the society and in the family, the loss of spouse are very strong risk factors for attempting suicide.
- Elderly men are in the highest risk group in terms of age and gender for committing effective suicide.

Case History

Mr. K is 70 years old. He is widowed. His wife died 4 years ago. They have a 40 year-old daughter. Mr. K is retired since 2013 (for 5 years). During his life, he was a physical activity teacher in primary school and a boxing coach in a local sports club. In the past, he trained boxers for 15 years, when he had numerous head injuries connected with boxing fights. Mr. K always had many friends and he was actively involved in the local community. He enjoyed his life in these years. He was rarely ill and was appreciated by his colleagues. Before his wife died they were very close to each other.

On 15th of August 2018 Mr. K was taken to the emergency department by the ambulance service after his daughter found him in his home trying to commit suicide by hanging. A timely medical help was given and he was rescued. He did not have a history of depression or other psychiatric disorder and there was no history of suicidal behaviour or psychiatric disorder among his relatives. However, since several years Mr. K had complained to his daughter about increasing difficulty in maintaining all kinds of daily events. In addition, he complained more often about headaches and troublesome back pain. For this reason, he often met the general practitioner and regularly took strong painkillers (paracetamol with tramadol, ketoprofen). Shortly after retirement, Mr. K slowly started withdrawing from the local community events. At the moment of his wife's death, he stopped leaving the house and meeting with friends. Moreover, patient started to complain about memory disturbances consisting of forgetting names and names of people he knows, forgetting daily plans and shopping lists.

The family thought that majority of Mr. K's problems were related to aging process and mourning after the death of his wife. Nevertheless, he became more and more passive and sometimes he started presenting aggressive behaviours.

Diagnostic process: The psychiatric consultation was organized in order to assess if Mr. K has mental disorder and if he needs psychiatric treatment. Mental state examination found him in logical, laconic verbal contact. Psychomotor drive was slightly reduced. Patient was in depressed mood, confirmed complaints about difficulties with memory, difficulties in concentration, problems with functioning on a daily basis, and resignation thoughts. There were no psychotic symptoms. At the time of the assessment he had no suicidal ideas or plans although he was pessimistic about the future, had no appetitie and complained of insomnia. He did not remember when he last read anything or met friend.

There were no significant somatic disorders except well-controlled hypertension, mild level of hypercholesterolemia and mild prostatic hypertrophy. There were no symptoms of substance or alcohol abuse.

Investigations
- Full blood count including differentials,
- Electrolytes and renal function,
- Liver function,
- Thyroid function tests,
- C-reactive protein (CRP), and
- Electrocardiogram.

No abnormalities detected.

Differential Diagnosis
- Severe depressive episode without psychotic symptoms (F32.3 according to ICD-10 classification).

Management Plan

- Mr. K refused the proposal to be treated on inpatient psychiatric ward and there was no indication to involuntary admission.
- The consultant gave a referral to the mental health outpatient clinic with the recommendation to perform neuropsychological tests, to start psychotherapy and recommended the use of mirtazapine 15 mg at night until starting the treatment in the clinic.
- The patient's daughter was informed about the current health situation of her father with the recommendation to take care of him until he was treated in the outpatient psychiatric clinic and improvement of his mental condition.
- A simultaneous contact with the primary care physician was proposed to let him know that the psychiatric treatment Mr. K had begun.
- A daily psychiatric ward with daily medical care, psychotherapy and rehabilitation was proposed as an alternative to hospital treatment.
- Mr. K decided to go to the psychiatrist, who prescribed him sertraline (50 mg at morning for 4 days, then increasing to 50 mg twice daily) and continuation of mirtazapine (15 mg late evening), which improved his sleep after few days. Usage of mirtazapine allowed the patient to get some sleep relief and tranquillity before sertraline started to work (usually it takes 2–3 weeks in proper dosages).
- After several control visits in outpatient psychiatric clinic, Mr. K continued his treatment with his GP. Mirtazapine was discontinued after improvement of mood and activity as well as sleep (6 weeks of regular antidepressive treatment).
- Psychosocial intervention: The psychiatrist convinced him to use stress management techniques, such as relaxation techniques, psychosocial intervention, as well as to persuade him to consider sports, change perception of the environment and avoid negative habits in life and nutrition in CBT therapy.

Outcome

- The patient made a lot of progress and recovered.
- His family motivated Mr. K to sign up for the universities of the third age that aim to improve the lives of older adults through a range of educational activities such as learning basic English or social sciences, and favours establishing and maintaining social contacts.
- Therapeutic work will be based primarily on coping with losses (retirement and death of the wife), which the patient has experienced recently and on the patient's adaptation process to its current reality/life.

Wider Lessons

- The above example describes the socially significant occurrence of depressive symptoms in older people, especially in those who have experienced different losses.
- It draws attention to the importance of analyzing the smallest changes in the behaviour, even if it seems to family that these changes may be related to age.
- This example demonstrates that holistic approach to each patient and working in interdisciplinary collaboration (GP, psychiatrist, and psychologist) is essential in terms of diagnosis but also in terms of providing adequate post-diagnostic interventions.

References

1. Hayes SL, Mann MK, Morgan FM, Kelly MJ, Weightman AL. Collaboration between local health and local government agencies for health improvement (Review). Cochrane Database Syst Rev. 2012;10:1–138.
2. Institute for Healthcare Improvement. How to improve. 2018. http://www.ihi.org/resources/Pages/HowtoImprove/ScienceofImprovementTestingChanges.aspx.
3. Prince M, et al. Dementia UK: update second edition report produced by King's College London and the. London: School of Economics for the Alzheimer's Society; 2014.
4. Alzheimer's Society. Dementia facts for the media. https://www.alzheimers.org.uk/about-us/news-and-media/facts-media
5. Department of Health. Dementia: a state of the nation report on dementia care and support in England. London: Department of Health; 2013.
6. Kasteridis P, Mason AR, Goddard MK, Jacobs R, Santos R, McGonigal G. The influence of primary care quality on hospital admissions for people with dementia in England: a regression analysis. PLoS One. 2015;10(3):e0121506. https://doi.org/10.1371/journal.pone.0121506.
7. Brown A, Kirichek O, Balkwill A, Reeves G, Beral V, Sudlow C, Gallacher J, Green J. Comparison of dementia recorded in routinely collected hospital admission data in England with dementia recorded in primary care. Emerg Themes Epidemiol. 2016;13:11. https://doi.org/10.1186/s12982-016-0053-z.
8. NHS Digital. Hospital accident and emergency activity. 2016–2017. https://digital.nhs.uk/data-and-information/publications/statistical/hospital-accident%2D%2Demergency-activity/2016-17.
9. NHS Digital. Hospital accident and emergency activity. 2017–2018. https://digital.nhs.uk/data-and-information/publications/statistical/hospital-accident%2D%2Demergency-activity/2017-18.
10. London Health Board. Better health for London. 2015. One year on https://www.london.gov.uk/sites/default/files/better_health_for_london_-_one_year_on.pdf.
11. Waltham Forest CCG. NHS Waltham Forest CCG Commissioning Strategic Plan 2016/17–2019/20. 2016.
12. Waltham Forest Health and Wellbeing Strategy. 2016–2020. https://search3.openobjects.com/mediamanager/walthamforest/fsd/files/waltham_forest_health_and_wellbeing_strategy_2016-20_1_1.pdf.
13. Closs E, et al. A evolução do índice de envelhecimento no Brasil, nas suas regiões e unidades federativas no período de 1970 a 2010. Rev Bras Geriatr Gerontol. 2012;15(3):443–58.
14. Silvestre JA, et al. Abordagem do idoso em programas de saúde da família. Cad Saúde Pública. 2001;19(3):839–47.
15. Neto JBF. Carta Aberta à População brasileira. https://sbgg.org.br//wp-content/uploads/2014/12/R19.pdf. Accessed 19 Jan 2019.
16. Veras RP, et al. Desenvolvimento de uma linha de cuidados para o idoso: hierarquização da atenção baseada na capacidade funcional. Rev Bras de Geriatr e Gerontologia. 2013;16(2):385–92.
17. Stern TA, et al. Massachusetts general hospital handbook of general hospital psychiatry. 6th ed. Amsterdam: Elsevier; 2010.
18. Arie T. The development in Britain. In: Copeland JRM, Abou-Saleh MT, Blazer DG, editors. Principles and practice of geriatric psychiatry. Chichester: John Wiley; 1994. p. 6–10.
19. Philpot M, Banerjee S. Mental Health Services for older people in London. London's Mental Health. London: King's Foundation; 1996. p. 46–64.
20. Wertheimer J. Psychogeriatric organisation in the medico-social network: the experience of the canton of Vaud, Switzerland. Dement Geriatr Cogn Disord. 1997;8:143–5.
21. Mental Health Law. Monitorul oficial al Romaniei, XIV, Nr. 589, Chapter 4. 2002.
22. Tătaru N. Chapter 20: services for people with dementia: a world wide view – Romania. In: Burns A, Ames D, O'Brien J, editors. Dementia. 3rd ed; 2005. p. 296–8.
23. Tătaru N. Chapter 6 practice of dementia care: Romania, standard in dementia care. In: Burns A, editor. EDCON. Milton Park: Taylor & Francis Group; 2005. p. 41–8.
24. World Health Organization, Division on Mental Health and Prevention of Substance Abuse and World Psychiatric Association. Management of mental and Brain Disorders-Reducing stigma and discrimination against older people with mental disorders. A Technical Consensus Statement. Geneva: WHO; 2002.
25. Polish Central Statistical Office. Size and structure of population and vital statistics in Poland by territorial division. December 31, 2014. Warsaw, Poland. 2014. Retrieved from http://stat.gov.pl/en/.
26. Eurostat. Mortality and life expectancy statistics. 2013. Retrieved from http://epp.eurostat.ec.europa.eu/statistics_explained/index.php/Mortality_and_life_expeancy_statistics.
27. World Health Organization. Preventing suicide. A global imperative. Geneva: WHO Library Cataloguing-in-Publication Data; 2014.
28. Polish Central Statistical Office. Suicide in 2016. September 8, 2017. Warsaw, Poland. 2017.
29. Leszko M, Zając-Lamparska L, Trempala J. Aging in Poland. The Gerontologist. 2015;55(5):707–15.

Printed in the United States
By Bookmasters